THE PINEAL ORGAN

THE PINEAL ORGAN

The Comparative Anatomy of Median and Lateral Eyes,
with special reference to the Origin of the Pineal Body;
and a description of the Human Pineal Organ considered
from the Clinical and Surgical Standpoints

BY

REGINALD J. GLADSTONE

M.D., F.R.C.S., F.R.S.E., D.P.H.

FORMERLY READER IN EMBRYOLOGY AND LECTURER ON ANATOMY, AT KING'S COLLEGE,
UNIVERSITY OF LONDON, AND LECTURER ON EMBRYOLOGY AT THE MEDICAL
COLLEGE, MIDDLESEX HOSPITAL, LONDON; MEMBER OF THE ANATOMICAL
SOCIETY OF GREAT BRITAIN AND IRELAND; FORMERLY FELLOW OF
THE ROYAL ANTHROPOLOGICAL INSTITUTE, AND FELLOW
OF THE ZOOLOGICAL SOCIETY OF LONDON

and

CECIL P. G. WAKELEY

D.Sc., F.R.C.S., F.R.S.E., F.Z.S., F.A.C.S., F.R.A.C.S.

FELLOW OF KING'S COLLEGE, LONDON, AND LECTURER IN APPLIED ANATOMY AT KING'S
COLLEGE, UNIVERSITY OF LONDON; SENIOR SURGEON, KING'S COLLEGE HOSPITAL
AND THE WEST END HOSPITAL FOR NERVOUS DISEASES; CONSULTING
SURGEON TO THE MAUDSLEY HOSPITAL AND TO THE ROYAL NAVY;
HUNTERIAN PROFESSOR ROYAL COLLEGE OF SURGEONS
OF ENGLAND

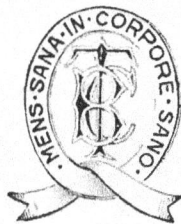

LONDON

BAILLIÈRE, TINDALL AND COX

7 AND 8, HENRIETTA STREET, COVENT GARDEN, W.C.2

1940

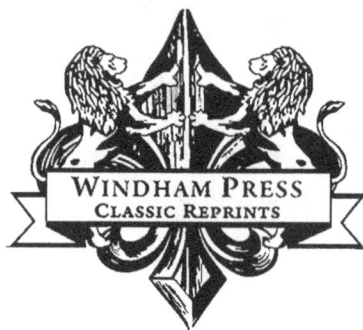

Initium sapientiæ timor Domini.

For a thousand years in Thy sight are but as yesterday when it is past, and as a watch in the night.—*Psalm* xc. 4.

FOREWORD

By Sir Arthur Keith, F.R.S.

I should mislead readers were I to assure them that this book, written by an anatomist who has given half a century to the elucidation of the human body and by a surgeon who stands in the forefront of his profession, reads as easily as a work of fiction. Books which are fundamental in character are not easy reading, and this is a work of the kind. And yet the story which Dr. Gladstone unfolds is a romance. To trace the origin and evolution of the human pineal body or epiphysis, he has had to go back to an early stage of the world of life, one some 400 millions of years removed from us, when median as well as lateral eyes had appeared on the heads of our invertebrate ancestry. His search has not been confined to the geological record; he has brought together from the literature of comparative anatomy and from his own observations what is known of median eyes and the pineal organ in all types of living forms, both invertebrate and vertebrate.

If Dr. Gladstone's story begins in a past which is very distant, that which Mr. Wakeley has to tell belongs to the present and the future. His story opens a new chapter in surgery, that which is to deal with the diagnosis and treatment of disorders of the pineal body.

It is many years since Dr. Gladstone and I became students and friends at the University of Aberdeen, and friends and students we have remained ever since. We have in that time seen strange changes in the anatomy of the human body—structures such as the pituitary, thyroid, and adrenal, which we counted negligible, soar to positions of dominance; we have seen parts of the brain such as the hypothalamus, which we regarded as mere wall-space of the third ventricle, become the seat of fundamental and vital processes; and we have seen some structures dethroned. Although the " pineal gland " had fallen from its high estate long before Gladstone and I became students, it is of interest to compare the opinion which Descartes formed of it in the seventeenth century with the conclusions reached by our authors in the twentieth century.

Those who are familiar with *The Life and Opinions of Tristram Shandy* will recall Mr. Shandy's wish to discover " that part where the soul principally took up her residence." Let me quote from the original:

vii

" Now from the best accounts he had been able to get of this matter, he was satisfied it could not be where *Des Cartes* had fixed it upon the top of the pineal gland of the brain, which, as he philosophized, formed a cushion for her about the size of a marrow pea ; this to speak the truth, as so many nerves did terminate all in that one place, it was no bad conjecture."

Readers will remember how Uncle Toby knocked the bottom out of Descartes' theory by relating the case " of a Walloon officer at the battle of Landen, who had one part of his brain shot away by a musket ball— and another part of it taken out after by a French surgeon, and after all, recovered and did his duty very well without it."

I need not anticipate the conclusions reached by our authors regarding the nature and function of the pineal body of the human brain ; they will be found in the concluding chapter of this book. In spite of all their labours, much remains enigmatic concerning the pineal body ; but they have laid a basis from which those who would go further must set out.

I must not be like a too loquacious chairman and abuse the privilege the authors have given me, in writing the foreword, by intruding my own opinions. Yet at the risk of sinning in this respect, there are one or two observations I have picked up in my recent reading, which seem to throw light on some of the problems discussed by them. There is first an observation made by Wislocki and King (*Amer. Journ. Anat.*, 1936, **58**, 421), who on injecting a solution of trypan blue in the live animal, found that it stained certain nuclear structures in the hypothalamus and also the cells of the pineal body—an outgrowth from the epithalamus. There are structural resemblances in the parts so stained. Such an observation fits easily into the final conclusions drawn by our authors. Hypothalamus and epithalamus, so widely separated by the thalamus in the human brain, were anciently close neighbours, both being associated with olfactory tracts and connections. Both are constituent parts of that cavity of the brain from which the lateral eyes as well as the median or parietal eye are developed.

Our authors find that the evidence which attributes a sex function to the pineal body is confused and contradictory, and rightly in my opinion bring in, on this head, a verdict of " unproven." Before we finally reject the evidence, however, it seems well to remember that through our retinæ, there are transmitted to the brain not only stimuli which give rise to vision but also " light reflexes." It seems probable that the median as well as the lateral eyes had this double function. Through centres in the hypothalamus and pituitary, light reflexes can bear in upon the gonads and regulate their times of ripening. Prof. Le Gros Clark and his colleagues (Proc. Roy. Soc., 1939, 126 (B), 449) by cutting the optic nerves of the ferret and thus cutting off light reflexes, altered the onset of the period of heat. One can best explain the connection of the habenular ganglia of the pineal with the hypothalamus (through the striæ medullares) by supposing that the median or parietal eye did exercise an influence on the hypothalamus and pituitary. Nor is it unreasonable to suppose that, in connection with sex-function, there arose in the basal part of the diverticulum which gives rise to the pineal organ an area or segment of nerve-cells, which, like certain groups in the hypothalamus, are neuro-secretory in nature. With the disappearance of the parietal eye in birds and mammals, this basal part embedded in the epithalamic system, persisted in them to form the pineal body.

I count it a privilege to have had the opportunity of reading this work while it was still in proof-form. I have learned much from it and I am sure others will benefit from its study as much as I have done. I would especially endorse a sentence in the first chapter, which reads :

" As one branch of medicine advances it becomes repeatedly necessary to fall back on the fundamental sciences for help and guidance, and realizing that the investigation of these pineal tumours proved rather barren some years ago, the authors determined to investigate the whole question of the nature of the pineal organ from the lowest to the highest forms in the animal kingdom."

By so doing they have shown themselves to be true disciples of John Hunter.

ARTHUR KEITH.

BUCKSTON BROWNE RESEARCH FARM,
    DOWNE, KENT,
        October 28th, 1939

PREFACE

THIS book is the outcome of a desire to study the pineal body from the broad standpoint of comparative anatomy, and to correlate as far as possible the structural appearance and connections of the mammalian epiphysis with the conflicting views which are held with regard to its origin and functions.

It was originally intended to deal with the subject mainly from the practical standpoints of diagnosis and operative technique, based upon the exact anatomical relations and connections of the pineal organ in the human subject. It soon became evident, however, that the study involved a much wider basis than the purely anatomical and clinical, and in order to assess the true significance of the facts which have been observed in connection with the mammalian epiphysis it would be necessary to investigate the history of the pineal body and parietal sense-organ from the standpoints of embryology, comparative anatomy, and geology. This, study raises further questions which are of great biological importance such as the influence which heredity appears to have in causing the retention for millions of years of an organ which in the majority of living vertebrate animals has completely lost its original function of a visual sense-organ ; also the problems that are raised by the recent hypothesis that the pineal body of the higher vertebrate classes is evolving as an endocrine organ by transformation of the vestigial parietal sense-organ into a gland of internal secretion, or the alternative supposition, that the mammalian epiphysis is a genetically distinct structure which has arisen independently of the parietal eye of fishes and reptiles. Another problem which has engaged the attention of previous investigators, and which we have discussed in the light of recent palæontological work, is the explanation of the coexistence of a general similarity in structure of the pineal eyes of vertebrates and the median eyes of invertebrates along with certain differences in detail, which also exist, and which were formerly considered to exclude any possibility of the two systems being genetically connected. One of the first fruits of this inquiry was the definite confirmation which we found is afforded by palæontology and comparative anatomy of the primarily bilateral origin of the parietal sense-organ ; and a second the conviction which was gained of the extreme antiquity of the pineal system—this seems not only to have evolved before the evolution of the

xi

roof-bones of the vault of the skull but in some types of primitive fish to have already entered the regressive phase of its ancestral history at the time when the dermal bones of the skull had first completely covered over the brain and formed a protective investment for the principal sense-organs, namely the olfactory, visual, and static.

The authors hope that the book will be of interest to readers outside as well as within the medical profession and that it will stimulate the study of other organs and systems of the human body from the stand-point of comparative anatomy, in addition to the purely practical aspect. We feel assured that the wider outlook which is gained by the investigation of any particular structure by the embryological and comparative methods well repays the additional time which is spent in acquiring this know-ledge. It not only greatly increases interest in the particular organ which is being studied but it also gives a better insight into the special functions of the system both in health and disease.

Special care has been taken in selecting and making the illustrations, each of which has an independent explanatory legend. They have been assembled from various sources ; some are original drawings made specially for this work or which have previously been published by either one or both of us in the *British Journal of Surgery*, the *Journal of Anatomy*, or the *Medical Press and Circular*. Others have been reproduced from blocks, redrawn from lithographic plates, photographs, or drawings illustrating original papers, or from well-known standard works. The source of the latter has in each case been duly acknowledged, and the authors desire to take this opportunity of expressing their gratitude to the publishers and authors who have generously allowed us to make use of these figures ; and we desire specially to thank the publishers of those journals and books from which certain of the illustrations have been reproduced : John Wright and Sons, Bristol ; Baillière, Tindall and Cox, London ; *Quarterly Journal of the Microscopical Society*, London ; Cambridge University Press ; Macmillan and Co., London ; Contribu-tions to Embryology, John Hopkins University.

The authors also wish to acknowledge their indebtedness to the published works of all those writers whose names appear in the biblio-graphy and in the following list. These works have been of the greatest value in determining the general trend of the book and an aid in coming to the conclusions which we have been enabled to draw from our own observations and experience. We wish especially to mention the names of the following authors : Achucarro, Agduhr, Ahlborn, Altmann, Amprino, Bailey, Badouin, de Beer, Béraneck, Berblinger, Bernard, Bertkau, Bourne, Brown, Cairns, Cajal, Calvet, Cambridge Natural History,

Cameron, Cushing, Dandy, Dendy, Dimitrowa, Eycleshymer, Favaro, Foa, Gaskell, Globus, Goodrich, Grenacher, Harris, Haswell, Hill, C., Howell, Huxley, T., Huxley, J., Izawa, Kiaer, Kappers, Kerr, Kishinouye, Klinckostroem, Kolmer, Krabbe, Lang, Lankester, Leydig, Lereboullet, L'Hermitte, MacBride, MacCord, Marburg, Nicholson, Nowikoff, Parker, G. H., Parker and Haswell, Pastori, Patten, Penfield, Quast, Rio de Hortega, Schwalbe, Spencer, Stensiö, Stormer, Strahl and Martin, Studnička, Tilney and Warren, van Wagenen, Watson, Woodward, A. S., Zittel.

We desire, further, to gratefully acknowledge the help which we have received from Professor Doris L. MacKinnon of the Department of Zoology, King's College, London, and Dr. J. A. Hewitt, Lecturer on Physiology and Histology, King's College, London, for permission to make use of the specimens of *Geotria* and *Sphenodon* which belonged to the late Professor Arthur Dendy, and specimens from the Department of Histology from which some of the illustrations have been drawn. We also wish to thank Professors A. Smith Woodward, D. M. Watson, and W. T. Gordon, for valuable help with respect to references to literature, and Mr. Walpole Champneys and Margaret M. Gladstone for assistance in drawing some of the illustrations.

We also wish to express our thanks to Mr. E. J. Weston, Mr. Charles Biddolph, and Mr. Denys Kempson for the valuable assistance they have given in the preparation of serial sections of embryos and microphotographs. Lastly, we would like to thank Miss Milward Smith and Miss Mary Popham, who between them have typed the whole of the manuscript.

R. J. G.
C. P. G. W.

London,
November, 1939

CONTENTS

THE PINEAL ORGAN

CHAPTER I

INTRODUCTION

THE pineal organ has interested scientific investigators from the earliest times and much speculation has been expended in attempts to discover what its function might be. But it is only in very recent years that the medical profession has realized that it has a practical importance and that tumours may occur in this small piece of cerebral tissue. It was little more than fifty years ago that the late Sir Rickman Godlee performed the first operation for the removal of a cerebral tumour, yet in the comparatively short period of time which has elapsed since then great advances in both the diagnosis and treatment of such tumours have been made, and among the various types of cerebral tumour which have been distinguished and surgically treated are those which originate in or near the pineal body. The first real discussion on pineal tumours took place at the Royal Society of Medicine in London in 1909, when the subject was introduced by Hinds Howell. At this meeting Gordon Holmes stated that in his opinion surgical removal of pineal tumours arising in the pineal gland was feasible, and Sir Victor Horsley said that he would operate on the first case that came his way, by a supratentorial route. History, however, does not relate whether Horsley ever did operate upon a pineal tumour. Since the first discussion many cases of pineal tumour have been published, and in this short monograph we record nine cases.

The pineal organ after puberty frequently becomes calcified and its shadow can be seen on an X-ray film (Fig. 1). As the organ is a midline structure it is liable to be shifted from this central position if any pressure is brought to bear upon it from either side. Hence a cerebral tumour in the right hemisphere will shift it towards the left, and this " pineal shift " can easily be demonstrated in an antero-posterior skiagram. This in itself, apart from any pathological condition of the pineal body, may be a valuable localizing sign in the diagnosis of cerebral tumours. We have found the pineal gland to be calcified in 65 per cent. of patients over 16 years of age. This occurred in the examination of over 300 adult skulls, and there can be no doubt that with improved technique and better X-ray apparatus the percentage of calcified pineals which are visible and are recorded will gradually rise.

The pineal organ is thus of considerable importance in general medicine, and as the years go by and pineal lesions are more frequently recognized, this importance will become more marked.

As one branch of medicine advances it becomes repeatedly necessary to fall back on the fundamental sciences for help and guidance, and

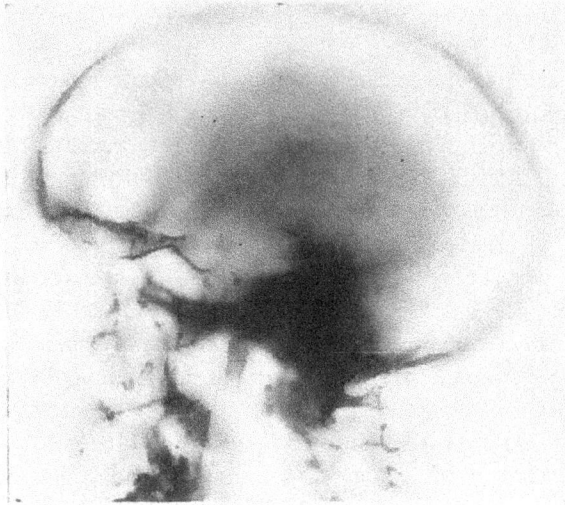

FIG. 1.—CALCIFICATION OF PINEAL ORGAN.

realizing that the investigation of these pineal tumours proved rather barren some years ago, the authors determined to investigate the whole question of the nature of the pineal organ from the lowest to the highest forms in the animal kingdom and see if this would shed any light on these interesting and little-known tumours of the pineal which so often are not diagnosed in the early stages when complete removal would be much easier than if left to grow large and involve neighbouring structures.

CHAPTER 2

HISTORICAL SKETCH

THE existence of the pineal organ was known by the ancient Greeks and Romans. Galen (A.D. 131–201) spoke of it as " scolecoid," or worm-like. His dissections were carried out on oxen, sheep, apes, and other animals, and he mentioned that it had been named by other writers the *epiphysis*. He also emphasized its intimate connection with the great vein which to this day is known all the world over by his name. Other classical writers who were impressed by its conical, pine-like form named it the *conarium*. Various ideas were held as to its function, among which was the notion that it acted as a valve or flood-gate, and regulated the quantity of spirit (? cerebro-spinal fluid) necessary for the psychological requirements of the individual. The theory that it functions as a gland seems to have originated with the Romans, who described it as the *glandula pinealis*. Little advance was made in the knowledge of the pineal organ in the centuries which followed, and in 1637 René Descartes taught that the human body was an earthly machine which was presided over by the " rational soul," which was situated in the pineal gland, " the little gland in the middle of the substance of the brain." This idea was ridiculed by Voltaire, who suggested a coachman sitting on his seat and holding the reins of the horses—which were supposed to be represented by the peduncles of the gland.

William Cowper (1666–1709), who considered the pineal to be a lymphatic gland, wrote " the glandula pinealis which we take to be a lymphatic gland, receiving lympha from the lymphe ducts which pass by way of the third ventricle of the brain to the infundibulum and glandula pituitaria." This idea of the lymphatic nature of the pineal body was shared by some others, among whom we may mention that pioneer histologist Jacob Henle (1809–85), who, being impressed by a general resemblance of its microscopic structure to that of a lymphatic gland, considered that it might also function as a lymphatic node. With modern microscopes and improvement in histological technique, however, the distinction between lymphatic tissue and the peculiar structure of the normal adult pineal organ has been rendered easy, and its developmental history coupled with a more exact knowledge of its comparative anatomy have shown that this conception of the nature and function of the organ is quite untenable.

3

The work on the pineal region in the latter part of the nineteenth century and the commencement of the present century was attended by a marked advance in our knowledge of the true nature of the pineal apparatus in all its aspects—geological, zoological, embryological, and phylogenetic. It is to this period that we owe the conception, which was generally held at that time, of the vestigial nature of the pineal organ. It was thought that the " parietal organ " or " pineal eye," which was found to be most highly developed in certain living reptiles, amphibia, and cyclostomes, was the vestige of an unpaired median eye or the persistent member of a

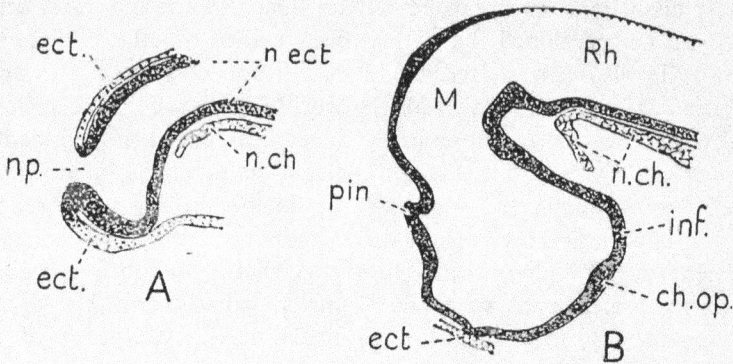

FIG. 2.—SAGITTAL SECTIONS THROUGH THE BRAIN OF ACANTHIAS EMBRYOS. (AFTER KUPFFER.)

A : 3·3 mm., showing the open neuropore. B : 10 mm., showing the cutaneous ectoderm still adherent to the neural ectoderm, at the site of the closed neuropore, which lies in front of the pineal diverticulum, *pin*.

ch. op. : optic chiasma.	*n.ch.* : notochord.
ect. : cutaneous ectoderm.	*n. ect.* : neural ectoderm.
inf. : infundibulum.	*np.* : neuropore.
M. : midbrain.	*Rh.* : rhombencephalon.

pair of median eyes one of which was rudimentary or had completely disappeared.

Before proceeding to the discussion of the more recent work on the pineal, we shall give a short account of some of the problems which arose during the period 1870–1915, and we shall mention in an approximately chronological order the names of a few of the principal authors, giving at the same time a brief note of the special contribution which each made to the general knowledge of the subject.

Among the first of these was Leydig (1872), who discovered the parietal organ in the embryos of *Lacerta agilis*, *L. muralis*, and *L. vivipara*. He described its general position above the interbrain in the region of the third ventricle ; the external appearance of the pineal plate ; the disposition of the pigment ; and the microscopical structure of the vesicle ; but was doubtful of its nature and even contended that it was not a sense-organ. Goette (1875), described the epiphysis in *Bombinator* and stated that the site of its out-growth from the brain was identical with the position of the anterior neuropore, or the point where the medullary folds finally unite with each other in the formation of the neural tube. It was, how-ever, shown by Mihalkovics that at the time of the first appearance of the evagination in birds (chick) (Fig. 200, Chap. 21), and in mammals (rabbit) (Fig. 208, Chap. 22), the medullary wall is separated by a considerable in-terval from the cutaneous ectoderm, and that the intervening space is filled in all amniote embryos by a layer of mesenchyme long before the pineal out-growth takes place; and it has also been shown by Kupffer in anamniota that the pineal evagination in *Acanthias* embryos lies behind the point of closure of the anterior neuropore and arises independently of it (Fig. 2).

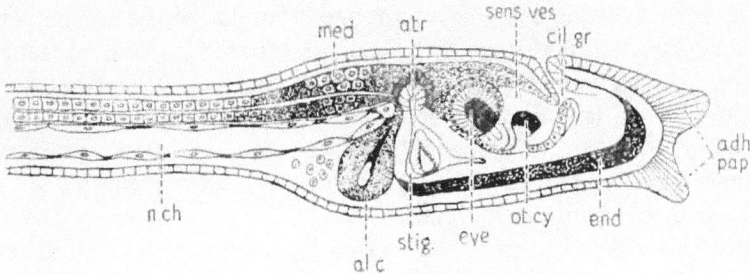

FIG. 3.—FREE-SWIMMING LARVA OF PHALLUSIA OR ASCIDIA MAMMILLATA, SHOWING THE SINGLE EYE AND OTOCYST ENCLOSED WITHIN THE CEREBRAL CAVITY (VENTRICLE).

adh. pap. : adhesive papillæ.	*med.* : medullary tube.
al. c. : alimentary canal.	*n. ch.* : notochord.
atr. : atrial opening.	*ot. cy.* : statocyst.
cil. gr. : ciliated groove or funnel.	*sens. ves.* : sensory vesicle.
end. : endostyle.	*stig.* : earliest stigmata.
eye : right eye.	

These specimens illustrate the production of a single eye or a single stato-cyst by the suppression (complete or incomplete) of one member of a pair of sensory organs.

(From Korschelt and Heider, after Kowalewsky.)

Götte's opinion with regard to the formation of the pineal diverticulum at the point where the roof of the brain remains latest attached to the external skin was also criticized by F. M. Balfour in 1885, who stated that he could find no indication in elasmobranchs of a process similar to that which was described by Götte, and that his observations had not been confirmed for other vertebrates. Balfour also alludes to Götte's com-parison of the pineal gland or diverticulum to the " long-persisting pore which leads into the cavity of the brain in *Amphioxus*," and he comments : " We might also add that of the Ascidians " (Fig. 3).

Rabl-Ruckhard, in 1886, put forward the interesting suggestion that the function of the organ was to estimate the heat of the sun's rays, and that it was a thermal sense-organ rather than visual. Spencer, who in '87 experimented on the sensitivity of the parietal organ to light, stated that " In lizards, whose paired eyes are closed, no result is obtained by focusing a strong beam of light on to the modified eye scale, and thus on to the pineal eye ; in fact, strong light focused into one of the paired eyes merely causes the lid to be drawn down, without any further apparent result, whilst in the pineal eye there is no protecting lid, and no movement whatever takes place to remove the eye from the direction in which the light is coming." Nowikoff experimented similarly with electric lights and magnesium wire on lizards without producing movements. Francotte in 1887 experimented with *Lacerta muralis* and *Anguis fragilis*. He constructed a cage consisting of six boxes arranged round a central rectangular space. Each box communicated with the central space by a small opening. In one box he placed an electric lamp ; and in the central space a lizard was placed, with its lateral eyes covered by a red material. The top was then closed in by a covering lid. The experiment, which was repeated several times, showed that in eight cases out of ten, after a quarter of an hour the lizard was found in the lighted box. The same experiment was also tried with a " blind worm," *Anguis fragilis*, under similar conditions, and the animal was found in the lighted chamber three times out of ten.

Francotte considered that the experiment, without being absolutely conclusive, allowed one to think that in the lizard, at any rate, the unpaired eye is still capable of perceiving light. He thought, however, that the experiment hardly proved that the lizard was attracted by the light only, but that it was also attracted by the warmth of the electric light. He accordingly modified the experiment by darkening one half of the terrarium and allowing a diffuse light to fall on the other half. After allowing a considerable period of time to elapse he found that the animals had shown no tendency to collect in the lighted half.

Experiments were also conducted with the object of ascertaining the influence of light in producing movement of pigment in the retina of the median eyes of both vertebrates and invertebrates. Thus Nowikoff in 1910 investigated the action of light on the median eyes of *Lacerta agilis* and *Anguis fragilis*. He divided the experimental animals into two groups, one of which he kept for 2 to 3 hours in absolute darkness, while the other group was exposed for a similar period to full sunlight. In the subsequent histological examination of the retina of those animals which had been exposed to the light, he found the pigment granules tended to accumulate in the inner ends of the cells nearer the source of light and central cavity ;

whereas in those animals which had been kept in the dark the pigment was found in the outer part of the retina, farther from the source of light. The subject of the presence of pigment in and around the pineal organ is of the very greatest interest with reference to (1) the origin of light-perceiving organs in general (Bernard) and (2) the occurrence of regressive changes and melanotic tumours in the human pineal organ. A more detailed description of the position of the pigment granules, their variations in type, and their significance will be given later in the appropriate places.

Another important period in the history of the pineal body is that in which its median situation between the two lateral eyes and the apparent similarity of its structure to that of the median eyes of invertebrates attracted the attention of some of the leading biologists and palæontologists of the time (1880–1910), more especially with reference to the light that its study might shed upon the problems of the ancestry of the vertebrates and the connection of the pre-vertebrate stock with that of the inverte-brates. Intimately bound up with this question was the controversy which arose as to whether the pineal body originated as a bilateral pair of light-percipient organs or whether as two separate median organs which arose serially one behind the other and belonged to two neural segments. Among those specially interested in these different problems we may mention : Baldwin Spencer, Lankester and Bourne, Kingsley, Beard, Gaskell, Patten, Dendy, Smith Woodward, Studnička and Klinckowström. As in the case of pigment, the detailed consideration of these questions will be most appropriately dealt with in the section on the morphology of the pineal system. It may be mentioned here, however, that although much speculation, based on preconceived notions and insufficient evidence, occurred during this period, some of the most important observations were made on the structure and nature of the pineal system during this period and in some cases arose as a direct result of investigation which was stimulated by the controversy.

Among the observations brought out in this way we may specially mention the discovery and accurate description of the nerves of the pineal eye by Nowikoff, Béraneck, Dendy, Klinckowström, and others, more especially in cyclostomes, fishes, amphibians, and reptiles. Moreover, it will be appropriate to draw attention here to the significance of the connection of the right and left pineal nerves, with the corresponding right and left habenular ganglia (Dendy), and also of the relation of the pineal nerves with the habenular and posterior commissures (Studnička). We may further emphasize the significance of the existence of a *nervus pinealis* during one phase of development and the disappearance of this nerve at a later stage as evidence of a regressive character being manifested in the ontogenetic history of the organ.

In recent years the interest shown in the pineal body has been revived, more especially in connection with its supposed endocrine function. This has led to a more exact study of its histological structure and experimental work on animals along the lines of extirpation, feeding with the whole gland or desiccated preparations of the gland, injection of extracts, and grafts. Details of this work will be discussed later, it being only necessary to mention here that although much has been learned by the use of special neurological methods of histological technique and from the clinical observations of pathological cases occurring in the human subject, the results recorded by various authors of the experimental work are often conflicting, and the clinical syndrome described by Pellizzi, namely macrogenitosomia præcox, does not always accompany destructive lesions of the pineal body, and the symptoms have sometimes been present but on post-mortem examination no abnormality of the pineal has been discovered. On the other hand, the careful observation and record of the special pressure-symptoms which are produced by enlargement of the pineal organ, accompanied by X-ray examination, has been of great value in the diagnosis of tumours originating in or near the gland.

Significance of the Pineal Body, considered from the Standpoint of Comparative Anatomy

Towards the end of the nineteenth century the opinion expressed by Dendy, Gaskell, Patten, and others, that the pineal eye of vertebrates was primarily bilateral in origin, led not only to further work on the pineal eye of vertebrates but also to a careful comparative study of the position and microscopical structure of the median (paired and unpaired) eyes of invertebrates ; and it was considered by Gaskell that the pineal system formed one of the most important clues to the origin of the vertebrates. These, he believed, originated from a pre-vertebrate ancestor which had affinities with one of the higher invertebrate phyla, and more particularly the Arthropoda. The similarity in general form of certain fossil fishes belonging to the class Ostracodermi—e.g. *Cephalaspis* and *Pteraspis*—to the living representatives of the Xiphosura, namely the king crabs (*Limulus polyphemus*), and also to some small living crustaceans, e.g. *Apus cancriformis* and *Lepidurus*, seemed to indicate that the whole vertebrate stock had arisen from a remote fish-like ancestor which was related to the arthropods and more particularly to the Xiphosura, Trilobites, and the gigantic " sea scorpions " *Eurypterus* and *Pterygotus*. Recent embryological and palæontological work has, as we shall show later, done much to confirm the view that the pineal organ was primarily a bilateral structure, but it is now believed that the vertebrate stock branched off from the invertebrate ancestors at a very remote period, before the special characters which are typical of the higher classes of invertebrates and vertebrates had been established. Many of the points of resemblance which have been observed between the higher types of invertebrates and vertebrates may be explained by assuming that certain fundamental characters, such as a general bilateral symmetry involving the nervous system and sense-organs, and certain common characters in the structure of the genito-urinary system, have been retained in both. While the differences between these classes may be accounted for on the assumption that a gradual differentiation has arisen in the course of time in adaptation to varying needs and possibilities of development, and that these changes, taking place along divergent lines, have eventually led to the formation of more fully evolved organs, which while retaining certain common characters inherited from the ancestral stock, yet differ in important respects, such as having eyes with an upright or an inverted type of retina. Some idea of the antiquity of the vertebrate kingdom and, by inference, the still greater antiquity of the common ancestor of the higher types of invertebrates and vertebrates may be gained by a consideration of the evidence which is afforded by the existence of the pineal organ in some of the most ancient types of fossil fish, e.g. *Cephalaspis*, *Pteraspis*, and other species. In these the small shallow pit which is situated between the orbits and believed to mark the position of the pineal organ is on the *inner* aspect of the cephalic shield. The existence of this depression on the **internal** aspect of the vault of the skull indicates that even in these archaic types of fish the pineal organ, although retaining its connection with the skull, must have already been withdrawn from its primary super-ficial position beneath the skin into the cavity of the skull, or that in the course of ontogeny the " parietal organ " or " pineal eye " had been severed from the stalk of the pineal outgrowth and that the distal end of the latter had caused the impression on the inner aspect of the vault of the skull, as is seen in many living types of fishes, Amphibia, and reptiles. In either case it is evident that the organ in these extinct fishes must have already reached a retrogressive or vestigial stage in its evolutionary history. Since the " parietal organ " had already been cut off from its connection with the brain as well as from the source of light, it is obvious that at this very remote period in the history of the vertebrates it must have ceased to function, at any rate as a light-perceiving organ.

CHAPTER 3

TYPES OF VERTEBRATE AND INVERTEBRATE EYES

By the study of the adult organ and different stages of its development in the various types of eye—" upright " or " inverted," " simple " or " compound," " single " or " composite "—it has been shown that the receptive or sensory cells of all these types have been evolved by modification of the surface layer of epithelium. In invertebrates the epithelium is derived from the " hypoderm " which lies beneath the cuticle (Fig. 4).

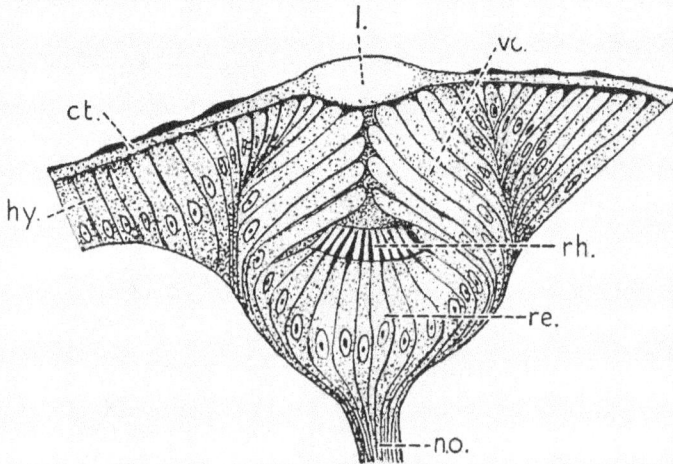

FIG. 4.—SECTION THROUGH THE OCELLUS OF A YOUNG DYTISCUS LARVA. (AFTER GRENACHER.)

ct. : chitinous cuticle.	*rh. :* rods.
vc. : cells of the vitreous body.	*re. :* retinal cells.
l. : cuticular lens.	*n.o. :* optic nerve.
hy. : hypodermis.	

In vertebrates the sensory epithelium originates from the medullary plate, or " neural ectoderm." This is at first spread out on the surface of the embryo and forms an elongated placode of thickened epithelium continuous at its edges with the surrounding cutaneous ectoderm, and in this respect it resembles the olfactory, otic, and branchial placodes

(Fig. 5, p. 11). A pit, the optic groove, then appears on each side in the situation of the future optic vesicle (Figs. 6, 7, 8). Later, when the medullary folds close in to form the neural tube, the optic pits appear as hollow evaginations springing from the sides of the neural tube. The

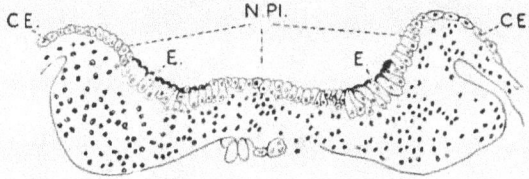

FIG. 5.—TRANSVERSE SECTION OF OPEN NEURAL PLATE OF RANA PALUSTRIS, NEAR ITS ANTERIOR END, SHOWING THE POSITION OF THE OPTIC RUDIMENTS. E., ALREADY MARKED OUT BY THE FORMATION OF PIGMENT.

CE. : Cutaneous epithelium.   *N.Pl.* : Neural plate.

(After Eycleshymer, 1895, *Textbook of Embryology*, Vol. II, Graham Kerr.)

expanded outer end of each outgrowth is known as the primary optic vesicle, and the constricted neck is the optic stalk. The stalk is at first a hollow tube which connects the cavity of the primary optic vesicle with

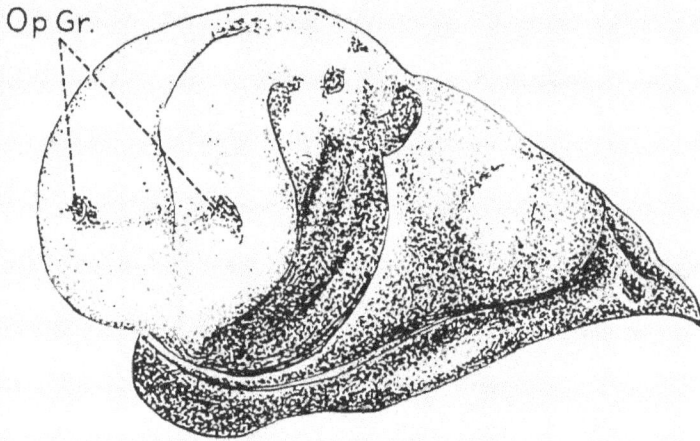

FIG. 6.—MODEL OF THE HEAD OF A PIG EMBRYO 4·7 MM. (16 DAYS), SHOWING THE OPTIC GROOVES ON THE SURFACE OF THE OPEN, NEURAL PLATE. THE MODEL IS VIEWED FROM THE FRONT AND LEFT SIDE. (AFTER FRORIEP.)

Op. Gr. : Optic grooves.

the third ventricle ; and its opening into the ventricle corresponds to the mouth of the original pit or groove which opened on the surface of the open medullary plate. The epithelium, which forms the outer part of the primary optic vesicle and later becomes invaginated to form the sensitive part of the retina, does not appear at this stage of development to differ markedly from that of the lens placode.

The invagination of the outer part of the primary optic vesicle into the ensheathing segment which becomes the pigment layer of the retina constitutes the essential structural difference between the " upright eye," typical of invertebrates, and the " inverted " eye which is characteristic

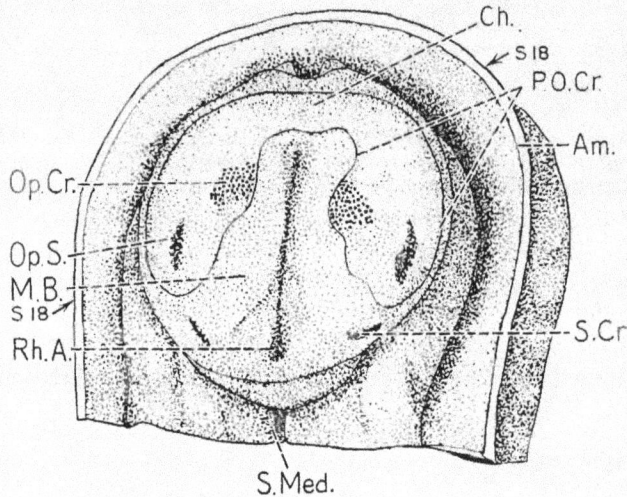

Fig. 7.—Dorsal View of the Head Region of a Human Embryo at an Early Stage of Development, showing the Optic Grooves before the Closure of the Neural Tube. (Legge embryo, 12 somites, after Bartelmez and Evans.)

> Am. : Cut edge of Amnion.
> Ch. : Site of the future optic chiasma, where the right and left halves of the primordium of the optic crest become continuous anteriorly.
> M.B. : Midbrain.
> Op. Cr. : Stippled area representing the region beneath which the cells of the optic crest originate.
> Op. S. : Optic groove.
> P.O. Cr. : Primordium opto-cristale.
> Rh. A. : Anterior segment of Rhombencephalon.
> S. Cr. : Sulcus cristale.
> S. Med. : Sulcus medullaris.
> S.18 : Arrows indicating the plane of section Fig. 8.

of the paired lateral eyes of all vertebrates. In the inverted eye the receptive end of the sensory retinal cells—rods and cones—is turned away from the source of light, entering the eye through the pupil. In those animals, however, such as the horse and ox, in which a *tapetum lucidum* is present on the retinal surface of the choroid coat and gives to this a metallic lustre, it is believed that light is reflected by it on to the outer

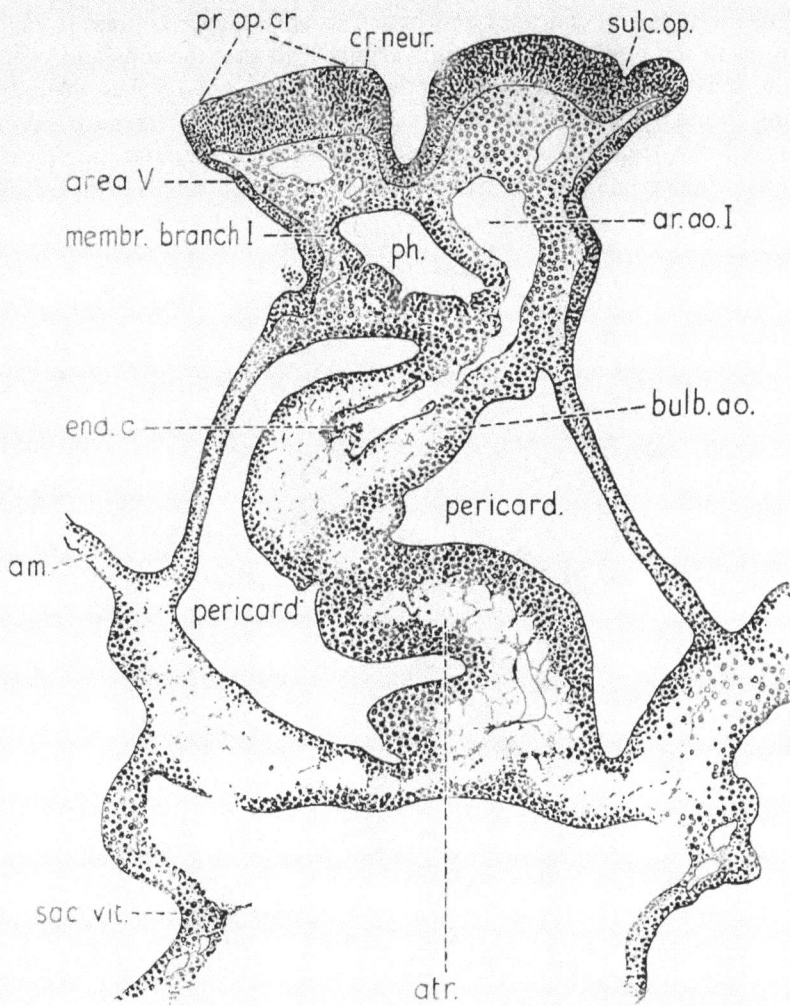

FIG. 8.—SECTION PASSING THROUGH THE OPTIC GROOVE AND OPTIC CREST IN THE PLANE WHICH IS INDICATED BY ARROWS AT S.18, IN THE PRECEDING FIG. 7.

am. : Amnion.
ar. ao. I. : arcus aortæ I.
area V. : area of fifth cranial nerve.
atr. : atrium.
bulb. ao. : bulbus aortæ.
cr. neur. : crista neuralis prosencephali.
end. c. : endothelial canal of bulbus aortæ.
membr. br. I. : membrana branchialis I.
pericard : pericardial cavity.
ph. : pharyngeal cavity.
pr. op. cr. : primordium opto-cristale.
sac. vit. : vitelline sac.
sulc. op. : sulcus opticus.

ends of the rods and cones ; but whether a tapetal layer is present, or is
absent as in the human eye, it is universally held that the rods and cones
are the sensitive elements of the retina and that light reaches them by
passing through the transparent anterior layers which intervene between
them and the refractile elements—cornea, aqueous humour, lens, and
vitreous. The relation of the nerve fibres to the sensory cells of the retina

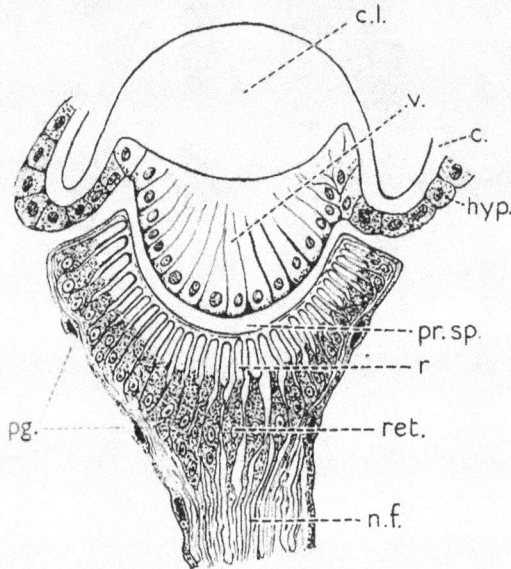

FIG. 9.—VERTICAL MEDIAN SECTION THROUGH ONE OF THE THREE FRONTAL
OCELLI, OR STEMMATA, OF A BLOW-FLY IMAGO. (AFTER T. B. LOWNE.)

c. : cuticle.	hyp. : hypodermi.
c.l. : cuticular lens.	n.f. : nerve fibres.

pg. : pigment cells forming fibrous sheath, continuous with the perineural sheath.

pr. sp. : preretinal space. r. : rods. ret. : retina.

v. : vitreous cells, continuous with hypoderm cells. These cells, which
are present in the imago as a layer of tall, columnar cells, degenerate
and in the mature animal exist only as a very thin stratum which is
easily overlooked.

is well seen in Fig. 9, which represents an invertebrate eye of the upright
type, and Fig. 10, A, B, the developing " inverted " lateral eye of a
vertebrate.

The retina of both " upright " and " inverted " eyes may be either
" simple " or " compound." The simple retina consists of a single layer of
sensory cells, as in Fig. 9 ; the compound retina of two or more layers of
sensory or neuro-sensory cells, as in the compound faceted or non-faceted

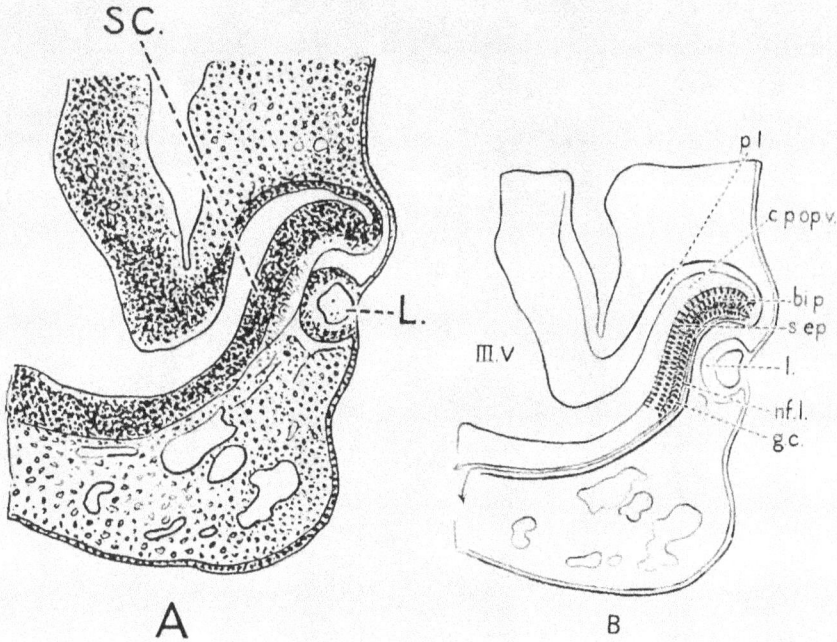

FIG. 10.

A—Section through the optic vesicle of a human embryo, 7 mm., showing continuity of the cavity of the primary optic vesicle with the cavity of the third ventricle.   The surface (SC.) of the invaginated layer of the optic cup was originally on the superficial aspect of the medullary plate.   *L. :* lens vesicle.

B—Schematic diagram of a vertical section of the optic cup of the 7-mm. human embryo shown in A, representing the positions of the retinal layers when these are fully differential, in order to demonstrate the relation of the rod-and-cone layer of sensory cells to the cavity of the primary optic vesicle, the lining epithelium of which was originally on the superficial surface of the neural-plate, and later formed the epithelium at the bottom of the optic groove, before the closure of the medullary folds.   The nerve-fibre layer of the retina corresponds to the deep surface of the neural plate.   When the optic cup is formed it becomes directed towards the outer surface of the cup by the inversion of the ventro-lateral segment of the primary optic vesicle.   The arrows indicate the direction of the decussating and tract fibres of the optic nerve in the region of the future chiasma.

bi.p. : bipolar cells.	*nf.l. :* nerve-fibre layer.
c.p.op.v. : cavity of primary optic vesicle.	*p.l. :* pigment layer of retina.
g.c. : ganglion cells.	*s.ep. :* sensory layer (rods and cones).
l. : lens.	III. V. : third ventricle.

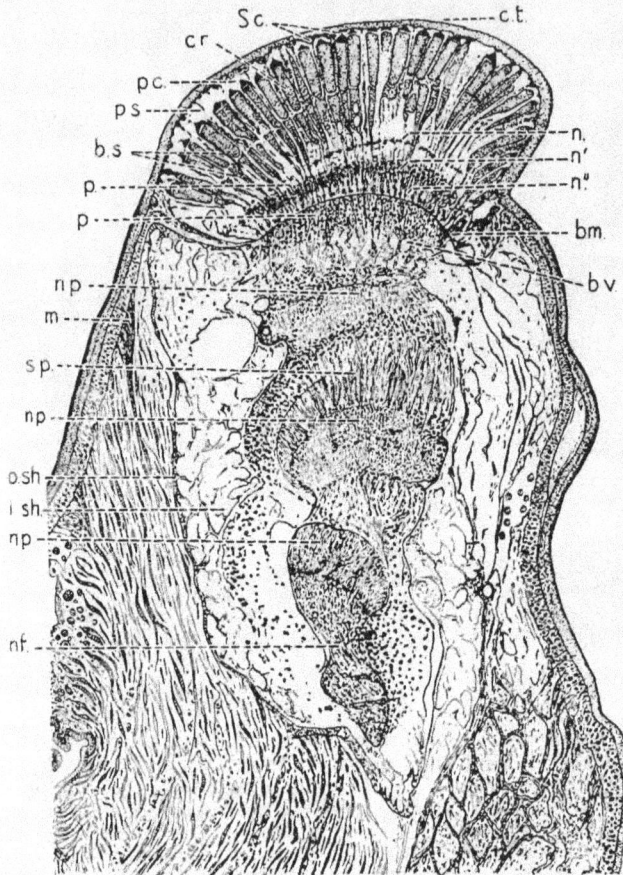

FIG. 11.—LONGITUDINAL SECTION THROUGH THE OPTIC STALK AND EYE OF A
CRAYFISH (ASTACUS FLUVIATILIS). (ORIGINAL.)

ct. : showing a smooth non-faceted cornea, continuous with the cuticle of the
stalk ; *Sc.* : Semper's cells partially concealed by pigment ; *pc.* : the
conical pigment caps continuous with the pigment sheath surrounding the
distal segments of the crystal rods *cr.* ; these are socketed in the cup-shaped
outer ends of the inner segments of these cells ; *n'.*, *n".*, *n.* : three zones of
retinal nuclei, the middle of which is obscured by pigment ; *bm.* : basement
membrane which is continuous at the margin of the retina with the basement
membrane beneath the hypoderm cells of the cuticle. The pedicle shows
four enlargements or optic ganglia, containing nerve cells, nerve fibres, a
reticulum of supporting fibres, the neuropil, *np.* ; and spirally or transversely
striated, refractile spindles, *sp.* ; *m.* : insertion of muscle fibres into the hypodermal membrane of the optic stalk ; *o.sh.* and *i.sh.*, outer- and inner-
fibrous sheaths of the pedicle between which is a loose layer of mesenchymal
tissue. There is a marked spiral twist of the central nervous axis of the
pedicle. *bv.* : blood vessels ; *nf.* : nerve-fibres.

eyes of certain crustaceans and the retina of the paired lateral eyes of mammals (Figs. 11 and 12).   Simple upright eyes are present in the lower and some of the higher invertebrates and are also found in the median paired eyes of both invertebrates and vertebrates (Figs. 9, 13, 14).   They may occur in the form of simple patches of modified epithelium, pits, or hollow vesicles.   From the inner ends of the epithelial cells elongated processes or nerve-fibres are given off.   These leave the deep surface of the plaque or vesicle and join a subepithelial nerve-plexus or cerebral ganglion. The sensory epithelial cells are often pigmented in one part, the rest of

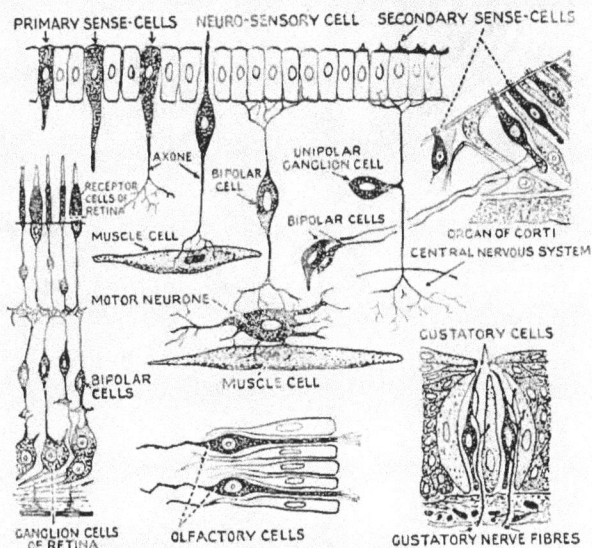

FIG. 12.—DIAGRAM ILLUSTRATING THE SUPPOSED MODE OF GROWTH OF PRIMARY AND SECONDARY SENSORY CELLS, AND THE CONVERSION OF THE FORMER INTO BIPOLAR OR UNIPOLAR NEURO-SENSORY CELLS.

(Redrawn with some modifications from Arien-Kappers and Retzius.)

the cell being clear, or specialized pigment-cells may lie between or around the receptive cells.   The outer end of a sensory or visual cell is frequently rod-like, and is termed the rhabdite.   This part of the cell is clear and refractile, and it is believed to transmit the rays of light to the body of the cell in which the nucleus is situated and which is continuous at its inner end with a nerve fibre.   In the more highly evolved types of upright eye, a circular fold of epithelium enclosing a layer of mesenchyme grows inward superficially and closing the mouth of an optic pit converts it into an optic vesicle (Figs. 33–35, Chap. 3, pp. 48, 49).   When in this way the optic vesicle has been cut off, the epithelium lying over it and the under-

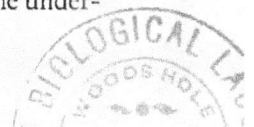

2

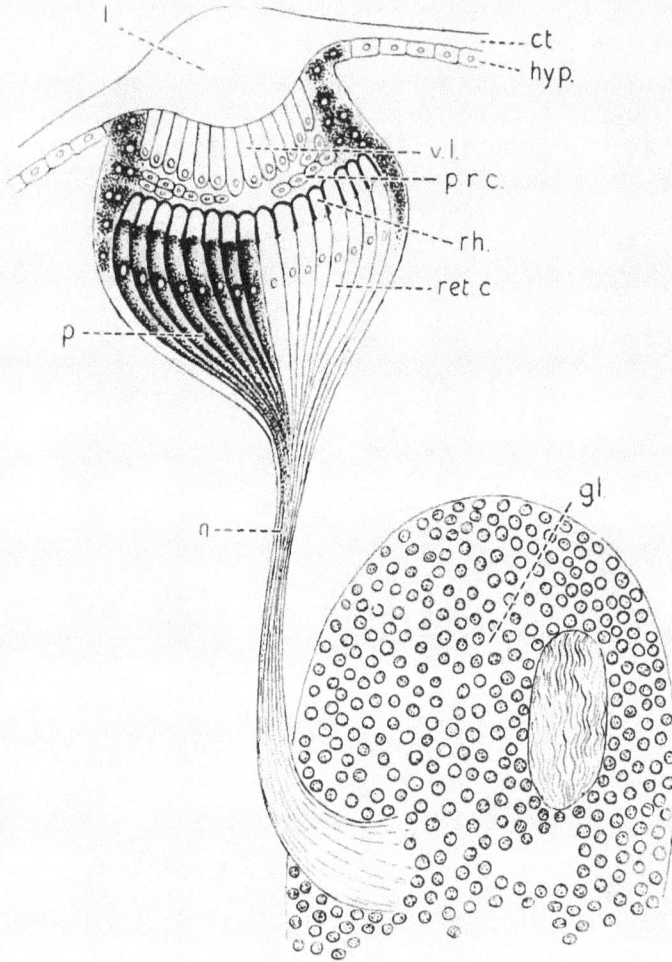

FIG. 13.—SECTION THROUGH EYE OF ACILIUS LARVA, SHOWING THE NATURAL
APPEARANCE WITH THE PIGMENT IN SITU ON THE LEFT, AND THE RETINAL CELLS
AS SEEN IN A SPECIMEN WHICH HAS BEEN BLEACHED ON THE RIGHT. (AFTER
GASKELL.)

ct. : cuticle.	*p. :* pigment.
gl. : cerebral ganglion.	*p.r.c. :* pre-retinal cells.
hyp. : hypodermis.	*rh. :* rods.
l. : lens.	*ret. c. :* retinal cells.
n. : optic nerve.	*v.l. :* vitreous layer.

Compare with Fig. 14.

Fig. 14.—Semidiagrammatic Section through the Right Pineal Eye, Pineal Nerve and Right Habenular Ganglion of Ammocœtes. (After Gaskell.)

Showing an optic vesicle of the simple upright type which resembles in some respects types found in certain of the invertebrates, e.g. *Acilius* (see Fig. 13). The outer or superficial segment of the vesicle consists chiefly of elongated clear cells which form an imperfect lens. The inner segment is the retinal layer, which on the right side of the diagram is represented as seen in a bleached specimen and on the left in the natural condition with the pigment *in situ*. It consists of elongated sensory cells, the distal segments of which are rodlike, while the proximal ends of the cells appear to be continuous with the component fibres of the main optic nerve, which ends in the right habenular ganglion. In addition to the sensory cells of the retina are certain oval and rounded cells which are peripheral in position and lie between the columnar cells of the retina and the capsule, and others between the retina and the lenticular cells. The pigment appears to lie partly within the substance of the sensory cells and partly in specialized intermediate pigment cells between the sensory cells. Superficial to the optic vesicle are the connective tissue fibres of the cranial capsule, above this but not shown in the diagram is the parietal plug, which intervenes between the vesicle and the sub-epidermal stratum of connective tissue, the latter corresponds to the substantia propria of the cornea of the lateral eyes of vertebrates in general.

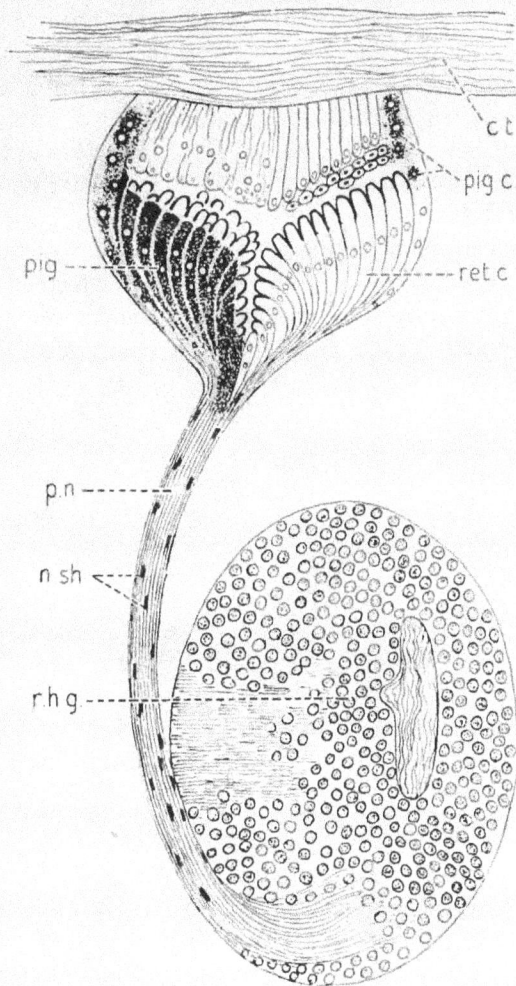

c.t. : connective tissue.	*p.n.* : pineal nerve.
n. sh. : nuclei of nerve sheath.	*ret. c.* : sensory cells of retina.
pig. : pigment.	*r.h.g.* : right habenular ganglion.
pig. c. : pigment cells.	

lying mesenchyme form a transparent layer termed the cornea; or in some cases this layer is called " secondary cornea," whereas the unpigmented superficial segment of the optic vesicle is called the " primary cornea " (Fig. 36, Chap. 3, p. 50). When a simple upright eye has only a single lens it is classed as an " ocellus," a term also applied to eye spots and other simple types of eye. The lens of an invertebrate eye may be non-cellular or cellular. The non-cellular type is most frequently formed by a thickening of the cuticle or chitin, cuticular lens; sometimes as a condensation of the secretion of vitreous cells (Figs. 33–35, 38, Chap. 3, pp. 48, 49, 53). The vitreous may be formed from a secretion of the cells lining the optic vesicle, but in some cases it appears to originate from two or more very large cells in the cavity of the optic cup or vesicle, which

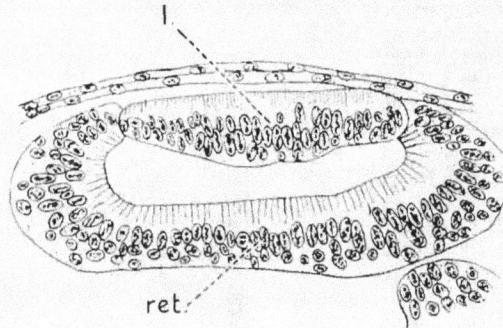

FIG. 15.—LONGITUDINAL VERTICAL SECTION THROUGH THE PARIETAL EYE OF AN ADVANCED EMBRYO OF ANGUIS FRAGILIS SHOWING DISTINCT BOUNDARY BETWEEN LENS AND RETINA. (AFTER J. BEARD, *Q.J. Micro. Sc.*, **29**, 1889.)

l. : lens.   *ret. :* retina.

degenerate and give rise to a clear viscous fluid, as in the eyes found on the back of *Onchidium* (Fig. 39, Chap. 3, p. 54).

Cellular lenses may be formed in invertebrates by elongation of the hypoderm cells, as in the median eyes of the blow-fly (Fig. 9) or the ocelli of the larva of a beetle (*Dytiscus*) which shows a transition from the surrounding hypoderm cells through the elongated " vitreous " cells of the lens to the sensory cells of the retina. This type of lens is frequently combined with a cuticular lens which forms a transparent thickening of the cuticle over the centre of the " vitreous " part (Fig. 4, p. 10). A cellular lens formed from the distal wall of the optic vesicle is well seen in the median or " pineal eyes " of some lizards, e.g. in the blind-worm—*Anguis fragilis* and *Sphenodon* (Fig. 15; and Fig. 183, Chap. 20, p. 259). A good example of a cellular lens is also present in the remarkable eyes arranged round the edge of the mantle in the *Scallop* (Patten) (Fig. 107,

Chap. 12, p. 149). Lastly, the " crystal cones " belonging to each component of the composite faceted eyes of certain Crustacea are partly " cellular," partly " vitreous," and will be described in the section dealing with the eyes of arthropods (Figs. 81, 95, Chap. 11, pp. 119, 133).

Single and Composite Eyes.—Groups of single eyes or ocelli, each with a separate lens, may be aggregated in a single organ which is best termed a composite faceted eye. These composite faceted eyes have to be distinguished from eyes having a compound retina, as in the lateral eyes of vertebrates, in which only one lens is present, but there are three layers of sensory cells : rod- and cone-cells, bipolar-cells, and ganglioncells. Unfortunately the term " compound " has been used by different writers to denote both the aggregate or composite faceted eyes and those in which the retina is made up of two or more layers of sensory cells. However, in many insects and crustacea the two conditions are combined, the eye being both composite and compound. Thus the confusion in terminology is not so great as it might have been if they were separate.

The Relation of Ocelli to Composite Faceted Eyes.—A considerable amount of interest has been taken in the relation which the simple eye having a single lens has to the composite lateral eyes which are typical of many adult insects and Crustacea. The two types of eye may be present together in a single adult individual, or ocelli may occur in the larva which are replaced or supplemented by composite faceted eyes in the adult. The ocelli may be lateral or median or may be both lateral and median in position. They may occur singly or in groups (Fig. 16). Fusion of a pair of median eyes to form a single unpaired median eye is common, or in some instances where two pairs of median eyes are close together the members of one pair, usually the

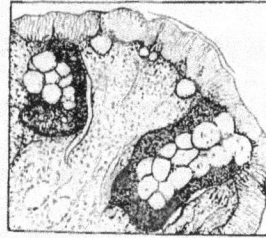

FIG. 16.—SOLITARY AND AGGREGATED EYES OF AN ANNELID—HÆMOPIS SANGUISUGA.

(AFTER ARIENS KAPPERS.)

anterior, will join, while the posterior pair of ocelli remain separate ; a group of three simple eyes thus arise from two pairs of such eyes, which originally were situated one behind the other, and between the lateral faceted eyes (Fig. 72, Chap. 11, p. 110 ; Fig. 249, Chap. 24, p. 361). The fused eyes frequently show regressive characters, being small and imperfectly developed as regards structure. Ocelli, moreover, are often present in the larval stage which disappear completely in the adult (Fig. 78, Chap. 11, p. 117). An interesting departure from the general rule that the median eyes are simpler in type and less developed than the lateral eyes is found in the scorpion, in which the lateral eyes (Fig. 94,

Chap. 11, p. 132) resemble the simple eyes or ocelli of insects (Fig. 9, p. 14) while the pair of larger median eyes differ from them in having the retinal cells arranged in groups, as in the composite eyes of certain insects and crustacea ; they resemble the simple eyes, however, in having a non-faceted single lens (Fig. 95, Chap. 11, p. 133). The whole question of the existence of the " median," " frontal," or " accessory " eyes in larval and adult insects and Crustacea, and the frequent disappearance of the larval eyes which takes place in the change to the adult form, is of the greatest importance in understanding the nature of the median or " pineal eyes " of vertebrates. We shall, therefore, attempt to give a brief sketch of some of the more essential points of these and of the lateral eyes in invertebrates, with the object of making a comparison between the two and showing the differences as well as the similarities in their structure and position.

Beside the median and lateral eyes of the head, eyes of different type appear in various parts of the body, e.g. on the margin of the umbrella in coelenterates, on the edge of the mantle in certain molluscs, and on the back in *Chiton*. The general form and connections also vary ; thus they may be stalked, sessile, or imbedded in a socket lined by a serous membrane. Some of the best examples of stalked eyes occur in the Crustacea, e.g. the crayfish and the shrimp ; among the Mollusca—snails and slugs ; and in vertebrates the " parietal-organ " or " pineal eye." In the lateral stalked eyes of the invertebrates, mobility is dependent on the movements of the stalk, which are carried out by muscle fibres within the stalk. The small pineal eye—" parietal organ "—of living vertebrates is usually immovably socketed in the parietal foramen, where it is surrounded by dense fibrous tissue. We have no direct evidence of its mobility in extinct animals ; the parietal foramen in many of the extinct reptiles and amphibia is, however, much larger than in any living species, and it is within the bounds of possibility that movements of the stalk or stalks similar to those which occur in the stalked eyes of invertebrates may have taken place.

In discussing these different types of eye it will be unnecessary to describe in detail certain varieties of eye, which although of considerable general interest, yet have no special bearing on the subject with which we are dealing. It is important, however, to note that a knowledge of the structure of certain atypical eyes, which owing to their position cannot be regarded as homologous with those of the head, although they have many points in common with these, is nevertheless of considerable value. The structural resemblances must have arisen in response to similar environmental factors and similar somatic conditions, e.g. the action of light on skin and pigment granules contained in the epithelium and subcutaneous tissue, and the existence of a structural basis for the transmission of impulses from sensory epithelial cells by afferent nerves to the central nervous system.   The existence of such close structural resemblances in organs which are not truly homologous may serve the purpose of putting us on our guard against drawing conclusions which are seen to be unwarranted when all relevant circumstances are taken into account.

Good examples of such structures are the " luminous organs " seen on the ventro-lateral aspect of certain deep-sea teleosteans, e.g. *Stomias boa* (Fig. 17) and the " photospheria " on the thoracic and abdominal appendages of *Nyctiphanes Norwegica*, a crustacean closely allied to the cuttle-fishes.   An interesting point in connection with these " photospheria," Fig. 18,[1] is that in addition to the thoracic and abdominal luminous organs, a pair which are similar in structure to these have been

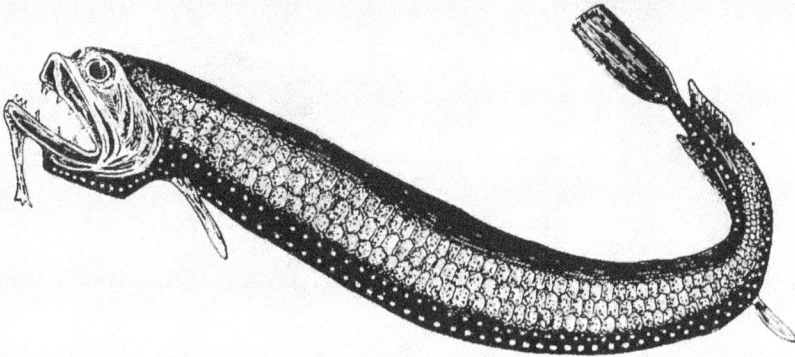

FIG. 17.—STOMIAS BOA—A DEEP-SEA TELOSTEAN FISH WHICH IS CHARACTERIZED BY A SERIES OF LUMINOUS ORGANS ARRANGED IN LONGITUDINAL ROWS ALONG THE VENTRO-LATERAL ASPECTS OF THE BODY.   (FROM HICKSON, AFTER FILHOL.)

shown by Vallentin and Cunningham to be present in the adult animal at the base of the stalk of each of the composite faceted eyes.   Incidentally the appearance of this luminous organ in close association with the faceted eye suggests the possibility of the latter having been evolved as a modification of the more simple type of organ which is situated at the base of the stalk.

Claus,[2] in an earlier paper on *Euphausia Mulleria*, a nearly allied species, speaks of these organs as " accessory eyes " of which some are median and unpaired, while others are lateral and paired.   He described them as ten small, globular, reddish organs, having a resemblance in many respects

---

[1] R. Vallentin and J. T. Cunningham, *Q.J. Micro. Sc.*, **25**, 319.
[2] Claus, " Ueber einige Schizopoden und niedere Malacostraken, Messinas " (1863), *Zeit. f. wiss. Zool.*, **13**.

to such eyes as those of vertebrates and some molluscs and chætopods. The pair of similar organs behind the two composite faceted eyes apparently escaped Claus's notice. Vallentin and Cunningham record that the light which is given off in " flashes " in response to stimulation is always intermittent in character, not continuous as in some " phosphorescent " organs, and they showed that the parts of the organ from which the light was emitted was the reflector (Fig. 18).

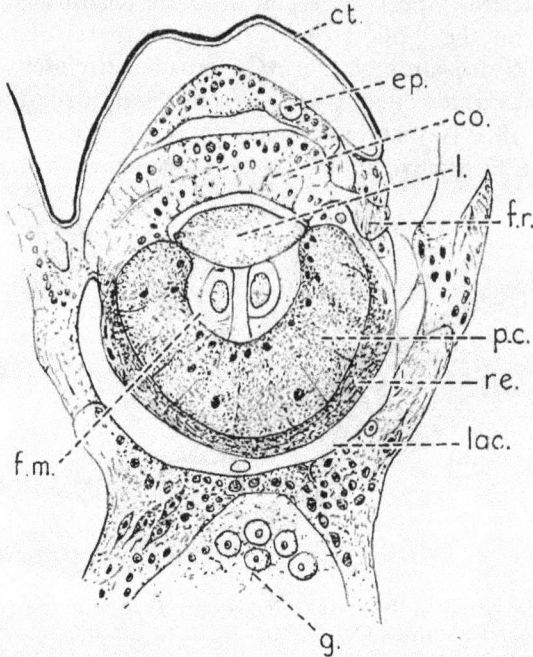

FIG. 18.—SECTION OF THE PHOTOSPHERION OF THE FIRST ABDOMINAL SOMITE OF NYCTIPHANES NORWEGICA. (AFTER VALLENTIN AND CUNNINGHAM.)

co. : cornea.	*g.* : ganglion.
ct. : cuticle.	*l.* : lens.
ep. : epidermis.	*lac.* : lacuna.
f.m. : fibrillar mass.	*p.c.* : posterior cellular layer.
f.r. : fibrous ring.	*re.* : reflector.

Two possible ways of obtaining a composite eye from ocelli suggest themselves : (1) groups of separate ocelli may fuse to form a composite organ ; or (2) the individual cells composing an ocellus may divide in such a way as to form groups of cells lying side by side.

The latter process has been shown to occur by Kingsley[1] in the development of the stalked eyes of *Crangon* (shrimp), and this has been

[1] J. S. Kingsley (1886), *Zool. Anz.*, **9**, 597.

confirmed by other workers in different species of Crustacea and insects. The compound faceted eye was found to develop from a single invaginated pit, a fact which proves that in these species the compound faceted eye is not to be regarded as derived from ocelli which have coalesced during ontogeny. Similar observations were made by Sedgwick, on *Peripatus*, and Locy, on spiders. The details of this development will be considered in the section on the eyes of crustaceans, and it will be only necessary to mention here that the fusion of ocelli to form a single median eye usually

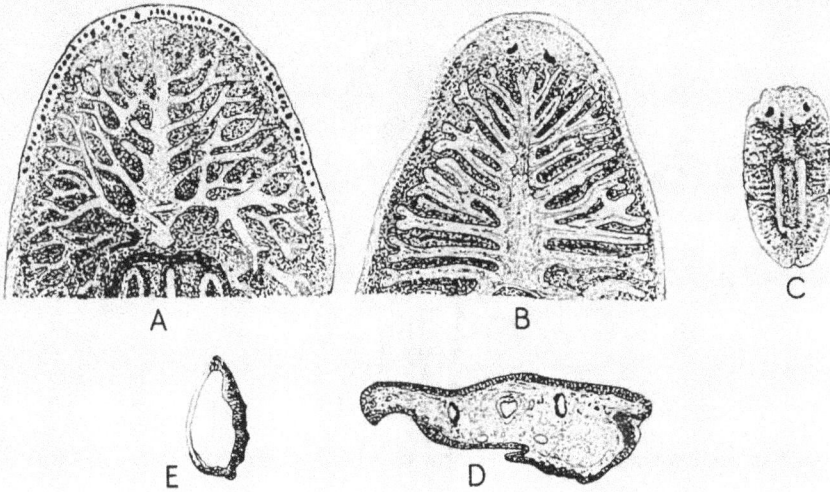

FIG. 19.

A—Freshwater Planarian. Pigment spots are situated on the dorsal aspect of the head region, along the margin in front and laterally, and also two pairs one behind the other on the top of the head near the middle line.

B—Freshwater Planarian having a single pair of pigment spots on the dorsal aspect of the head.

C—A marine Turbellarian (*Gunda*) showing a single pair of pigment spots.

D—Transverse section through the eyes of *Dendrocœlum lactea*.

E—Section through one of the eyes of *Dendrocœlum* more highly magnified. (R. J. G.)

results in an eye of a simple type which shows regressive characters rather than progressive evolution ; and the ontogeny of an organ which is highly differentiated both in structure and function, such as the compound faceted eyes, results from the subdivision of the individual cells of a simple eye. This subdivision may take place (a) in a direction vertical to the surface, producing (1) undifferentiated or slightly modified epidermal or hypodermal cells, (2) retinal cells, and (3) ganglionic cells, continuous with the cerebral ganglia ; and (b) transversely to the plane of the surface epithelium, thus giving rise to groups of cells arranged round a single axial cell continuous with a single nerve fibre, the whole constituting an ommatidium [1] or unit of the composite eye with its separate lens or corneal facet.

As previously mentioned, the fusion of two median eyes to form a single median eye is common in certain Insecta and Crustacea, and is frequently attended by regressive changes with diminution or loss of function ; and it will be useful at this stage of our description to consider the possible causes leading to (1) the approximation of a pair of eyes, and (2) their fusion and degeneration.

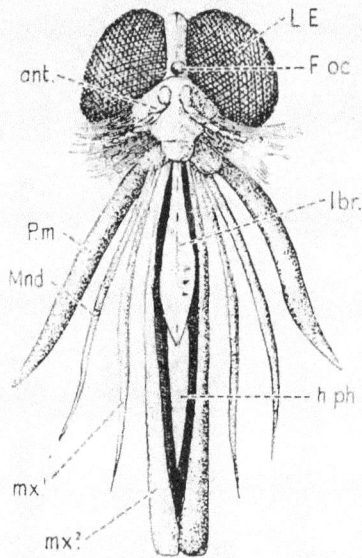

FIG. 20.—PAIRED LATERAL EYES AND SINGLE MEDIAN EYE OF A GAD FLY (TABANUS). (AFTER LANG.)

ant. : antenna.	*mx.*[1] : First pair of maxillæ.
F. oc. : frontal ocellus.	*mx.*[2] : proboscis which is formed
h. ph. : hypopharynx.	from the labrum which encloses
lbr. : labrum.	the mandibles and maxillæ.
L.E. : lateral or faceted eye.	*P.m.* : palp o the first pair of
Mnd. : mandible.	maxillæ.

If we examine the simple, pigmented eyes of certain species of flat worm, e.g. the *Planaria*, we find that in some the eyes are arranged in a semicircle around the front and sides of the head, the eyes being on the dorsal aspect of the head and near its edge (Fig. 19) ; in other species in addition to the eyes round the margin of the head there is a pair, sometimes two pairs, of eyes placed medially and farther back than the others (Fig. 19, A) ; while in a third group the marginal row of eyes is absent

---

[1] Ommatidium : ὄμμα, eye ; ὀμμάτιον, diminutive of eye.

and only the median pair is present (Fig. 19, B, C).   These appearances are suggestive of the median paired eyes having originated from the marginal eyes, two of the central members of which, having become shifted backwards, are left behind the others on the dorsal aspect of the head,

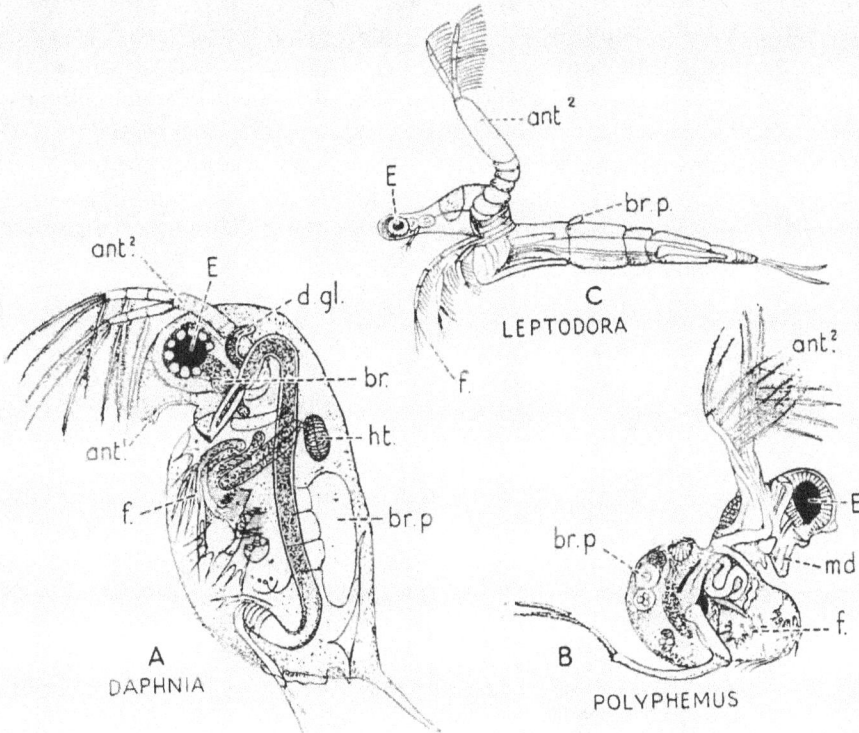

FIG. 21.—THREE SPECIMENS OF *Cladocera*, BELONGING TO THE SUB-ORDER BRANCHIOPODA OF THE CLASS CRUSTACEA.   THE LATERAL EYES ARE SESSILE AND JOINED TOGETHER IN THE MEDIAN PLANE TO FORM A SINGLE ORGAN.   THE *Cladocera* ARE GREATLY REDUCED IN SIZE (I TO 2 MM.) AND SEGMENTATION IS VERY IMPERFECT.

A—*Daphnia*.   B—*Polyphemus*.   C—*Leptodora*.

The eyes of *Daphnia* and *Polyphemus* are, relative to the size of the body, very large.

ant.[1] : antennule.	*d.gl.* : digestive gland.
ant.[2] : antenna.	*f.* : swimming feet.
br.p. : brood-pouch.	*ht.* : heart.
E : eye.	*md.* : mandible.

(A : after Claus.   B and C : after Gerstaecker.)

while the remaining marginal eyes are carried forward and laterally, following the general growth of this region of the head.   Whether paired eyes have arisen in this way or have been evolved independently, the foundation of a paired system of eyes is present in these simple Planarian worms. In higher types of invertebrates it is found that one such pair of eyes has become much more highly evolved and larger than the others, and constitutes the functional lateral pair of eyes, whereas the other pair or pairs remain small and simple in type. In some insects, e.g. the gad fly (*Tabanus*) (Fig. 20), the faceted lateral eyes having increased enormously in size and being directed forwards as well as laterally, have come so near together that the area which gives origin and nutriment to the median pair or pairs of eyes is encroached upon, and the whole area, including its vessels and nerves, being reduced, the median eyes also become reduced in size, approximated, and fused. It thus seems possible that a mechanical and nutritive as well as a functional preponderance of one pair of eyes over

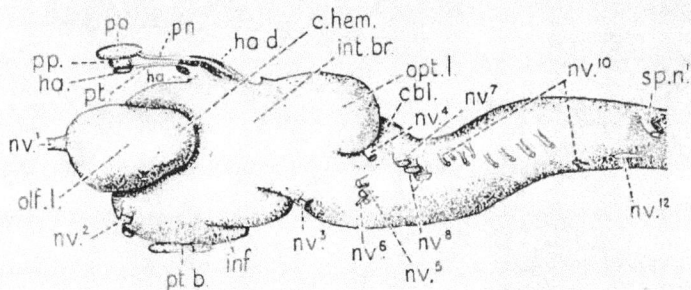

FIG. 22.—LEFT SIDE OF THE BRAIN OF PETROMYZON, SHOWING THE RELATIONS OF THE PINEAL ORGANS AND THE HABENULAR GANGLIA. (AFTER AHLBORN.)

cbl. : cerebellum.	*olf. l.* : olfactory lobe.
c. hem. : cerebral hemisphere.	*opt. l.* : optic lobe.
ha. : anterior and posterior segments of the left habenular ganglion.	*po.* : parietal organ.
	pn. : pineal nerve.
ha. d. : right habenular ganglion.	*pp.* : parapineal organ.
inf. : infundibulum.	*pt.* : pineal tract.
int. br. : interbrain.	*pt. b.* : pituitary body.
nv.[1–12] : cranial nerves.	*sp. n.*[1] : first spinal nerve.

the other may come into play and contribute to the fusion and atrophy of the less developed pair. In other invertebrates, e.g. some of the low-type crustaceans, more particularly *Daphnia*, *Polyphemus*, and *Leptodora* (Fig. 21), it is the lateral paired eyes which become fused. The underlying principle which is involved, however, is the same as in the fusion of the median eyes. There is, with the adoption of a parasitic life, a general reduction in the size of the animal and more particularly of the head, and with the loss of the necessity for using the eyes along with atrophy of the interocular tissues, the eyes are brought in contact with each other and fuse into a single organ.

The substitution of a single unpaired organ for the earlier paired median eyes is exemplified also in the pineal organ of the vertebrates.

The earlier pair of median eyes appear to have been supplanted by the more highly evolved lateral eyes, and thus undergo regressive changes. The vestigial median eyes are seen to arise in certain cases from a common stalk. This divides into two terminal swellings, which are often of unequal size. In some cases the smaller vesicle lies beneath the larger, as in Ammocœtes (Fig. 22); in other cases one organ, which is the less highly developed of the two, is shifted behind the other and the two vesicles in the adult animal lie approximately in the median plane, as in *Sphenodon* (Fig. 248, Chap. 24). These relations and their significance will be discussed in detail in the sections on the eyes of fishes and of reptiles (pp. 187, 242). The consideration of the geological evidence of the bilateral origin of the pineal organ in vertebrates and the fusion of the two parietal organs into a single median structure will also be postponed until later. It will be convenient, however, at this stage to describe the condition of cyclopia, which is produced by a process which is similar to that of the fusion of the median eyes of invertebrates and of the pineal organs in the vertebrates.

Cyclopia

The occurrence of one-eyed monsters has excited the curiosity not only of men belonging to our own period but also of the ancients. Among the latter Homer stands out pre-eminently, and his tale of the adventures of Ulysses and his fellow travellers with the giant Polyphemus has fascinated and stimulated the imagination of all students of mythology.

The questions which these ancient lays suggest, are :

1. Is there any foundation in fact for the classical myths of a race of giant cyclopes living apart from the world in insular seclusion ?

2. Is it possible for human cyclopes to reach maturity and have normal vision ?

Both these questions may be answered in the negative. Among the records of mammalian cyclopean monsters we have not found any authentic cases of such having survived their birth by more than a few hours. Many cases of cyclopia are combined with a high degree of agnathia, in which the jaws are absent or imperfectly developed. In many of these cases the nasal cavities are completely shut off from the pharynx, and in some the pharynx ends blindly.[1] In the latter, the young would quickly die from suffocation, while in the former the infant would be prevented from breathing during the act of suction, and the process of sucking would

[1] R. J. Gladstone, " A Cyclops and Agnathic Lamb " (1910), *Brit. Med. J.*, **2**, 1159.

have to be carried out by alternate respiratory and suction movements. In many cases, also, there are grave defects in the development of the brain, and the young are apt to die suddenly in convulsions soon after birth, as in cases of anencephaly. With regard to the possibility of a cyclops possessing normal vision, we find that in nearly all the published cases in which a dissection has been made of the median eye, the interior of the eyeball is almost completely filled with choroid and no mention is made of either retina or vitreous. Moreover, the lens has been found in some instances to be double, or if single it has usually shown signs of its composite nature. It is extremely improbable, therefore, that if it were possible for a human cyclops to reach maturity, he would possess normal vision.

The cause of cyclopia and the frequently associated defect agnathia has been investigated by many authors and experimental embryologists, and numerous theories have been advanced in explanation of the defect. The more important of the earlier contributions were summarized by Schwalbe, who gives full references to the literature up to the year 1905. Since this period the various theories with regard to the nature of cyclopia and of the malformations which are usually associated with it have been profoundly modified by the conception of the regulation of growth by the action of an organizer—more particularly at centres of cell-proliferation such as the " apical bud " of a growing stem or the " dorsal lip " of the blastopore. Some of the more recent publications on the nature of cyclopia are referred to in a paper which was published by us jointly in the *Journal of Anatomy* (1920) on a " Cyclops Lamb (Cyclops rhinocephalus)." In this communication we pointed out that a distinction may be drawn between those cases of cyclopia which occur in primarily double-headed monsters as the result of the fusion of the outer segments of eyes derived from two heads, and those which occur in single-headed monsters, the cyclops eye being due in these cases to the fusion of the temporal halves of the eyes belonging to one head in which the central region of the head, including the nasal halves of the two eyes, has failed to develop. As a type of the former we may select an example of the well-known class Cephalo-thoracopagus monosymmetros, in which the two heads are united in such a way that two " secondary faces " are formed (Fig. 23, A and B). One of these faces may be regarded as looking forwards and the other backwards. The secondary face in A is apparently complete, whereas the secondary face on the opposite side of the double-head seen in B is incomplete, there being neither nose nor mouth, and there being but one palpebral aperture, *p.ap.*, in the situation of a cyclops eye which is hidden from view by the fusion of the outer segments of upper and lower eyelids belonging to the two heads. The difference in the two heads is accounted

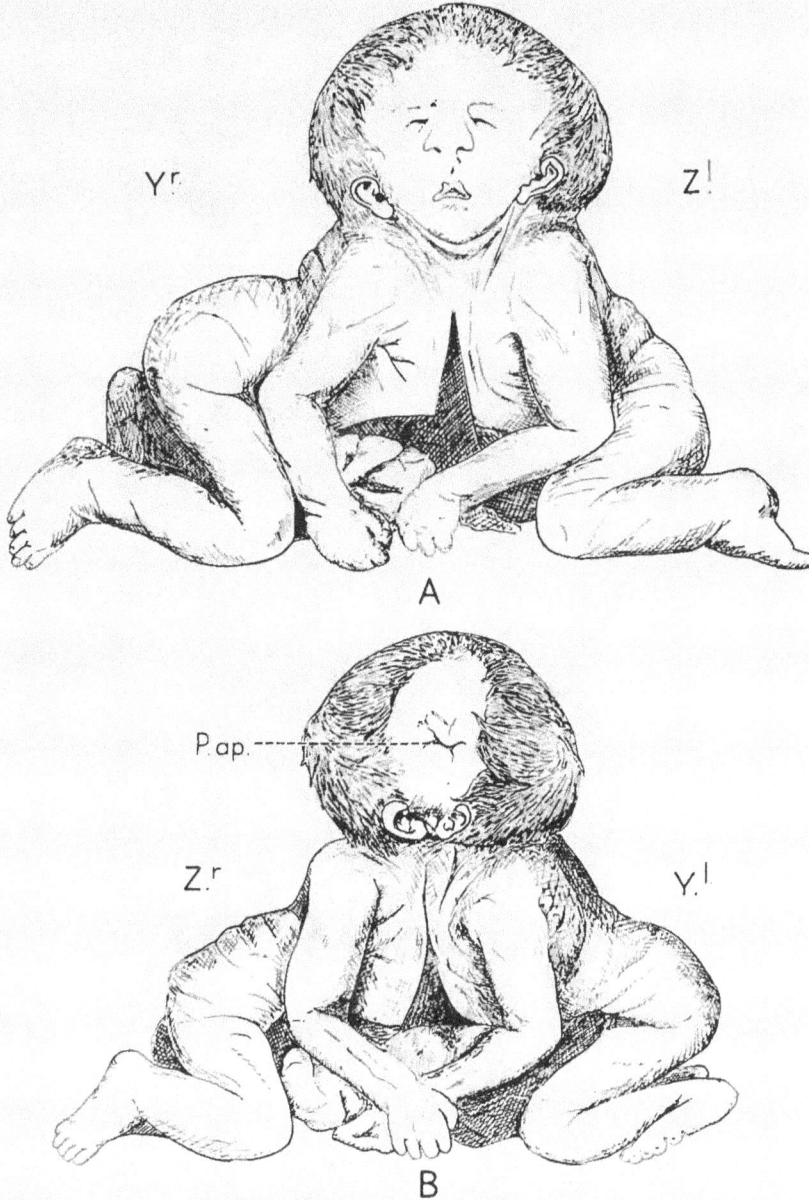

FIG. 23.—CEPHALO-THORACOPAGUS MONOSYMMETROS (DUPLICITAS POSTERIOR).
(REDRAWN FROM SCHWALBE.)

A and B, the same specimen viewed from opposite sides. The letters Y and Z
denote the individual components of the twin monster, and the letters l and r
the left or right side. A, complete " secondary " face, Y^r Z^l; B, incomplete " secondary " face Z^r Y^l showing a single palpebral aperture and
fused eyelids covering a cyclops eye. The nose and mouth are absent and the
ears approximated.

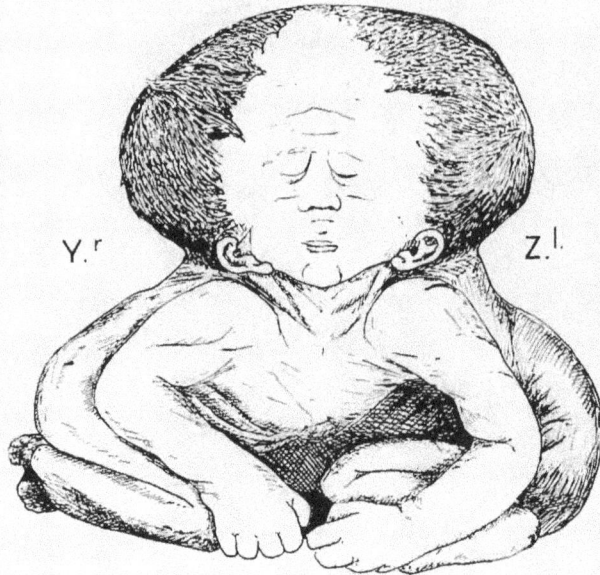

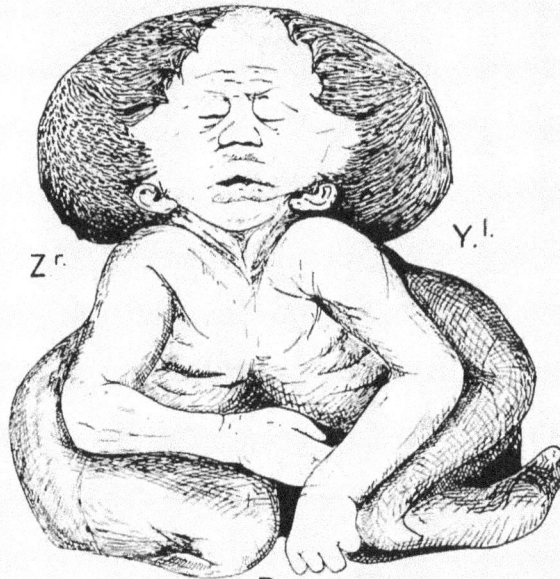

FIG. 24.—A JANUS-HEADED MONSTER, CEPHALO-THORACOPAGUS DISYMMETROS (DUPLICITAS POSTERIOR). (REDRAWN FROM SCHWALBE.)

The two " secondary " faces $Y^r + Z^l$ and $Z^r \cdot Y^l$ are almost identical, and look in a direction which is away from and at right angles to the median dorsoventral planes of the two fœtuses. In the disymmetrical type of Cephalo-thoraco-pagus these planes coincide.

for by the obliquity of the primary median antero-posterior axis of the two heads. If these had been in the same plane and at right angles to the primary dorso-ventral median planes of the two conjoined embryos, each secondary face would have been complete and similar, as in the Janus-headed monster shown in Fig. 24, A and B. In this example each "secondary face" has two eyes, one of which belongs to the fœtus designated Y, the other to the twin fœtus Z.

Another type of double-headed monster—Duplicitas anterior (Diprosopus)—in which cyclopia sometimes occurs is shown in Fig. 25. In this form the two faces look forward in the same direction and the cyclops eye

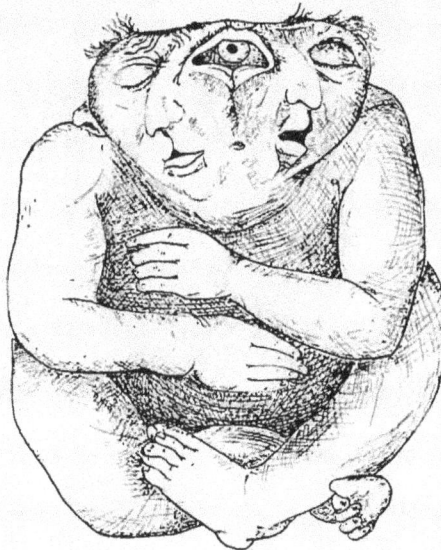

FIG. 25.—DIPROSOPUS. DUPLICITAS ANTERIOR.
Median eye formed by the union of the nasal half of the left eye of the right fœtus, with the nasal half of the right eye of the left fœtus.
(After Sömmering, from *Die Morphologie der Missbildungen* : Schwalbe.)

is bounded by the inner or nasal segments of four eyelids (two upper fused together, and two lower). The eye itself is formed by the growth in contact with each other of the inner or nasal halves of the opposed organs, the temporal halves being suppressed. The auricles of the external ears on the opposed sides are also suppressed, but a small opening below the palpebral aperture and at the same level as the mouths represents the common external auditory meatus. An X-ray photograph showed two vertebral columns extending as far as the single pelvis, where fusion took place in the sacral region. There was complete absence of the arms and legs on the opposed sides. Notwithstanding the marked difference

3

in general form between the Cephalo-thoracopagus and the Diprosopus
types, the principles which are concerned in the development of the cyclops
eye belong to the same category, although in the one case (Fig. 23, B)

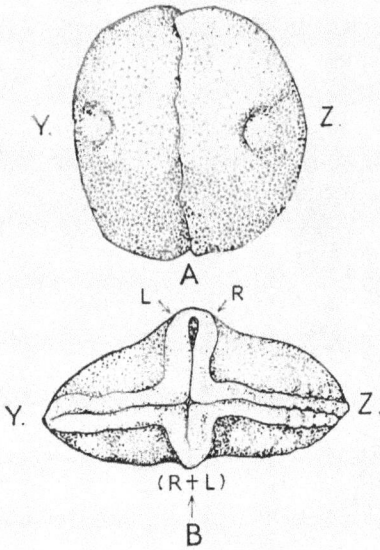

FIG. 26.

A—The dorsal halves *Y* and *Z* of two
Triton gastrulæ grafted together so
that the directions of invagination
at their blastopores are directly
opposed to each other.

B—The resulting embryo showing
crossed doubling—duplicitas
cruciata—each half gastrula has
developed a single posterior trunk
region with spinal cord and two
"secondary" head regions. These
are formed at right angles to the
longitudinal axis of the trunks.

L R, region which will give rise to the
L and R eyes of one "secondary"
face; (R+L) region which will
give rise to the cyclops eye of the
other secondary face.

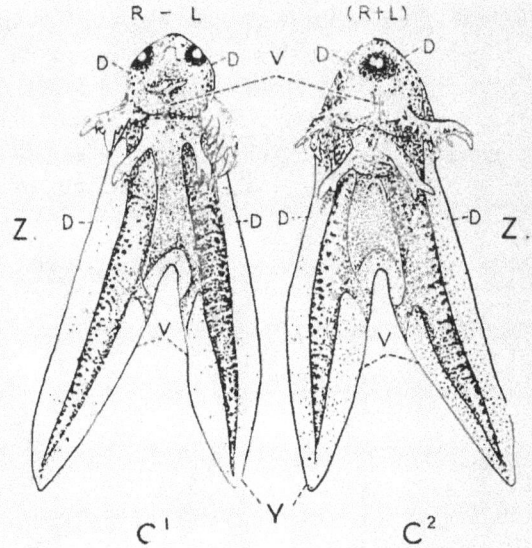

FIG. 27.

C¹—A later stage of the duplicitas
cruciata larva, viewed from the
direction of the arrows *L R* seen
above the drawing in B, Fig. 26.

In C² the same larva is viewed from
the direction of the single arrow
(R+L) in B, Fig. 26, which points
to the region which will give rise to
the cyclops eye, seen in C². In
both C¹ and C² the trunk and tail
regions are viewed from the side.
The two "secondary faces" are
developed so that each is directed
at a right angle away from the
dorso-ventral plane of the bodies
of the larvæ.

Y, Z : the component larvæ. D :
dorsal. V : ventral.

(After Spemann.)

the cyclops eye is formed by the union of the temporal halves of the
opposed eyes and in the other (Fig. 25), by the union of the nasal halves
of the two opposed eyes.   In both instances the segments of the developing

eyes which have grown in contact with each other have been suppressed, or, more correctly, have failed to develop. In Cephalo-thoracopagus monosymmetros it is the inner parts of the developing facial regions which first come into contact with each other on the cyclopic side, and these consequently fail to develop, whereas the outer parts of the face, being deflected, remain free, and thus undergo development; this will be explained later when dealing with the regulation of growth by the influence of an organizer, namely the dorsal lip of the blastopore, as when the normal course of development is interfered with by growth contact, in the experimental grafting of two gastrula-halves together and the formation of a Duplicitas cruciata, as described by Spemann (Figs. 26 and 27).

In the second type of cyclops, namely that occurring in single-headed monsters (Figs. 28, 29, and 30), the cyclops eye is formed by the more or less complete fusion of the outer or temporal segments of the right and left eyes of a single individual. It is accompanied by absence or defective growth of the median parts of the head, including the inner or nasal segments of the eyes and eyelids, the nose and mouth, the frontal region of the cranial part of the skull, and the corresponding parts of the brain. It is common in domestic animals—cats, dogs, sheep (Fig. 28), and cattle (Fig. 28 A, B)—and frequently occurs in artificially reared fish, amphibian and reptilian larvæ, and also in artificially incubated eggs. The injurious agents which have been employed in the experimental rearing or the artificial incubation that have resulted in the formation of these anomalies are : (1) mechanical injuries, e.g. separation of the blastomeres, incision, excision, and destruction of growing parts ; (2) the addition of magnesium, lithium, and other salts to the water in which the larvæ are reared ; (3) raising or lowering the temperature above or below the normal ; (4) variations in the amount of oxygen or carbon dioxide ; (5) narcotics and poisonous drugs such as chloroform, chloretone, and potassium cyanide. The results obtained by such treatment vary not only with the degree of the injury inflicted and the part injured, but also with the particular stage of development reached at the time when the experiment is made. Thus the production of normal or of cyclops eyes in *Triton* or *Amblystoma* larvæ appears to depend on the presence or absence of the anterior part of the entodermal gut-roof, which acts as a regulator or organizer on the presumptive eye-region in the neurula stage of development. If the anterior and central region of the entodermal gut-roof is injured there is a liability to cyclops formation, owing to interference with the normal organization of the optic vesicles and cerebral hemispheres from the overlying neural ectoderm. If the whole eye-region is destroyed, anophthalmia will result.

One of the most important deductions to be made from these experiments is, that since they have been carried out on fertilized embryonic material which was primarily normal, the anomalies have been produced

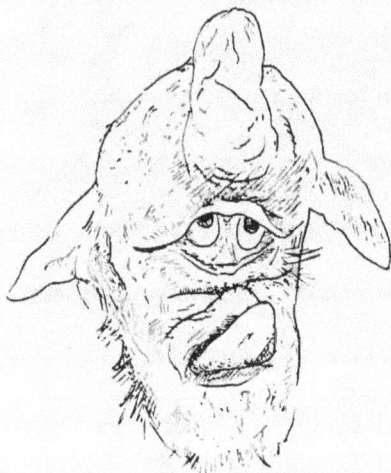

FIG. 28.—A CYCLOPS LAMB (C. RHINO-CEPHALUS) VIEWED FROM IN FRONT.

The tubular projection which springs from the frontal region is the " proboscis "; the single nasal orifice showed traces of its bilateral origin by fusion of the right and left nostrils. In the centre of the face is the single palpebral aperture, and the median eye, which was formed by the fusion of the outer parts of the right and left eyes. There were two corneæ and two lenses, but a single optic nerve. All the median structures, the septum of the nose, the internal orbital muscles and their nerves, were absent.

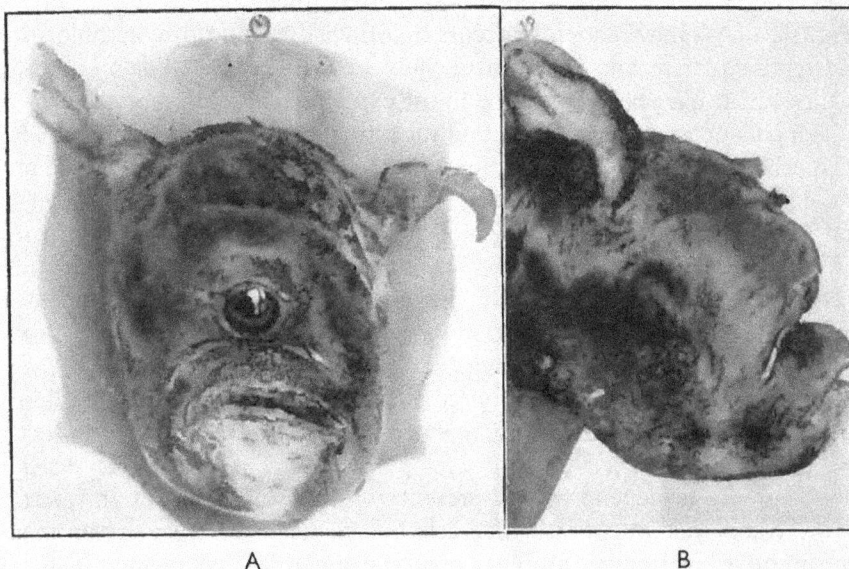

A   B

FIG. 28A, B.—HEAD OF CYCLOPS CALF.

A—View from the front.

B—Seen from the side.

(An artificial glass eye has been inserted into the eye-socket of the cyclops.)

by environmental factors; and so far as the experimental material is concerned are not due to germinal variations—in other words, the defects have not been inherited and are not due to defects in either of the two germinal cells. Moreover, it seems probable that the occurrence of identical defects in mammals and in the human subject may also be attributed to injury or faulty nutrition affecting the embryo in the very early stages of development, although obviously it does not exclude the possibility of a defective condition of either of the germinal cells being the cause of a defect in the subsequent growth of the embryo.

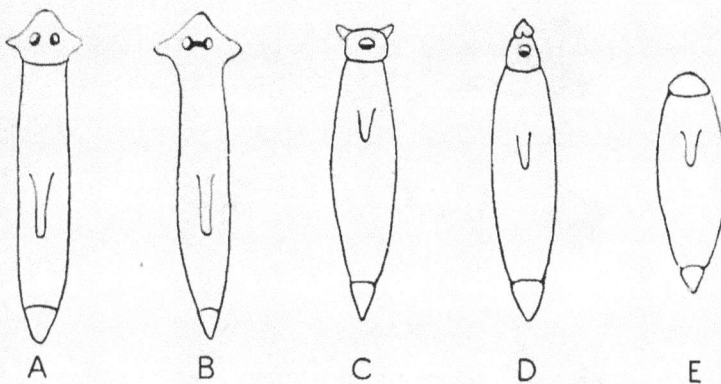

FIG. 29.—VARIOUS DEGREES OF REGENERATION AND HEAD DIFFERENTIATION AFTER AMPUTATION OF THE HEAD REGION IN PLANARIA. (AFTER CHILD.)

A—normal; B—partial fusion of eyes; C—cyclops eye, lateral sensory projections approximated and directed forwards; D—cyclops eye, lateral sensory projections fused; E—anophthalmos, head reduced in size.

The experiments carried out by Child on *Planaria* (Fig. 29) and by Stockard on *Fundulus* (Fig. 30), both indicate that the use of depressant agents produces what is known as " differential inhibition " on growth processes. Thus the most actively growing parts at particular periods of development are the most susceptible to the influence of the drug and suffer most. One of these areas, namely, the interocular and adjoining regions, may be specially mentioned as being a zone where active proliferation and differentiation is taking place, and as being more affected or susceptible to injury than the rest of the head, both in the regenerating head after amputation of the head region in *Planaria* and in the intact ova of developing *Funduli* during the gastrular stage of development.

Incidentally it may be mentioned here, with reference to the discussion which follows on the nature of double-monsters, that two-headed *Planaria* may be produced experimentally by splitting the anterior end of an early larva and preventing the two halves from uniting. Each head will show bilateral symmetry and develop the normal pair of eyes and sensory organs.

Thus two organizing centres may be obtained after the stage when a single normal organizer has already been established. Further, it is well known that twin or even multiple gastrulæ may occur in normal ova ; as for example, in the Texas armadillo, which has four primitive streaks, and a South America species of armadillo, which has eight, and normally

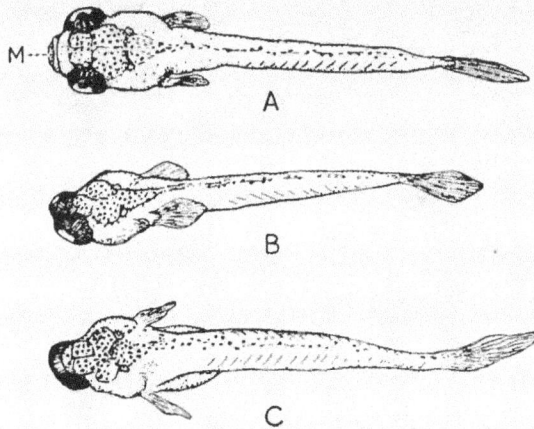

FIG. 30.—LARVÆ OF FUNDULUS HETEROCLITUS.

A—Normal larva with anteriorly placed mouth.

B—Incomplete cyclopean larva ; the two eyes are joined, and occupy the position usually taken by the mouth.

C—Complete cyclopean larva, with antero-median eye. Dorsal aspect.

M : mouth.

(After Stockard, from Dendy's *Outlines of Evolutionary Biology*.)

eight offspring at a single birth. These are believed to arise by the subdivision of a single blastoderm, and to be comparable with the artificial dichotomy of a growing bud and possibly also the induction of twinning in lower animals by merely separating the primary blastomeres ; or the production of separate embryonic axes in the eggs of fishes by lowering the temperature or reducing the oxygen supply during the early stages of segmentation.

There is, in fact, abundant proof of the uniovular origin of true twins. Further, the occurrence of multiple births arising from a single ovum, as in the case of the two species of armadillo, is well known to be an inherited condition. Moreover, that multiple growth-centres, twin and single monsters may occur as the result of alterations in the environmental conditions has been irrefutably demonstrated by experimental methods in the lower types of animals, and their occurrence appears to be extremely probable as a result of injury, disease, or toxic conditions of the blood circulating in the placenta in mammalia.

These conclusions, as we shall see hereafter, have a very definite bearing on the development and inheritance of the single median-eyes of both invertebrates and vertebrates, and their study with special reference to cyclopia is, therefore, not irrelevant to the general purpose of this book. Both types of cylopia, namely, that occurring in double-headed monsters and that arising from a defective growth of the interocular region in single monsters, are brought about by the growth in contact with each other of apposed parts of two eyes, while the development of the remaining parts of the eyes which are situated in the interval between them is suppressed. The principle which is involved is the same whether the cyclops eye is developed from the outer or temporal segments of two eyes growing in apposition with each other, as in one of the two secondary faces of a Janus-headed monster, or whether the cyclops eye is formed from the inner or nasal segments of two apposed eyes, as in the double-faced (Diprosopus) monster, in which the two faces look in the same direction and all eyes are to the front ; moreover, it is evident that, whatever other causes may be at work, this same principle, of the suppression of the growth of the intervening parts, is concerned in the development of a cyclops eye in single monsters.

The following questions arise in connection with the causes of the suppression or arrest of development ; namely, is it due to :

1. A lack of building material from which to form the missing parts ?
2. A lack of or defect in the organizing power of a growth centre ?
3. A displacement or arrest of development due to the growth of two parts in apposition with each other ?

Finally, is the arrest to be considered as due to a combination of any two or all of these three factors ?

Before attempting to answer these propositions we will pass on to the general question of the production of double-monsters and give a brief historical sketch of the earlier conceptions of the problems which are involved, one of which held that a double monster was the result of a splitting of the early embryonic rudiment, either at the head-end— " anterior dichotomy "—or at the tail-end—" posterior dichotomy " ; the other that two embryonic rudiments appeared in a single embryonic area and that these rudiments afterwards came into contact and grew

together, the corresponding parts uniting with each other so as to form a
" duplicitas anterior " or a " duplicitas posterior."

Each of these two hypotheses has assisted in the proper comprehension
of the various conditions which are presented in the whole series of
anomalies involving duplication of parts, and both are necessary, although
in a modified form, in order to appreciate fully the way in which according
to the newer conceptions an organizer has the power at an early stage of
development to determine from the outset the mode of development of a
particular part ; or at a later stage, of overriding the previously determined power of a particular part of the embryonic area to form a particular
region or organ, such as that of the eyes, nose, and mouth. The older
observations and records of blastoderms showing two separate embryonic
axes and the explanations which were put forward to account for these
were of great value in solving some of the general problems arising from
the occurrence of twin or multiple births and double monsters, and they
have in many instances formed the basis on which the more recent work
of Spemann and others has been founded. The new conceptions, therefore, must be regarded as supplementary to rather than as replacing the
older conceptions. The latter cleared the way for the newer work by
establishing the distinction between uniovular and biovular twins ; the
origin of double monsters from a single ovum, in which two gastrular
invaginations and embryonic axes were present ; many of the details with
regard to gastrular invagination and the formation of the primitive streak
and head-process, and other important points, relating to relative rate
of growth of particular parts, and also dominance of one part over
another.

Beginning with what is known as the " radiation theory " of Rauber,
Fig. 31, A, B, C, represents in a schematic manner three stages in the
development of a Duplicitas anterior in the blastoderm of a bony fish.
Rauber considered that the occurrence of double monsters was due to the
formation of two embryonic buds at the thickened margin of the embryonic
disc in place of one. These buds grew towards the centre of the disc in
a radial direction. In those cases in which the embryonic axes were
exactly opposite to each other the germinal disc would be divided by a
vertical plane passing through the longitudinal axis of each embryonic
bud, comprising an area including 180 of the whole. If, however, the
embryonic buds arose close to each other, as represented in Fig. 31, A,
the part of the germinal ridge *mn* between them, which he termed the
" inner intermediate zone," would be much shorter than the rest of the
circumference, *ystz*, which he called the " outer intermediate zone " ;
in the formation of the head-regions of the double-monster, the segments
mn and *yz* of the germinal ridge will be added to the original ingrowing

embryonic buds as represented in Fig. 31, B; whereas when the whole of the inner intermediate zone *mn* had been utilized, the remaining segments of the ridge *st* would come in contact and give rise to the single

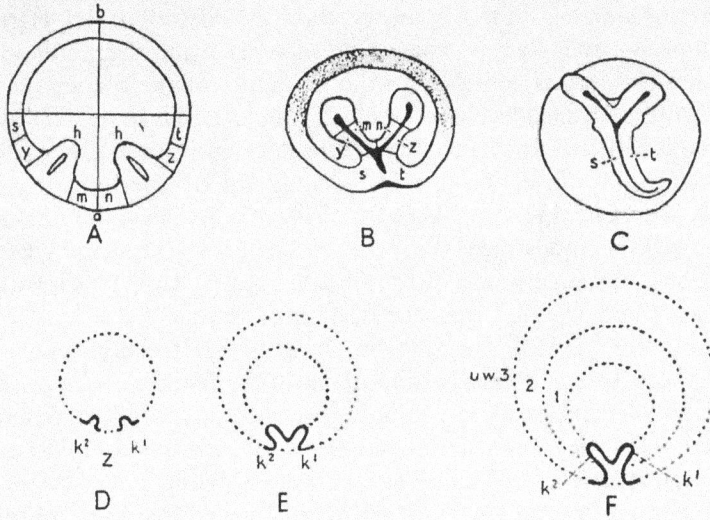

FIG. 31.

A, B, C—Scheme indicating the mode of formation of Duplicitas anterior according to Rauber's theory. *ab* : vertical or antero-posterior diameter dividing the germinal disc or blastoderm into right and left halves and corresponding to the principal, or dorsoventral, longitudinal axis of the body of the future larva; *hh* : head-ends of the embryonic " outgrowths "; *mn* : the right and left halves of the inner intermediate segment. These, with the corresponding parts of the embryonic outgrowths, will give rise to the internal or opposed halves of the two head-regions of the double monster; *yz* : the corresponding outer segments of the margin of the germinal disc; these will form the external (left and right) halves of the twin head and neck regions; *st* : the remaining parts of the germinal ring, which by uniting directly with each other will form the right and left halves of the single body and tail of the abnormal embryo.

D, E, F—Figures illustrating the formation of Duplicitas anterior in the salmon's egg from two gastrular invaginations, after Hertwig, in accordance with the " concrescence theory " of His. This conception differs from Rauber's in that Hertwig considered that the multiple formations are due to multiple gastrular invaginations at the margin of a single germinal disc, whereas Rauber considered the whole germinal ring as being the boundary of the gastrula-mouth or blastopore. *Z* : intermediate segment between the two gastrular invaginations; k^1, k^2 : right and left head rudiments of a double monster; uw^1, ^{2}, ^{3} : interrupted lines indicating the expansion of the germinal disc.

body and tail, by fusing with each other in the median dorso-ventral plane, as appears in C, in which a complete Duplicitas anterior is represented. In this and the preceding drawing it will be seen that when all the available inner intermediate zone has been utilized in the formation of the anterior end of the embryo, the remaining parts of the outer zone, *st* will come into apposition and fuse so as to form the right and left halves of the single body and tail.

A modification of Rauber's theory was later described by Hertwig, who pointed out that Rauber was wrong in considering the whole extent of the germinal ring as constituting the boundary of the blastopore, and that multiple neurulæ developed from a single gastrula. Hertwig, on the contrary, believed that multiple growths develop from several gastrular invaginations, in confirmation of which standpoint he cited the discovery of double gastrulæ in *Amphioxus* by Wilson and the observations of Schmidt, who demonstrated the existence of two separate gastrular invaginations in the germinal discs of young trout ova. In explanation of his theory he suggested the modification of Rauber's theory which is illustrated in Fig. 31, D, E, F. In D he shows two gastrular invaginations, k^2, k^1 close together and growing inward from the margin of the germinal disc. Between them is a short " inner intermediate zone " as described by Rauber, and the rest of the circumference corresponds to Rauber's " outer intermediate zone." In E it is seen how, as the disc enlarges, the adjoining parts of the ring are gradually transformed into the " primitive mouth " (or, in other words, become included in the boundaries of the two blastoporic openings which now open by a single common orifice). It is obvious that the nearer the embryonic rudiments or axes are to each other, the sooner will the inner intermediate zone be used up in the formation of the embryo, and the right and left halves of the outer intermediate zone come into contact ; and that as a result the two primarily separate gastrular cavities will form posteriorly a single common gastrular cavity, as shown in E and F. In the further course of development the margins of the blastopore or primitive streak can only be increased by additions from the lateral intermediate zones, which meet one another in the median plane, as in the formation of a normal single embryonic axis. Hertwig further emphasized the important point that multiple formations probably arise at the time of gastrula-formation, or even before the time when a gastrula is actually present.

Fischel also criticized Rauber's " radiation theory " ; he recognized that a generalization of this theory was in many instances met by grave difficulties, and further that it was even insufficient to explain the development of a Duplicitas anterior, for which Rauber had first postulated the theory as affording a solution. Making use of the schematic diagrams, Fig. 32, A, B, C, which were employed by Kopsch to illustrate the development of Duplicitas anterior according to the " concrescence theory " of His (see legend), Fischel and Kopsch point out that only a very small part of the cellular material of the germinal ring is utilized in the formation of the head-region, and that the greater part of the ring contains the material for the lateral and ventral parts of the body of the embryo. During the expansion of the germinal disc there occurs in the first place

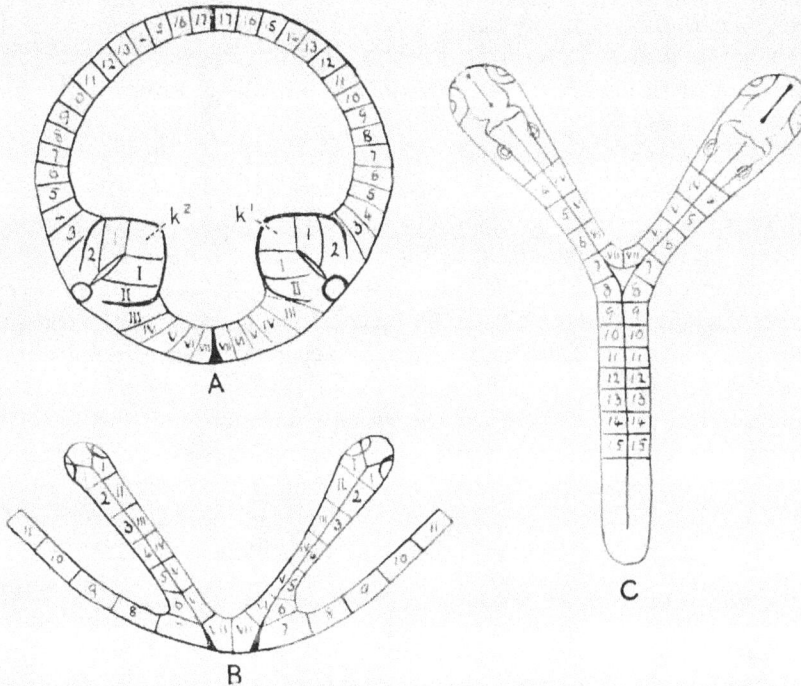

FIG. 32.—SCHEMATIC DRAWINGS ILLUSTRATING THE FORMATION OF A DOUBLE-HEADED MONSTER, DUPLICITAS ANTERIOR, ON THE BASIS OF THE CONCRESCENCE THEORY. (AFTER KOPSCH.)

A—Germinal disc with two embryonic rudiments at the "lozenge-shaped" stage of development and situated close together. The inner intermediate segment is indicated by Roman figures ; the outer segment by Arabic figures. k^2, k^1 : head-ends of the embryonic rudiments.

In B the whole of the intermediate segment has been utilized in the formation of the opposed sides of the twin head-ends of the Duplicitas anterior.

In C the " inner " intermediate zone, no longer being available for the formation of the embryo, the outer segments of the growing margin of the germinal disc meet and fuse to form the single body and tail-end, as in normal development.

If the two embryonic rudiments were situated directly opposite each other, it is assumed that two completely separate uniovular twins would be formed—the so-called " inner " and " outer " intermediate segments being equal in extent and sufficient to form two whole embryos.

a drawing together of the head-forming regions from which, by union in the median axis of the embryo, the right and left halves of the head are produced. The projecting embryonic bud contains the canalis neurentericus in the region of Hensen's node, and later there is formed, by a

backward growth from this point, the body and tail of the embryo, during
which the remaining section of the germinal ring surrounds the yolk
and contributes the lateral and ventral parts of the embryo. As a result
of his observations on the development of a series of double-monsters,
Fischel emphasizes the limitation of the zone which will give rise to the
embryonic rudiment to a relatively small region of the germinal ring,
and also the downward (ventral) direction of this growth. He admitted,
however, that fusion played an important rôle in the production of many
forms of duplicity.

Marchand, with whom Dareste may be included, may also be regarded
as a supporter of the fusion theory. He held that by far the greater
number of symmetrical double-monsters were formed by an extensive
union of originally separate embryonic rudiments on a germinal vesicle,
although in cases of incomplete anterior doubling he accepted an origin
by means of bifurcation. The incomplete Duplicitas posterior he thought
most probably arose from two originally separate rudiments (primitive
streaks). Schwalbe dissents from Marchand's view and more particularly
with reference to the bifurcation theory in connection with the posterior
variety. He further points out a group of cases which has to be considered,
and which can neither be regarded as belonging to the category of fusion
nor in the strict sense of the word to the cleavage theory, and which he
refers to under the designation " theory of incomplete separation." Now
Ahlfeld defined the controversy between the cleavage and the fusion
theories in the following words : " the one assumes that at first a common
rudiment was present which in the course of development divided ; while
the supporters of the other theory believed that from the very first two
separate rudiments can be observed on the germinal vesicle, which in
the course of development become united." The theory of incomplete
separation coincides with neither of these two theories exactly, and
Kaestner contended that the theory of incomplete separation was in reality
a modified cleavage theory dressed up in new clothes, and asserted that
incomplete double-monsters were not in any particular case one part
simple, one part doubled, but were one part completely doubled, the other
incompletely doubled ; also that in his opinion those cases in which,
instead of there being one primitive streak, two primitive streaks are
present, the whole germinal disc to the most distant parts of the embryonal
region, into which neither the primitive streak nor the head process has
yet penetrated, is already determined or adapted for the development
of two embryonal rudiments. Also that all cases of double-monsters
which hitherto have been completely examined, proved to be in reality
double in all parts ; and where in a general view organs appeared to be
simple, these showed on section more or less distinct traces of duplicity.

This statement is, however, challenged by Schwalbe, who gives as an example to the contrary cases of slight Duplicitas anterior (Diprosopus) in which some parts are not incompletely doubled. It may be noted, however, that in the case of Duplicitas anterior (Diprosopus) shown in Fig. 25, although the body on superficial inspection appears to be single, an X-ray photograph showed two vertebral columns extending as far as the pelvis. According to Kaestner's view, this case would represent incomplete doubling.

Kaestner states that if two primitive streaks are present, the axes of two medullary grooves will also be laid down and the position of two fore-gut grooves determined. If the two primitive grooves are not sufficiently separated from each other to allow of all the organs of the two embryonic rudiments to be infolded, an arrest of development occurs which may be compared with the interference of two wave-systems and the changed conditions of wave-form occasioned by this. Thus if two primitive streaks are sufficiently far apart, two complete medullary grooves will be formed, with a notochord situated below the floor of each groove. If the primitive streaks are very close together there will be one double medullary groove which is wider than normal, and shows two subsidiary grooves lying parallel with each other in its floor. The subsidiary grooves indicate its composite double character, and beneath each of these is a notochord. When the medullary folds which flank the main double medullary groove unite, a single neural tube will be enclosed. This is, however, not a simple tube, but is compound in nature. At the extreme anterior end a double bud is present which has the power to form two separate forebrains. If the embryonic axes are still more closely approximated, a single forebrain will be formed, although developed from two embryonic axes. Kaestner states that many authors would describe the latter condition as due to the fusion of two medullary tubes, but " no— they are, on the contrary, incompletely separated."

Rabaud puts a slightly different interpretation on this process, namely that in dual or twin developments we have a differentiation within a common region of two developmental centres.

This view is very similar to the modern conception of two organizers dominating a region which has not yet been completely determined, and which would under normal circumstances give rise to a different structure. Where the spread of the two centres is interfered with by mutual contact, as in Fig. 26, B, further growth in that direction is arrested or proceeds in a different direction. If the primary dorso-ventral planes of the two embryonic axes are in the same plane, the resulting double-monster will be symmetrically developed ; but if the primary dorso-ventral planes of the two embryonic axes are disposed in different planes, so that when the two axes meet the primary dorso-ventral planes form an angle with each other, the resulting secondary surfaces will be unequal, as in Fig. 23, A and B, and there will be a tendency towards the suppression of the central parts on one side, with the production of such deformities as cyclops and synotia. Asymmetry or inequality may also arise from a difference in the size or vitality of the two growth-centres. Finally, as is suggested by experimental interference with the development of normal ova, the blastomeres or the organizing centre may be divided into two or more growth-centres by constriction or other means and the developmental rudiment of a double organism initiated. Moreover, as previously conjectured, it seems likely that alterations in the physico-chemical environment of the ovum in the gastrular or pre-gastrular stages due to injury or disease may produce similar defects under natural or non-experimental conditions in both non-placental and placental animals.

The next question which it is necessary to consider is, Can the causes of these general defects be limited in their action to the development of particular organs? And more particularly with reference to our present thesis; Can primarily paired organs such as the nose, eyes, or ears lose their function, atrophy, and either become fused into a single organ or disappear altogether? These questions involve another, namely, the inheritance of general and localized defects, such as albinism and hæmophilia on the one hand and the inability to complete the development of particular organs on the other hand. As examples of the latter, we may mention the rudimentary teeth which have been found in the jaws of fœtal whales and in the curious duck-billed Platypus (*Ornithorhynchus*); or, again, the vestigial limbs found in certain snakes, the vestigial wing-bones of the kiwi, the New Zealand *Apteryx* ; or Stiedas organ in *Rana temporaria* (Figs. 162, 163, and 167, Chap. 19, pp. 228, 229, 233), and the median eyes of many invertebrates.

Associated with these questions is also that of change of function. Of this we have fewer examples than is generally supposed, for although a forelimb may be modified for use as a paddle, a leg, or a wing, its use as an organ of locomotion has not been altered ; perhaps one of the best-known instances of change of function is the conversion of the swim-bladder of fishes, a hydrostatic organ, into the air-breathing lungs of terrestrial animals. Now it sometimes happens that it is easier to build an entirely new structure than to improve and adapt an old one ; the latter is either destroyed in order to make room for the new building or is allowed to fall into decay. The latter alternative seems to have happened in the replacement of one organ by another in the course of evolution which sometimes happens in the animal kingdom, e.g. in the replacement of the median eyes of invertebrates by the lateral eyes, but as we shall see later, both median and lateral eyes seem to have been evolved from the simple ocellus.   In other cases a particular organ having lost its original function is gradually moulded or transformed so as to fulfil a different purpose.   In the case of the pineal organ, or epiphysis, of birds and mammals, opinion is still divided upon the question as to whether this structure is being transformed into a secretory gland or is being left as a derelict vestige, which is gradually disappearing or has already disappeared, as seems to be the case in crocodiles.

That causes of general defects of development may be limited in their action to the development of particular organs is a proposition that may be answered in the affirmative both with respect to ontogenetic and phylogenetic development.   Thus if diminution or loss of function of an organ be taken as an example, it is obvious that the full development of an organ such as a muscle or sense-organ will be curtailed by want of function during the life of an individual, and it may also be inferred that the poorly developed muscles of domestic animals living in confined spaces, such as rabbit-hutches, as compared with those of wild animals, are defects of development which are inherited, because the stimulus—exercise or light —which brings about the full development of the organ has been absent in many successive generations.

Also, as we shall see later, primarily paired organs such as the olfactory or visual, if their function is curtailed or actually ceases, may in the course of phylogeny be reduced in size, displaced, fused into a single organ, and finally disappear.   As examples of this we need only mention : (1) the fusion which has taken place of the paired olfactory organs in the class Monorhina, which includes among its living representatives the degenerate hag-fishes and the lampreys ; and (2) the formation of a single median eye by the fusion of paired vestiges of median eyes whose function has been usurped by the gradual evolution of highly differentiated lateral eyes, as has occurred in many of the arthropoda.

The inheritance of a grave defect such as cyclopia which is commonly associated with other defects, such as absence of the mouth and nasal passages and defective growth of the brain, is obviously excluded, as the individual is not viable ; moreover, the cause of the defect, as we have seen, is in many cases due to injury, defective nutrition, poisons, or other environmental conditions acting in a deleterious manner on the already fertilized ovum and more particularly during the gastrular and neurular stages of its development.

Development of the Lens and other Refractile Elements of the Eye

These may be derived from :

1. The cutaneous ectoderm or epidermis, including the cuticle and the hypoderm cells (Figs. 4, 9, and 10).

2. The superficial epithelial stratum of the retina, by a special modifica-

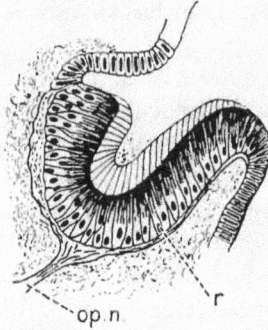

FIG. 33.—SIMPLE OPTIC PIT OF A LIMPET (PATELLA).

The pit is lined by pigmented epithelium, which is continuous at the margin of the pit with the cuticular epithelium.   The outer ends of the cells are clear and rod-like.   The nuclei are deep to the pigment layer, and the inner ends of the cells are continued into the fibres of the optic nerve.   *op. n. :* optic nerve ; *r. :* retina.

(*Cambridge Natural History*, after Helger.)

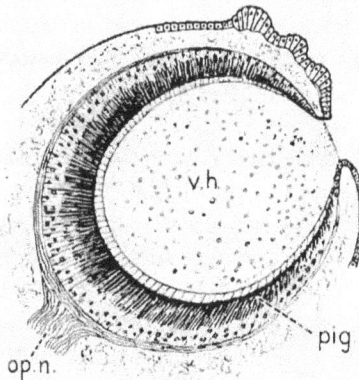

FIG. 34.—OPEN OPTIC VESICLE OF TROCHUS.

The cavity of the vesicle is filled with a semi-fluid secretion, the vitreous humour, *v.h.* ; *op. n.*, optic nerve ; *pig.*, pigment.

tion of certain cells or parts of cells belonging to the retinal segment of the optic cup or optic vesicle (Figs. 33, 36).

3. The distal or superficial wall of the optic vesicle—hypoderm cells in invertebrates or neural ectoderm in vertebrates (Figs. 37, 10).

4. A condition intermediate between 1 and 3 in which the elongated hypoderm cells on the sides of the optic cup form a tube of clear refractile cells, having a very narrow lumen in front of the retina. These cells are continuous superficially with the hypoderm cells lying beneath the cuticle and proximally with the retinal cells (Fig. 38).

5. Mesodermal elements which become included in the dioptric apparatus of the more complex eyes. For instance, the substantia propria

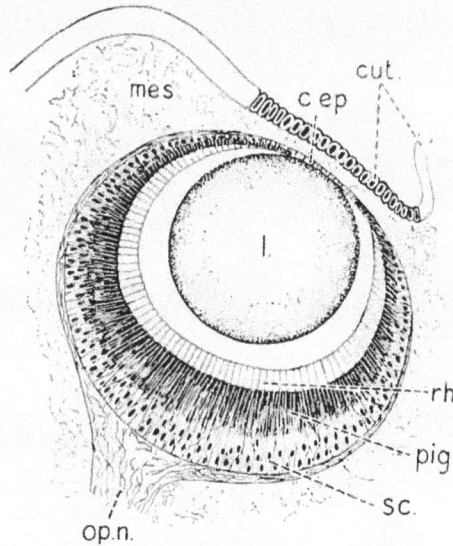

FIG. 35.—CLOSED OPTIC VESICLE OF MUREX, COMPLETELY SEPARATED FROM THE SURFACE EPITHELIUM BY A LAYER OF MESENCHYME.

A spherical non-cellular lens of the vitreous type is separated by a space from the sensory cells of the retina.

c.ep. : corneal epithelium.	pig. : pigment.
cut. : cuticle.	sc. : sensory cells of retina.
l. : lens.	rh. : layer of rods formed of parts
mes. : mesenchyme.	of the retinal cells.
op. n. : optic nerve.	

The clear cylindrical cells lining the vesicle after having secreted the vitreous become differentiated in their inner parts as refractile rods, while their outer parts function as receptive sensory cells.

of the cornea in the lateral eyes of vertebrates, or in the form of a supporting tissue in the vitreous humour, or accessory structures such as the elastic laminæ of Bowman and Descemet and the capsule of the lens.

6. A semi-fluid or gelatinous secretion from cells derived from :

    (a) The hypoderm cells or cutaneous ectoderm.
    (b) The retinal epithelium.
    (c) The mesenchyme.

4

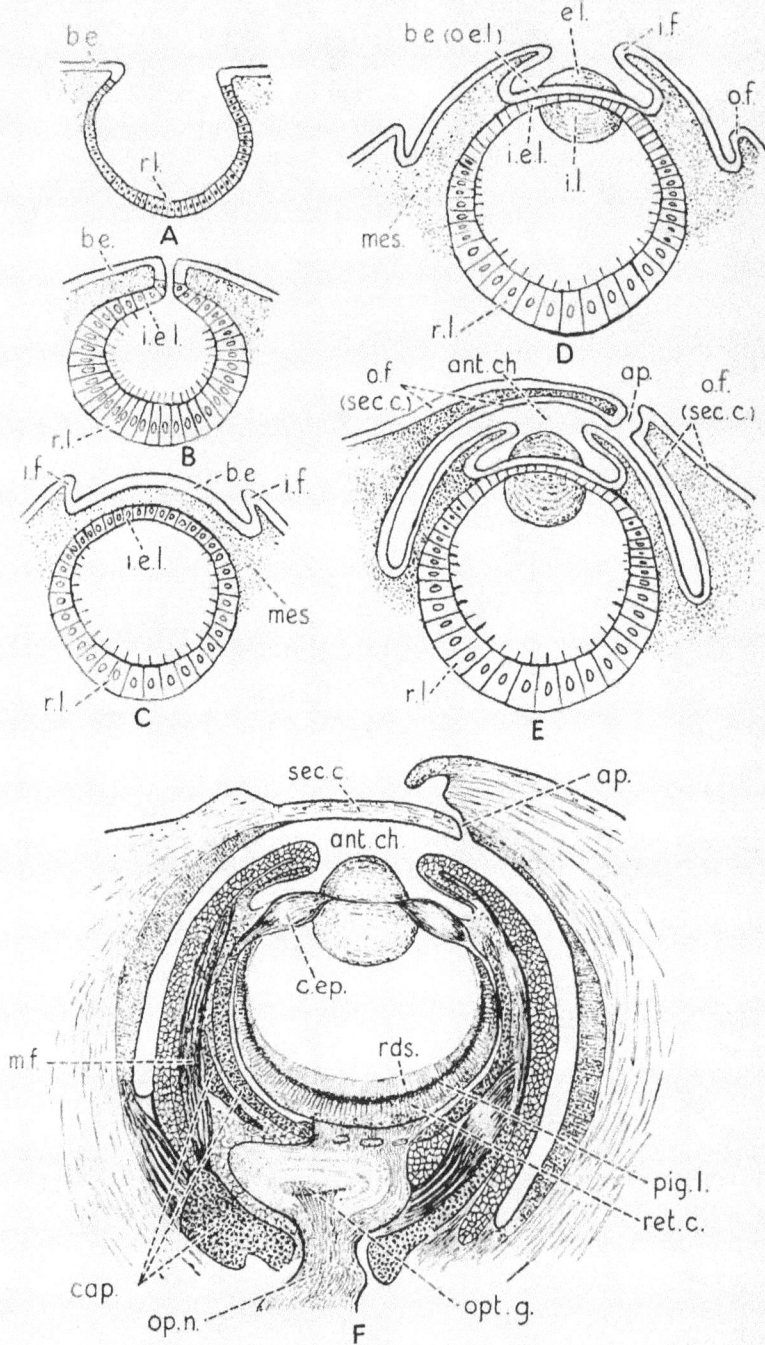

FIG. 36.—DIAGRAMS REPRESENTING THE DEVELOPMENT OF THE EYES IN DECAPODA
AND OCTOPODA.

[Continued at foot of next page.

The refractile fluid or substance may be first formed in the substance of the cells, appearing as droplets in the cytoplasm ; thereafter it may be retained in the substance of the cells, either in a semi-fluid condition or a more solid state, as in the clear refractile rods or " rhabdites," or the " crystal cones " of some types of simple or compound eyes ; or it may be discharged as a secretion into the vitreous cavity. In some cases the whole cell degenerates, the cell boundaries and nuclei disappear completely, and adjacent cells coalesce to form a viscous mass which afterwards consolidates and assumes a lens-like form. In other cases two or more cells may become enormously enlarged so that they fill the greater part of the optic vesicle ; these become clear and highly refractile and may then function as a lens or vitreous humour (Fig. 39). Considerable importance has been attributed to the distinction between lenses which are cellular and lenses which are non-cellular ; and also to the type of epithelium which enters into their composition. The distinction is of importance more especially with reference to the type of lens found in the lateral eyes of vertebrates, which is cellular and epidermal in origin, and the lens of the " pineal eye," which is also cellular but originates from the distal wall of the optic vesicle, and is therefore derived from the ectoderm

A—Cup-like depression of the body epithelium which forms the *primary optic pit*.
B—Constriction of the mouth of the pit to form the *primary optic vesicle*.
C—Formation of the *iris fold* and *primary cornea*.
D—Development of the two halves of the non-cellular lens and the rampart-like outer fold which gives rise to the *secondary cornea*.
E—Further development of the secondary cornea, and formation of the *anterior-chamber*.
F—Section of the fully developed eye of *Sepia officinalis*, showing the retina, optic ganglion, optic nerve, various parts of the cartilaginous capsule, muscle-fibres, anterior chamber and the opening of the latter to the exterior :

  ant. ch. : anterior chamber.
  ap. : opening of anterior chamber to the exterior.
  b.e. : body epithelium, which becomes the outer epithelial layer (Corpus epitheliale externus).
  cap. : cartilaginous capsule.
  c. ep. : Corpus epitheliale.
  e.l. : part of lens formed by the outer epithelial layer.
  i.e.l. : outer wall of optic vesicle, which becomes the inner epithelia layer (Corpus epitheliale internus).
  i.f. : circular fold which becomes the iris.
  i.l. : part of lens, formed by the inner epithelial layer.
  mes. : mesenchyme.
  m.f. : muscle fibres.
  o.f. : circular fold which forms the secondary cornea.
  opt.g. : optic ganglion.
  op.n. : optic nerve.
  pig. l. : pigment layer of retina.
  rds. : rods.
  r.l. : inner wall of the optic pit, which becomes the retina.

  (Redrawn from Lang's *Comparative Anatomy*.)

of the " neural plate." The distinction is also of importance with reference to the comparison of the type of lens found in the pineal eye of vertebrates with the forms of lens found in invertebrates, whether in the

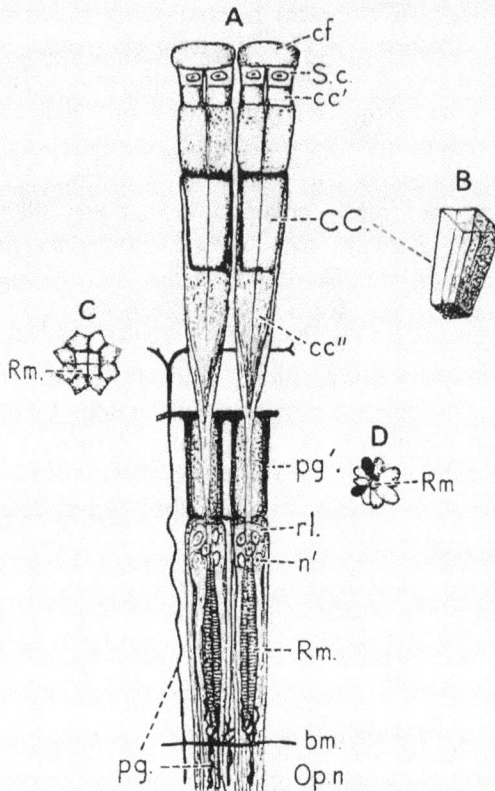

FIG. 37.

A—Two isolated retinulæ from the compound eye of a prawn, *Palæmon squilla*.
(After Grenacher.)

cf. : corneal facet.	*rl.* : retinula.
Sc. : Semper's cells.	*n'.* : nuclei of retinular cells.
cc'. : outer crystalline cone.	*bm.* : basement membrane.
CC. : middle crystalline cone.	*Op. n.* : optic nerve.
cc". : inner crystalline cone (hollow).	*Rm.* : rhabdome.
pg. pg'. : pigment.	

B—An isolated " crystal cone."
C—Transverse section of a retinula about its middle, bleached.
D—Transverse section of the posterior or inner end of the retinula.

median or lateral eyes. It was maintained by some authors that the existence of a corneal or cuticular type of lens in the central eyes of certain arthropods and other classes of invertebrates put completely out of court any comparison of the " pineal eye " of vertebrates with the central eyes

of invertebrates.　A reference to the central eyes of *Euscorpius* (Fig. 95,
Chap. 11, p. 133) or a section through an ocellus of a *Dytiscus* larva
(Fig. 38) will show, however, that one type of lens formation can pass into
the other ; and it is obvious that if the optic vesicle is withdrawn away
from the surface ectoderm, as has occurred in the phylogenetic history
of the pineal eyes of vertebrates, the cutaneous ectoderm or epidermis
can no longer form or participate in the ontogenetic development of the
lens of the " pineal eye," although it may have done so primarily.　With
reference to the ontogenetic development of the " pineal eye," Beard,
who studied the pineal organ in the *Ammocœte* or larval form of *Petromyzon*,

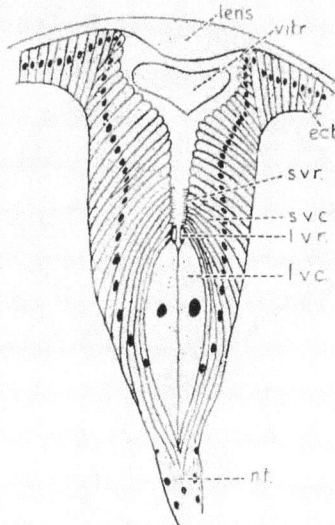

FIG. 38.—VERTICAL SECTION THROUGH OCELLUS OF LARVA OF DYTISCUS MAR-
GINALIS, ACROSS ITS SHORTEST DIAMETER.　(AFTER GÜNTHER.)

ect. : unaltered ectoderm.	*s.v.c.* : short visual cell.
l.v.c. : large visual cell.	*s.v.r.* : short visual rod.
l.v.r. : long visual rod.	*vitr.* : vitreous mass secreted by
n.f. : nerve fibres.	perineural cells at mouth of pit.

thought it possible that a portion of the cutaneous ectoderm might be
included in that part of the neural tube which gives rise to the pineal
organ, these cells being cut off at the time when the neural tube becomes
separated from the surface, or cutaneous ectoderm.　Whether this explanation is valid or not, it is quite certain that phylogenetically the neural
ectoderm has been derived from the cutaneous ectoderm ; moreover,
ontogenetically the neural ectoderm is continuous with the cutaneous
ectoderm in the early stages of embryonic development.　Further, there
exist not only transitional forms between the types of lens developed from
the optic vesicle and those derived directly from the hypodermal cells,

but also it is quite frequent to find a cuticular or corneal lens combined
with a vitreous lens formed from hypodermal cells in one and the same
eye, e.g. in the larvæ of *Dytiscus* or *Acilius* (Figs. 38 and 13).

In this connection it will be interesting to consider the capabilities of
lens-formation from the cutaneous or surface layer of ectoderm and
from the optic cup that have been demonstrated by experimental embryologists ; and also the influence of light and darkness on the contraction

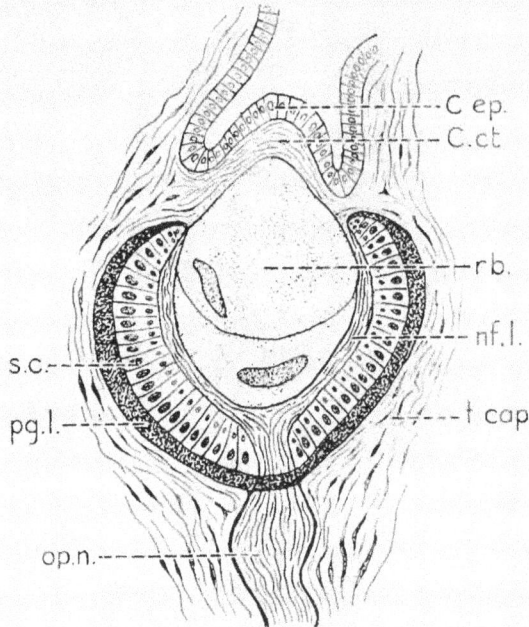

FIG. 39.—SCHEMATIC SECTION THROUGH A DORSAL EYE OF ONCHIDIUM, SHOWING
THE OPTIC NERVE PIERCING THE RETINA, AND ITS FIBRES SPREADING OUT ON
ITS INNER SURFACE AS IN THE LATERAL EYES OF VERTEBRATES.

C. ep. : epithelium of cornea.
C. ct. : connective tissue layer of
  cornea.
f. cap. : fibrous capsule of eye.
n.f.l. : nerve-fibre layer of retina.

op. n. : optic nerve.
pg. l. : pigment layer of retina.
r.b. : refractile body consisting of
  two very large cells.
s.c. : sensory cells of retina.

or expansion of melanophores and on the movements of pigment granules
and pigment cells. Moreover, the multiplication of pigment cells that
takes place in fish reared on a dark background as contrasted with others
reared on a white background has a definite bearing on this subject.

1. *Dependent differentiation of the lens vesicle.*—An example of this is
furnished by the differentiation of the lens from epidermis, which is dependent on the influence of the optic cup (Fig. 40).[1]   See p. 174, Chap. 15.

[1] O. Mangold (1929), *Arch. Entw. mech.*, 117.

A piece of presumptive brain region from a *Triton* larva at the mid-gastrula stage was grafted into another *Triton* embryo at the same stage of development. The graft developed by self-differentiation into parts of the brain and an optic cup. This induced the formation of a lens from

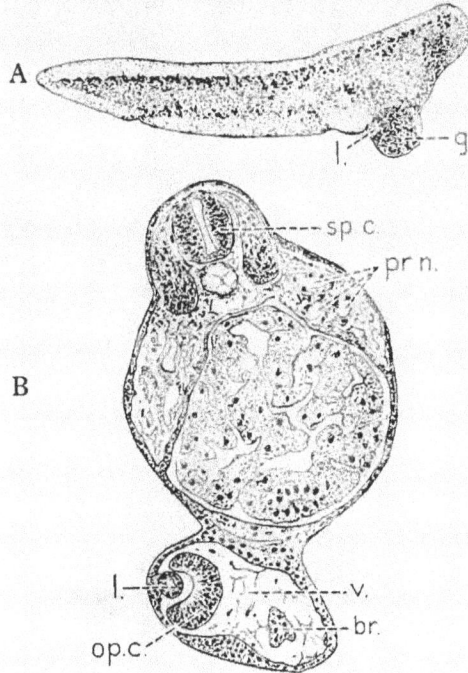

FIG. 40.—DEPENDENCE OF THE DEVELOPMENT OF THE LENS ON THE PRESENCE OF THE OPTIC CUP.

A—*Triton* larva into which a piece of presumptive brain region was grafted from another embryo of the same age. *g.*: graft which developed by self-differentiation into parts of the brain and an optic cup, which induced the formation of a lens *l.* from epidermis derived from the abdominal region of the host.

B—Transverse section through the same larva, showing the vesicle produced from the tissue of the host, *v.*; a portion of the grafted brain, *br.*; the optic cup, *op. c.*, derived from grafted tissue; *sp. c.*: spinal cord; and *pr. n.*: pronephric tubules.

(After O. Mangold, from *Elements of Experimental Embryology*: Huxley and de Beer.)

epidermis which was continuous with that covering the ventral part of the trunk of the host.[1]

2. *Self differentiation.*—The same author describes independent differentiation of the lens in *Rana esculenta* after extirpation of the presumptive eye rudiment at the early neurula stage (Fig. 41). The drawing

[1] O. Mangold (1931), *Ergebn. der Biol.*, 7, after Spemann.

shows a transverse section through the larva fourteen days after the operation. In other cases negative results were obtained or a small lens-

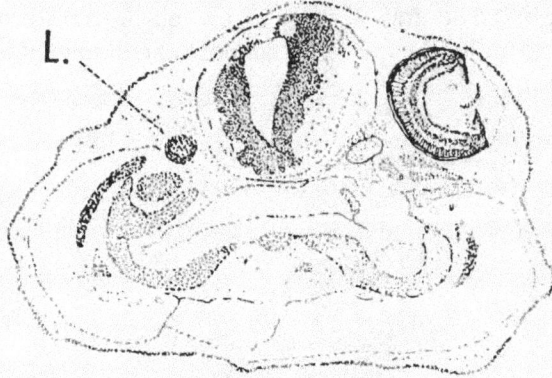

FIG. 41.—SELF-DIFFERENTIATION OF THE LENS.

Transverse section through larva of *Rana esculenta*, fourteen days after extirpation of the presumptive eye-rudiment. A lens *L*. has developed, although no optic cup was present.

(From Huxley and de Beer, after Spemann.)

like thickening of the epidermis occurred in the situation in which the lens should have been developed if the optic cup had been present.

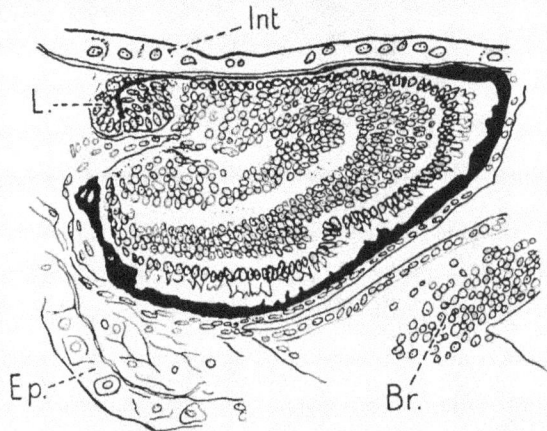

FIG. 42.—LENS FORMED FROM THE MARGIN OF THE OPTIC CUP.

The presumptive eye-rudiment of an embryo of *Triton* was grafted into the side of the body of another embryo. The optic cup, not being in relation with epidermis, has formed a lens from its own margin.

Br. : portion of grafted brain tissue.   L. : lens.
Int. : wall of intestine.   Ep. : epidermis of ventral wall.

(From Huxley and de Beer, after Adelmann, *Arch. Entwmech.*, 113, 1928.)

3. *Lens formation from the edge of the optic cup.*—The presumptive eye-rudiment of an embryo of *Triton* was grafted into the side of the body

of another embryo and developed by self-differentiation deeply beneath the epidermis. Under these circumstances it gave rise to a lens which developed from the edge of the optic cup, as in cases of regeneration of an extirpated organ or part of an organ [1] (Fig. 42).

The latter experiment is of particular interest with reference to the normal formation of a lens from a part of the optic vesicle as is the case in the eyes of many invertebrates and in the " pineal eye " of some fishes and reptiles ; although it must be born in mind that in the latter the lens is developed from the distal or superficial wall of the optic vesicle, which in the lateral eyes of vertebrates is invaginated to form the sensitive part of the retina. In the experimental *Triton* embryo the regenerated lens originated from the margin of the optic cup at the junction of the invaginated layer with the ensheathing or pigmented layer of the retina, and in the same situation as the vitreous or cellular, hypodermal lens of the *Dytiscus* or *Acilius* larvæ (Figs. 4 and 13). Incidentally it may be noted that the pigment layer of the retina is in the same situation relative to the " regenerated lens " as the zone of pigmented hypodermal cells beneath the cuticle is to the vitreous lens of *Dytiscus*.

The Influence of Light in the Formation of Pigment and the Production of Physico-chemical Changes in the Superficial Layers of Epithelium.

The whole question of lens formation and the specialization of refractile-elements in relation with the receptive or sensory cells of the retina appears to be linked with the action of light on the cuticle and hypodermal cells of invertebrates and on the epidermis and the neuro-epithelial cells of the retina in vertebrates. This action is associated with the formation of pigment granules, also with chemico-physical changes and movement of the pigment granules within the cell-bodies and of the cells themselves. As is well known, the skin and subcutaneous tissues tend to become pigmented when exposed to light and pigment granules or pigment cells as a whole tend to move towards the source of light. This movement has been demonstrated in the pigmented cells of the retina in both vertebrates [2] and invertebrates.[3] H. M. Bernard in 1896 suggested that eyes first arose as local modifications of tissue induced by the crowding of pigmented granules at spots in the skin which were most frequently and brilliantly illuminated. In the *Q. J. Micro. Sc.* (1896–7), **39**, 343,

---

[1] H. B. Adelmann (1928), *Arch. Entw. mech.*, 118.

[2] L. B. Airey, *J. Comp. Neurol. and Psychol.*, **25**, 1915 ; **30**, 1918. S. R. Detwiler, *J. Comp. Neurol. & Psychol.*, **30**, 1924. M. S. Mayou, *Brit. J. Ophthalm.*, 1932, p. 227, and 1933, p. 477.

[3] H. M. Bernard, *Q. J. Micro. Sc.*, **39**, 43, 47. G. H. Parker, 1899, *Bull. Mus. Comp. Zool.*, **35**, No. 6, p. 143.

he discussed differences in the structure of the median and lateral eyes of vertebrates and assumed that these different types of eyes of vertebrates must have arisen as modifications of two types of skin—the vestigial " pineal eye " being formed originally from a type of skin similar to that of the invertebrates, consisting of a single layer of palisade or hypodermal cells beneath the cuticle, which was supported internally by a layer of connective tissue ; whereas the lateral, paired eyes arose from the neural ectoderm and the stratified layers of squamous epithelium which form the epidermis of vertebrates, combined with the connective tissue components forming the outer tunics of the eyeball. He suggested also that the " pineal eye " " developed first as an optic pit from the skin of the ancestors of the vertebrates before that skin had assumed the vertebrate

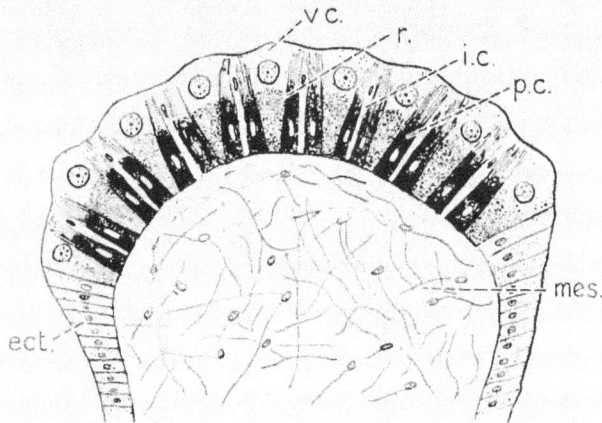

FIG. 43.—SECTION OF AN EYE OF ARCA BARBATA. (AFTER RAWITZ.)

ect. : ectoderm.
i.c. : interstitial cell.
mes. : mesoderm.
p.c. : pigment cell.

r. : inner segment of cell containing rod-like elements.
v.c. : visual cell of retina.

type, i.e. before the palisade layer had become protected externally by the mucous and horny layers." He also assumed that :

1. The retina is but a specialized portion of the epithelial layer of the skin, between the cells of which the pigment granules from the subjacent chromatophoral layer stream outwards under the influence of light.

2. The retina and the chromatophoral layer must have been in intimate and inseparable association through all the stages of evolution of the eye.

He believed that simple eyes first arose in pigmented areas on exposed surfaces of the body in invertebrates, and that the action of light not only produced and caused movement of pigment granules, but that the irritation of the hypodermal cells resulted in the formation of slime. This slime, secreted as droplets either in the substance of the cell-body or making its way to the surface, was the first step towards lens-formation. Later certain of the hypoderm-cells became elongated and their cytoplasm becoming clear, they formed a cellular lens of the vitreous type (Fig. 43), or the clear viscous secretion of the cells formed a non-cellular vitreous lens of the type seen in certain molluscs : e.g. the limpet (*Patella*), in which a simple optic pit is present the cells of which secrete a viscous fluid into the hollow of the pit ; *Trochus*, in which the pit is converted into an unclosed vesicle, completely filled with highly refractile secretion ; and *Murex* (Venus's comb), in which the secretion has become consolidated and shrunk away from the retina, thus forming a non-cellular spherical lens ; and the optic vesicle has become closed (Figs. 33–35). A " primary cornea " formed from the unpigmented distal segment of the optic vesicle and a " secondary cornea " derived from the superficial covering layer of hypoderm-cells and subjacent mesenchyme have also been evolved (Fig. 36, p. 50, and Fig. 121, Chap. 12, p. 164). These eyes, moreover show the differentiation of an outer clear refractile zone, a middle pigmented, and an inner nuclear-zone in the cells of the retina. In higher types of eye a specialization of individual cells of the retina is observed into refractile, pigment, and sensory cells (Figs. 11, 81, pp. 16, 119), and in many of the arthropods and insects these cells are grouped together into the separate units or ommatidia of a faceted eye (Fig. 37, p. 52).

The Pigment-cells of the Pineal Body

The occurrence of pigment in the pineal body is of interest not only from the light which it throws on the nature of this organ, but is of practical importance to the surgeon, as cases have occurred in which melanotic sarcoma [1] and other pigmented tumours have arisen in or in association with the pineal organ. The nature of the pigment contained in the human and mammalian pineal organ and its exact situation have been studied in detail by Quast [2] ; and pigmentation in the pineal organ of vertebrates in general, but more particularly cyclostomes and reptiles, by Beard, Dendy, Gaskell, and Studnička.

As is well known, the colour of the skin in man depends chiefly on the presence in the skin of the pigment melanin. This is deposited as fine granules which are found in the cells of the stratum germinativum, more especially in its basal layer next the derma. As, in course of time, these deeper cells move towards the surface to replace the more super-

[1] C. Ogle, " Sarcoma of the Pineal Body : Diffused Melanotic Sarcoma of the Surface of the Cerebrum." *Trans. Path. Soc., London*, **50**, 4–6, 1898.
[2] P. Quast, " Beiträge zur Histologie und Cytologie der normalen Zirbeldrüse des Menschen," *Zeitschr. f. mikr. anat. Forsch.*, Bd. **23**, s. 335, 1931.

ficial cells, the pigmentation becomes less pronounced, so that only a diffuse colouring of the epidermis is present in the stratum corneum. Besides the pigmented basal cells of the epidermis, large multipolar pigment-cells called melanoblasts are found beneath the epidermis in the superficial layers of the true skin. Their pigmented processes may extend for a considerable distance outwards between the cells of the epidermis, and the cells are characterized by a special staining reaction with the " dopa " reagent—3.4-dioxyphenylanilin [1]—while the pigment cells of the stratum germinativum or Malpighian layer, and the dermal chromatophores do not react. It is generally believed that the melanoblasts are modified epidermal cells, that they elaborate the melanin, and that this passes from them into the cells of the epidermis.

In addition to the melanoblasts, cells bearing pigment and called

[1] *The Origin of Melanin.*—Bloch, in 1917, demonstrated that the cells of pigmented regions contain a specific intracellular oxidase. He isolated from the embryo of the broad bean a substance, 3.4—dihydroxyphenylanilin, which he called " dopa," and showed that it was readily changed by this oxidase into melanin. When this substance is added to the epidermal cells of skin in frozen formalin-fixed sections granules of melanin are formed—the " dopa " reaction. Bloch concluded that the colourless " mother-substance," or melanogen, is almost certainly closely related or identical with " dopa."

A large number of groupings in the protein molecule form coloured products on oxidation—tyrosine, tryptophane, phenylaniline—and it seems obvious that melanin is formed as an end-product from one of these chromogen groups. The colourless mother-substance is brought to the cell by the blood-stream ; here it meets the " dopa-oxidase " and is turned into the coloured pigment melanin.

Melanin is closely allied to adrenaline, and it is probable that the two substances are derived from the same precursors and form alternative end-products in metabolism. When the cells are stimulated to proliferate, so that there is an increase of the oxidative ferment, a pigmented tumour is the result or a general melanomatosis. When owing to cachexia or some dyscrasia of the adrenals these glands fail to utilize the chromogenic substance for the manufacture of adrenaline, an increase of pigment is the result, as is seen in Addison's disease, the effects of which are seen in the skin and even in the epithelial cells of the cornea ; and if there is no enzyme at all present, pigment cannot be formed and the condition of albinism results.

There is considerable difference of opinion with regard to the kind of cell in which pigment arises, thus : Recklinghausen believed that the pigmented cells of nævi arise from the endothelium of the vessels. Unna held that pigmented cells were confined to the epithelia, and that the uveal pigment migrates from the retinal epithelium. Also, that malignant pigmented tumours are carcinomatous. Kornfeld showed that in the skin of frog embryos the subepithelial pigment sheet is formed by the migration of epithelial cells through the basement membrane into the corium. Krompecher held that the epithelial cells not only became morphologically similar to connective tissue elements, but also assumed their function, producing collagenous fibrils, a change which he termed " desmoplasia." Ribbert, on the contrary, contended that the pigmentation depended on a specialized connective tissue cell, the chromatophore, which was mesoblastic, and maintained that pigmentation and the formation of pigmented tumours were functions of the mesoderm. Pigment produced artificially by ultra-violet light appears in the deeper germinal layers of the epidermis. (Sir Stewart Duke-Elder, Extract from *Recent Advances in Opthalmology*, J. and A. Churchill, 1934, London.)

dermal chromatophores are present in the connective tissue of the derma, and the areolar subcutaneous connective tissue. These are capable of amœboid movement and are believed to serve as carriers of pigment which is formed elsewhere, e.g. in the melanoblasts. The pigment granules in these cells are larger and more irregular than in the basal epidermal cells and melanoblasts. Moreover, their distribution in the cell-body is not so even as in the epidermal melanoblasts. Pigment cells containing melanin which has actually been formed in the cell-body are, however, said by Maximow to occur, although rarely, in the derma, and have been named by him " dermal melanoblasts."

Like the pigment of the skin, the pigment of the eye may be considered under two headings, viz. (1) epithelial pigment and (2) the pigment present in connective tissue or mesenchyme cells. Thus both in invertebrates and vertebrates the pigment is chiefly found in the sensory receptive cells or in specialized epithelial cells of the retina, which either surround individual receptive sensory cells, as in the ommatidia of a composite faceted eye, or form a layer such as the external layer of hexagonal pigment cells in the retina of vertebrates. The connective tissue type of pigmented cell is found either in the form of " intrusive " mesenchyme cells among the sensory cells of the retina, as in the central eyes of the king crab (*Limulus polyphemus*), or in a definite layer in one of the tunics of the eyeball, e.g. the lamina chorio-capillaris, in which the spaces between the vessels contain a large number of branched cells of the chromatophore variety, or again in the anterior mesodermal layer of the iris. One of the principal functions of this pigment appears to be to screen off or to absorb superfluous rays of light. In the case of the iris in the lateral eyes of vertebrates, the pigment contained in the epithelial cells of the pars iridica retinæ and the mesodermal anterior layer serves by means of the sphincter and dilator pupillæ muscles to regulate the amount of light entering the eye through the pupil. The iris thus serves as a movable curtain which not only prevents oblique or circumferential rays entering the eye but controls the number of rays which fall upon the central part of the lens and more sensitive portions of the retina. In those animals in which the eye is not provided with a movable iris, pigment is nevertheless deposited in a circular zone round a transparent area of the skin or cuticle, which area serves as a cornea (Fig. 107, Chap. 12, p. 149). The clear area surrounded by a rim of pigment will allow the passage of a beam of light to any particular part of the retina, from approximately one direction only, and an indistinct image will be formed, the direction of which is well indicated, but there is often no means of focusing this image or regulating the amount of light entering the eye : such eyes are represented by the eye of Nautilus (Fig. 112, Chap. 12, p. 152), or the eyes round the edge of the pallium in the Scallop (*Pecten*) (Figs. 106, 107, Chap. 12, pp. 148, 149).   The same type of simple upright eye is also seen in the " pineal eyes " of cyclostomes and reptiles, in which a clear area free from pigment lies immediately over the pineal organ.   Incidentally, it may be mentioned that pigment is sometimes present in the part of the pineal vesicle which gives rise to the lens, both in cyclostomes and in some reptiles, e.g. the blind worm, *Anguis fragilis*.   The pigment found in this situation is probably a degenerative product, and indicates the vestigial nature of the " pineal eye."

Quast distinguishes two kinds of pigment in the pineal gland of man. Yellow pigment, present in the cells of the parenchyma, which results from the wear and tear or breaking down of the parenchyma cells— " Abnützungspigmente " ; and black pigment, or melanin, which is found in the interstitial tissue.[1]   The characteristic features of these are contrasted in the following table :

Yellow Pigment	Black Pigment
Parenchymal pigment. Waste pigment.	Pigment of the membranes and of the interstitial tissue. Melanin.
1. Irregular masses of granules of different size often clumped together.	1. Granules almost always of approximately the same size, and of uniformly spherical form.
2. Granules rather coarse.	2. Fine granules.
3. Clear, glistening, yellow-brown colour (though in aged subjects it may take on a deeper tone which does not differ much from the pigment of the interstitial tissue).	3. Dark brown colour.
4. Feebly stainable.	4. Relatively deeply stainable.
5. Stains with basic dyes, especially after the removal of fat or bleaching.	5. Does not stain with basic dyes, either before or after bleaching.

Quast describes varying degrees of pigmentation of the parenchyma cells, and emphasizes the extreme fineness of the pigment granules found in the interstitial tissues, more especially in some of the branched pigment cells and elongated cells following the course of the larger vessels in the connective tissue septa and in the connective tissue of the membranes (investing layer of pia mater).   Quast, referring to a case of primary melanotic sarcoma in the epiphysis of a woman aged 32, states that Ogle described the normal pineal gland as containing only a very small amount

[1] With reference to the use of the term " interstitial tissue " as denoting the supporting tissue of the " parenchyma cells," it is necessary to state that this is a complex tissue composed largely of a glial reticulum which is epithelial in origin, but also containing connective tissue elements, derived from the pia mater investing the pineal organ and carried into its substance by the vessels.

of melanin pigment, but not so small as to exclude the growth of a primary melanotic tumour. In the case described the pigment was of a brown colour and distributed in the parenchyma cells of the gland. The primary presence of pigment in the epiphysis, according to Ogle, is otherwise only to be seen in cases of cystic degeneration. Although pigment is scanty in the normal pineal body in man, it is abundant in the cells and connective tissue of the pineal in the horse and ass.

Quast concludes by stating that " the pigment cells of the interstitial tissue are, on morphological grounds, to be regarded as chromatophores. The chromatophores contain only one kind of pigment, melanin. The pigment of the interstitial tissue of the pineal considered from every aspect, namely from its morphological, physical, and optical characters, including its microchemical and staining reactions, belongs to the mesodermal, melanin type."

With reference to the parenchyma pigment he states that the older the patient the greater the pigment content of the parenchyma.

The morphological significance of the type of pigment found in the pineal body of mammalia lies in the indications that it may give, first, as to whether its presence may be regarded as evidence of its vestigial nature, namely, whether a particular kind of pigment indicates the derivation of the epiphysis from the " pineal eye " of lower types of vertebrates ; or, secondly, whether it throws any light on the view, maintained by some authors, that the mammalian epiphysis is a newly evolved glandular structure, which differs in structure and in function from the parietal organ of cyclostomes, reptiles, and Amphibia. Again, whether the presence of pigment in the organ is merely incidental, being derived from the pia mater covering the organ, or results from degenerative processes occurring in the parenchyma cells of the gland, which processes are comparable to the katabolic products of actively secreting glands.

Like Quast, who studied the pigment of the mammalian epiphysis, Leydig, working on the " pineal eye " of reptiles and cyclostomes, distinguished two kinds of pigment. The one present in small amount and having the dark (brown-black) type of granule, the other when seen with transmitted light having the dusky-yellow granule, which corresponds closely to the guanin-containing pigment of the skin. With reflected light these granules in the retinal cells of the " pineal eye " of cylostomes appear white. The latter type of pigment was in Leydig's opinion comparable with pigments containing uric acid. Studnička confirmed Leydig's opinion of there being two types of pigment in the "pineal eye " of cyclostomes : there being a small amount of pigment consisting of fine granules widely separated from one another and of a dark brown colour found in the supporting tissue of the retina, this latter type being

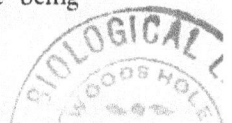

clearly seen in preparations from which the " white pigment " had been removed.

Concerning the nature of the white pigment seen in the " pineal eye " of cyclostomes, there is a considerable difference of opinion with regard to its true nature. Thus, according to Studnička, Mayer in 1864 stated that the epiphysis of *Petromyzon* contained many concretions of lime. Ahlborn considered the small white corpuscles to be a special white substance, which he described as white pigment somewhat similar to the " brain sand " of higher vertebrates, and thought that the substance with which they were dealing might be calcium phosphate.

These small corpuscles compactly fill the retinal cells, and they give, with reflected light, a snow-white appearance to the organ. When it is deposited in large masses, so as not to be transparent, it appears on examination with the microscope by transmitted light to be a deep black, which circumstance has, according to Studnička, given rise to many erroneous statements, certain authors having described the retina as being filled with black pigment. The substance, however, was observed by Gaskell and also Studnička to be completely removed from specimens fixed in Perenyis fluid, which contains nitric acid, and also from specimens fixed with picric acid. Under high magnification, Studnička observed the material in the form of separate pigment granules. These varied in size, were round or oval in form, with well-defined, sharp contours. In his opinion they are present in the protoplasm of the retinal cells and not on their surface, as maintained by some authors. These granules are present also in the ganglion cells, which, when they are completely filled, have the appearance of irregular clumps of pigment. Finally, in the deepest part of the retina, many of the pigment corpuscles are found in the intercellular tissue, in the wall of the atrium, and prolonged into the pineal nerve. The pigment is absent in the larval form, or ammocœtes, when smaller than 50 mm. in length. In older ammocœtes it is generally present, and it is always present in the adult animal. The absence of the pigment in the young ammocœtes and its absence in specimens prepared with acid fixatives have given rise to the view expressed by certain authors that the pigment is present in some species of *Petromyzon*, but is absent in others. Gaskell maintained that the " brain sand " so commonly present in the human pineal organ was not only an indication of its vestigial nature, but that it also pointed to the mammalian " epiphysis " being derived from the " pineal eye."

It will be of interest to mention here that white pigment has also been described in the eyes of invertebrates. Thus G. H. Parker figures in *Gammarus* " accessory " retinular cells, which lie outside the pigment cells that surround the clear axial rod or rhabdome. These cells are said to contain white pigment, which Parker believed had the function of reflecting rays of light back to the central part of the rhabdome, when this was exposed by retraction of the black pigment away from the central segment of the rhabdome (Fig. 44). It may be presumed that this action

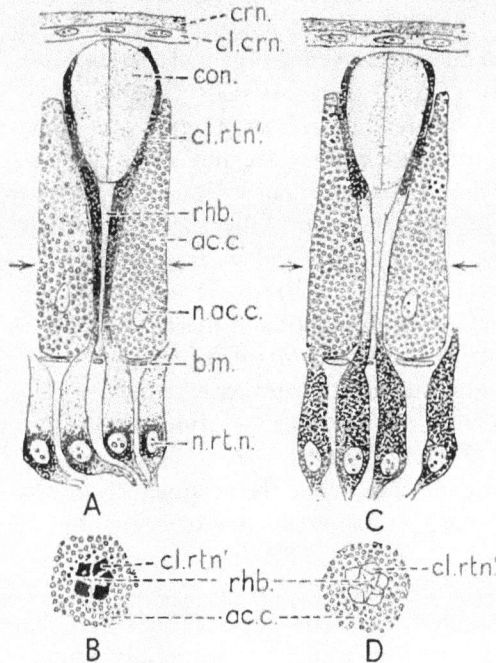

FIG. 44.—GAMMARUS ORNATUS (FRESHWATER SHRIMP). PHOTOCHEMICAL CHANGES IN THE RETINAL PIGMENT OF GAMMARUS. (AFTER G. H. PARKER.)

Changes due to exposure to light are limited to the black pigment in the middle and proximal portions of the retinular cells, they are not observable in the accessory pigment cells (white pigment).

A—Specimen fixed after exposure to light. The pigment has left the body of the cell and has accumulated round the rhabdome.
B—Transverse section of retinula through region of rhabdome.
C—Longitudinal section through the retinula when light has been excluded.
D—Transverse section through the retinula when light has been excluded.

ac. c. : accessory retinal cell.	*crn.* : cornea.
b.m. : basement membrane.	*n. ac. c.* : nucleus of accessory cell.
con. : crystalline cone.	*n. rt. n.* : nucleus of retinal nerve-
cl. crn. : corneal cell.	cell.
cl. rt. n. : central retinal nerve cell.	*rhb.* : rhabdome.

- - - Arrows indicating the level of the transverse sections B and D.

of the white pigment would come into play when the eye was exposed to a dim light, and compensate in a measure for the loss of a bright illumination. Whether it is of the same nature as the white pigment of the " pineal eye " of *Petromyzon* has not been demonstrated, but the presence

5

of " white pigment " and " black pigment " in well-defined and constant positions in the cells composing the retinulæ of the compound eyes of the same animal indicates that the appearance of black pigment in *Gammarus ornatus* is not merely due to the deposit in the retinal cells of concretions of phosphate of lime, which on examination with the microscope by transmitted light appear black, as has been said to be the case with the white pigment in the pineal sense-organ of *Petromyzon*. In *Gammarus* the white pigment of the " accessory cells " when viewed by transmitted light appears as glistening refractile granules, not black. These " granules," according to Parker, are not subject to the photochemical changes which occur in the pigment cells which ensheath the colourless rhabdome, and he suggests that " the accessory [white] pigment cells probably act as reflecting organs and in very dim light turn such rays as have escaped laterally from the rhabdome back again into that structure, thus aiding in an effective stimulation of this organ." Parker's description of these two kinds of pigment contained in separate cells lying adjacent to one another, one subject to physico-chemical changes produced by exposure to light and the other merely serving as a reflecting mechanism, suggest that the " black " granules in the dark cells are true pigment granules containing melanin, while the granules of the " white " accessory cells are possibly due to a fine crystalline or crystalloid deposit in the cell substance.

The variability in the colour of eyes is a subject of great interest and importance. The eyes of many invertebrates are red. Thus in the Protozoan *Euglena viridis*, which is commonly found floating on the water of ponds and gives to this a bright green colour, the eye-spot or " stigma " is a vivid red, in contrast to the general green colour of the body. The red colour is said to be due to a pigment allied to chlorophyll and called hæmatochrome. In some orders of the cœlenterates, the ocelli or eye-spots, arranged round the umbrella, appear as brilliant dots of colour, orange or red, sometimes phosphorescent.

Among the Annelida, or ringed worms, Andrews [1] has described in *Tubicola potamilla* highly differentiated compound eyes of a bright orange-red colour on the sides of the branchiæ. This animal lives in a leathery tube which is seen projecting from holes in gasteropod and bivalve shells. From the end of this tube cephalic, branchial plumes expand as a circular series of radiating stems, each bearing two rows of branchial filaments which are in the fully expanded state, directed forward. The eyes are on the posterior or outer sides of the main stems, there being rows of three to eight on each of the 20 stems. Each eye is a convex hemispherical protuberance on the outer side of the main stem. On section the eyes are

[1] E. A. Andrews, *J. Morph.*, 5, p. 271, 1891.

seen to consist of radiating groups of cells, resembling the ommatidia of compound eyes of insects and crustacea. The cells are differentiated into sensory cells and pigment cells, the former, in relation with clear refractile elements, ending distally in a conical inclusion of vase-shaped form, similar to the " crystal-cone " of certain composite eyes, e.g. the paired eyes of *Apus*. The eyes lie in close relation to nerve fibres and ganglia, and although a direct connection between the sensory cells and the nerve fibres has not been traced with certainty, the eyes have been shown experimentally to be very sensitive to light. Thus the shadow of a hand held over an aquarium containing the *Tubicola* will cause instant retraction of the filaments. These eyes have been found in other species, e.g. *P. oculifera*, and it is thought that they may be of some interest in interpreting the mode of development of the eyes of arthropods.

The Pigment in the Eyes of Insects, Arachnids, and Crustacea

The deposit of pigment in the form of small, dark-brown granules of approximately uniform size in the hypoderm or epithelial cells and of coarse granules in branched mesenchyme cells is very like that found in the eyes of vertebrates. Moreover, in the more highly differentiated eyes of species belonging to these three classes, there is a differentiation into separate sensory-cells and pigment-cells. There is also frequently a more abundant deposit of pigment in the immediate neighbourhood of the eyes, but absence or reduction of pigment in the region of the lens. On the other hand, in the composite eyes each rhabdite or crystalline-rod or crystalline-cone is usually surrounded and isolated from its fellows by specialized pigment cells. Further, the pigment cells of the retina in many species are of two types, namely, (1) epithelial, and (2) pigment-bearing, " intrusive " mesenchyme cells, which are elliptical or multipolar in form and are believed to have wandered into the retinal zone from the exterior, as in the medial or central eyes of *Euscorpius* and *Limulus polyphemus* (Fig. 95, Chap. 11, p. 133 and Fig. 87, p. 125).

Pigmentation of the Eyes of Molluscs

The same characteristic features are present with regard to the deposit and distribution of pigment in the eyes of molluscs as in the arthropods and vertebrates, namely (1) a uniform deposit of small, deep-brown granules in the epithelial cells—including the hypoderm cells and inner layer of columnar retinal cells ; (2) an irregular deposit of granules of unequal size in branched or fusiform mesenchyme cells. The deposit in the tall columnar cells of the retina is, moreover, usually confined to the middle third of the cell, while the inner end of the cell which is turned towards the light is clear, as in the eyes of *Patella*, *Trochus* or *Murex* (Figs. 33–35). This distribution of the pigment in the cells of the retina is similar to that found in the retina of the parietal eye in some reptiles, e.g. *Anguis* and *Pseudopus Pallasii*. It must be borne in mind, however, that although the resemblance in the distribution of pigment and the general disposition of the cells of the retina in the examples given is very close, these eyes differ in other respects and cannot be regarded as homologous. But the close resemblance in minute structural details, with regard to the deposit of pigment in two types of cell and the similarity of its disposition in the eyes of widely different classes of animals, does point to a general homology with regard to histological structure among these classes—a point which is fully corroborated by resemblances in histological structure which occur in other tissues.

Pigmentation of the Eyes of Vertebrates

This subject may be considered under two headings :

    1. Pigmentation occurring in the pineal organ.

    2. Pigmentation of the lateral- or paired-eyes.

Pigmentation of the pineal apparatus may further be considered in two sections, namely :

    A. Pigmentation of the parietal sense-organ, or " pineal eye," and the accessory structures connected with it.

    B. Pigmentation of the " epiphysis," conarium, or " pineal gland."

Commencing with the description of the pigment found in the pineal eyes of cyclostomes, we have to distinguish between the pigment found in the retina of the parietal sense-organ and that which is found in the tissues surrounding this. The pigment cells of the retina are distinct from the sensory cells and have been accurately described by Dendy in the late velasia stage of the New Zealand lamprey—*Geotria* (Fig. 45). They are long, tapering cells, having a wide inner end directed towards the cavity of the vesicle. The free end of this inner segment is rounded in form and marked off from the body of the cell by a clear line which corresponds in position to a limiting membrane ; this membrane can be clearly seen in depigmented specimens. The nucleus is oval and situated near the outer end of the cell ; beyond this, where the cell divides into thin tapering processes, pigment granules are absent. The granules are almost uniform in size and appear dark-brown or black by transmitted light. Pigment cells are not found in the left parietal sense-organ—" parapineal organ " of Studnička—and they are absent in the single parietal sense-organ of the hag fish, *Myxine glutinosa*.

The appearance of the pineal region of an adult lamprey, *P. planeri*, as seen from above is indicated in Fig. 47, after Studnička. This author describes the whole triangular area shown in the figure as the " parietal cornea " or " Scheitelfleck " (parietal-spot). He defines the cornea as comprising all the layers between the pineal organ and the surface of the head. It has a " glass-like transparency " and consists of, first,

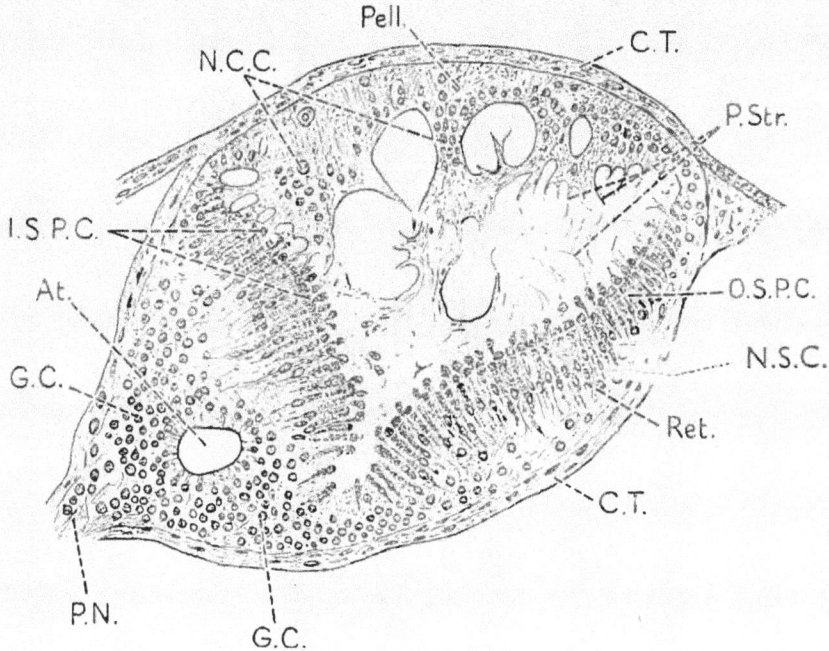

FIG. 45.—PARIETAL SENSE-ORGAN OF GEOTRIA, THE NEW ZEALAND LAMPREY. THE STAGE REPRESENTED IS OF THE SEXUALLY IMMATURE FORM, " VELASIA STAGE." (AFTER DENDY.)

Sagittal section of the right parietal eye (slightly diagrammatic) showing the general structure of the organ.

At. : atrium.
C.T. : connective tissue.
G.C. : ganglion cell.
I.S.P.C. : inner segments of pigment cells.
N.C.C. : nuclei of columnar cells of pellucida.
N.S.C. : nuclei of sense cells.
O.S.P.C. : outer segments of pigment cells.
P.N. : pineal nerve.
P. Str. : protoplasmic strands in interior of vesicle.
Pell. : pellucida.
Ret. : retina.

a thin fibrous layer, continuous with the cranial wall, and, next, the eye. This is convex towards the surface. Superficial to it is a conical mass of transparent mucoid tissue—the " parietal plug " of Dendy (Fig. 134, Chap. 17, p. 188). Over the mucoid tissue lie the corium and epidermis. The branched pigmented cells of the surrounding corium are completely absent over the pineal organ, and the pigment cells of the epidermis are much reduced here both in size and number (Fig. 134, Chap. 17, p. 188). The whole area thus appears pale as compared with the surrounding skin. In the middle of the parietal cornea is a circular white spot (" weissen Scheitelfleckes ") produced by the retina of the parietal organ which is

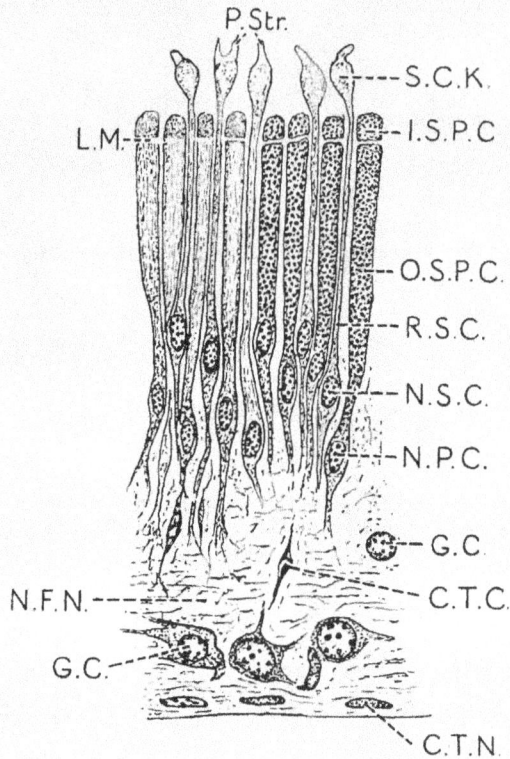

FIG. 46.—PARIETAL SENSE-ORGAN OF GEOTRIA, AS IN FIG. 45.

Diagram showing the minute structure of the retina ; on the right side the pigment is represented, on the left the cells as seen when the pigment has been removed. Lettering as in Fig. 45, in addition :

C.T.C. : connective tissue cell.	N.S.C. : nucleus of sense-cell.
I.S.P.C. : inner segment of pigment cell.	O.S.P.C. : outer segment of pigment cell.
L.M. : limiting membrane.	R.S.C. : retinal sense-cell.
N.F.N. : network of nerve-fibres.	S.C.K. : terminal knobs of sensory cells of retina.
N.P.C. : nucleus of pigment cell.	

seen shining through the cornea. Dendy describes the appearance of this minute central area in the New Zealand lamprey, when seen from above (Fig. 47), as a white rim enclosing a central spot, the latter lying directly over the " pellucida " or " lens." The white rim is due to the white pigment of the retina (? phosphate of lime) shining through the transparent cornea.

The appearance of a central spot inside the white rim is due to the interposition of the lens between the cornea and the retina, obscuring a direct view of the central part of the retina. In reviewing these points we may note that : when the pineal eye is removed and the parietal cornea is then viewed from above, the central white area has disappeared ; and if the parietal cornea is held up to the light, the area is seen to be translucent. When sections of the pineal eye are examined with the microscope by transmitted light, the white pigment contained in the retinal cells of older specimens is found to be absent in young specimens or specimens which have been fixed in acid-containing fluids. In adult specimens or late larvæ fixed in alcohol or other preservative not containing acid, the "granules (? phosphate

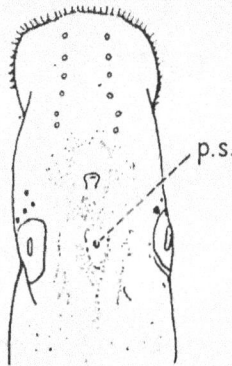

FIG. 47.—THE HEAD OF AN ADULT LAMPREY, *Petromyzon planeri*, SEEN FROM ABOVE ; SHOWING THE PARIETAL AREA AND PARIETAL SPOT (*p.s.*) (AFTER STUDNIČKA, 1893.)

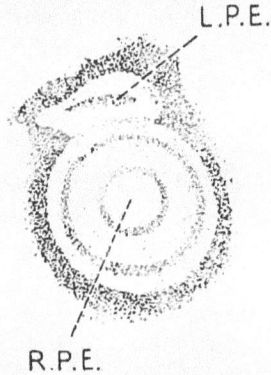

FIG. 48.—THE PINEAL AND "PARAPINEAL ORGANS" (RIGHT AND LEFT PARIETAL EYES), AS SEEN FROM ABOVE UNDER A DISSECTING LENS. (AFTER DENDY, 1907.) *R.P.E.*, *L.P.E.* : right and left parietal eyes. Geotria.

of lime) appear as minute spherical bodies evenly distributed through the inner and greater part of the outer segment of the cells " (Dendy).

The inheritance of a negative character, such as the generalized absence of pigment in albinism or the absence of a particular constituent of the blood or of a ferment such as prothrombin in cases of hæmophilia, is well known ; but the inheritance in living animals of a localized absence of pigment in connection with the vestige of what presumably was once, in animals belonging to the palæozoic period, a functional organ, is a problem of the greatest interest, and the solution of this problem appears to be as difficult and as remote as many other problems relating to pigment distribution and the inheritance of pattern.

A significant exception to the absence of pigment in the region of the " parietal scale " occurs in the wall-lizard (*Lacerta muralis*), in which pigment has been shown by Leydig not only to lie beneath the parietal or corneal scale but even to encroach on the clear central spot which lies immediately over the pineal organ. This change is evidently a secondary one, and is probably due to the need for pigment in this situation in a type of animal frequently exposed to the heat of the sun and lacking any protective covering in the way of hair or feathers. The present needs of the animal in this case have apparently overcome the inherited bias towards lack of pigment formation in the pineal region, but it is possible or, indeed, probable that the pigment figured by Leydig is not actually formed in or under the corneal scale of the lizard, but has been carried into the region by chromatophores from the surrounding tissues ; if this is the case, the hereditary lack of pigment formation in the area still exists, but it has been countered by the migration of pigment cells into the deeper layers of the cornea.

Pigmentation of the Pineal Region in Fishes

The parietal sense-organ, or " pineal eye," is generally thought to be absent in living classes of fishes ; though it is possibly represented in some by the expanded end-vesicle of the pineal organ. Notwithstanding the absence of the parietal sense-organ, there is frequently a parietal foramen, or a parietal canal or pit, closed externally but opening into the cranial cavity internally (Fig. 49). This lodges the " end-vesicle " and distal part of the stalk of the pineal organ. Over this area is a pigment-free area of the epidermis and corium. In the spiny dog-fish (*Spinax niger*), the " Scheitelfleck " is very conspicuous, although no true parietal cornea is present, like that of the cyclostomes and certain reptiles. It appears as a pale area in the parietal region, which contrasts sharply with the deeply pigmented skin surrounding it. This area is separated by a considerable thickness of loose, subcutaneous tissue containing the tubular organs, or ampullæ of Lorrenz, and it is completely separated from the pineal organ by the cartilage closing the parietal canal.

In some fishes, e.g. *Raja clavata*, the stalk of the pineal organ is accompanied throughout its whole length by a sheath containing blood-vessels ; this shows an intensive degree of pigmentation, especially around the large dorsal vein, which is wider than the diameter of the end-vesicle itself.

In the spoonbill, *Polyodon* (Fig. 50), a lozenge-shaped parietal plate is present over the end-vesicle of the pineal organ, and the skin over this, as in *Spinax*, is destitute of pigment. The general relations of the pineal organ to the cranial wall are very similar to those of *Spinax*.

Very few allusions are made with reference to the existence of pigment in the cells of the end-vesicle or the stalk of the pineal organ of fishes, and it seems probable that pigment is not generally present in the end-vesicle of fishes. Although from the developmental standpoint the end-vesicle appears to represent the part of the primary pineal diverticulum

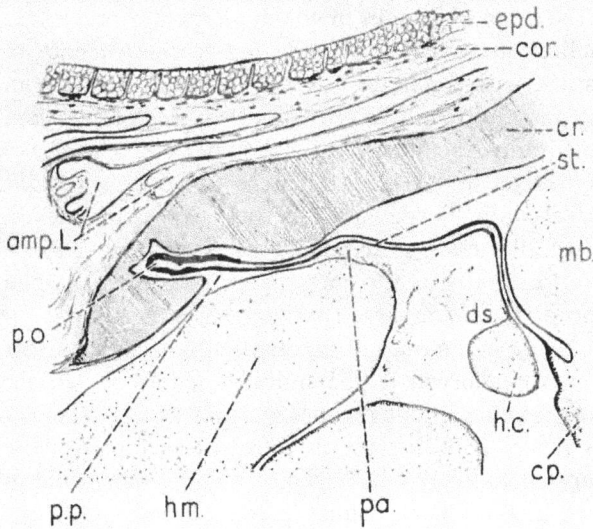

FIG. 49.—THE PINEAL ORGAN OF AN ADULT SPINAX NIGER, SEEN IN LONGITUDINAL SECTION, AND SHOWING THE RELATIONS OF THE SURROUNDING STRUCTURES.
(FROM STUDNIČKA.)

amp. L. : ampulla of Lorrenz.
cor. : corium.
cp. : posterior commissure.
cr. : cranial wall.
ds. : dorsal sac.
epd. : epidermis.
h.c. : habenular commissure.
hm. : hemisphere.
mb. : midbrain.
pa. : paraphysis.
po. : end-vesicle of pineal organ.
p.p. : mouth of parietal pit.
st. : stalk of pineal organ.

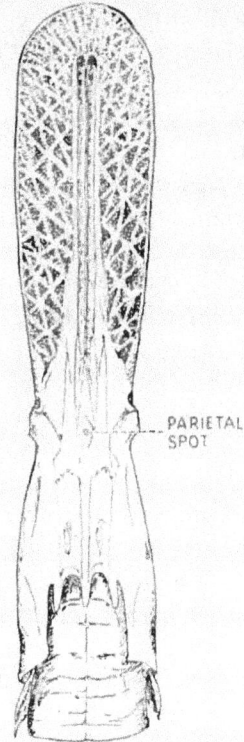

FIG. 50.—DORSAL ASPECT OF THE HEAD OF A SPOON BILL, OR PADDLE FISH (POLYODON FOLIUM), A NORTH - AMERICAN FRESH-WATER FISH OF PRIMITIVE TYPE ALLIED TO THE STURGEONS AND SHOWING A WELL-MARKED PARIETAL PLATE AND PARIETAL SPOT. (R. J. G.)

which gives origin to the " pineal eye " of cylostomes, and of certain Amphibia and reptiles, it evidently does not differentiate so far as to represent the parietal sense-organ of these animals, and a retina with sensory, ganglionic, and pigment cells is not differentiated.

Pigmentation of the Pineal Region of Amphibia

Little has been recorded about the presence of pigment in the pineal organ of Urodeles. Eycleshymer (1892), however, alluded to the presence of pigment in the inner ends of the cells, forming the many-layered inner wall of the hollow epiphysis in *Amblystoma mexicanum*, and according to Galeotti (1897), in *Proteus anguineus* pigment granules are present in its very small pear-shaped epiphysis. The pigment granules are situated in special cells in the neighbourhood of the nucleus, and he states that this is the only place in the brain of Proteus in which pigment is present.

In the Anura, or tailless amphibians, the allusions to the presence of pigment and its situation with reference to the parietal sense-organ (Stieda's frontal organ) and the epiphysis are much more definite than is the case with the tailed amphibians. Thus, the " parietal spot " was accurately described by Stieda in 1865 : " There is to be seen a slight bulging of the skin on the top of the head, between the lateral eyes. When the skin lying over the organ is removed, the spot is seen to be transparent ; this being principally due to the absence of pigment. The corium surrounding the pigment-free area (parietal cornea) contains an abundance of pigment. A small amount of pigment is, however, present in the epidermis over the frontal organ. The epithelial glands are absent or are reduced in size and number in this region."

The parietal spot is not equally distinct in different examples of the same species and it is absent in many allied species. Thus, according to Leydig, it is best marked in *Rana fusca*, whilst in *Rana arvalis* and *Rana agilis* only traces are visible and in some specimens it is entirely absent.

The position of the end vesicle in Bufo is indicated by a clearly defined white spot. In *Bombinator* the pigment layer and glands are totally absent in the corium over the vesicle ; the epidermis here is, however, strongly arched upwards and its outermost layer is prolonged into a long, deeply pigmented black horn. In *Alytes obstetricans*, the midwife-frog, the pigment layers of the corium and epidermis over the vesicle are as well developed as in the surrounding skin.

With regard to pigment in the " frontal organ " (Stirndrüse, end-vesicle), Leydig states that the organ contains pigment in *Bombinator*, but that in frogs the frontal organ is devoid of pigment.

Pigmentation of the Pineal Organs of Reptiles

The highest degree of development and differentiation of the parietal sense-organ and " pineal sac " in living animals is preserved in this class, more particularly in *Sphenodon* and certain lizards, in which the general structure of the organ has been mostly minutely studied, and in which it is believed to function at any rate as a light-percipient organ and possibly be of some use to the animal. On the other hand, both parietal sense-organ and pineal sac are absent in the Crocodilia, although habenular and posterior commissures are present. The pigment, as in other classes of vertebrates, is of two types : (1) epithelial, in the form of fine, dark-brown granules, present in the cylindrical cells of the retina, and in the large, round ganglion cells (pigment balls) and also in the epidermis of the skin, except directly over the parietal scale ; (2) mesodermal, the granules of which are contained in branched cells, around the sheaths of the parietal organ and pineal sac, more especially in relation with the blood-vessels and in the subcutaneous tissue. The details of distribution of the pigment in the cells of the retina will be dealt with later in the description of the pineal eyes of *Sphenodon* and of different types of lizard, and it will only be necessary here to allude to certain general points :

1. The variability in the degree and distribution of the pigment in different orders within the same class.
2. The similarity in the distribution of the pigment within the retinal cells to that in the eyes of many invertebrates.
3. The presence of pigment in the wall of the pineal sac or end vesicle of the epiphysis in the same situations as in the retina of the parietal sense-organ (" pineal eye ").
4. The presence of pigment in " accessory parietal organs " in the same situation, e.g in *Pseudopus Pallasii*, with other evidence suggests the primary double nature of the organ—the apical part of one member of the pair being ordinarily suppressed, but occasionally appearing as an incompletely differentiated sense-organ ; this organ, however, possesses structural peculiarities which agree even in such details as the distribution of pigment in the cells of the retina, and render its identification as a parietal sense-organ almost certain.

Pigmentation of the Pineal Region in Birds

Klinckowstroem (1892) described a peculiar pigmented outgrowth from the surface of the head, opposite the epiphysis, in certain swimming birds, which he considered to indicate the site of a former parietal spot.

He found this vestige of a parietal spot in only 12 cases out of 200 embryos examined by him. These were in : *Sterna hirundo*, the swallow-tern (1 ex.) ; *Larus marinus*, the black-backed sea-gull (4 ex.) ; *Larus canus*, the common gull (2 ex.) ; *Larus glaucus*, the green gull (4 ex.) ; and *Anser brachyrhynchus*, the pink-footed goose (1 ex.). In the adult birds he found nothing special in the region of the parietal spot.

The outgrowth consists of a small, dome-shaped projection on the surface of the head, which appears before the development of the feather-papillæ, opposite the point towards which the apex of the pineal diverticulum is directed. The epidermis is raised above the level of the surrounding skin. In this situation there appears at the same time a remarkable accumulation of pigment, both in the epidermis and the subcutaneous mesenchyme. The cupola-like projection later divides into two small hillocks. Still later, the parietal spot becomes surrounded by a circle of feather-papillæ. Finally, the area is invaded by the ingrowth of small feather-papillæ and it eventually disappears. Studnička, in commenting on these observations, mentions that he has himself heard of a case in which a parietal foramen was present in the skull of an adult goose, and that a round hole closed by connective tissue is found in the roof of the skull of adult geese, more especially in those varieties which possess a crest. This hole lies just in front of the point where the epiphysis ends, and he states that it can have no other significance than that of a parietal foramen.

The occasional appearance of this embryonic vestige in the above-mentioned varieties of sea-gull and allied species of bird and of the parietal foramen in the skull of adult geese is especially interesting as the parietal foramen is usually absent in the skulls of birds, notwithstanding the high degree of development of the pineal body. The pigment spot and the occasional presence of a parietal foramen in these birds serve as an indication of the previous existence of a parietal sense-organ in the ancestors of birds and of the identity of the avian epiphysis, or proximal part of the pineal apparatus, with the more fully evolved organ which is present in certain living reptiles, such as *Varanus* and *Sphenodon*.

Pigmentation of the Pineal Organ in Mammals

We have already referred to the work of Quast, p. 62, on the pigment of the human pineal organ. All authors appear to be agreed that in the mammalian pineal organ pigment is contained in two types of cell: (1) the parenchyma cells, (2) branched or elongated cells which are present in abundance in the capsule and interlobar septa following the course of the vessels. The latter often appear to be stretched out over the vessel walls and to lie in the perivascular spaces. There is, however, considerable difference of opinion with respect to the colour of the pigment granules in the two types of cell, and it seems probable that considerable variations occur in the depth of colour between pale yellow and dark brown, or even black, which are due in part to age and in part to different methods of preparation. The close association of the branched or elongated pigment cells with the blood-vessels, which is especially evident in the horse, has given rise to the opinion that the situation of the pigment often in fine streams resembling nerve-fibres, along the course of the vessels, may indicate the route which is taken by secretions leaving the gland, it being suggested that these make their way from the spaces of the reticulum into the perivascular spaces and veins along the course of the pigment granules.

The pigment which occurs in eyes, whether vertebrate or invertebrate, is concerned not only in the reflection or absorption of light, or, as in the iris, the screening off of superfluous rays, but it may also be developed in other situations than the eye or its immediate neighbourhood as a means of attraction or sometimes detraction. An example of the latter is found in the spots of dark pigment known as " false eyes " seen on the sides of certain fishes near the tail, which probably serve to distract attention from the true eye and more vital parts of the body. Pigment, moreover, is not always developed for a useful purpose, but may be formed as a waste product in a degenerating organ, as is the case in the lens of the pineal eye of certain lizards, e.g. the blind-worm (*Anguis fragilis*). Moreover, the deposition of pigment in the retinal cells of the pineal organ may occur as an inherited character, although the need for this pigment has, according to geological evidence, ceased millions of years ago. The clinical importance of the occurrence of pigment in the pineal body in the human subject lies, as previously mentioned, in the possibility of a melanotic sarcoma arising in this organ. The presence of light brown or yellow pigment granules in cells of glial type or the branched connective tissue cells around the vessels and in the capsule or the interlobar and interlobular septa appears to be one of many indications of the vestigial nature of the organ, more especially as the amount of this type of pigment is greater in specimens obtained from aged individuals than in the pineal bodies of young children or infants.

Pigmentation of the Lateral Eyes of Vertebrates

The situation and types of pigment found in the lateral eyes of vertebrates are so well known that we do not propose to do more than allude to this aspect of the general question. Broadly speaking, the two types of cell in which pigment is deposited or formed, namely (1) epithelial and (2) mesodermic, resemble the same two types of cell in the pineal organ and in the eyes of invertebrates. There are some points of interest, however, with reference to the development of pigment in the lateral eyes which have a bearing on pigmentation in the pineal organ, and we shall therefore give a brief account of the development of pigment in the human eye. This subject has been recently studied by Ida Mann.[1] Minute

[1] Ida Mann, *Development of the Human Eye*, Cambridge University Press, 1928.

pigment granules of a golden-brown colour first appear in the neuro-epithelium which forms the outer wall of the optic cup in human embryos at the 8–10-mm. stage of development. They are deposited at first in patches or small groups in the cytoplasm between the nucleus and the inner margin of the cell, namely the border of the cell next the cleft between the outer and the inner walls of the optic cup, which represents the original cavity of the primary optic vesicle. By increase in number of the granules they soon completely fill the inner part of the cell, whereas in the outer part of the cell the granules are fewer in number and with low-power magnification this part of the cell appears clear. A significant circumstance is that the deposit of pigment in the outer wall of the cup appears at the same time as the development outside it of the plexus chorio-capillaris. At first the plexus is in close relation with the neuro-epithelium ; later, however, at the 14-mm. stage of development, a continuous clear membrane, the membrane of Bruch, is formed between the epithelium and the choroid. It is probable that this membrane would prevent the passage of pigment granules from choroid to epithelium, but would act as a dialysing membrane with reference to the fluid constituents of the pigment, namely tyrosin, which has been shown to be converted into melanin by the action of the ferment tyrosinase. Little is known with regard to the formation of pigment granules, but it seems probable that these are developed in the cytoplasm of epithelial cells (Fig. 51), and grow to a definite size and shape ; and that the relation of the colouring matter to the granule is much the same as that of hæmoglobin to a blood corpuscle—that is to say, under ordinary circumstances the colouring material is carried by the granule, but it may under certain conditions escape from the granule and become diffused in the cytoplasm or intercellular spaces. Returning to the further development of the pigment layer of the human retina : this continues and remains throughout life as a single layer of cells, which in the definitive form are seen to be hexagonal when viewed in tangential sections and of an oblong quadrangular shape in sections made vertical to the surface. The inner end is prolonged into delicate, tapering processes which surround the outer ends of the rods and cones. These are specially well seen in the retina of certain fishes and Amphibia, in which the pigment granules appear as minute oval plates arranged in series and in parallel rows, their colour when seen by transmitted light being a resinous-brown or amber tint. The two layers of the optic cup are each carried forward as a single layer of cells beyond the ora serrata, on to the inner or posterior surface of the ciliary region and iris, as the pars ciliaris retinæ and pars iridica retinæ. The outer or anterior layer of the pars ciliaris retinæ only is pigmented, and this is the case in the early stages of development of the pars iridica retinæ, the outer layer being pigmented, the inner posterior layer being at first destitute of pigment, but gradually becoming pigmented between the end of the third month and the seventh month. The deposit commences at the margin of the pupil extending from the anterior layer round the marginal sinus, and then outward in the posterior layer as far as the bases of the ciliary processes ; beyond this the pigment ceases to extend, and in the adult the posterior layer of the pars ciliaris retinæ is unpigmented.

The mesodermal pigment of the choroid appears later than the ecto-

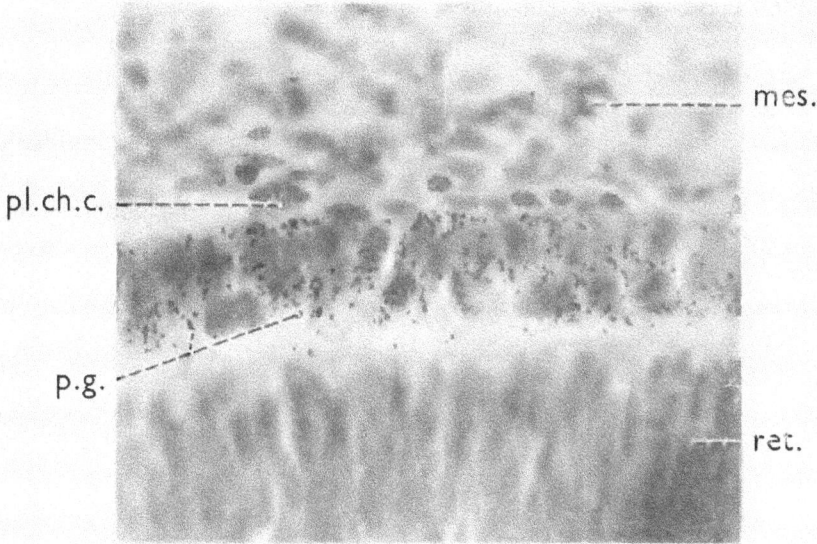

FIG. 51.—SECTION OF THE RETINA OF A 12-MM. HUMAN EMBRYO. (R. J. G.)
    p.g. : pigment granules lying in the epithelium which forms the outer
      wall of the optic cup.
    ret. : retina.
    pl. ch. c. : plexus chorio-capillaris, containing vessels filled with erythro-
      blasts.
    mes. : mesoderm.

dermal retinal pigment, about the beginning of the fifth month. The pigment is found in irregularly branched cells—chromatophores—which appear first in the outermost layer next the sclera and gradually spread inwards. The same type of branched pigment cells are found in the mesodermal layers of the ciliary region and iris. The development of pigment in the stroma of the iris appears after birth and to a very variable extent, being scanty in blue and grey eyes, but in brown eyes there is a thick deposit in the superficial layers which obscures the view of the vessels of the iris. In albinos pigment is diminished or absent in both the retinal epithelium and the mesodermal layers of the eye.

The pigmentation of the lateral eyes in lower types of vertebrates does not vary in any essential manner from that in the human eye. In all cases, whether in the choroid or in the retina, we find the same kind of deep coloured pigment (melanin), which when viewed *en masse* in thick sections appears black. In making a comparison of this actively functional dark pigment in eyes which when in use are exposed to bright light with the pigment of the pineal body (basal epiphysis) which in the higher types of vertebrates is enclosed in the cranial cavity and is never exposed to light, one may note, as has been pointed out by Quast, that the pigment found in the parenchymal cells is of a yellow-brown colour and resembles the type of pigment which is found in degenerating nerve cells either in disease or in advanced age. Where the pigment is darker in colour, as in the membranes and in the supporting tissue, the explanation is probably to be found in the nature of the blood supply, which like that of the suprarenal body approaches the sinusoidal type. It may be assumed that owing to a slowing down of the circulation, any chromatophores or pigment-producing substances would tend to be deposited either in the meshes of the reticulum or in the substance of the cells. The deposit of dark pigment in the retina of the parietal organ is obviously an hereditary condition.

CHAPTER 4

EYES OF INVERTEBRATES

Cœlenterates

THE simplest type of sense-organ which has been proved experimentally to be sensitive to light is represented by the eye-spots or " ocelli " situated between the bases of some of the tentacles in certain forms of Medusæ, e.g. the jelly-fish, *Aurelia aurita* (Fig. 52, A). They consist of specialized groups of ectoderm cells containing red or black pigment, which are

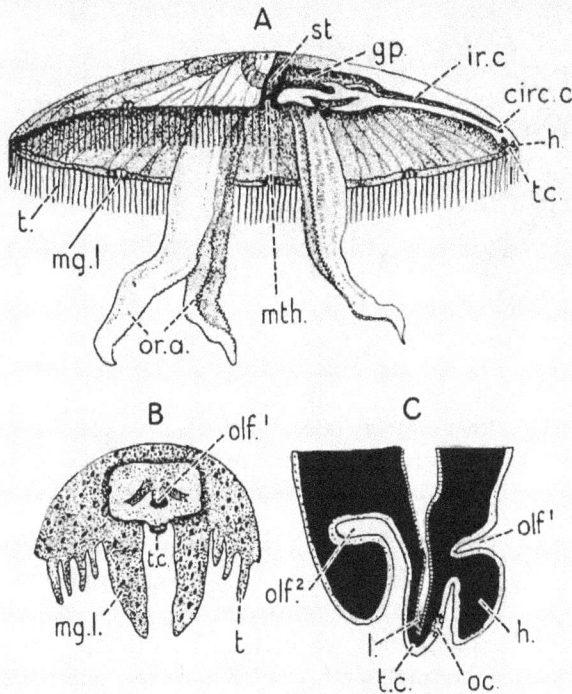

FIG. 52.—DIAGRAM SHOWING THE POSITION OF THE EYE-SPOTS OF A JELLY FISH, AURELIA AURITA.

A—Side view. A segment of the umbrella has been cut away to show the interior.
B—A small part of the edge of the umbrella to show the position of the tentaculo-cyst and marginal lappets.
C—Vertical meridional section showing the position of the eye-spot.

[Continued at foot of next page.

sometimes phosphorescent, or luminous in the dark, and are arranged round the margin of the umbrella.   They are found on the outer side of a hollow, club-shaped process called the tentaculo-cyst (Fig. 52, B, C), which lies between each pair of marginal lappets.   These marginal lappets, of which there are eight, are situated between the tentacles around the edge of the umbrella (Fig. 52, A, B).   They lie in relation with the outer end of each " radial " and " per-radial " canal and between each pair is a prolongation of the " circular " canal, namely the tentaculo-cyst.

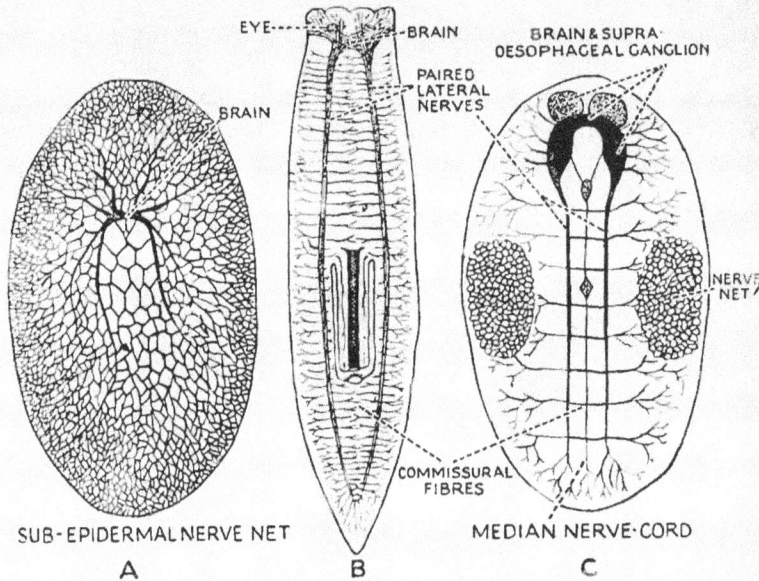

FIG. 53.—DIAGRAM SHOWING THE ORIGIN OF THE CENTRAL NERVOUS SYSTEM AND PRIMARY NERVE TRUNKS FROM A SUB-EPIDERMAL NERVE NET.

A—Low type of flat worm ; B—Higher type (Planaria) ; C—Arthropod.

(After Jijima Hatschek, and Stempel.)

Another type of sense-organ which must be considered along with the ocelli is the " statocyst."   These frequently contain calcareous particles which are supported on cilia and constitute one of the earliest types of equilibrating organs, such as are represented in vertebrates by the paired systems of semicircular canals and vestibules of the internal ear.   Such

circ. c. : circular canal.	*oc. :* eye-spot.
gp. : gastric pouch.	*olf.¹, olf.² :* olfactory pits.
ir. c. : interradial canal.	*or. a. :* oral arms.
h. : hood.	*st. :* stomach.
l. : lithite.	*t. :* tentacles.
mg. l. : marginal lappet.	*tc. :* tentaculo-cyst.
mth. : mouth.	

(After Lankester, from *A Textbook of Zoology*, Parker and Haswell.)

equilibrating organs are found in *Hormiphora plumosa*, one of the comb-bearing free-swimming cœlenterates. The class Ctenophora to which this species belongs is, moreover, of special interest in tracing the history of the sense-organs owing to the occurrence in these animals of a definite bilateral symmetry, as indicated by right and left tentacles and more especially, as in *Hydroctena*, by the presence of an ampulla at the apex containing *two* lithites supported on spring-like epithelial processes. Pigment spots are arranged as in the more primitive cœlenterates circum-ferentially round the body. Moreover, the development of a definite sub-epithelial plexus of nerves in connection with the sense-organs beneath the general surface of the body and in the tentacles is worthy of note, as this sup-epithelial plexus of nerve-fibres and cells is the precursor of the central nervous system of the higher types of invertebrate animals (Fig. 53), and it is generally supposed that the central nervous system of the prevertebrate ancestors of the vertebrates arose in the same way.

CHAPTER 5

THE EYES OF FLAT WORMS—PLATYHELMINTHES

IN the flat worms, e.g. the fresh-water Planaria or Dendrocœlum, there is very evident bilateral symmetry. At the anterior or head-end of the body are a pair of rounded or kidney-shaped black spots—the eyes, or ocelli. They are situated on the dorsal surface of the body and are

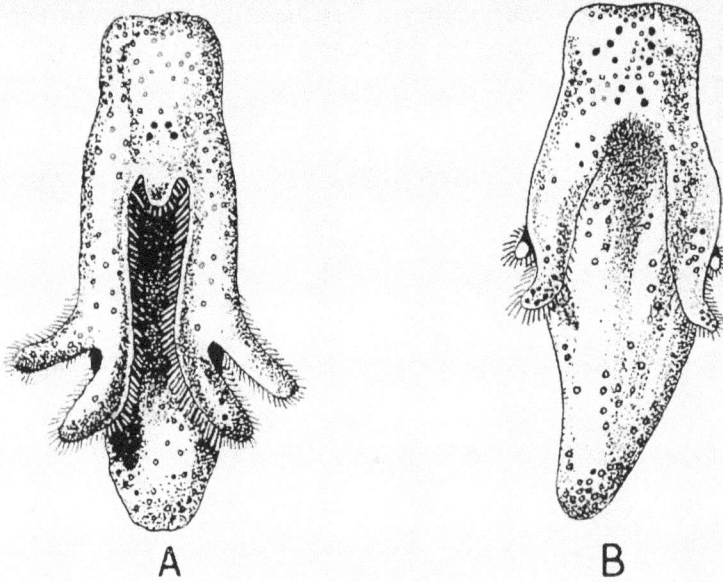

A   B

FIG. 54.—VENTRAL ASPECT OF LARVÆ OF YUNGIA AURANTIACA.

A—commencement of metamorphosis.   B—Metamorphosis almost completed.

In A, two pairs of ocelli have appeared in the region occupied by the apical cells of the earlier embryo (Muller's larva).   In B, additional pairs of eye-spots have appeared in the same region.   A pair of temporary eye-spots not shown in the figure also appear on the dorsal aspect of A near the base of the ciliated lobe which overhangs the mouth.

(After Lang, from MacBride.)

connected by nerve-fibres with the anterior commissure or cerebral ganglion which joins the right and left longitudinal nerve cords (Fig. 53, B). The eye-spots consist of two or more pigmented epithelial cells which enclose a cup-shaped cavity filled with a clear, refractile substance. Nerve-fibres leave the deep surface of the organ and join the cerebral ganglion. In some marine forms the eyes are multiple and are found on the dorsal aspect of the head, arranged round its anterior margin and sides. In others both marginal and paired eyes are present in the same individual (Fig. 19, p. 25).

In the liver-fluke, *Fasciolia hepaticum*, which is sometimes found in the larger bile-ducts of the sheep, no eyes are found in the adult form. This is what might be expected during the parasitic phase of the animal's existence, and it is interesting to note that in its free-swimming larval stage, two pigmented eyes are present and that remnants of these eye-spots are still found in the sporocyst stage of its existence in the body of a snail.

Eye-spots are also present in the region of the embryonic apical cells on the larva of *Yungia aurantiaca* (Fig. 51). Two pairs appear first on the ventral aspect, near the median plane ; later, at the period of meta-morphosis, other pairs appear farther forward and situated more laterally.

Well-developed paired eyes are present in the Triclad forms of Turbellaria, and an eye-spot is found in the anterior segment of *Micro-stomium*, a simple type of Turbellaria which reproduces by an asexual process of budding.

In the tape worms eyes are completely absent, these animals being endoparasitic in all stages of their existence.

CHAPTER 6

THE EYES OF ROUND WORMS,
NEMATHELMINTHES

MANY of these, such as *Ascaris lumbricoides, A. suilla, A. megalocephala, Dochmius duodenalis, Oxyuris, Trichina spiralis, Filaria medianensis*

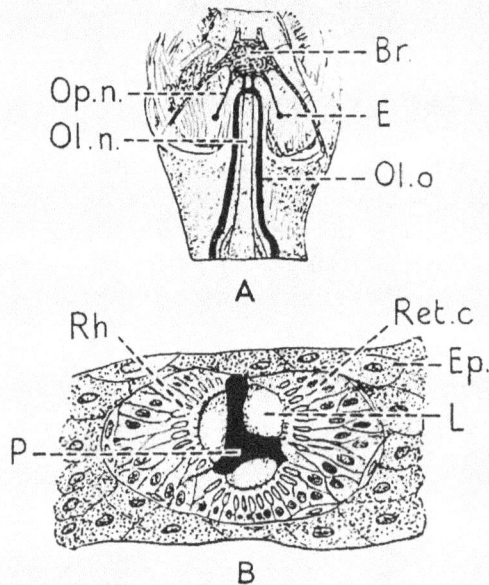

FIG. 55.

A—Dorsal aspect of head of *Sagitta bipunctata*, showing paired eyes connected by optic nerves with the brain.

E. : eye.	*Ol. n.* : olfactory nerve.
Op. n. : optic nerve.	*Br.* : brain.
Ol. o. : olfactory organ.	

B—Section through eye of *Sagitta hexaptera*, after O. Hertwig.

Ep. : cutaneous epithelium.	*Rh.* : rods.
L. : lens.	*Ret. c.* : retinal cells.
P. : pigment.	

(guinea worm), *F. sanguinis hominis*, and *Trichocephalus dispar*, are parasitic and have no eyes. Among the non-parasitic round worms, which live in fresh-water near the sea-shore or on the surface of the ocean, we may mention the arrow worm, *Sagitta hexaptera*, which has two eyes placed laterally on the dorsal surface of the head. Each eye is rounded in form and contains three biconvex lenses ; these are separated by a tri-radiate pigment zone and are surrounded by converging rod-like sensory cells. The latter end in nerve fibres which are grouped together into a pair of optic nerves which end in the cerebral ganglion (Fig. 55). This tri-radiate arrangement of the pigment zone, and of the refractile elements and sensory cells of the paired eyes of *Sagitta hexaptera*, is very similar to that which is seen in the median triplacodal eyes of arthropods (Figs. 248, 249, 250), and like these it appears to have originated by the fusion of 3 separate ocelli, see pp. 360, 361, 362.[1]

[1] Hertwig, O., 1880, *Die Chaetognathen*. Gustav Fischer, Jena.

CHAPTER 7

THE EYES OF ROTIFERS (WHEEL ANIMALCULES)

In tracing the homology of different groups of animals it often appears that although the adult forms of these have undergone marked differentiation along divergent lines, so that they show little resemblance to each other, yet the larval forms are so like that the possibility of the two groups having sprung from a common ancestor is at once apparent. In this

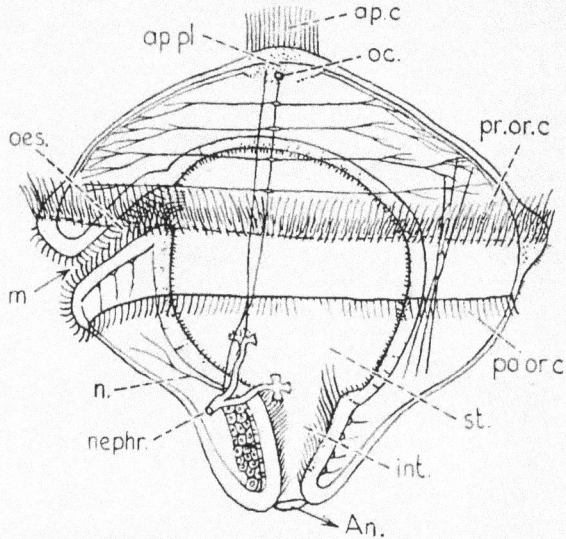

FIG. 56.—TROCHOPHORE LARVA OF A ROTIFER SHOWING APICAL PLATE AND EYE-SPOT, OF WHICH THERE ARE USUALLY TWO. (AFTER HATSCHEK.)

An. : anus.	*nephr.* : nephridium.
ap. c. : apical cilia.	*oes.* : œsophagus.
ap. pl. : apical plate.	*oc.* : eye-spot.
int. : intestine.	*po. or. c.* : post-oral circlet of cilia.
m. : mouth.	*pr. or. c.* : preoral circlet of cilia.
n. : nerve.	*st.* : stomach.

respect the study of the larva or trochophore of the rotifers is of the very greatest interest. This trochophore (Fig. 56) is a pear-like structure which in many respects resembles the Tornaria of *Balanoglossus* (Fig. 124, Chap. 13, p. 170, and Fig. 125, Chap. 14, p. 172). Thus in the trochophore we recognize a pear-shaped organism with the broad end uppermost, having an apical plate bearing a tuft of vertical cilia. This plate has a pair of short tentacles and eye-spots which lie over the nerve-centre or ganglion. There are, moreover, usually two circlets of vibratile cilia which surround the body, one lying above or in front of the mouth—preoral—the other below or behind the mouth—postoral. The mouth is placed on one side of the body, namely the ventral aspect, and the anus is at the lower pole or posterior extremity. A pair of tubes, the excretory organs or nephridia, are present and in the female adult an ovarium is connected by an oviduct with the cloaca.

Taking the adult form of *Brachionus rubens* as an example, we find

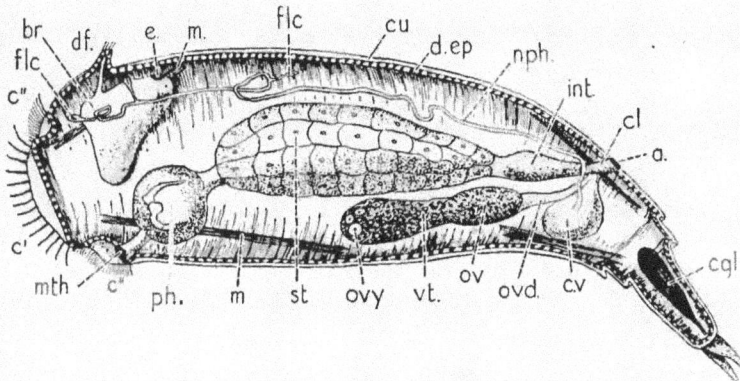

FIG. 57.—DIAGRAM OF A ROTIFER, SHOWING THE RELATIVE POSITIONS OF THE BRAIN, MEDIAN EYE, AND OTHER VISCERA.

a. : anus.	*e.* : single red eye-spot.
br. : brain.	*fl. c.* : flame cells.
c' : pre-oral circlet of cilia.	*int.* : intestine.
c'' : post-oral circlet of cilia.	*m.* : muscles.
c. gl. : cement gland.	*mth.* : mouth.
cl. : cloaca.	*nph.* : nephridial tube.
cu. : cuticle.	*ovd.* : oviduct.
c.v. : contractile vesicle.	*ovy.* : germarium.
d. ep. : deric epithelium.	*ph.* : pharynx.
df. : dorsal feelers.	*st.* : stomach.
	vt. : vitellarium.

(Redrawn from Parker and Haswell.)

that in spite of its minute size there is a high degree of differentiation. As regards the nervous system, a large cerebral ganglion is present at the anterior end of the body which lies above or dorsal to the alimentary canal. Where the cerebral ganglion comes into contact with the body-wall, there is a median eye-spot of small size and red. Three other organs considered to be sensory are known as tactile-rods ; one of these, bearing stiff hair-like organs, projects from the dorsal surface just behind the " wheel " or " trochal disc " ; the other two are paired and situated on the dorsal surface of the glass-like cuticle or " Lorica " ; in a few cases there is in addition to the dorsal ganglion (which is supra-œsophageal in position) a small ventral ganglion which is infra-œsophageal. Compare Fig. 57, showing a longitudinal section of a typical rotifer, with Fig. 68, Chap. 11, p. 106, which represents a similar view of *Lepidurus*. It may be noted that in *Lepidurus* there are paired lateral eyes in addition to the median eyes.

CHAPTER 8

THE EYES OF MOLLUSCOIDA

THE Molluscoida are marine animals comprising three classes, the Polyzoa, Brachiopoda, and Phoronida. The Polyzoa form colonies known as " sea-mats " or " coral-lines." The Brachiopoda are characterized by the possession of bivalve shells which differ from those of the molluscs in being dorsal and ventral with regard to the animal instead of right and left

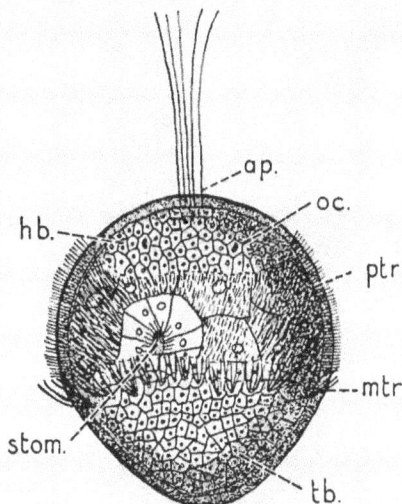

FIG. 58.—TROCHOPORE LARVA OF PHASCOLOSOMA VULGARE, SHOWING THE TYPICAL POSITION OF THE PAIRED EYE-SPOTS IN THE PODAXONIA (SIPUNCULOIDEA).

ap. : apical tuft of cilia.   oc. : eye-spots.
h.b. : head blastema.   stom. : stomodæum.
mtr. : metatroch.   tb. : trunk blastema.
ptr. : prototroch.

(From McBride, after Gerould.)

as is the case in molluscs. A typical example of the class is the common " lamp shell." The Phoronida are worm-like animals enclosed in leathery tubes. They live in associations composed of numerous individuals each of which possesses a number of tentacles springing from a horse-shoe-shaped pedicle, the lateral horns of which are often spirally coiled. The body is strongly flexed in a dorsal direction, so that the mouth and

91

anus are brought near together at the anterior end of the body. The dorsal surface or back of the animal is thus markedly reduced in length. The adult animals of all these three classes are fixed and no sensory organs are present, but the ova give rise to free-swimming larvæ of the trochophore type which in some species have a typical apical plate, bearing a vertical tuft of cilia and lying over a cerebral ganglion. In close relation with this, e.g. in the Phoronida, Phascolosoma (Podaxonia) (Fig. 58),

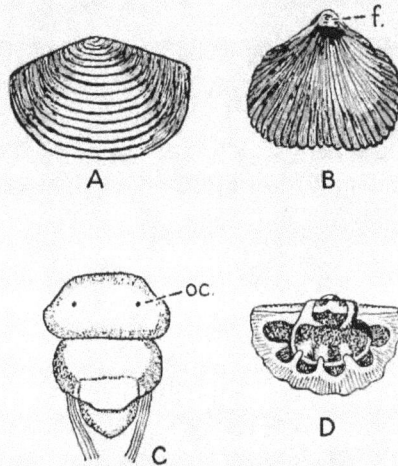

FIG. 59.

A—*Paterina*. Simple ancestral fossil form of Brachiopod—enlarged; lower Cambrian rocks, America.

B—*Rhynchonella*. Dorsal aspect of shell, showing foramen, *f.*, in beak which transmitted the stalk. Fossil shell. Lower Cretaceous.

C—Young larva of *Cistella*, showing two eye-spots, three segments, and two bundles of setæ.

D—Interior of dorsal valve of *Cistella*, which closely resembles the fossil types of Brachiopoda shown in A and B. The simpler species have presumably persisted with little change in their form or mode of development since the lower Cambrian period (see Fig. 324, p. 479).

there are two pigmented eye-spots which lie right and left of the median plane ventral to the plate. Bilateral eye-spots are also present in the free-swimming larva of Cistella. When the larvæ become fixed the eye-spots disappear. A point of great interest with regard to the presence of paired eyes of simple type, in the larvæ of the Brachiopods is that the more primitive forms of this class, judging from the characters of the shell, have existed almost unchanged from the palæozoic period represented by the lower Cambrian rocks of America, e.g. the hinged bivalve brachiopod *Paterina*, which is regarded as the ancestor of the living brachiopods (Fig. 59).

CHAPTER 9

THE EYES OF ECHINODERMATA

THIS phylum includes the star-fishes, Asteroidea; the sea-urchins, Echinoidea; feather-stars, Crinoidea; and sea-cucumbers, Holothuroidea.

Eye-spots are found at the bases of the terminal tentacles, which spring

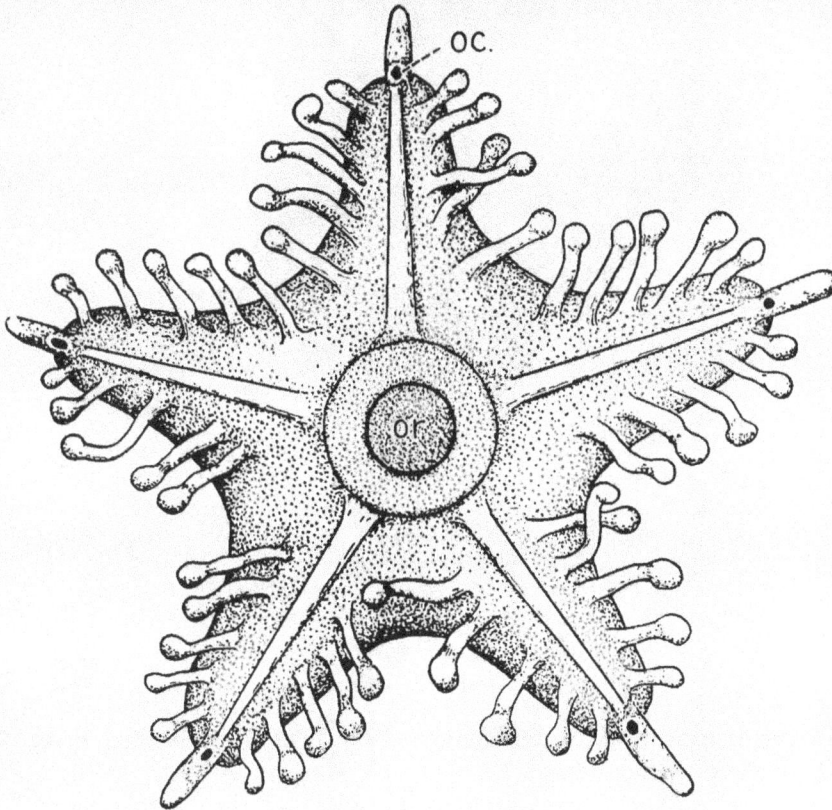

FIG. 60.

Semi-diagrammatic drawing of a very young Asteroid, showing the positions of the optic cushions—*oc.*—at the base of each terminal tentacle. *or. :* mouth. Each eye-spot is connected by the superficial or epidermal radial nerve of the corresponding arm with one of the angles of the " nerve pentagon " which surrounds the mouth. The ocelli are of a bright red colour.

(From Arnold Lang, *Textbook of Comparative Anatomy.*)

from the tip of each of the five rays of a starfish (Fig. 60). They are of a bright red colour and form a slight elevation which is called the optic cushion (Fig. 61). On microscopic examination, the cuticular epithelium is seen to be specially modified in this area, and to line a series of small conical pits or ocelli. The cells are elongated and form a single layer. Their outer ends are directed towards the hollow of the pit, and are clear and rod-like. The middle portion of each cell is deeply pigmented, while the outer part which contains the nucleus is in relation with a subepidermal plexus of nerve-fibres ; this is continuous with the radial nerve of the

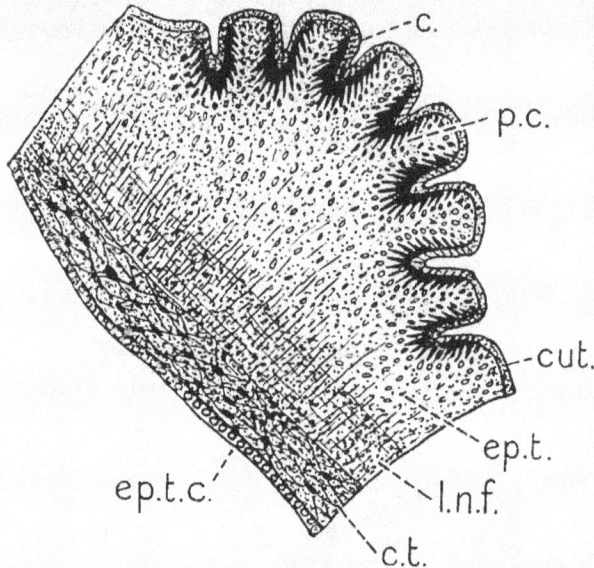

FIG. 61.—SECTION THROUGH THE OPTIC CUSHION AT THE BASE OF THE TERMINAL
TENTACLE OF AN ASTEROID.

c. : cuticle of the optic cup.	ep. t. : epithelium of tentacle.
p.c. : pigment cells.	l.n.f. : layer of nerve fibres.
cut. : cuticle of the epithelium of the tentacle.	c.t. : connective tissue.
	ep. t. c. : epithelium of tentacle canal.

corresponding arm which terminates in the central pentagonal nerve-ring surrounding the mouth.

In the sea-urchins slight elevations are present on the " ocular plates." These are situated in a position which corresponds to that of the " optic cushions " of star-fishes, namely at the tips of the five ambulacral zones of the shell, in the " periproctal " region, round the anus. The ambulacral zones are homologous with the rays of a star-fish ; the rays having, as it were, been bent backwards towards the anal or aboral pole, which lies opposite the oral pole on which the mouth is found.

The small elevation on the " ocular plate," although it was at one time thought to be a rudimentary eye, has, however, been shown to be a vestigial tentacle. This vestigial tentacle, however, corresponds to the " terminal tentacle " of the star-fish at the base of which the " optic ganglion " is developed.

CHAPTER 10

THE EYES OF ANNULATA

THE phylum Annulata includes the earthworms; fresh-water worms; marine annelids; the primitive Archi-Annelida (Polygordius); certain parasitic and tube-worms, and the leeches.

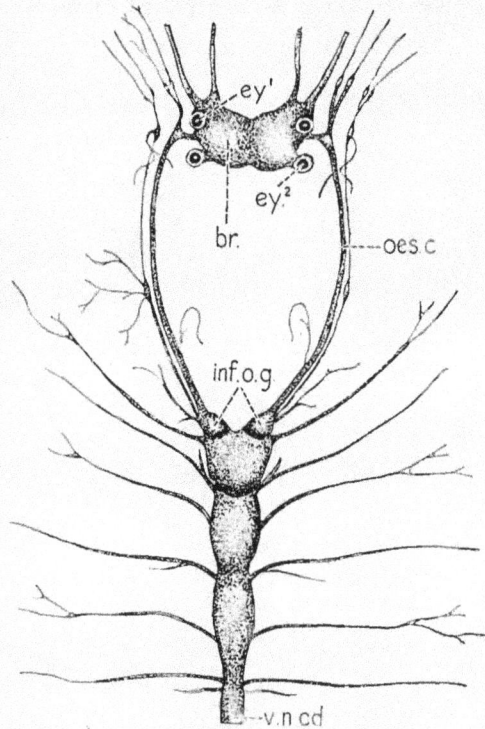

FIG. 62.

Anterior part of the nervous system of *Nereis*, showing two pairs of eyes, *ey.*¹, *ey.*²; which are connected by short stalks, the optic nerves with *br.*, the supra-œsophageal ganglion or brain; the brain is connected by two nerve cords, the œsophageal connectives, *œs. c.*, with the infra-œsophageal ganglion, these pass ventrally one on each side of the œsophagus; *inf. o. g.*, the infra-œsophageal ganglia, are continuous behind with the ventral chain of fused bilateral ganglia, and nerve cords, which supplies the viscera and posterior segments of the body. (After Quatrefages—Parker and Haswell.)

96

The eyes of these different classes of " ringed worms " are mostly of the simple upright type ; and when present in the adult animal are mostly borne on the anterior segment of the head (prostomium) ; they are usually paired and near the median plane. The eyes in some species are exceptional in position and also in structure. Thus among the Polychæte worms, *Polyophthalmos*, in addition to the prostomial eyes, has pairs of luminous organs on many segments of the body ; while *Leptochone* has a pair on each segment and in *Fabricia* there is a pair on the anal segment. Moreover, in many species of *Sabella* and all the

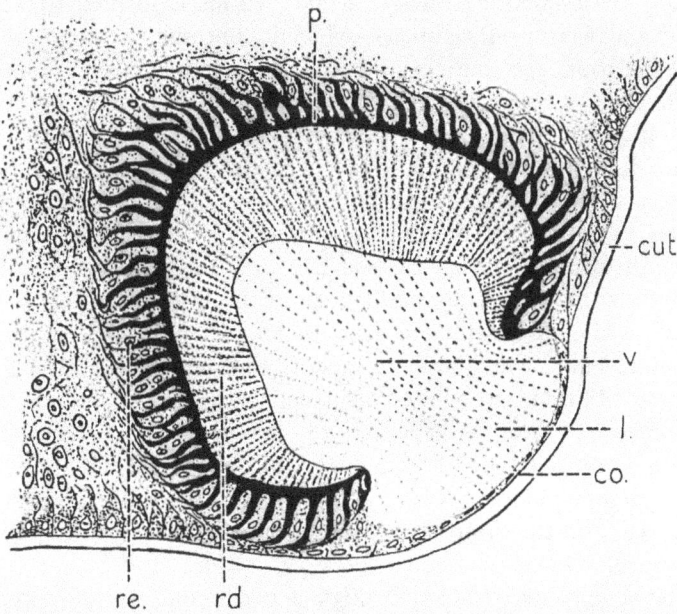

FIG. 63.—SECTION THROUGH ONE OF THE EYES OF NEREIS, SHOWING A VITREOUS, NON-CELLULAR TYPE OF LENS, WHICH IS CONTINUOUS WITH THE VITREOUS BODY CONTAINED IN THE OPTIC CUP. (AFTER ANDREWS.)

co. : cornea.   *rd.* : layer of rods.
cut. : cuticle.   *p.* : pigment.
l. : lens.   *re.* : sensory cells of retina.

species of *Dasychone*, eyes are present on the branchial filaments. These are highly differentiated compound eyes. The eyes of leeches are peculiar in structure, being formed of a number of large refractile cells lining a tubular pit and surrounded by a pigment layer. Moreover, the nerve fibres and cells, instead of being situated on the outer side of the pigment layer, are on the inner side of the refractile cells and lie in the central axis of the tube in what appears to be its potential cavity (Fig. 66). Eyes are absent in many of the adult animals, e.g. the earth-worms and certain of the parasitic and fixed forms, such as *Terebella* and *Serpula*. The

7

free-swimming larvæ, however, in the trochophore stage are in some species characterized by the presence of one or two eye-spots, placed near the apical plate, as in the trochophore larvæ of some of the echinoderms and many of the arthropods and molluscs.

Taking *Nereis*, a marine worm, as an example of the class Polychæta, or worms with many bristles, we find a distinct head bearing on its dorsal aspect two pairs of eyes. Each of these is connected with the superior œsophageal ganglion or brain by a separate optic nerve (Fig. 62). The eyes lie near the median plane, and consist of a cup-shaped vesicle closed superficially by a smooth cornea (Fig. 63). This is formed superficially by a non-cellular layer—the cuticle—which is continuous circumferentially with the surrounding cuticle; beneath this is a layer of flattened hypoderm cells. The optic cup is filled with a viscous, non-cellular material—the vitreous. This is divided by a constriction at the mouth of the cup into a superficial lens-like structure, lying outside the cup, immediately beneath the cornea, and the true vitreous which occupies the cavity. The wall of the cup is formed by tall columnar cells, the inner ends of which are clear and rod-like. These converge towards the centre of the vitreous. The middle zone of the wall of the cup is deeply pigmented, while externally are seen the nuclei of the cells and their tapering outer ends, which are continued into a nerve-fibre layer and the optic nerve. The mouth of the cup is constricted so as to form a pupil of the immovable type, there being no iris or pupillary muscles. No special ocular muscles are developed around the eyes and there would thus be no independent movement of the eyes, the separate fields of vision would overlap and the brain would receive impulses from a combination of two binocular fields of vision.

The larva of *Nereis* passes through a trochophore stage in which a typical " apical plate " is formed, beneath which is the rudiment of the cerebral ganglion. In the dome-like, upper segment of the trochophore near the apical plate a pair of pigment spots, the larval eyes, are developed. These are succeeded at a later stage by the appearance of another pair.

An interesting feature in the further development of *N. dumerilii* is its conversion by metamorphosis into a second form called *Hetero-nereis*, in which one of the principal changes is a great increase in the size of the eyes. This is associated with a change in the habits of the animal, from a slow, creeping life at the bottom of the sea to one in which it swims actively through the water.

In a recent communication by R. S. Brown to the *R. Soc. Edin.* on the anatomy of the Polychæte *Ophelia cluthensis*, he describes the eyes in this species as being three in number (Fig. 64) : two anterior, right and left, and one posterior on the left side, the right member of the posterior pair being absent. He also notes that the eyes are imbedded in the substance of the brain. They are slightly flattened spheres about 20μ in diameter, and consist of a lens surrounded by a large number of closely aggregated pigment granules. The worms examined were found in a limited area in fine-grained sand, occupying the upper third of the neap-tide range, in a belt which crossed the outflow of a small stream into Kames Bay.

A comparison of these with other Polychæte worms indicates that, as in other animals which burrow in the sand or earth, there is a tendency for the eyes to degenerate and be reduced in number. Thus in *Polynoid* and *Syllid*, two pairs of eyes are visible on the prostomium ; in *Eunice* and *Phyllodoce* one pair ; and in *Nephthys* and *Trophonia* the eyes are absent altogether (Fig. 64).

No eyes are present in the earthworm (*Lumbricus*), but these worms have been shown to be sensitive to bright light, the sensation being perceived by the agency of large epidermal cells which are devoid of pigment.

The commensal, parasitic, and tube-forming chætopods, as previously mentioned, also have no eyes. Among the latter, however, there are certain notable exceptions. Thus, Andrews [1] has described in certain of the tube-forming Polychæta eyes of a highly differentiated compound type ; these he found on the branchiæ of *Potamilla*, and he considered that they might give some aid to the interpretation of arthropod eyes. In the species *P. reniformis* the number of eyes may be as many as seven or eight on each branchia. This animal lives in a leathery tube which may be found projecting from holes in the shells of Gasteropods and from bivalve shells. At the end of the tube the cephalic branchial plumes are expanded in a circular series supported by radiating stems, each bearing two rows of branchial filaments, all of which are directed anteriorly in the fully expanded condition. In this state the eyes are on the outer or posterior sides of the main stems of the branches, there being a row of three to eight on each of the twenty radiating stems. Each eye appears as a convex, hemispherical protuberance on the outer or convex side of the main branchial stem. The diameter of one of these eyes is about 92μ, but it varies much ; smaller eyes being often found towards the tip or even interpolated between some of the larger ones along the stem. Their colour is a uniform dark red, but in strong sunlight the reflected light is golden yellow. On section the eye is seen to be covered by a smooth cuticle continuous at the base with the surrounding cuticle ; beneath this the cells forming the eye are likewise seen to be continuous at the base with the hypoderm cells surrounding it. The cells in the centre are

[1] E. A. Andrews, " Compound Eyes of Annelids, *T. Potamilla*," *J. Morph.*, 5, 271, 1891.

greatly elongated, and are differentiated into sensory cells and pigment cells. The outer ends of the sensory cells are expanded by a refractile vase-shaped inclusion, the " crystal cone." The inner end contains an

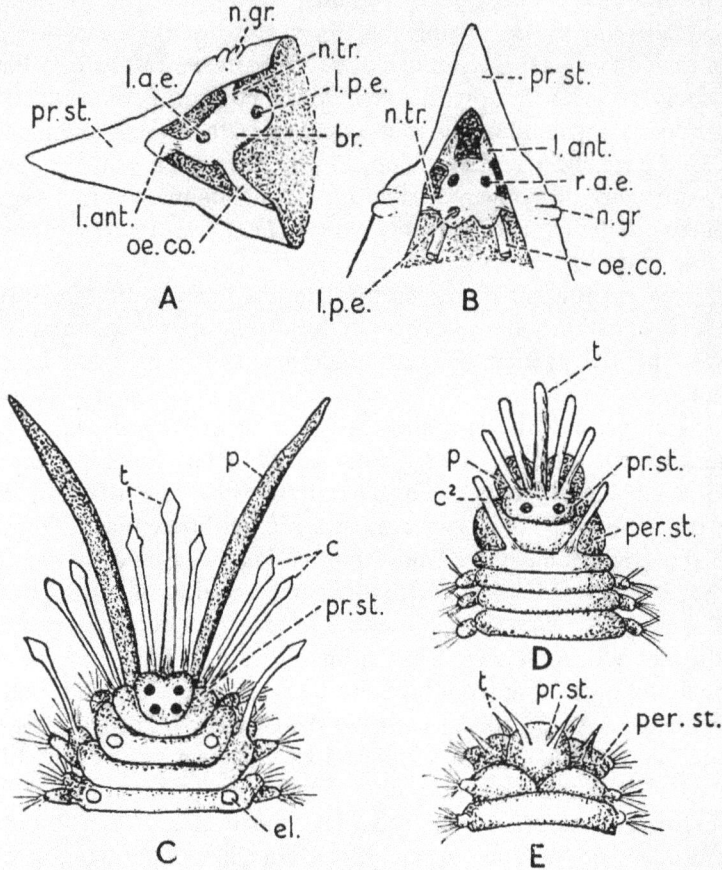

FIG. 64.—EYES OF POLYCHÆTE WORMS, SHOWING VARIATIONS IN THE NUMBER OF OCELLI.

A, B— Lateral and dorsal views of the brain and eyes of *Ophelia cluthensis*. (After R. S. Brown.)

C, D, E—Heads of *Polynoid*, *Eunice*, and *Nephthys* (*Cambr. Nat. Hist.*). In the species *Ophelia cluthensis* the right member of the posterior pair of ocelli is absent. In *Eunice* only one pair is present, and in *Nephthys* the eyes are absent.

br. : brain.	*n. tr.* : nuchal lobe.
c. : cirri.	*œ. co.* : œsophageal commissure.
c.^{2} : cirrus of first body segment.	*p.* : palp.
el. : point of attachment of elytron.	*per. st.* : peristomium.
l.a.e. : left anterior eye.	*pr. st.* : prostomium.
l. ant. : lobus anterior.	*r.a.e.* : right anterior eye.
l.p.e. : left posterior eye.	*t.* : tentacle.
n. gr. : nuchal groove.	

oval nucleus and tapers into a delicate process which comes into close relation with branches of the two longitudinal nerves of the branchial stem, but a direct continuity of the branches could not be demonstrated with certainty. Transitional hypodermal cells are present around the base of the eye, which show the continuity of the retinal type of cell with

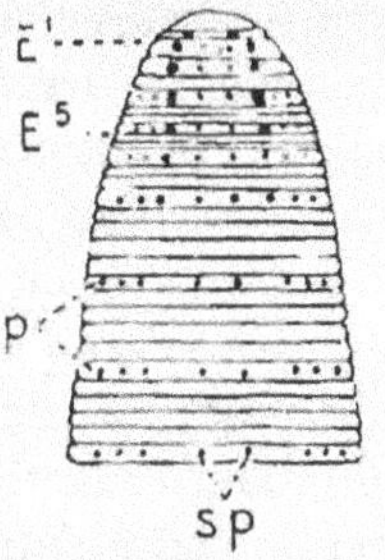

FIG. 65.—HEAD OF HIRUDO MEDICINALIS, SHOWING THE CONTINUITY OF THE FIVE PAIRS OF EYES, WITH THE ROWS OF SEGMENTAL PAPILLÆ.

E^1 to E^5 : pairs of eyes.   s.p. : segmental papillæ.

(From *A Textbook of Zoology* : Parker and Haswell.)

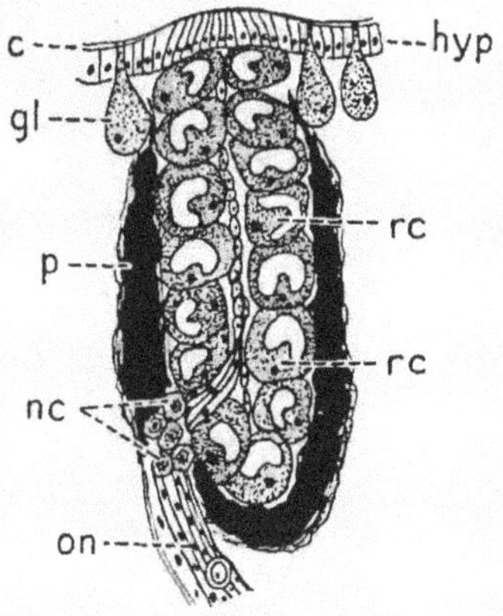

FIG. 66.—SECTION OF AN EYE OF A LEECH.

c. : cuticle.   o.n. : optic nerve.
gl. : glandular cell.   p. : pigment.
hyp. : hypodermis.   r.c. : refractile cells.
n.c. : nerve cells.

(From Lang's *Comparative Anatomy.*)

the hypoderm cells. Andrews examined several other allied species, including *Sabella microophthalmia* and *Hypsicomus*, and he mentioned that the compound eyes of *Branchiomma Kollikeri* are so sensitive to light that the movement of a hand in the air at a distance of a metre from the water containing the animals would cause all the animals to withdraw into their tubes as soon as the shadow fell upon them.

THE EYES OF LEECHES.—The general structure of the paired eye-spots of leeches has already been alluded to, and it will only be necessary to mention here that in *Hirudo medicinalis* (Fig. 65) there are five pairs placed symmetrically in series on the dorsal aspect of the anterior sucker ; and that their arrangement in series with the sensory papillæ which occupy the same position behind them indicates that they are formed as special modifications of these. The papillæ are arranged in rows extending backward from the head to the tail-end of the body. Two of these rows are placed one on each side near the median plane. These are continuous in front with the most anterior pair of eyes on the 1st segment. The other papillæ on the body are arranged serially in groups of three on the dorsolateral aspect and on the middle ring of each successive segment. The innermost row of these is continuous with the eye-spots from the 2nd to the 5th segment. The number of eyes is subject to considerable variation in different species. They may be developed on the posterior sucker or may be absent altogether.

CHAPTER II

THE EYES OF ARTHROPODA

THIS great class comprises the Crustacea, Onychophora (Peripatus), the centipedes and millipedes, insects, and arachnids. Hitherto the eyes with which we have been dealing have been chiefly of the simple type. We have now to consider, in addition to the simple eyes of the ocellar type, the laterally placed, paired, compound eyes. These attain a very high degree of differentiation and specialization in certain insects and Crustacea, and their structure has attracted the attention of some of the most distinguished pioneers in the domain of microscopical zoology. Owing to the vastness of the subject, the account which we are able to give will be only in the way of a brief sketch ; this, however, we hope will indicate the lines along which devolution and evolution of the simple median type of eye and the highly complex lateral eyes of this class have taken. Although many of these changes and developments, when considered from the standpoint of the genealogical history of eyes in general must be regarded as having occurred in types of animal which have branched off very widely from the vertebrate stem, they nevertheless help us to understand something of the history of the " pineal eye," and incidentally many interesting points of general biological interest.

Eyes of Crustaceans

One of the most interesting Orders of the Class Crustacea is that which includes the species *Apus* (Fig. 67) and *Lepidurus* (Fig. 68). In these small fresh-water animals the back is covered by a shield which resembles the dorsal shield or carapace of *Limulus polyphemus*, the king crab (Fig. 69). In both, median paired eyes and lateral paired eyes are present. The median paired eyes are of simple type ; the lateral eyes are compound.

In *Apus* the median eyes consist of 3 or 4 groups of large, clear sensory cells surrounding a mass of pigmented tissue (Figs. 247, 248, Chap. 24, pp. 350, 360) ; together they appear under a low magnification as a single black spot and hence are often described *en bloc* as " the median eye." The compound lateral eyes which have been described by Bernard are covered by a transparent cuticle forming the cornea, beneath which is a narrow space, the water sac, which opens on the exterior by a pore. The eye itself is composed of a large number of radially arranged units called ommatidia, each of which consists of an outer and an inner segment. The outer segment is formed of clear cells enclosing within them a conical vitreous body, the crystal cone. The inner segment is formed by a group of sensory cells enclosing a clear axial rod, the rhabdite and forming with the former a retinula. The retinula is the actual sensory part of the ommatidium, and its cells are comparable in this respect, although not in details of structure, with the sensory cells of the retina in vertebrates. The retinulæ of adjacent ommatidia are separated from each other by a circumferential zone of cells, containing black pigment.

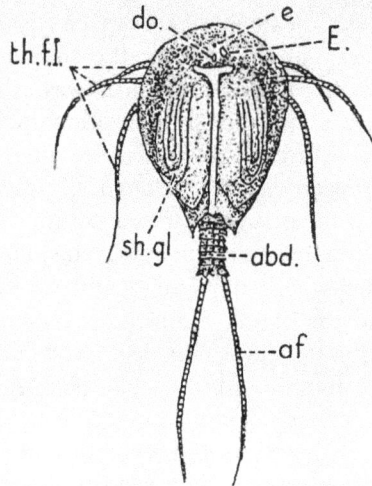

FIG. 67.—DORSAL ASPECT OF APUS CANCRIFORMIS, A SMALL FRESH-WATER CRUSTACEAN OF PRIMITIVE TYPE, POSSESSING A SINGLE MEDIAN EYE AND PAIRED COMPOUND LATERAL EYES.

abd. : abdomen.	E. : paired lateral eye.
af. : caudal style.	e. : median eye.
d.o. : dorsal organ.	th.f.l. : endites of first thoracic foot.

(From Bronn's *Thierreich*.)

The sensory cells of the retinulæ appear to be continuous with corresponding separate fibres of the optic nerve and since each ommatidium is surrounded by pigment cells and is thus isolated from its fellows, it would be able to transmit one part only of the whole field of vision to the particular nerve fibres which are directly connected with its sensory cells. The development of the median eye of *Apus* is similar to that of *Cyclops*, in which a deeply pigmented and bilobed eye-spot is developed (see description by Patten alluded to in Chap. 24, p. 360).

In *Cypris* the nauplius or larval form of *Lepas fascicularis* (allied to *Lepas anatifera*, the common barnacle) (Fig. 70), both median and lateral compound eyes are present at one period of its development and both have disappeared in the fully developed adult animal. In *Apus* and *Lepidurus* both types of eye are retained in the adult animal, as in *Limulus*, and it appears probable that many types of Crustacea, which in the adult state are parasitic or becoming attached by a pedicle to rocks, lead a fixed existence, have descended from ancestors who possessed both median and lateral eyes and made use of them in their free-swimming adult life.

In the Cladocera, as previously mentioned, the paired lateral eyes have fused into a single median organ, as in *Daphnia*, *Polyphemus*, and *Leptodora* (Fig. 21, p. 27), while in *Cyclops*, the water-flea (Fig. 71), it is the simple, median pair of eyes which have fused into a bilobed eye-spot, no compound eyes being developed in this form.

In the parasitic *Eucopepods*, or fish lice, both median (simple) and lateral (compound) eyes are present. The median eyes in the adult animal are represented by a composite organ which appears as a three-lobed structure in the median line, considerably behind the plane of the two compound eyes. In the centre is a Y-shaped pigmented area which separates three clear lens-like bodies. The anterior of these is probably formed by the complete fusion of two eyes, while the fusion of the hinder pair is incomplete. The arrangement is somewhat similar to the fusion of ocelli which takes place in *Sagitta hexaptera* (Fig. 55, p. 86), but in *Sagitta* the ocelli which have fused, presumably correspond to the lateral paired groups of ocelli in the larval stages of higher types. In the Phyllosoma larva (*Palinurus*) (Fig. 72) the median eye is bilobed, and it is probable that one of two median pairs of eyes has degenerated or completely disappeared. In this crustacean there is a very high degree of development of the stalked compound eyes and optic ganglia.

The structure of such a compound eye is well seen in *Caprella acutifrons*, belonging to the Order Amphipoda. If a whole specimen is viewed from above under a low power of the microscope by transmitted light from below, it presents the appearance shown in Fig. 73, and if the equator of the eye is focused each retinula is seen to be covered by a transparent corneal or cuticular facet. The central ommatidia show a star-like, five-rayed, central axis, which transmits the light upwards from below. Each of these stars corresponds to a retinula with its central rhabdite and crystal cone (see Fig. 44, showing longitudinal and transverse sections of the eye of *Gammarus ornatus*, the fresh-water shrimp, a nearly allied species). Surrounding the clear area are five pigment cells filled with black pigment, while the intervening spaces are occupied by interstitial tissue, and in *Gammarus* also by the white pigment cells already referred to (p. 65).

The compound eyes and optic ganglia of the crayfish, *Astacus*

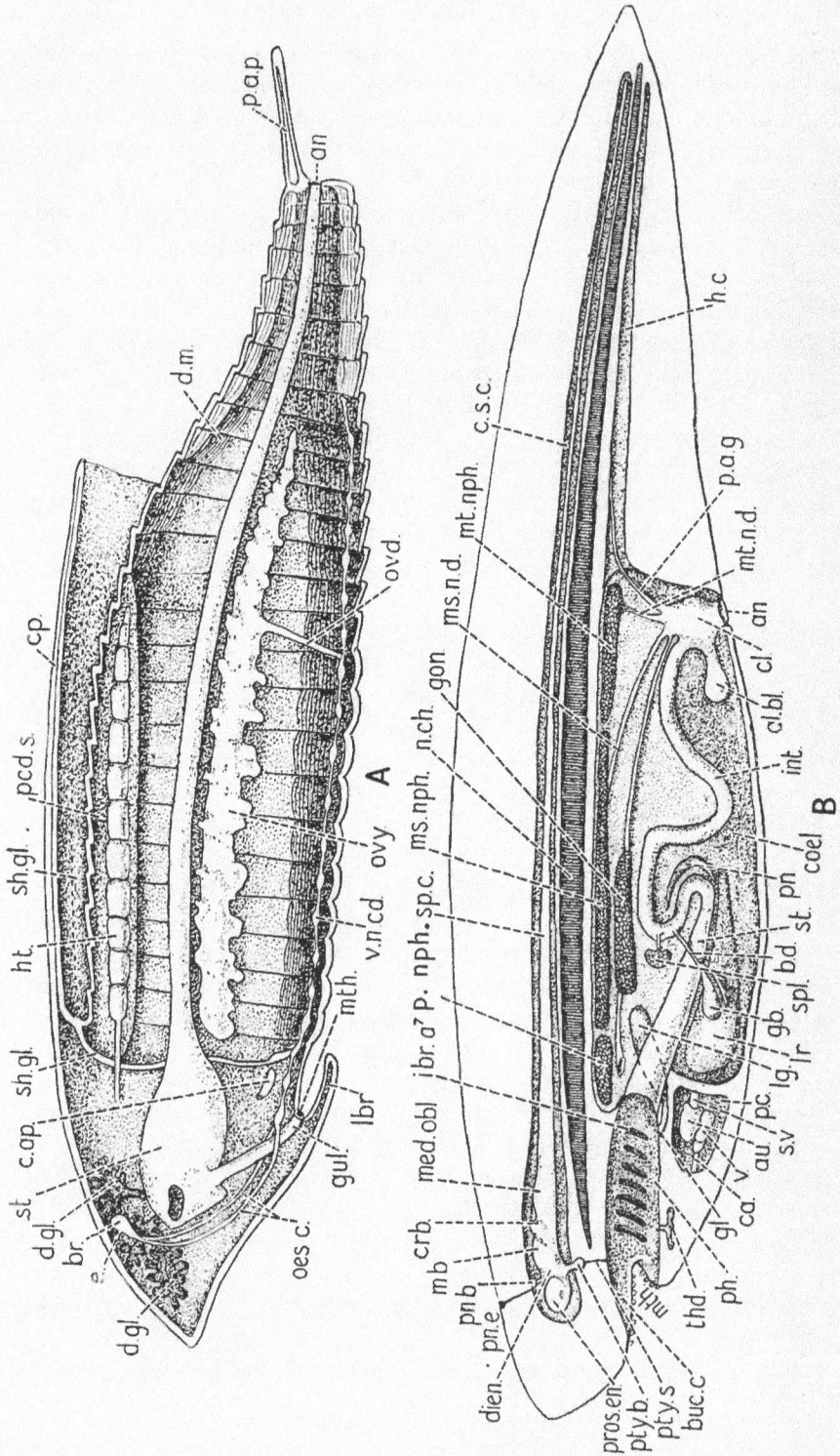

A

p.a.p
an
d.m.
cp.
ovd.
pcd.s.
sh.gl.
ht.
sh.gl.
c.ap.
st.
d.gl.
br.
d.gl.
oes c.
gul.
lbr.
mth.
v.n.cd.
ovy.

B

[See foot of next page.

h.c
c.s.c.
p.a.g
mt.nph.
ms.n.d.
mt.n.d.
an
cl.
cl.bl.
int.
gon.
n.ch.
coel
ms.nph.
pn
st.
bd.
gb.
spl.
lr.
pc.
lg.
s.v.
au.
v.
ca.
gl.
ph.
thd.
mth
buc.c.
pty.s
pty.b.
pros.en.
dien.
pn.e.
pn.b
mb
crb.
med.obl.
ibr.a² P.
nph.
sp.c.

fluviatilis, the shrimp, *Crangon*, and the prawn, *Palæmon*, exhibit an extra-ordinary complexity and diversity of structure, and they afford a most valuable insight into the relation of the sensory receptive cells to those of the ganglia in the central nervous system. The early stages of development of *Astacus* were first studied by Reichenbach (Fig. 74), who showed that the superficial cells which will give rise to the future eye are at first indistinguishable from those of the cerebral lobe and appear to be continuous with them. Further, it is believed by Kappers and others that the cells of the cerebral lobes have been derived from the superficial

FIG. 68.

A—*Lepidurus Kirkii* : semi-diagrammatic, sagittal section showing the median eye and its relation to the supra-œsophageal ganglion or brain ; also the relation of the œsophageal connectives to the gullet and of the heart and genital gland (r. ovary) to the alimentary canal.

an. : anus.	*mth.* : mouth.
br. : brain.	*œs. c.* : œsophageal connective.
c. ap. : cephalic apodeme.	*ovd.* : oviduct.
cp. : carapace.	*ovy.* : ovary.
d. gl. : digestive gland.	*p.a.p.* : post anal plate.
d.m. : dorsal muscles.	*pcd. s.* : pericardial sinus.
e. : median eye.	*sh. gl.* : shell gland.
gul. : gullet.	*st.* : stomach.
ht. : heart.	*v.n. cd.* : ventral nerve-cord.
lbr. : labrum.	

B—*Ideal Craniate* : sagittal section of a typical vertebrate for comparison with A.

al. bl. : allantoic bladder.	*ms. nph.* : mesonephros.
an. : anus.	*mt. n. d.* : metanephric duct.
au. : auricle.	*mt. nph.* : metanephros.
b.d. : bile duct.	*nch.* : notochord.
buc. c. : buccal cavity.	*p.a.g.* : post-anal gut.
c.a. : conus arteriosus.	*pc.* : pericardium.
cœl. : cœlome.	*ph.* : pharynx.
crb. : cerebellum.	*pn.* : pancreas.
c.s. c. : cerebro-spinal cavity.	*pn. b.* : pineal body.
dien. : diencephalon.	*pn. d.* : pronephric duct.
g.b. : gall bladder.	*pn. e.* : pineal sense organ.
gl. : glottis.	*p. nph.* : pronephros.
gon. : gonad.	*pros. en.* : prosencephalon.
h.c. : hæmal canal.	*pty. b.* : pituitary body.
i. br. a. : internal branchial aper-tures.	*pty. s.* : pituitary sac.
int. : intestine.	*sp. c.* : spinal cord.
lg. : lung.	*spl.* : spleen.
lr. : liver.	*st.* : stomach.
m.b. : midbrain.	*s.v.* : sinus venosus.
med. obl. : medulla obloingata.	*thd.* : thyroid.
ms. n. d. : mesonephric duct.	*v.* : ventricle.
mth. : mouth.	

(Redrawn from Parker and Haswell's *Textbook of Zoology*.)

epithelium, the cells of the latter having sunk down into the subepithelial tissue, where they develop dendritic- and axonal-processes, thus becoming bipolar.   These cells which retain at first their direct connection with the surface are called the primary receptor cells.   Their place on the surface

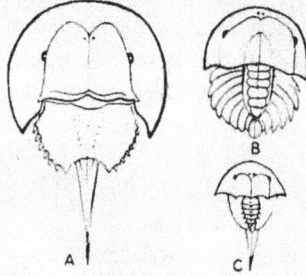

FIG. 69.

A—*Limulus polyphemus* (dorsal aspect).
B—Larval form of *Limulus* (Trilobite stage).
C—Prestwichia rotunda.
The position of the paired median and the paired lateral eyes is indicated.
(After H. Woodward.)

is afterwards taken by the formation of new cells which later also send processes into the subepithelial tissue.   The primary receptor cells now losing their connection with the surface are termed secondary or bipolar

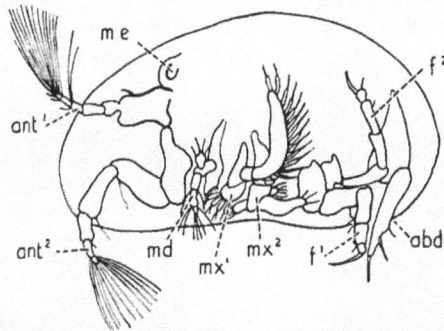

FIG. 70.—THE LEFT SIDE OF CYPRIS, EXPOSED BY THE REMOVAL OF THE LEFT
    VALVE OF THE SHELL, SHOWING THE MEDIAN EYE AND APPENDAGES.   (AFTER
    GERSTAECKER AND ZENKER.)

abd. : abdomen.	*md.* : mandible.
ant.[1] : antennule.	*m.e.* : median eye.
ant.[2] : antenna.	*mx.*[1], *mx.*[2] : maxillæ.
f.[1], *f.*[2] : thoracic feet.	

neurones.   By a repetition of the process a third layer of cells is formed, so that eventually the retina consists of three principal layers of cells with their communicating processes (Fig. 12, Chap. 3, p. 17).   Such a retina is known as a compound retina, and is comparable in this respect with the compound retina of the lateral eyes of vertebrates, which also consist essentially of three layers of sensory elements :

1. Receptor cells . . . . Rod- and cone-cells.
2. Secondary neurones . . . Bipolar cells.
3. Tertiary neurones . . . Ganglion cells.

There is this difference, however, between the lateral invertebrate eyes under consideration and the lateral eyes of vertebrates, namely, the

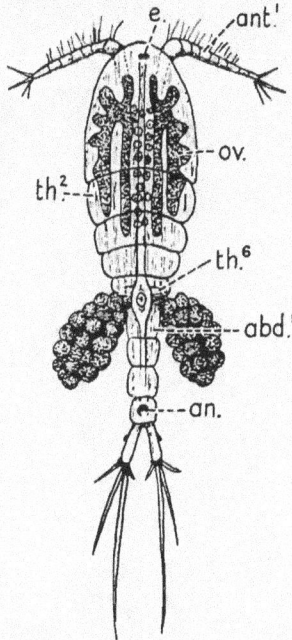

FIG. 71.—DORSAL VIEW OF CYCLOPS, A FREE-SWIMMING EUCOPEPOD (CLASS CRUSTACEA), SHOWING A SINGLE MEDIAN EYE, FORMED BY FUSION OF A PAIR OF SIMPLE MEDIAN EYES.

abd. : first abdominal segment.   ov. : ovary.
an. : anus.   th.² : thoracic segments.
ant.¹ : antennule.   th.⁶ : thoracic segments.
e. : median eye.

retina of the invertebrate eye is upright, whereas the vertebrate retina is inverted.

Between the receptor cells and the secondary neurones in both vertebrate and many invertebrate retinæ is a plexiform layer, formed by the communicating axonal and dendritic branches of these cells, and another plexiform layer is formed between the axonal branches of the bipolar neurones and the dendritic branches of the ganglion cells. Also in invertebrates, as in vertebrates, the fibres of the optic nerve are carried

inwards as a tract to the central nervous system.   In invertebrates, however, the optic tract is formed by a series of ganglia, with intervening
plexiform zones, the tissue of which is known as the neuropil or punctate
substance.   The ganglia appear as localized swellings in the stalk of the
eye, which differ in number in different types of Crustacea.   In *Astacus*,
if the retinal ganglia are included, there are four ganglia ; in others there
are three or two.   Thus in *Astacus* we have a *compound* retina and a
continuation of the nerve-chain as a tract in the form of a series of ganglia.

The compound retina of crustacean eyes is, moreover, complicated by

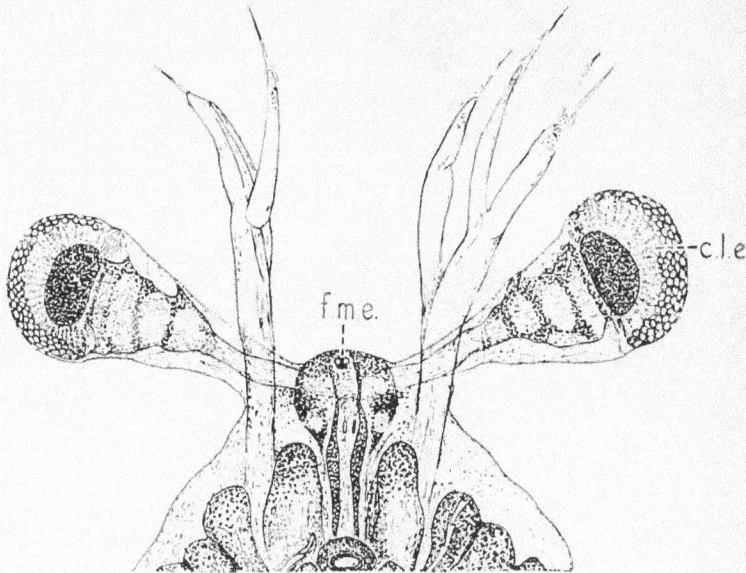

FIG. 72.—HEAD OF PHYLLOSOMA LARVA, SHOWING LATERAL AND MEDIAN EYES
(PALINURUS) (R. J. G.).

c.l.e. : compound lateral eye.
f.m.e. : fused median eyes.

the modification of the outer ends of certain of the cells to form refractive
elements, namely, the crystal-cones—cylinders or prisms which are isolated
by separate pigment cells.   Moreover, there is a further modification both
in the retina itself, as in *Palæmon* (Fig. 37, p. 52), and in the optic stalk
beyond the basement membrane in the form of spindle-shaped swellings
which are highly refractile and are either transversely striated or show
spiral markings.   These were named " rhabdomes " by Grenacher, and
are especially well seen in the retina of *Palæmon*, which besides the corneal
facets or lenses and the principal crystal cones *CC*, which are intermediate,
has distal *cc'* and proximal refractile elements *cc"*.   This type of eye is

described as an upright compound eye, and since it consists of many retinulæ or ommatidia, arranged in a radiating manner side by side, it is also a composite eye. It will be unnecessary to attempt a full description of the detailed structure of the eyes of *Astacus* and *Palæmon*, as this has been so admirably achieved by Grenacher in his great work on the *Eyes of Arthropods*. It is worth noting, however, with reference to Fig. 11,

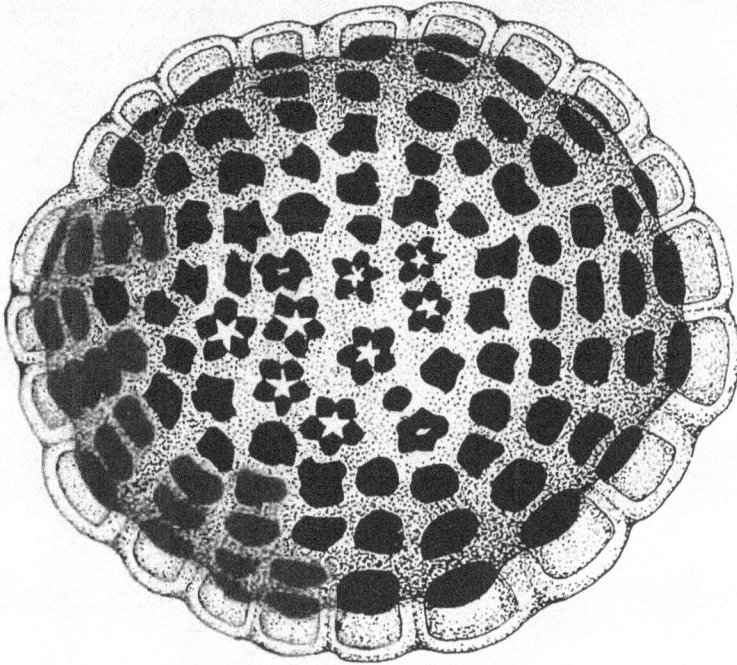

FIG. 73.

Compound eye of *Caprella acutifrons*, viewed from above and seen by transmitted light under a low-power magnification of the microscope. The drawing shows how light can pass upwards through the central axes of a particular group of retinulæ, towards the eye-piece of the microscope; and it may be presumed that in the natural condition the direction of light passing in the reverse direction would be transmitted by definite groups of retinulæ, whose sensory cells would be those chiefly affected. By varying the position and direction of the source of light, different groups of retinulæ would be affected and different fibres of the optic nerve would carry impulses to the brain. (R. J. G.)

that the smooth outer layer of the eye is continuous with the surrounding cuticle and that the cells of the retina and its basement membrane are directly continuous with the hypoderm cells and basement membrane of the stalk; also that the optic ganglia and fibres of the optic nerve are enclosed in a loose, double-layered sheath, which will permit of free movement of the stalk without injury to the optic nerve, and that this movement can be brought about by the bands of striped muscle-fibre, some of which are seen to be inserted into the basement membrane of the skin. These movements can be made in all directions, including rotation, as

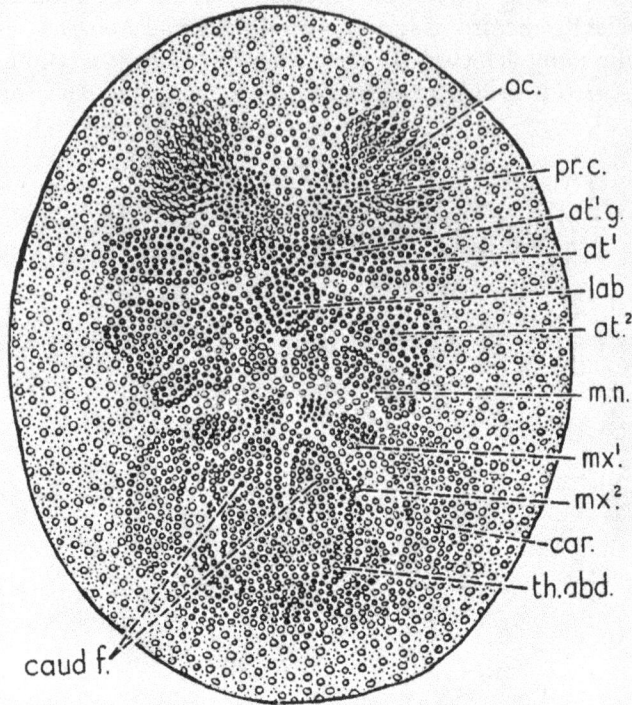

FIG. 74.—EARLY STAGES IN THE DEVELOPMENT OF ASTACUS FLUVIATALIS, SHOWING THE RELATION OF THE OCELLI TO THE PROTOCEREBRUM.

at.[1] : antennule.	*lab.* : labrum.
at.[2] : antenna.	*m.n.* : mandible.
at.[1] *g.* : ganglion of antennule.	*mx.*[1] : first maxilla.
car. : fold which becomes edge of carapace.	*mx.*[2] : second maxilla.
	oc. : ocellus.
caud. f. : forked extremity of abdomen.	*pr. c.* : protocerebrum.
	th. abd. : rudiment of thoraco-abdomen.

(From MacBride after Reichenbach.)

evidenced by the transverse direction of some of the fibres cut in cross-section and the spiral twist of the optic nerve.

THE EYES OF PERIPATUS (ONYCHOPHORA)

Peripatus is a caterpillar-like animal which, although generally classed among arthropods, differs from these in certain important respects and it is regarded as intermediate in type between the Arthropoda and Annulata. The paired lateral eyes of *Peripatus* (Fig. 75) are very similar to those of

Nereis (Fig. 63, p. 97), and they also resemble the lateral eyes of spiders. They are of the simple, upright type, there being : (1) a corneal lens, formed by cuticle and hypoderm cells ; (2) a central vitreous body ; (3) a retina consisting of an outer, clear, bacillary layer, an intermediate pigment zone, and an inner nerve-fibre layer containing the nuclei of the sensory cells. The optic nerve passes directly into the central neuropil of the supra-œsophageal ganglion or brain.

The development of *Peripatus* was investigated by Sedgwick, who showed that the eyes are formed at the antero-lateral ends of the two cerebral grooves, which later become closed off from the exterior and form for a time hollow outgrowths (optic stalks) from the brain (Fig. 76) ;

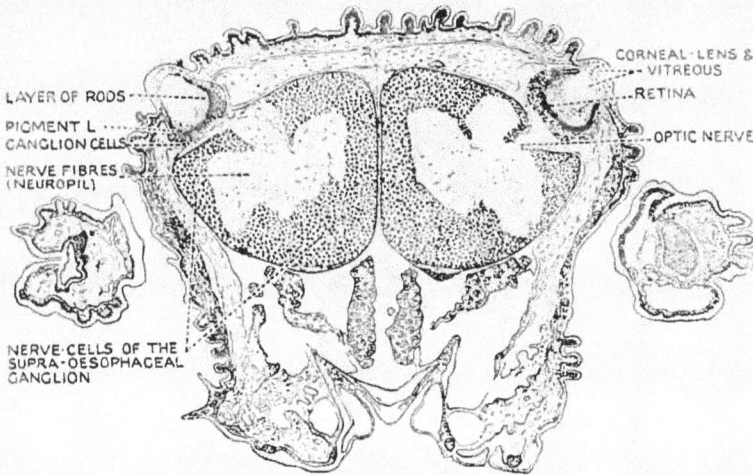

FIG. 75.

TRANSVERSE SECTION THROUGH THE HEAD OF PERIPATUS, A PRIMITIVE TYPE OF ARTHROPOD, SHOWING THE GENERAL ARRANGEMENT OF NERVE CELLS IN THE " BRAIN " OR SUPRA-ŒSOPHAGEAL GANGLIA OF INVERTEBRATES. (R. J. G.)

later the cavity disappears and the optic nerve becomes solid. In *Agelena* (cellar spider) the posterior ends of these cerebral grooves give rise to the central or median pair of ocelli (Kishinouye).

The development of *Peripatus*, which was described by Balfour in 1881, is extremely interesting from the morphological standpoint, since in many ways it resembles that of vertebrates. The importance of the comparison of invertebrate development with vertebrate development becomes still more obvious when the details of development of other arthropods such as that of certain insects, e.g. *Hydrophilus*, and of arachnids are taken into consideration. To do this it will be necessary to recall some well-known points of resemblance between the early stages of embryonic development of arthropods and vertebrates in order to

8

understand the general position of the cephalic area of certain arthropod embryos with reference to the development of the brain and that of the median and lateral eyes.

In *Peripatus*, when the early superficial segmentation of the ovum has been completed, the central mass of yolk is covered by the blastoderm, except at one part on the ventral aspect, where an invagination of cells takes place. This is the blastopore, and the floor of the depression, which is bounded by its thickened, involuted lips, is formed by the underlying yolk. Later, the blastopore appears as an elongated groove; the sides of the groove then join in the middle part, leaving an aperture at

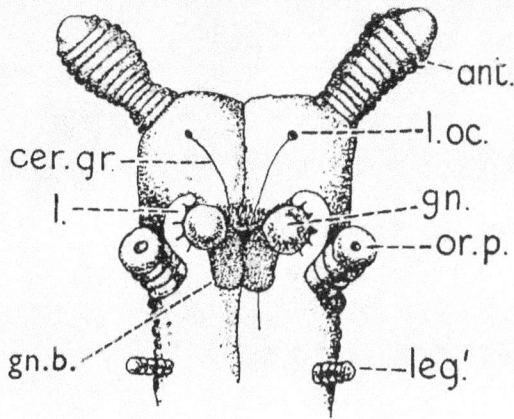

FIG. 76.—VENTRAL ASPECT OF HEAD OF A PERIPATUS EMBRYO, SHOWING THE
CEREBRAL GROOVES AND ANTERIOR OCELLI.

ant. : antenna.	*l.* : lip enclosing buccal cavity.
cer. gr. : cerebral groove.	*l.oc.* : lateral ocellus.
gn. : gnathite or jaw.	*leg ¹.* : first leg.
gn. b. : swelling at base of jaw.	*or. p.* : oral papilla.

" The anterior ocelli which were primarily posterior in position are carried forward by the forward growth of the head."—After Sedgwick, from MacBride : *Textbook of Embryology*, Vol. I.

either end. The anterior opening becomes the mouth, the posterior the anus. On each side of the blastoporic groove a series of hollow meso-dermic somites are formed, the cavities of which give rise to the internal vesicles of the nephridia and genital ducts. At the anterior end in front of the mouth is a crescentic area which gives rise to the cerebral lobes and head.

A rounded process which will give rise to the labrum is situated in front of the mouth, and it is from the base of this that the two cerebral grooves, previously mentioned, diverge towards the roots of the antennæ.

In *Hydrophilus* (Fig. 77), before the appearance of the cerebral grooves, however, the whole area, including the blastoporic groove, somites, and cephalic region, is enveloped in an amnion fold which grows up over the ventral plate and becomes cut off from the superficial layer of the amnion fold or serosa, in the same way as in vertebrates, but on the ventral aspect of the body instead of on the dorsal aspect. Another interesting point is that in the scorpion the covering of the dorsal surface of the embryo with skin is effected by the lateral growth of the ventral plate, its right and left edges carrying with them the lines of origin of the amnion on each side, round the dorsal aspect of the ovum, until they meet in the median line. The further study of the development of arthropods, more especially

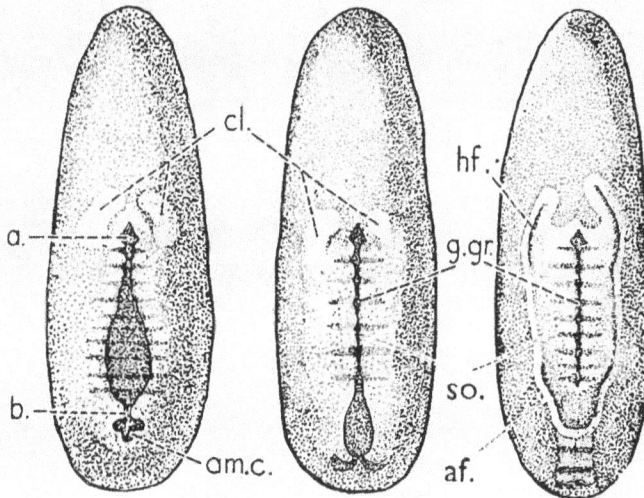

FIG. 77.—VENTRAL VIEW OF THREE STAGES IN THE DEVELOPMENT OF HYDROPHILUS.
(FROM LANG, AFTER HEIDER.)

a. and b. : points at which the blastopore first closes.
af. : edge of the amnion fold.
am. c. : rudiment of amnion cavity commencing at caudal end of embryo.
c.l. : procephalic lobes.
g. gr. : linear groove marking the line of invagination of gastral endoderm.
hf. : head fold of amnion.
so. : somites.

of spiders, scorpions, and *Limulus*, emphasizes the importance of our knowledge of their relation to each other and to their remote ancestors of the Silurian epoch, such as *Hemiaspis*, and still further back to the ancestors of the Trilobites. The whole subject is, however, very intricate, and it will be impracticable to discuss here the problem of the origin of vertebrates without diverging from the main subject of this part of our treatise, namely an inquiry into the origin and nature of the median eyes of vertebrates.

It will suffice to state here that the study of the median eyes of invertebrates does throw light on this question and also that the solution of the problem is assisted by a general knowledge of the essentials of comparative embryology of invertebrates, in addition to that of vertebrates. The net result of such a study appears to indicate that the common ancestral stock of living vertebrates and invertebrates must have lived in a very remote geological period ; and although that part of the brain which is connected with the principal sense-organs, along with the alimentary canal and sympathetic nervous system, appears to have an origin which is common to both ; the spinal cord and vertebral column of the vertebrates seem to have been evolved as an entirely new structure which has grown backward in a caudal direction from the head-end of the animal and with its somatic system of nerves and musculature has become incorporated with the primary parts which pre-existed in the prevertebrate stock.

If this view is accepted in principle, the possibility of the derivation of the parietal sense-organs or " pineal eyes " of vertebrates from the simple eyes of invertebrates appears to be not only possible, but in our opinion very probable, and any divergence in structure between the two types of eye, are only what might be anticipated in view of the extremely long period of time which has elapsed since the vertebrate stock branched off from the common ancestral stock of the two great Classes.

The Eyes of Insects

In the more highly evolved types, such as the dragon fly, the bees, wasps, and ants, or the butterflies and moths, there are two large, upright, lateral eyes of the compound faceted type, and frequently there are also one or two pairs of median eyes of the simple, upright type. These may be fused or separate and are usually small and degenerate (Fig. 20, p. 26). In the wingless insects, Apterygota, compound eyes and ocelli are sometimes present and sometimes absent. In the Order Collembola, which includes the spring-tails, compound eyes are never present. Ocelli or simple eyes with a non-faceted cornea are sometimes placed laterally, especially in the larval condition, where they may precede or co-exist with the rudiments of the compound eyes. The facets on the surface of a compound eye are usually hexagonal, and it is stated that in the dragon-fly there may be as many as 28,000. When seen in longitudinal section each ommatidium is found to consist of a cornea-lens formed by a modification of the cuticle which corresponds to one of the hexagonal facets seen on the surface ; beneath this is a crystalline cone or a group of four crystal cells. In the central axis is a clear, glass-like rod, the rhabdome ; the sensory cells of the retinula end in nerve-fibres which pierce a fenestrated basement membrane, beneath which is a plexus of nerve-fibres. The retinulæ and crystal cones are surrounded and isolated from one another by pigment cells.

The simple eyes, or ocelli, have been described by Grenacher, Lowne, Günther, and others, and their structure has already been alluded to in the description of the ocellus of a young larva of the beetle, *Dytiscus* (Fig. 4,

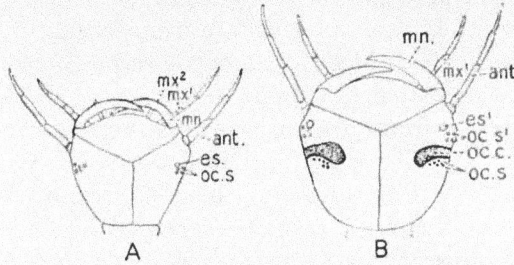

FIG. 78.—THE HEADS OF LARVÆ OF DYTISCUS MARGINALIS, SHOWING TWO STAGES OF DEVELOPMENT.

A—Aquatic larva.
B—Larva about to pupate.

ant. : antenna.
es. : eye-spot of larva.
es.[1] : lens of eye-spot carried away by loosening of the cuticle.
mn. : mandible.
mx.[1] : first maxilla.

mx.[2] : second maxilla.
oc. c. : rudiment of compound eye.
oc. s. : simple ocelli.
oc. s.[1] : lenses of the simple eyes, carried away by the loosening of the cuticle.

(After Günther, from MacBride.)

Chap. I, p. 10) ; in this a biconvex " corneal-lens " is formed by a thickening of the cuticle which lies over the elongated distal ends of specially modified hypoderm cells. These converge to the central axis

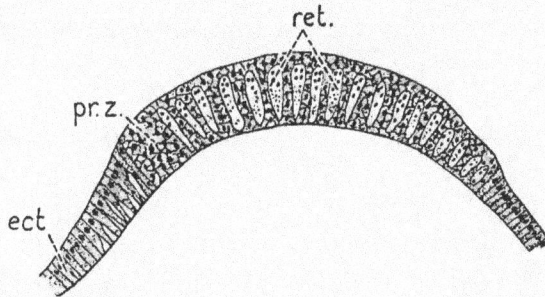

FIG. 79.—VERTICAL SECTION THROUGH RUDIMENT OF COMPOUND EYE— " IMAGINAL DISC "—OF DYTISCUS MARGINALIS, SHOWING FIRST DIFFERENTIATION OF RETINULÆ. (AFTER GÜNTHER.)

ect. : unaltered ectoderm.
pr. z. : proliferating zone of cell elements at margin of disc.
ret. : retinulæ.

or potential cavity of the eye and they form a refractile vitreous body. Deep to the vitreous is the retina composed of elongated sensory cells, which are continuous laterally with the cells of the vitreous and thus with the surrounding hypoderm cells. The outer ends of the retinal cells are clear and rod-like; in the middle portion of each cell is the nucleus and the inner end is continuous with a fibre of the optic nerve.

According to the description given by Günther in 1912 of the development of the eyes of *Dytiscus marginalis*, a water-beetle, the young larva has six ocelli on each side of the head and a rudimentary eye-spot. In the early stage of development only ocelli are present; at a later stage a crescentic area lies in front of these, which is the rudiment of the compound eye (Fig. 78). In section each ocellus is seen to be formed as a slit-like depression of the epithelium. The cells at the base of the pit end in visual rods; each rod consists of two semicylindrical segments adherent to each other and appearing to consist of a mass of agglutinated

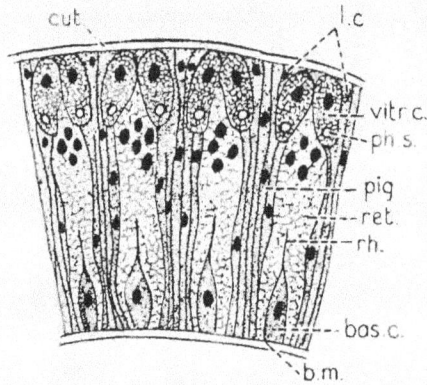

FIG. 80.—LATER STAGE IN THE DEVELOPMENT OF THE COMPOUND EYE OF DYTISCUS MARGINALIS, AS SEEN IN VERTICAL SECTION. (AFTER GÜNTHER.)

bas. c. : basal cell.	*pig.* : pigment cells.
b.m. : basement membrane.	*ret.* : retinula.
cut. : cuticle.	*rh.* : rhabdome.
l.c. : lentigen cells.	*vitr. c.* : crystalline cone-cell.
ph. s. : vacuole or phæosphere.	

fibrillæ. The cells lining the sides of the lower part of the pit bear horizontally directed rods which are similar to the rods of the larger basal cells, but are much smaller (Fig. 38, Chap. 3, p. 53). Nearer the mouth of the pit are some cells which secrete a gelatinous, non-cellular vitreous body. When the larva leaves the water and undergoes its pupal moult, a fine, pigmented line surrounds each group of ocelli. This line, which is horse-shoe shaped, afterwards thickens, and when the moult takes place the lenses of the ocelli are torn away from the deeper pigmented portions, since the lenses belong to the larval cuticle which is shed off from the deeper pigmented parts. The horse-shoe pigmented portion has now widened out and increased in breadth so as to form a crescent, the pigmented ocelli lying close behind its concave border. The cuticle covering the eye-spot is also carried forward with the lenticular parts of the ocelli. Before the final moult to form the imago is completed, the remnants of the ocelli recede from the surface, and the pigment area which is the

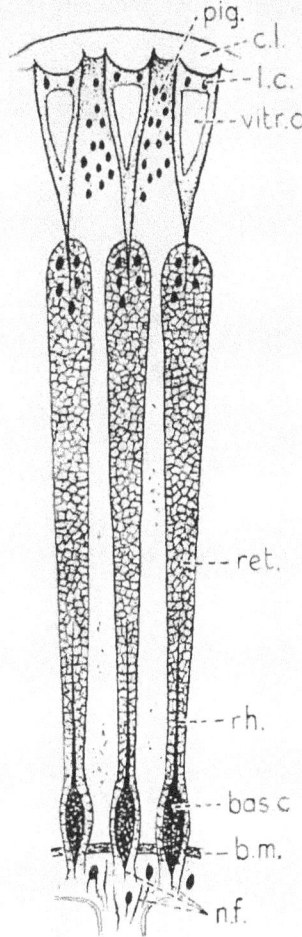

FIG. 81.—VERTICAL SECTION THROUGH A SMALL PART OF AN ADULT COMPOUND EYE OF DYTISCUS MARGINALIS. (AFTER GÜNTHER.)

bas. c. : basal cell.	*pig.* : pigment cells.
b.m. : basement membrane.	*ret.* : retinula.
c.l. : corneal lens.	*rh.* : rhabdome.
l.c. : lentigen cell.	*vitr. c.* : crystalline cone.
n.f. : nerve-fibres.	

rudiment of the compound eye, becomes circular in outline, spreading over the place which was originally occupied by the ocelli. These do not disappear completely, but remain through life as closed pigmented vesicles which are attached to the optic nerves.

The epithelium of the now disc-like pigmented area consists of tall, columnar cells which differentiate into basal and retinular cells from which the rhabdomes are formed ; cells which form the lenses, and crystalline cones, and inter-retinular pigment cells. At one end of the area there is a part where cells boundaries are indistinguishable and the

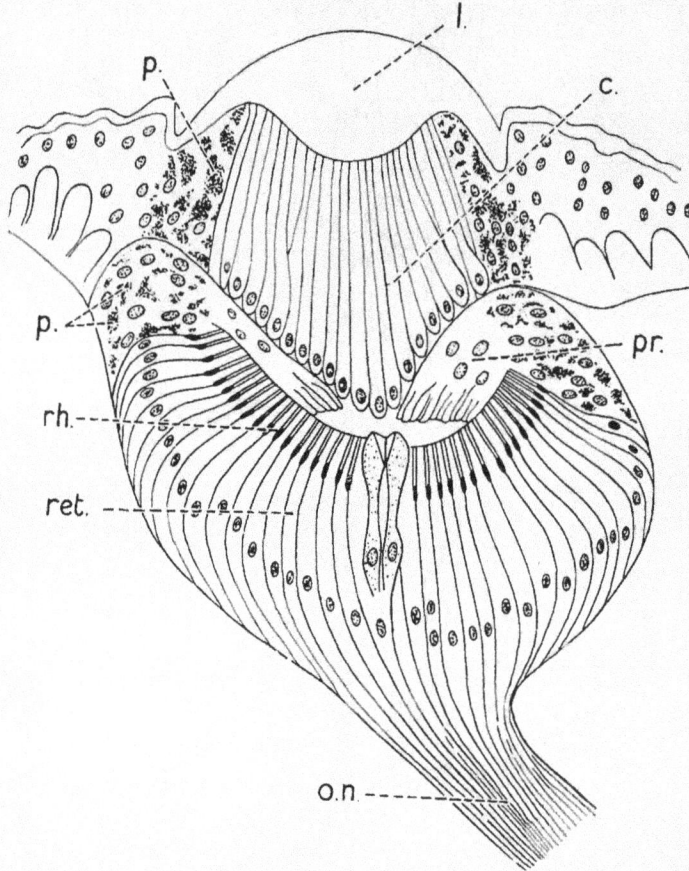

FIG. 82.—EYE OF ACILIUS LARVA. (AFTER PATTEN.)

l. : chitinous lens.
c. . corneagen, or hypoderm cells, forming the vitreous portion of the lens.
o.n. : optic nerve.   *p. :* pigment.   *pr. :* pre-retinal layer.
               ret. : retina.   *rh. :* rhabdomes.

epithelium appears to consist of a mass of protoplasm containing numerous nuclei irregularly distributed through it ; this is the proliferation zone from which for a considerable time new ommatidia are added to those which are already formed (Fig. 79). The ommatidia consist of two parts, namely, the crystalline cone and the retinula. The crystalline cone is formed by four superficial cells in which clear vesicles appear. The four cells cohere to form the cone, the vesicles in them also coalescing to form a single refractile body. The cells which will form the retinula retreat from the surface, each group of these consisting of eight cells, one central

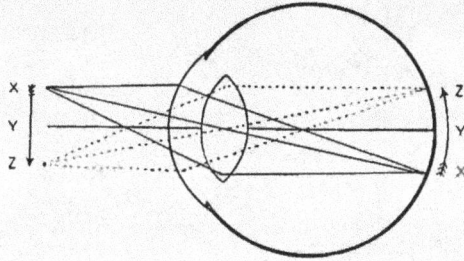

FIG. 83.—DIAGRAM SHOWING THE FORMATION OF AN INVERTED IMAGE ON THE RETINA OF A TYPICAL LATERAL EYE OF A VERTEBRATE.

and seven peripheral. One of these peripheral cells is squeezed out from between the rest, while the central cell and the remaining six peripheral cells co-operate in forming one long visual rod or rhabdome. The lower end of the rod has the form of a flask-shaped basal cell, while its upper

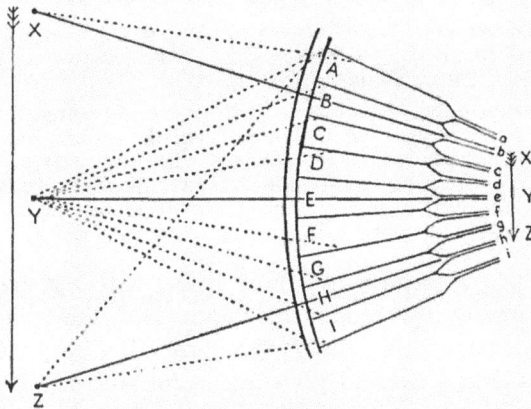

FIG. 84.

Diagram showing the course of rays of light from three points—x, y, z—through nine visual rods (supposed to be empty tubes) A to I, of a compound eye; a to i: nerve-fibres connected with the visual rods. The arrows have been inserted to indicate that the retinal image would not be inverted as in the vertebrate eye (Fig. 83).

(Slightly modified after T. H. Huxley.)

end thins out into a tapering process before reaching the upper limit of the retinula cells (Fig. 80).

In both ocelli and in the adult compound eyes (Fig. 81), the nerve fibres of the optic nerve originate as basal outgrowths from the retinal cells.

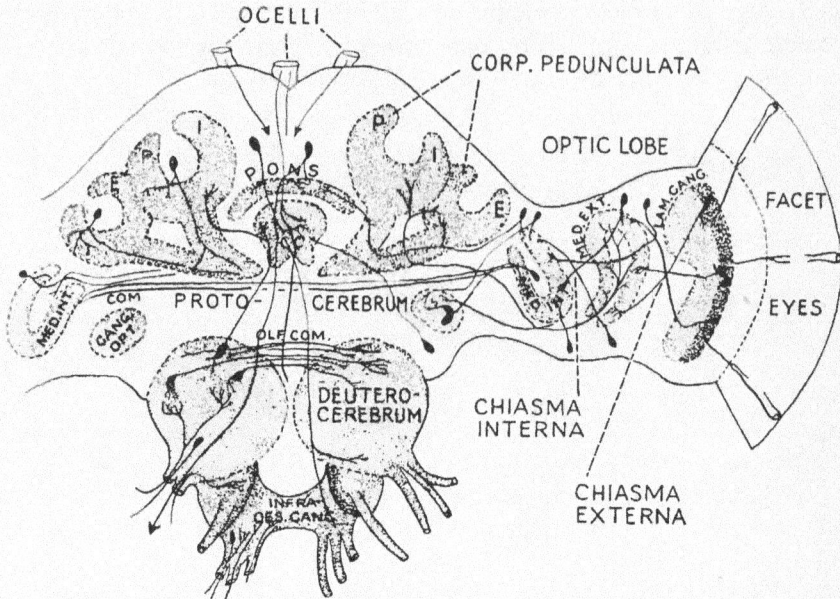

FIG. 85.—DIAGRAM SHOWING THE CONNECTIONS OF THE OCELLI AND THE FACET-
EYES WITH THE BRAIN IN THE HONEY BEE. (AFTER KENYON, JONESCU, AND
FORTUYN, FROM ARIËNS KAPPERS.)

The protocerebrum of insects is connected with two optic systems, the ocelli and
the compound facet-eyes. Of the three ocelli the middle one is connected
with the pons and central corpuscle (*c.c.*), where it acquires relations from
optic impressions from the compound eyes, and also with impressions from
the deutero-cerebrum in which the olfactory antenna ends. The corpora
pedunculata also receive optic impulses, but from the facet eyes only.

The same types of larval simple and adult compound eyes are found
in *Acilius*, the large central cells of the retina, with the long rods, being
especially well-developed in the larval form (Fig. 82). It was this
example which Gaskell selected for comparison with the " pineal eye "
of Ammocœtes. The principal objection which was raised at the time to
the validity of the comparison was that the lens of the *Acilius* larva is
formed by a thickening of the cuticle, whereas in the case of the " pineal
eye " of Ammocœtes the lens is formed as a modification of the anterior
or distal wall of the vesicle and is cellular in type (Figs. 13 and 14, Chap. 3,
pp. 18, 19). Another objection to the theory was that the ocellus of the
Acilius larva was formed as a depression of the hypoderm cells, whereas the
" pineal eye " is an evagination from the roof of the thalamencephalon
after the brain has been separated from the cutaneous ectoderm. The
evidence in favour of and against these objections will be considered on
p. 358.

It may be noted here that in the course of evolution of the inverted types of eye there has been a change not only in the position and direction of the retinal cells with respect to the incidence of light, but in the vertebrate or inverted types of eye, owing to the evolution of a single biconvex lens in a position which will cause an inverted image to be thrown upon the retina, as indicated in Fig. 83, the rays coming from the upper part of the object fall upon the lower part of the retina, whereas in the upright, aggregate type of eye, of insects and Crustacea, the retinal image is not inverted (Fig. 84), since each ommatidium can only transmit those rays of light which fall upon the surface of the eye in the direction of its longitudinal axis, and the retinal image is not inverted.   A decussation of the fibres of the optic nerve, however, takes place in the chiasma externa in the higher arthropods (Fig. 85), and in the Cephalopods (Fig. 122, Chap. 12, p. 166), whereby the cortical impressions received in the optic lobe form, it may be presumed, a mental picture which is in the same position as the object viewed—this picture, it is believed, being similar as regards orientation to that formed in the visual cortex of the human brain.

In the higher Mollusca the lateral eyes resemble the vertebrate type with regard to the position of the lens and iris relative to the retina, but differ in having an upright retina and in other respects which will be mentioned in Chapter 12.

The Eyes of Spiders—Arachnida

The Class Arachnida includes, in addition to the various forms of spider, the scorpions, mites and ticks, king crabs and the extinct Eurypterida.   The Class is much less homogeneous than the Insecta, and there is considerable variety in the number of eyes present in each animal and in the type of eye.   As in insects, many of the spiders have both median and lateral eyes.   The lateral eyes of the adult animal are, however, not compound, as in many of the insects, but are of the ocellar type, having a single, non-faceted cuticular or corneal lens.   As a rule the upright eye is simple in type with respect to the retina, but the central eyes of the scorpion differ in having the sensory cells grouped together in a form resembling somewhat the retinulæ of the compound eyes of insects and crustaceans.   Compound eyes are also present in *Limulus*, in which the retinulæ of the lateral pair of eyes (Fig. 86), are barrel-shaped and lie beneath papilliform downgrowths of the cutis, each of which is believed to serve as a separate lens for the retinula which lies beneath it.   The central eyes of *Limulus* (Fig. 87) also show a grouping of the sensory cells into units which have been described as resembling retinulæ, and have a marked general resemblance to those found in the central eyes of *Euscorpius*. These tulip-like buds (Figs. 86 and 87), however, differ markedly from the compact cylindrical retinulæ of the eyes of insects and Crustacea, and although they may be regarded as intermediate in type do not indicate a close relationship. The eyes of the ordinary garden and house spiders

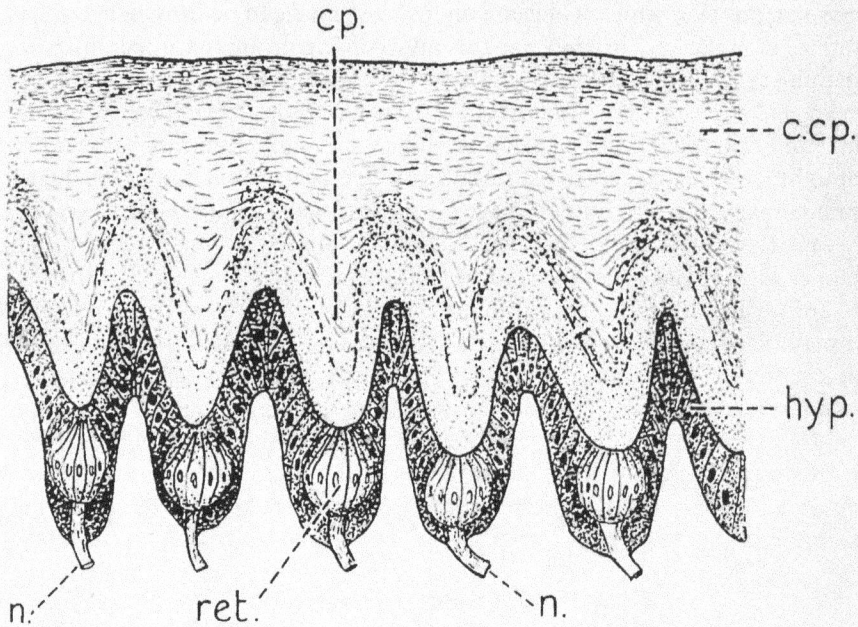

FIG. 86.

Part of a section through the composite lateral eyes of a king crab (*Limulus*), showing *c. cp.* : the chitinous carapace ; *cp.* : the ingrowing papilla-like thickenings of this which lie over the retinulæ, or separate eyes ; *ret.* : retinula ; *hyp.* : hypodermis, the cells of which are modified opposite the papillæ to form the sensory cells of the retinulæ ; *n.* : nerves of the retinulæ.
(After Lankester and Bourne.)

are also very remarkable. They vary in number from one to six pairs, four pairs being present in the leaping spider, *Salticus scenicus*, shown in Fig. 88, in which they are seen to be situated on the carapace, the central or frontal pair being the largest. The frontal eyes of *Epeira diaderma* are of the simple, upright type ; whereas the posterior or lateral eyes show what is described as an " inversion " of the constituent parts of the retinal cells. The posterior eyes vary more particularly with respect to the position of the nuclei of the retinal cells, relative to the refractile rods or bacilli ; instead of being proximal or posterior to the rods, they are in front of these, as in the lateral eyes of vertebrates. This position of the nuclei of the retinal cells was termed by Graber " præ-bacillary," in contrast to their " post-bacillary " situation in the simple, upright eye. It must be borne in mind, however, that the retina in the inverted lateral eyes of vertebrates is compound, whereas the lateral eyes of spiders, although inverted with respect to the constituent parts of the cells, are still simple in type, i.e. the retina consists of a single layer of sensory cells. In some types there is a definite tapetal layer which reflects the light on to

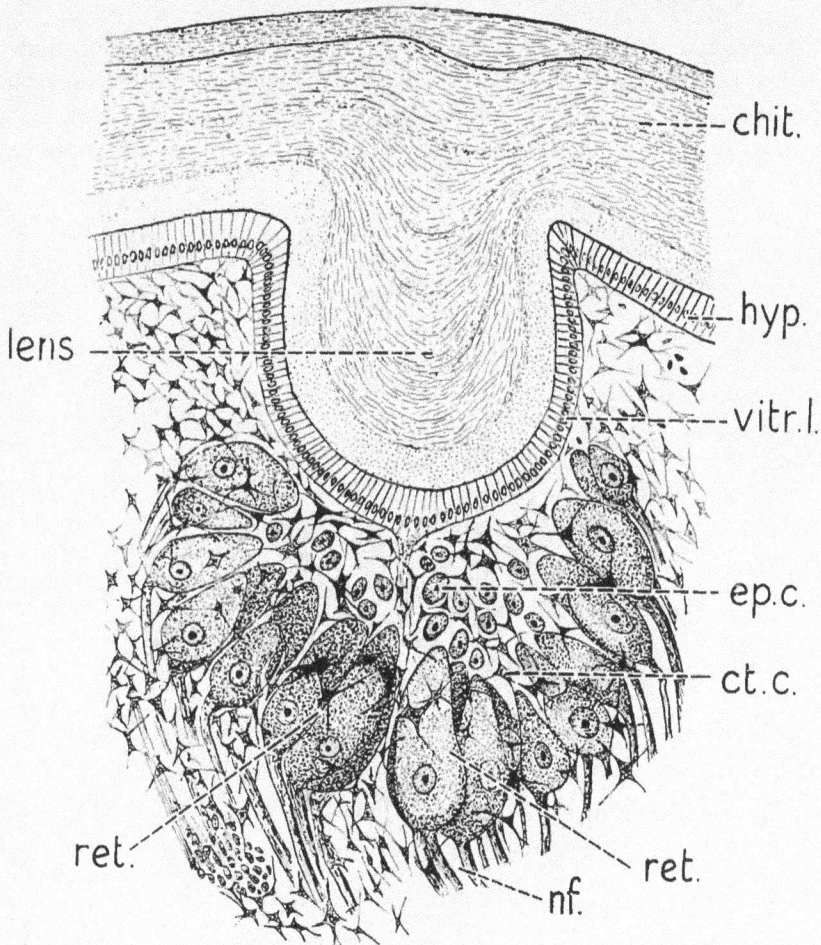

FIG. 87.

Section of one of the median eyes of the king crab, *Limulus polyphemus*, showing the transparent chitinous lens, which fills the optic pit and is continuous with the surrounding chitin which forms the head-shield or carapace. The optic pit is lined by a layer of columnar cells (vitreous layer), which are continuous with the surrounding hypodermal cells. Immediately beneath this layer is a loose tissue consisting of branched connective tissue cells (*ct.c.*), some of which contain pigment, and a few rounded or oval cells of an epithelial type (*ep.c.*). Embedded in this tissue are the retinulæ (*ret.*), which consist of groups of five to seven large pear-shaped, epithelial cells arranged round a refractile axial rod, called the rhabdome. Each retinular cell is continuous with a nerve fibre (*n.f.*), which joins with similar nerve fibres to form the main optic nerve of the median eye of the same side.

the rods as in the eyes of many vertebrates, e.g. certain fishes and carnivores, also the horse and ox.

The position which the refractile body (rod or cone) bears to the nucleus of the cell is probably not of so much importance with regard to the reception and transmission of impulses through the cell as one might be led to infer from the examination of specimens prepared with nuclear stains such as hæmatoxylin : these give the impression of the nucleus being an opaque, dark, oval body lying in the substance of clear cytoplasm,

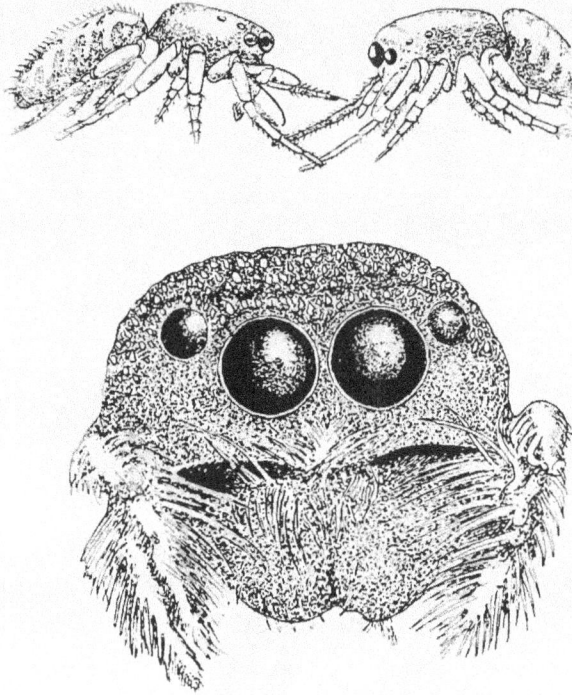

FIG. 88.

Above—side view of two spiders, *Salticus scenicus*, showing the four pairs of eyes.
Below—female of the same species more highly magnified, viewed from in front.
(After F. P. Smith, *By-paths in Nature*.)

whereas in living tissues the nuclei of cells are transparent and probably would not interfere greatly with the passage of light through them to reach a refractile body or rhabdite situated deep to or beyond the nucleus.

In the central eyes of the scorpion a refractile vesicle or phæosphere lies deep to the nucleus of each retinal cell, while superficial to it, that is, nearer the lens, is a well-developed rhabdite, and it is probable that rays of light traversing the cell would be refracted by both these bodies and would give rise to an impulse which would be transmitted to the nerve fibre arising from the proximal end of the cell. Since both of these bodies appear to be developed as a modification of or a secretion into the cell substance, it seems probable that either one or the other could be further developed so as to form the main refractile element or be suppressed, thus giving rise to differences in the position of the rhabdite relative to the nucleus without there being any inversion of the cell.

A true inversion of the layers of the retina, however, occurs in the early stages of development in the median eyes of the scorpion (G. H. Parker) and in the median eyes of the spider *Agelena* (Kishinouye). These will be described in Chap. 24, Figs. 249 and 250.

Development of the Eyes of Agelena

Agelena is a cellar-spider, the development of which has been studied by Kishinouye (1891–4). He describes the formation of a thickening in the wall of the blastocœle, namely the ventral plate, on which the first rudiments of the future organs make their appearance. The plate soon shows a series of transverse grooves, indicating a metameric segmentation. In front there is an undivided cephalic lobe, behind there is a caudal lobe, and between these is a region which is divided into five segments of which the first bears the pedipalpi, the remaining four giving origin to the walking legs. The cephalic lobe gives rise to two semi-circular lobes on each of which a crescentic groove is formed by an invagination of the ectoderm ; this resembles the grooves already described in *Peripatus* (Fig. 76), which are developed also in the scorpion and *Astacus*. The ectodermal invaginations become closed off from the surface by union of their edges, and they give rise to the greater part of the brain. The inner segments of the two crescentic tubes now unite to form the stem of a T, the transverse arms of which are formed by the outer portions of the grooves. The central eyes (Fig. 89, A, B) arise as two pits at the posterior ends of the grooves, which when united form the stem of the T and belong therefore to the hindermost segment. The lateral eyes on each side originate as a simple ring-like pit in the ectoderm (Figs. 89, 90), which becomes divided by a continuance of the process of invagination into several deeper secondary pits, each of which becomes closed off from the exterior by constriction of its opening. The floors of these pits are converted into retinulæ, their component cells becoming the visual cells. Between the upper or distal ends of the visual cells refractile rods or rhab-domes are developed, while their proximal ends become continuous with the constituent fibres of the optic nerve. The roofs of the pits are formed by the overfolding of the ectoderm and form the vitreous or hypoderm cells, while over all is formed a lens-like thickening of the cuticle, which is continuous with the surrounding cuticle.

The median eyes (Figs. 89, 90, A and B) are formed also as ectodermal pits which become closed off from the surface by constriction of their openings. The opening of each vesicle is situated behind, and when closed each vesicle has an upper and a lower wall between which is a slit-like cavity. From the upper of the two layers the visual cells arise, while the lower wall gives origin to what Kishinouye describes as the " post-retinal " layer (Fig. 250 B, Chap. 24, p. 362). The vitreous, as in the

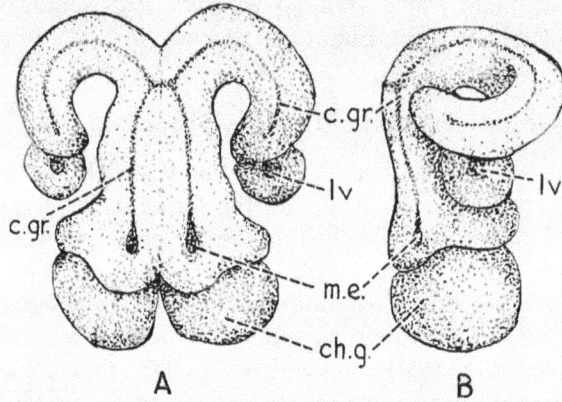

FIG. 89.—BRAIN OF EMBRYO OF AGELENA SHOWING THE POSITION OF THE MEDIAN EYES AND LATERAL VESICLES. (AFTER KISHINOUYE.)

A—Seen from in front.
B—Seen from left side.

> *c. gr.* : cephalic groove, now closed.
> *ch. g.* : cheliceral ganglion.
> *l.v.* : lateral eye vesicle.
> *m.e.* : median eye.

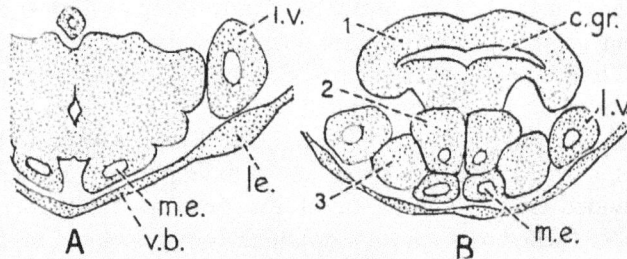

FIG. 90.—FRONTAL SECTIONS THROUGH BRAIN OF EMBRYO AGELENA. (AFTER KISHINOUYE.)

> *c. gr.* : cephalic groove.
> *l.e.* : thickening of ectoderm, which will form the lens of the lateral eyes.
> *l.v.* : lateral vesicle.
> *m.e.* : median eye.
> *v.b.* : vitreous body (lens of median eye).
> 1, 2, 3 : the three segments of the brain.

lateral eyes, is developed from the covering hypoderm or ectoderm cells, and a thickening of the cuticle gives rise to the superficial corneal lens. The early stage of the development of the median eyes is thus one which corresponds to the development of an inverted retina such as is found among the Mollusca, in the *Scallop* or *Pecten ;* and since the median eyes of adult spiders are as a rule of the simple upright type, it would be interesting to obtain further information with regard to the later stages of development and the structure of the adult eyes of *Agelena.*

The Eyes of Hydrachnida

A description of the eyes of freshwater mites was published by P. Lang in 1905, which affords a most instructive demonstration of widely divergent developments of the eyes of closely allied species : more especially with regard to transitions between eyes which are fixed in

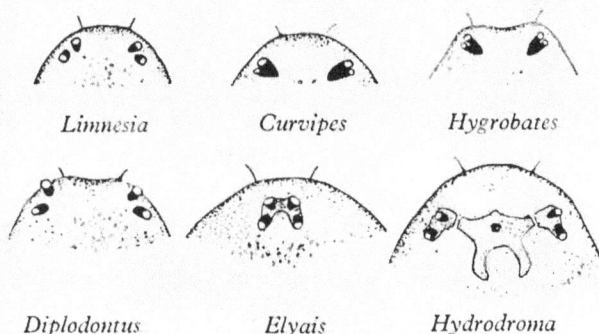

Limnesia   *Curvipes*   *Hygrobates*

Diplodontus   *Elyais*   *Hydrodroma*

FIG. 91.—DIAGRAMS SHOWING THE POSITION AND DIRECTION OF THE OCELLI, OR SIMPLE EYES, OF DIFFERENT SPECIES OF HYDRACHNIDA (FRESH-WATER MITES). IN THE GENUS HYDRODROMA A " FIFTH " MEDIAN EYE IS PRESENT ON THE DORSAL ASPECT OF THE HEAD SHIELD. (AFTER P. LANG.)

definite positions—the cuticular lens being continuous with or connected to the adjacent cuticle—and eyes which are enclosed within a chitinous covering, within which they are capable of movements produced by muscles arising from the wall of the cavity and inserted into the eyeball ; a condition which is somewhat similar to that of the lateral eyes of vertebrates, which being enclosed and protected by the walls of an orbital cavity are capable of movements within the capsule of Tenon, which are produced by special ocular muscles.

The eyes vary in number in different species of the Hydrachnida, which species were originally classed by Müller in three subdivisions : (*a*) oculis binis ; (*b*) oculis quator ; (*c*) oculis sex. Lang describes the eyes of *Limnesia undulata, Curvipes carneus,* and *Hygrobates longipalpis* as lying completely inside the cuticle. In *Limnesia* (Fig. 91) the eyes of the two sides are widely separated—the optic axes of the anterior pair are

9

directed forward and laterally, while the axes of the posterior pair are directed backwards and laterally. Approximately the same directions of the optic axes are present in *Diplodontus, Eylais,* and *Hydrodroma* as in *Limnesia*. These four species have, therefore, fields of vision corresponding to the four quarters of the compass.

In *Curvipes carneus* the anterior and posterior eyes on each side are united in a double eye, of which the posterior eye on each side is the smaller. The same type of fusion, of the anterior and posterior eyes of each side, takes place sometimes in *Hygrobates longipalpis*.

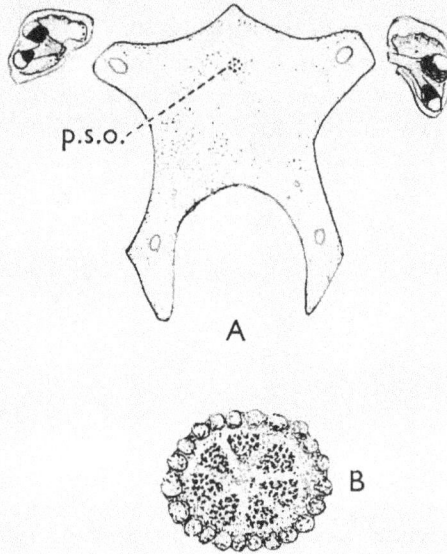

FIG. 92.

A—The dorsal-shield of *Hydrodroma,* seen from above, and showing the pigmented sense-organ *p.s.o.,* called the "fifth" or "median eye". On each side of the shield are the lateral eyes enclosed in a chitinous capsule.
B—The "median eye" highly magnified, showing seven radially arranged pigment-cells, surrounded by a circle of papillæ, of the cutis.

In *Eylais extendens* all four eyes, which are close together near the median plane, are enclosed in a so-called "spectacle frame"; while in the genus *Hydrodroma* the two eyes on each side are enclosed in a chitinous capsule, which is separated from its fellow of the opposite side by the whole width of the dorsal shield. In the centre of this shield is an organ which has been described as a "fifth median unpaired eye" (Fig. 92). It consists of a minute, disc-like body containing seven radially disposed pigmented areas in which, according to Schaub's description, there is to be seen a rhabdome formation. Lang, however, who examined specimens of the organ prepared by modern technique and under an immersion lens, expresses the opinion that the structure cannot be regarded as an eye in the strict sense of the word, and prefers to speak of it as simply a " pigmented sense-organ." Whether this remarkable organ is a vestigial eye or belongs to any other type of sense-organ, its presence in the centre of the dorsal shield in the median plane between the two pairs of laterally placed eyes is of very considerable importance, and it would be interesting to learn if further research reveals the presence of such an organ in related species.

It may be noted here that in the Linguatulida or Pentastomida, which are degenerate and parasitic Arachnida, the nervous system is greatly reduced and the organs of special sense have entirely disappeared. One species, *Pentastomum tænioides*, has been found in the frontal air sinuses and maxillary antra of the dog and wolf. Its embryos, escaping and falling on grass or other herbage, are eaten by hares and rabbits, perforate the walls of the stomach and intestine, become encysted in the liver, and undergo a metamorphosis. If the hare or rabbit should be eaten by a dog, the young pentastoma may find their way into its frontal air sinuses or antra.

In the Tardigrada or " bear animalcules," which are soft-skinned animals about 1 mm. in length living on damp moss or in fresh or salt water, there is also a reduction of the central nervous system and the sense-organs are represented merely by a couple of eye-spots at the anterior end of the body.

The Eyes of Scorpions

These have been studied by Lankester and Bourne (1883) and J. S. Kingsley (1886). The lateral eyes are placed on the margin of the prosomatic shield in a group on each side (Fig. 93). The number of separate lenses differs in various subgenera, and each lens indicates a separate eye. In *Androctonus* the eyes are more numerous than in other scorpions, each lateral group in *A. funestus* showing as many as five lenses—three larger and two smaller.

The lenses are of the cuticular or corneal type, and are highly convex on the inner or deep surface (Fig. 94). The hypoderm cells beneath the surrounding cuticle are continued on to the circumferential aspect of the cuticular lens, where they form the vitreous " marginal body " or the " perineural epidermic cells " ; whereas beneath the central part of the lens the hypoderm cells are specially modified to form the retina. This consists of elongated sensory cells the inner ends of which are continuous with the fibres of the optic nerve. In the body of each sensory cell deep to the large spherical nucleus is a refringent globule, called the postnuclear phæosphere, and in relation with the outer ends of the sensory cells are elliptical refractile elements termed rhabdomes. Interneural epidermic cells and some cells of a connective tissue type are also present.

The central eyes of scorpions resemble the central pair of *Limulus* in having a single biconvex, cuticular lens beneath which is a continuous

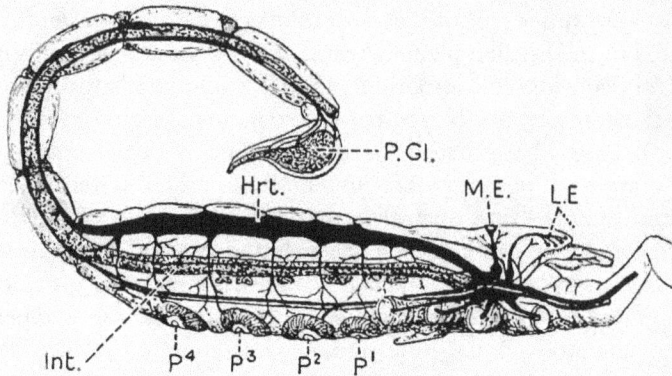

FIG. 93.—DIAGRAM SHOWING THE MEDIAN AND LATERAL EYES OF A SCORPION, AND THEIR CONNECTION WITH THE "BRAIN," OR SUPRA-ŒSOPHAGEAL GANGLION.

Hrt. : heart.
Int. : intestine.
L.E. : group of lateral eyes, connected by a common optic nerve with the supra-œsophageal ganglion.
M.E. : median eye, also connected with the supra-œsophageal ganglion.
P. Gl. : poison gland.
P¹ : pulmonary sacs.
P² : pulmonary sacs.
P³ : pulmonary sacs.
P¹ : pulmonary sacs.

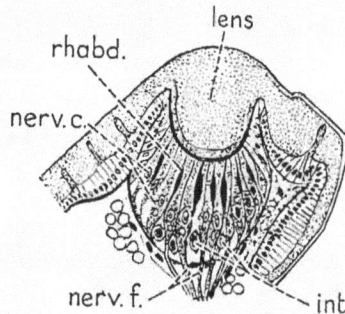

FIG. 94.—SECTION THROUGH A LATERAL EYE OF EUSCORPIUS ITALICUS.

int. : intermediate cells.
lens : single cuticular lens.
nerv. c. : nerve-cells.
nerv. f. : nerve-fibres, of optic nerve.
rhabd. : rhabdomes.

layer of columnar cells (Fig. 95). The retina is, however, composed of retinulæ disposed in groups, as in the composite eyes of insects and crustaceans. The retinulæ in the median eyes of scorpions differ, however, in being much less compact and cylindrical and less highly organized than in the higher types of insects and Crustacea. They consist of sensory cells which terminate at their proximal end in one of the fibres of the optic nerve ; at the outer ends of these cells are elliptical refractile elements, the rhabdomes, and there are also interstitial connective tissue cells containing pigment and an outer layer of epidermal cell-elements next

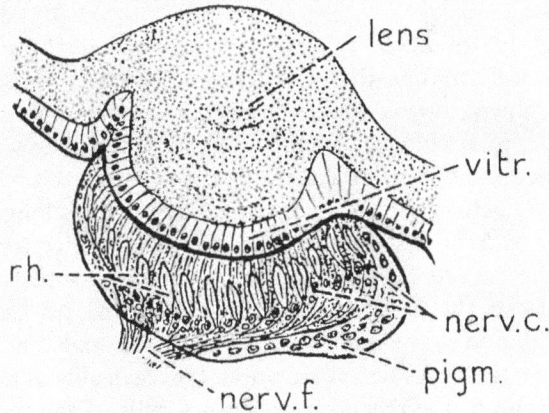

FIG. 95.—SECTION THROUGH MEDIAN EYE OF EUSCORPIUS.

A single lens is present in both the central and lateral eyes of *Euscorpius*. In the central eye the hypodermal cells are continued across the eye as a vitreous layer which lies between the retinulæ and cuticular lens.

lens : cuticular lens.
nerv. c. : terminal nerve cells.
nerv. f. : fibres of optic nerve.
pigm. : cells containing pigment.
rh. : rhabdomes.
vitr. : vitreous layer.

(After Lankester and Bourne.)

the basement membrane. The eyes are generally regarded as intermediate in type between the simple, upright eye of the ocellar type, with a single cuticular lens, and the composite and compound faceted types such as are found in certain Crustacea. Lankester considered that the resemblance of the scorpion's eyes, both lateral and medial, to those of *Limulus* was important evidence in favour of the latter being more closely related to the arachnids than to the crustaceans.

The Eyes of Limulus Polyphemus

Limulus, or the American king crab, is the only known living representative of the extinct palæozoic forms of the gigantic marine scorpions such as Eurypterus and Pterygotus which inhabited the sea in the Silurian period. The body consists of two parts separated by a movable articulation, namely, the cephalothorax, covered by the dorsal shield or carapace ; and the abdomen, also covered by a carapace. The body terminates in a tapering sword-like tail, which has given origin to the name " Xiphosura " applied to the Order to which these animals belong (Fig. 69). Beneath the head-shield are placed two pairs of eyes which were especially investigated by Lankester and Bourne [1] in 1883, who pointed out the fundamental resemblance of the central and lateral eyes of *Limulus* to those of the scorpion.

Each lateral eye of *Limulus* is covered superficially by a continuous transparent corneal stratum, the under-surface of which presents a series of papilliform downgrowths which lie over a corresponding number of barrel-shaped retinulæ (Fig. 86, p. 124). The papilliform downgrowths are believed to function as separate lenses for the separate retinulæ which lie beneath them. Each of the latter consists of a group of elongated sensory cells, the inner ends of which are continuous with the constituent fibres of the retinular nerve. The papilliform downgrowths forming the separated lenses of the composite eye were believed by Lankester and Bourne to correspond to the numerous two to seven small lenses belonging to the groups of lateral eyes which are present on each side of the scorpion's head. In addition to the receptive or sensory cells of the retinulæ, there are refractile elements or rhabdomes which on transverse section are seen to be arranged in a radial manner and also " intrusive " connective tissue cells containing pigment.

Each central eye consists of a single cuticular lens which is almost spherical in form and is continuous with the surrounding cuticle ; beneath this is a vitreous layer which consists of refractile columnar cells which are continuous circumferentially with the hypoderm cells beneath the general cuticle. We thus have an immovable cuticular lens of the corneal type, which is supplemented by a vitreous layer of hypoderm cells (Fig. 87). Beneath this is the receptive portion of the eye, which is composed of groups of large sensory cells, the inner ends of which are continuous with fibres of the optic nerve ; outside there are from five to seven fluted rhabdomes and between the sensory cells and around the retinulæ a considerable number of " intrusive " connective tissue pigment cells. The retinulæ differ from the retinulæ of the lateral eyes in their more open character, as contrasted with the compact barrel-shaped retinulæ of the lateral eyes. This loose character of the retinulæ of the central eyes, coupled with the large amount of intrusive connective tissue, was considered by Lankester and Bourne to be an indication of loss of function and degeneration of the central eyes as compared with the lateral.

[1] Lankester and Bourne, " The Minute Structure of the Lateral and the Central Eyes of *Scorpio* and *Limulus*," *Q.J. Micro. Sc.*, **23**, 1883.

The Eyes of the Extinct Eurypterida

The Eurypterida were extinct Arachnida. They were often of gigantic size and they inhabited the sea in the Silurian and early Devonian periods. Specimens of Pterygotus (Fig. 96) have been found which measure over 6 ft. in length. They agree with *Limulus* in many points, and more especially in the possession of a pair of both median and lateral eyes.

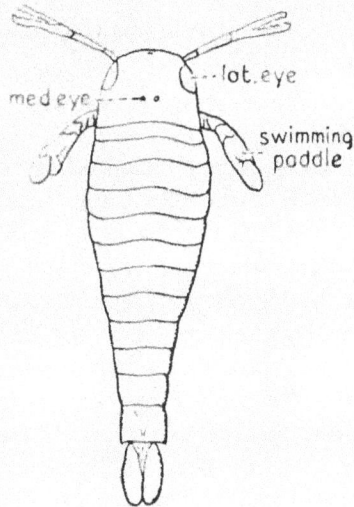

FIG. 96.—PTERYGOTUS OSILIENSIS. DORSAL VIEW, REDUCED. AN EXTINCT ARTHROPOD, FOUND IN UPPER SILURIAN STRATA, AND SHOWING PAIRED PITS IN THE SITUATION OF THE PAIRED MEDIAN EYES OF LIMULUS AND EUSCORPIUS.
(From Wood's *Palæontology*, after Schmidt.)

These were situated in the dorsal shield or carapace in the same position as in the king crab, and also in the same position as in the ancient mailed fishes, the Ostracodermata. The resemblance of *Limulus* to the latter is striking, but there are also important differences in the general structure of the body and limbs, which will be discussed in Chapter 23, on the geological evidence of the antiquity of the pineal organ.

The structural resemblances between the Eurypterids and certain living Arachnida, the Trilobites, and *Limulus* may, however, be alluded to at this stage. It is obvious that in the enormous period of time which has elapsed since the extinct Eurypterids and Trilobites existed, divergent changes in structure will have been evolved. These will be most evident in the adults of animals which have descended from the original stock and there will be less difference in the larval forms ; secondly, although the larval forms may be expected to resemble the ancestral stock more closely than do the adult forms, we may also expect very considerable differences in these. Thus, the likeness of the larval form of *Limulus* to the Trilobites is so close that the resemblance was regarded as unquestionable evidence of the origin of *Limulus* from a Trilobite stock. The resemblances are chiefly in the anterior part of the body, and concern the structure and general form of the head-shield and the relative position of the sense-organs, including the median and lateral paired eyes ; on the other hand, the contrast between the appendages of the prosoma and those of the abdomen which is so marked a feature in *Limulus*, is absent in the Trilobite, and *Limulus* shows no trace of the antennæ of the Trilobite. Thus, according to MacBride, the so-called trilobite larva of *Limulus* represents not a Trilobite but an Arachnid, which is not very unlike the adult animal, but with segments which are free from one another and without the long tail. Such Arachnids are known to have existed in the Silurian epoch (Hemiaspis), but the stock from which the Arachnids and Trilobites diverged must have been still farther back. The conclusion to be drawn from these premises is that the head region, with its important sense-organs, although it has undergone adaptational changes, has remained in its general form essentially the same since the early palæozoic periods ; and it was thought that the Protostraca, a name suggested by Korschelt and Heider for the precursors of the Palæostraca, were the ancestors of the Arachnids, Trilobites, and possibly also of the Ostracodermata, or ancient mailed-fishes ; further, that they possessed sense-organs, visual and static situated in the head-shield in the same relative positions to one another as in *Apus*, *Limulus*, certain insects, spiders, and vertebrates.

The Eyes of Trilobites

The existence of eyes has been demonstrated in most of the Trilobites, and they present great variations in form and size. By far the greater number are of the composite, faceted type ; they are placed laterally, and are supported by the movable cheeks ; the visual area is usually crescentic, but it may be rounded or oval in form. The adjoining part of the fixed cheek is often raised in the form of a lip or palpebral lobe. Their size varies ; they may be quite small, as in Encrinurus and Trimero-cephalus, or very large as in Æglina (Fig. 97, A), in some species of which, nearly the entire area of the movable cheeks is faceted and the visual surface extends right round the outer edge of the head-shield. In one species, *Remopleurides radians*, the number of facets has been estimated to be 15,000. In some Trilobites the eyes appear to be absent altogether, e.g. *Conocoryphe* and *Agnostus*, and in others they are so difficult to detect that for a long time they remained unrecognized—*Agraulus*, *Sao*, *Ellipso-cephalus*.

The paired lateral or composite eyes of Trilobites are of two types :

(1) Holochroal (Fig. 97, A) : the visual area being covered with a continuous horny cuticle or cornea, which may be either smooth, so that
externally it gives no indication of its aggregate nature, or granular on

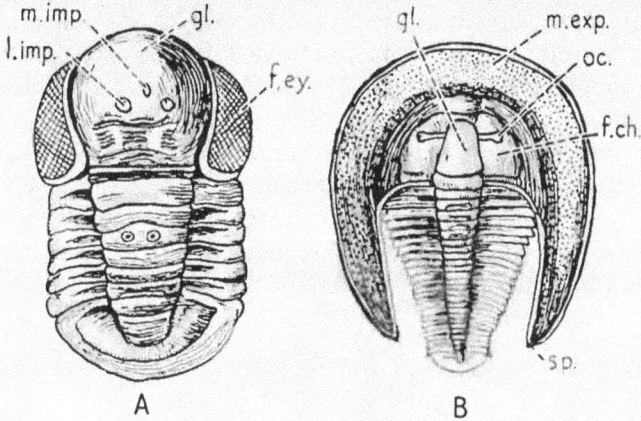

FIG. 97.

A—*Æglina prisca*. Ordovician ; Vosek, Bohemia. Glabella (*gl.*) large, showing a
median impression (*m. imp.*), and paired lateral impressions (*l. imp.*) ; the fixed
cheeks are suppressed and the facet eyes (*f. ey.*), which are very large, occupy
nearly the whole area of the free cheeks. (After Barrande.)

B—*Harpes ungula*, showing paired ocelli (*oc.*) on the fixed cheeks (*f. ch.*). The free
cheeks are ventral in position and there are no facet-eyes. The cephalon, or
dorsal shield, has a wide, pitted, marginal expansion (*m. exp.*), which is prolonged backward on each side into a pointed spine. Ordovician, Bohemia.
(After Barrande, from von Zittel.)

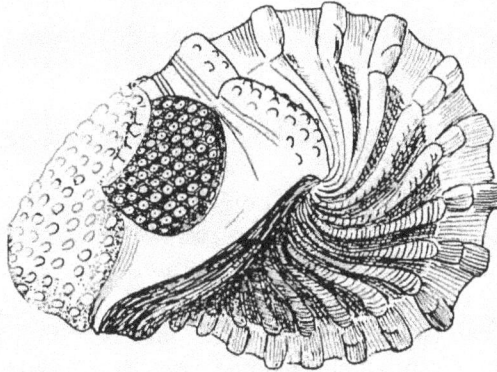

FIG. 98.—PHACOPS LATIFRONS. BRONN. DEVONIAN. GEROLSTEIN, EIFEL
DISTRICT. (FROM VON ZITTEL.)

The animal is rolled up and seen from the side. The prominent compound eyes
are of the schizochroal type.

account of the unevenness produced by the facets beneath. According
to von Zittel the lenses of the ommatidia are often visible by translucence.
(2) Schizochroal (Fig. 98) : this type is limited to the single family

Phacopidæ. The visual area consists of small round or polygonal openings occupied by separate corneal facets between which is an interstitial test or sclera.

But beside the faceted or lateral paired eyes of Trilobites there are indications in some of the more primitive types of eye-spots or ocelli. These are simple in type and may be paired or unpaired. The existence of such ocelli is indicated in *Harpes* (Fig. 97, B), and some specimens of *Trinucleus* (Figs. 100, 101, 102). They appear in the form of one to three simple elevations or small tubercles, on the fixed cheeks at the ends of the eye sutures, while the ordinary faceted eyes on the movable cheeks are absent. They are regarded as being correlated with the ocelli or median paired eyes which are present in many of the Crustacea and in *Limulus* ;

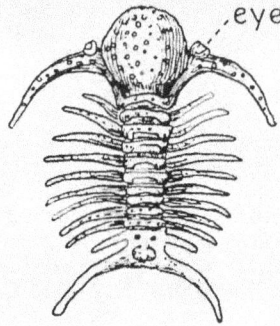

FIG. 99.—DEIPHON. SILURIAN. BOHEMIA. (AFTER BARRANDE.)
Glabella globular, without lateral furrows. Free cheeks minute. Fixed cheeks produced on either side into a long curved spine. Eyes small at base of spine.

and probably also those of Arachnida, Insecta, and other Classes of invertebrates.

The meaning of the impressions on the glabella of certain Trilobites is not certain, but the existence of two pairs of ocelli on the carapace of certain living crustaceans, Arachnida, and Insecta, either with or without lateral eyes, in the same relative position as in the Trilobites, suggests that there may have been two pairs of ocelli on some Trilobites and that either one or both of these pairs might in some cases have fused so as to form a single or median eye ; or that indications on the superficial surface of the glabella of either one or both pairs might have disappeared altogether. Further, that these median eyes were already degenerating in some of the earliest known examples of Trilobite and that they were being replaced by lateral paired eyes of the faceted type, the variations in size and complexity of which points to the great length of the period during which this differentiation had been taking place.

The possibility of there being more than one pair of median eyes—or even of lateral eyes—in trilobites is indicated by the distinct evidence of metamerism in the glabella and other parts of the head. There are

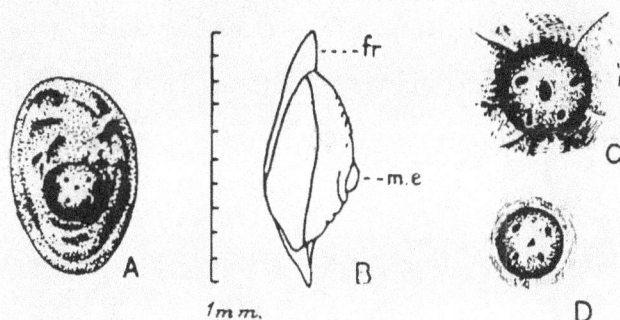

FIG. 100.—MEDIAN EYE TUBERCLE IN TRETASPIS SETICORNIS (HIS).

A, 80; B, 36; C, D, ×50. A, C, D showing five small pits on the tubercle. A–B: meraspid stage II. C–D: adult. B: lateral view of cephalon with the big median tubercle, *m.e.* A–B: from the Trinucleus shale Dalarne. C–D: from the upper Trinucleus limestone. *fr.*: pseudo-frontal lobe. Frogno Ringerike. (After L. Störmer.)

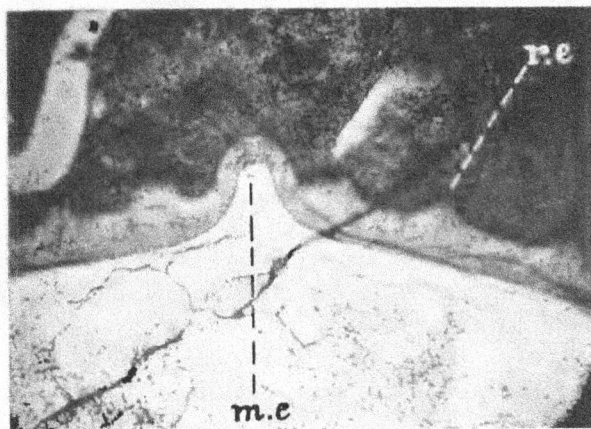

FIG. 101.—TRANSVERSE SECTION THROUGH THE MEDIAN EYE TUBERCLE (*m.e.*) OF AN ADULT SPECIMEN OF TRETASPIS KIÆRI N.SP. (AFTER L. STÖRMER.)

marked variations in the size and form of the glabella in different species of Trilobite. In the typical forms, however, it is seen to be composed of five segments (Figs. 103 and 104); these are separated by four transverse or oblique grooves. The anterior segment is known as the frontal lobe and sometimes bears a single median impression, or there may be three pits, one median usually in front and two lateral. The posterior segment is known as the occipital ring and is separated by an occipital or nuchal furrow from the fourth segment.

According to von Zittel the Trilobites differ from *Limulus* and all other arthropods in having compound (faceted) eyes supported on free cheek-pieces, which he believed represent the pleura of a head-segment, which is

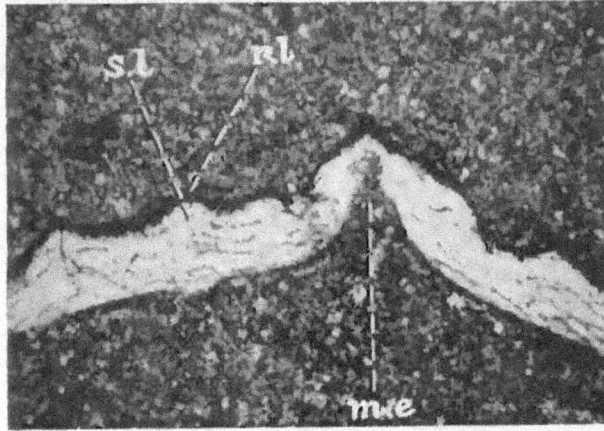

Fig. 102.—Longitudinal Section through the Median Eye Tubercle (*m. e*) of Trinucleus Bucculentus. Adult Specimen. (After L. Størmer.)

lost except in some forms with stalked eyes and in the cephalic neuromeres of later forms.

Since the publication of von Zittel's *Palæontology* in 1900 important recent work, which has been carried out with the employment of modern technique, has confirmed and supplied additional evidence of the presence of median eyes in the larvæ and adult specimens of trilobites. Thus Lief Störmer in 1930 demonstrated the presence of a hollow, slightly raised median-eye tubercle in several species of Trinucleidæ, Fig. 100 ; he also succeeded in obtaining sections of these, including a transverse section of the median eye of *Tretaspis Kiæri* (a photograph of which is reproduced in Fig. 101) and a longitudinal section of the median eye of *Trinucleus bucculentus* (Fig. 102). In Fig. 100, which shows the median eye tubercle of *Tretaspis seticornis* (seen from above—80 diameters), there are five small pits arranged like the ∴ of a playing-card, and a similar arrangement is seen in the meraspid stage II of *Tretaspis seticornis*. The explanation of the median pit has not been definitely settled, two or three alternative suggestions having been advanced. Thus in *Apus*, according to the accounts of Patten (1912) and Holmgren (1916), the median parietal eye consists of four distinct ocelli, which have migrated inward during development from the sides, and Patten states that they are enclosed in a common sac which opens to the exterior by means of a short duct or pore. Holmgren says that in the *Nauplius* eye there are, in his opinion, no less than five retinas. The five pits in *Tretaspis*, therefore, might be interpreted as representing two pairs of ocelli, one pair in front of and the other behind the central opening of the common sac. The central pit

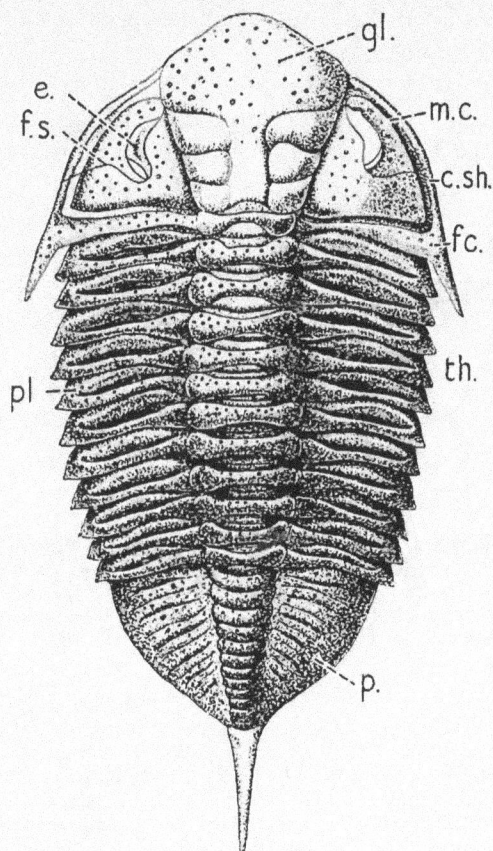

FIG. 103.

Dorsal aspect of a Trilobite, *Dalmanites socialis*, an extinct arthropod, peculiar to and characteristic of the palæozoic rocks, the class being especially abundant from the upper Cambrian to the Carboniferous.

c. sh. : cephalic shield.	*m.c.* : movable cheek.
e. : situation of eye.	*p.* : pygidium.
f.c. : fixed cheek.	*pl.* : pleura.
f.s. : frontal suture.	*th.* : thorax.
gl. : glabella.	

(After Gaerstaecker, redrawn from *Textbook of Zoology*, Parker and Haswell.)

may, however, represent a pair of ocelli which have fused in the median plane, as commonly occurs in the single median eyes of insects and some crustaceans. In this connection it is interesting to recall the conditions found in the freshwater mites (Hydrachnida) (see p. 129), more particularly the eyes of *Eylais extendens*, in which four eyes close together near the median plane are enclosed in a dense capsule shaped like a spectacle frame ; and the genus *Hydroma* in which two eyes enclosed in a chitinous capsule are separated by the whole width of the dorsal shield, in the centre of which is placed the organ which has been described as the 5th median unpaired eye (Fig. 92).

B. Hanström in 1926 published a full account of the genesis of the eyes and visual centres of the Turbellaria, annelids, and arthropods, and included in the latter some important observations on the eyes of

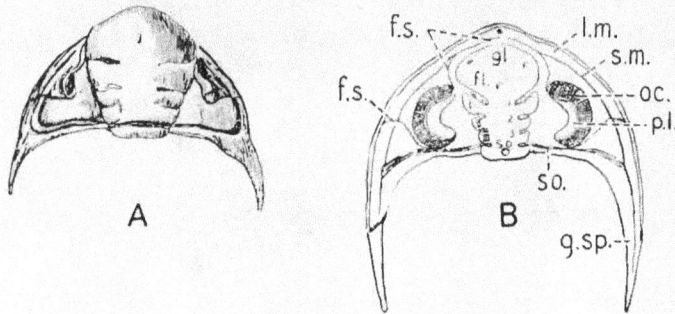

FIG. 104.

A—Dalmanites socialis 1 1. Dorsal aspect of cephalon, or head-shield, showing the glabella with single median impression ; three primary dorsal furrows and an occipital sulcus, which subdivide the glabella into five segments. There is a V-shaped fixed cheek and a triangular free cheek bearing a prominent facet eye ; the genal angles are prolonged backwards as strong, tapering spines.

B—Ordovician—Bohemia.   Diagrammatic representation of similar specimen.

f.l. : frontal lobe.	*p.l.* : palpebral fold.
f.s. : facial sulcus.	*s.m.* : marginal furrow.
gl. : glabella.	*s.o.* : occipital sulcus
g. sp. : genal spine.	I, II, III : lateral lobes.
l.m. : marginal furrow.	1, 2, 3 : lateral furrows.
oc. : compound eye.	

trilobites, Xiphosura, and Euryptera, in addition to those on living representatives of the class.   Commenting on the work of Barrande in 1872, he alludes to his illustration of the head of *Æglina prisca* (Fig. 97, A), showing three impressions on the glabella, which were regarded by Handlirsch (1905) as indications of the existence in it of three highly developed median eyes, corresponding to the three frontal eyes of insects. This interpretation of the three impressions on the glabella of *Æglina* is in Hanström's opinion correct.   For although the eyes of the trilobites have the closest connections with the simple nauplius eyes of the crustaceans, it would not be surprising if the median eyes of *Æglina*, which was distinctly a pelagic species, should have developed, as an adaptation to a pelagic mode of life, and for the completion of the dorsal field of vision in the form of three independent visual organs. The three pigmented cup-shaped ocelli of certain Copepods and Ostracoda have also developed in connection with a pelagic mode of life as three independent eyes, and in his opinion this also took place in the case of the eyes of the trilobite *Trinucleus*. Moreover, Woodward has interpreted the small depressions on the glabella of trilobites as median eyes; and in 1897 Beecher mentions ocelli as being " rarely present," although Hanström thinks it probable that he alluded to the stemmata of *Harpes*, which were also regarded by Kishinouye (1892–3) as indications of median eyes; but according to the more recent researches of Richter (1915–1920 and 1922), these are not median eyes but degenerated remnants of aggregated lateral eyes. Ruedemann (1916), referring to the median tubercle on the glabella of trilobites, writes that " In studying the structure of the tubercle it was found that the median eye presents all stages of development seen in other crustaceans from mere transparent thinner spots of the test to a lenticular body covered by a thin cornea," as in *Harpes*. The relation of the median eyes to the surface layers in fossil crustaceans is interesting in connection with the work carried out on living representatives of the extinct types, such as that by Lankester and Bourne on *Limulus* and by Margaret Robinson in 1892 on decapod arthropods, more particularly in adult specimens of *Palæmon serratus*, *Verbius varians*, and *Pandalus annulicornis*. Both in *Limulus* and in eight separate species of Carididæ, paired median eyes which are present in the nauplius stage have been demonstrated as persisting in the adult animals. In these they are covered over by a dense chitinous layer, lined on its under surface by an epithelial stratum. That is to say, they are deeply buried and can have little or no function. An idea of their general appearance and relations may be obtained by reference to Fig. 105, A, B, C, which shows in A the two median eyes exposed by removing the rostrum from a fresh specimen; C, a transverse section of the same, illustrating the structures lying superficial to the fused median eyes, namely, a chitinous layer, connective tissue and muscle, an epithelial layer and a blood sinus; it also shows the relation of the pigment cells to the nerve-end cells and the epithelial cords by which the eyes are suspended between the chitinous roof above and the cerebral ganglia below; B, a transverse section in front of C, shows the relations of the suspensory cords to the epithelium of the roof anterior to the median eye.

The general disposition of the parts will be realized if we quote in full Miss Robinson's description of her dissection of *Pandalus* : After removal of the rostrum, " the median eye can be seen as a black speck lying in the centre of the triangle formed by the brain and the stalks of the lateral eyes. The brain is covered by chitin which is lined by a thin layer of ectoderm ; if the dorsal part of this and a small part of the brain be removed, the eye can be seen lying in a blood space just dorsal to the brain.   It has the appearance of a black X which is slung on to the

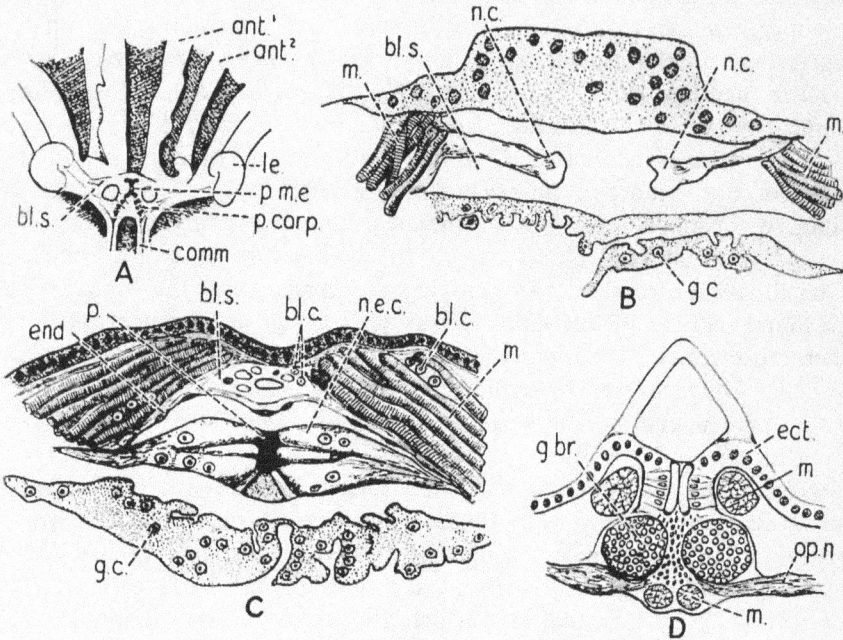

FIG. 105.—PAIRED MEDIAN EYES IN NAUPLIUS OF DECAPOD CARIDIDAE. (AFTER MARGARET ROBINSON.)

A : Median eyes of *Pandalus annulicornis*, viewed from dorsal aspect after removal of the rostrum.   The pigment appears as an X-shaped mass between two lateral groups of nerve-end cells.   B : Transverse section through region of median eyes of *Virbius varians*, showing ingrowth of suspensory ectodermal cords.   C : Transverse section farther back than B, showing the central mass of pigment cells, with the nerve-end cells on either side.   A median ventral group of nerve-end cells is also present.   D : Diagrammatic horizontal section through brain of *Virbius varians*.   The chitinous roof which covers the median eyes is not shown in the sections B and C.

ant.[1] and *ant.*[2] : first and second antennæ.	*g.c.* : ganglion cell.
	l.e. : lateral eye.
bl. c. : blood corpuscle.	*m.* : muscle.
bl. s. : blood space.	*n.c.* : ectodermal cord.
comm. : circumœsophageal commissures.	*op. n.* : optic nerve.
ect. : ectoderm.	*p.* : pigment.
end. : endoderm.	*p. corp.* : pigment corpuscles.
g. br. : nuclei of ganglion cells of brain.	*p.m.e.* : pigment mass of median eye.

ectoderm by two slender threads, which swell out in the concavities of the X and then narrow again as they approximate to each other.

   " The X consists of two large pigment cells, and the supporting strings are formed partly of ectoderm and partly of club-shaped nerve-end cells. No trace of a refractive body could be found in the eye. On the whole the resemblance to the eye of Branchipus, as described by Claus and more recently by Patten, also in the scorpion (Chap. 24, Fig. 350, p. 362, Fig. 246, p. 349), is very close."

Although Miss Robinson alludes to the eye as a single structure, it is obvious that in doing so she was following the customary designation at the time, and that she was well aware of the bilateral nature of the eyes in the nauplius phase of development. The interesting points, apart from the question of bilaterality, in the comparison of the median eyes of *Limulus* and the Decapod Arthropoda with the median eyes of trilobites, is the fact that in the adult stages of both the living and in many of the extinct forms the eyes lay deeply buried beneath the surface and presumably can have had little or no function. Judging from the appearances seen in many adult specimens of trilobite, the median eyes were already buried and presumably functionless even at the remote epoch, lower Cambrian, when some of the earlier and more simple types of trilobite were alive. On the other hand, indications of the existence of median eyes are present on the surface of the glabella in certain adult forms, e.g. *Æglina prisca*, as well as in the nauplius stages and afford valuable evidence of a transitional phase in the phylogeny of the median eyes, namely, an earlier stage when these eyes were superficial and presumably functional and a later stage when in the adult animal they became buried, their function having been taken over by the lateral eyes. Thus in many species, and more particularly those which are more recent and more highly evolved, no indications are present on the glabella of the frontal or median eyes. In view of the recent work by Günther on the ontogeny of the simple and compound eyes of the water-beetle *Dytiscus marginalis* (p. 117), in which he has shown that the eye-spot and the six ocelli which on each side precede the development of the compound eye sink beneath the surface, their remnants, however, remaining during life as closed pigmented vesicles attached to the optic nerve, the absence of indications of their presence on the superficial surface of the glabella in some species is not surprising. The replacement of the median eyes by the compound lateral eyes involves the whole problem of the evolution of the compound eye. For since, as pointed out by MacBride, *Peripatus*, Myriapoda, the lower insects and the larvæ of the higher insects agree in possessing only simple, pit-like ocelli, it is fairly clear that the massing together of these ocelli to form a compound eye must have occurred during the evolution of the arthropodan stock and presumably had not yet occurred in the primitive land Arthropoda. But primitive Crustacea, primitive Arachnida, and most Trilobita possess compound eyes. The

10

Insecta, therefore, must have been derived from a primitive arthropod
stock in which a compound eye had not yet been developed, and considering that a fully formed Orthopteran insect is already found in Silurian
strata, this is what we might naturally expect.

Intimately associated with the question of the origin of the compound
eyes in trilobites is that concerned with what are described as blind
trilobites, a problem which was investigated by Cowper Reed in 1898.
These he conceived as being divisible into two groups :

(1) those in which the eyes were not present, because of the low
    phylogenetical and morphological rank of the genera in question,
    as their general structure and stratigraphical appearance indi-
    cate ; and

(2) those which are genetically identical or closely allied to forms
    possessing eyes which are of high phylogenetic rank, and have
    lost their visual organs by a secondary modification, presumably
    as a result of adaptation to special conditions.

The first group he called the " primitive group " and the second the
" adaptive group." These will be described later in the section on
Geological Evidence of the Presence of Median Eyes in Extinct Animals,
Chapter 23. Quite apart from evidence of the existence of trilobites in
such ancient geological strata as the Upper Cambrian, the extreme
variability in the types of eye met with in trilobites (Figs. 97, 98, 99, 103)
as well as the marked differences in their general form point to the great
antiquity of these primitive arthropods and the probability not only of
evolutionary changes occurring in the direction of differentiation of more
complex eyes from simpler types, but also, as has been suggested by
Cowper and others, of degenerative or devolutionary changes taking place
in the eyes of certain species. The recognition of such degenerative
changes, as we shall see later, plays an important part in the interpretation
of the conditions which are found both in the median eyes of invertebrates
and in the pineal system of vertebrates.

CHAPTER 12

THE EYES OF MOLLUSCS

HAVING considered the geological evidence of the existence of median and lateral eyes afforded by the extinct Order of the Trilobites, which may be regarded as the precursors of certain living representatives of the Arachnida and Crustacea and which also have affinities with the Eurypteridæ, an extinct Order of the Arachnida and the Xiphosura, we will turn our attention to the Mollusca, in which phylum we meet with a great variety of types of eyes, from the simple epithelial pit (limpet) or simple camera type of eye without lens, as in *Nautilus*, to highly differentiated organs such as are found in the cuttlefish, squids, and octopus. In many of the Mollusca there is a hard shell which can be preserved in a fossil state ; and since many of the fossil shells resemble those of living species, they give a clear indication of the type of animal which was enclosed within the shell, notwithstanding the fact that many of these fossil shells have been found in Palæozoic strata as far back as the Cambrian period. Moreover, it is significant that living species possessing simpler types of eye, such as the limpet (*Patella*) and the pearly *Nautilus*, are represented by fossil shells found in the older Palæozoic strata, while the more highly evolved types of Mollusca, such as *Sepia* and the octopuses, having complex eyes, are represented by fossil relics which are found only in the more recent periods.

In the Class Pelecypoda (Lamellibranchiata), which includes the " right and left " bivalved shell-fish such as the mussels, cockles, oysters, and scallops, the sense organs are not highly developed. This is due to the fixed or non-motile condition of the adult animal, which usually lies on one side at the bottom of the water. In some, e.g. *Pecten* (Fig. 106), marginal eyes of a highly differentiated type are found round the edge of the mantle (Fig. 107). Nevertheless, whether eyes are present in the adult animal or not, their free-swimming larvæ pass through trochophore and veliger stages in which an apical plate, cerebral ganglia, cerebral pit, and statocyst are developed (Figs. 108 and 109). These resemble in their essential characters the veliger larvæ of other Classes of Mollusca, such as the Amphineura, which includes the Chitons—" coat-of-mail shells "—and the Class Gasteropoda, comprising the whelks, snails, and limpets, in which paired eyes of a simple upright type are found both in the adult and larval form of the animal (Figs. 110, 111).

The existence of the same types of shell—or parts of the shell, such as the operculum—in the living and fossil representatives of a species indicates a persistence of type which has gone on through countless ages,

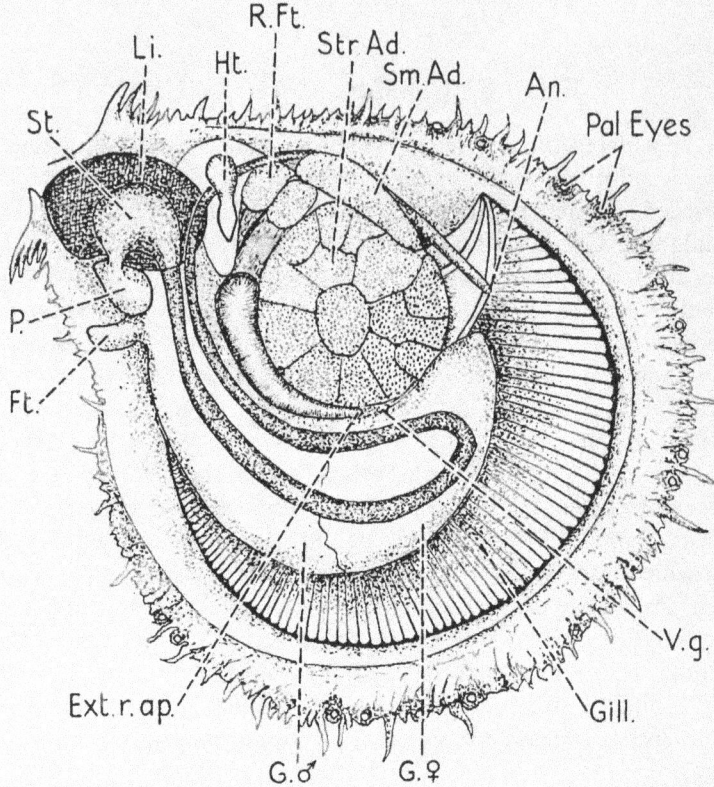

FIG. 106.—DRAWING OF A SCALLOP (PECTEN), SHOWING THE POSITION OF PALLIAL
EYES. (AFTER PELSENEER.)

An. : anal aperture.
Ext. r. ap. : external renal aperture.
Ft. : foot.
G.♂, G.♀ : male and female parts of gonad.
Ht. : heart.
Li. : liver.
P. : palp.
Pal. eyes : pallial eyes.
R. Ft. : right foot.
Sm. Ad. : smooth adductor muscle.
Str. Ad. : striated adductor muscle.
St. : stomach.
V.g. : visceral ganglion.

and also allows of the inference being made that the primary sense-organs, such as the paired ocelli and statocysts of the veliger larvæ of the living animals, were present also in the larvæ of the corresponding fossil representatives of these species. Further, it is from these simpler

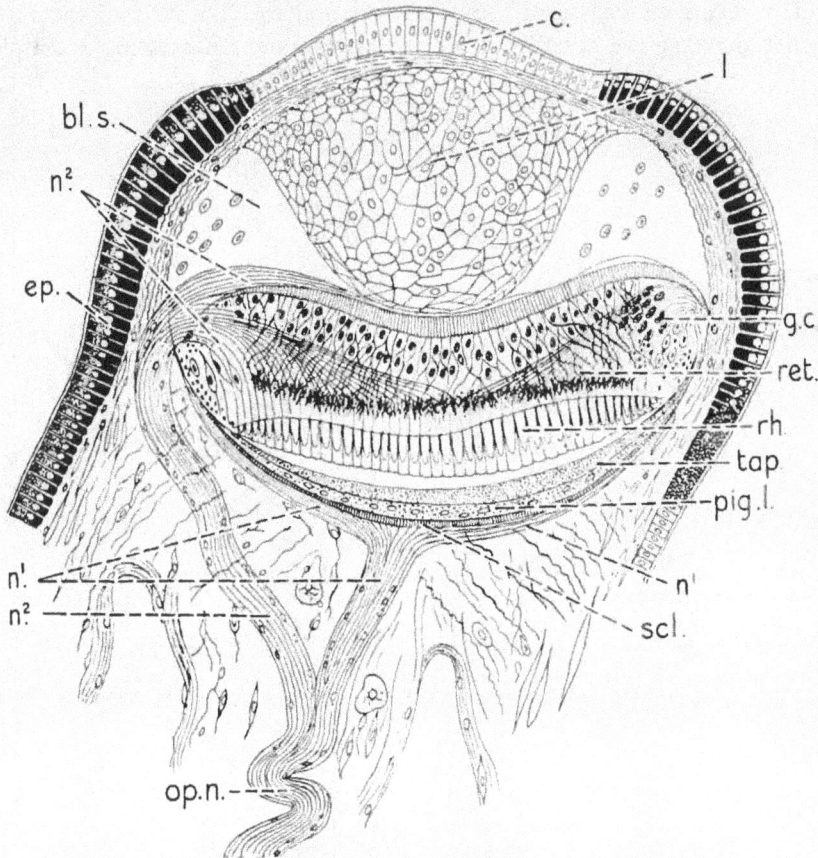

FIG. 107.—SECTION THROUGH ONE OF THE EYES ON THE OUTER MARGIN OF THE PALLIUM OF A SCALLOP (PECTEN). (AFTER PATTEN.)

The optic nerve divides into two branches, one of these passes to the inner, or posterior, pole of the eyeball, where it divides into fibres which spread out on the inner surface of the optic plate, and radiating in all directions pass to the peripheral margin of the plate. Here they turn round its edge and form a nerve-fibre layer containing ganglion cells, in front of the retinal cells, which they enter on their superficial surface. The other branch passes directly to the edge of the plate, having reached the margin it bends round this and breaks up into branches which form a superficial nerve-fibre layer containing ganglion cells in front of the retinal cells.

bl. s. : blood sinus.
c. : cornea.
ep. : epithelium.
g.c. : ganglion cells.
l. : lens of cellular type.
n.[1], *n.*[2] : branches and nerve fibres of optic nerve.

op. n. : optic nerve.
pig. l. : pigment layer.
ret. : retinulæ.
rh. : rhabdomes.
scl. sclera.
tap. : tapetum.

types of eye which are common to the trochophore and veliger larvæ of widely divergent Classes of Invertebrates and the Tornaria of the Protochordata that we must look for the parent stem possessing a simple

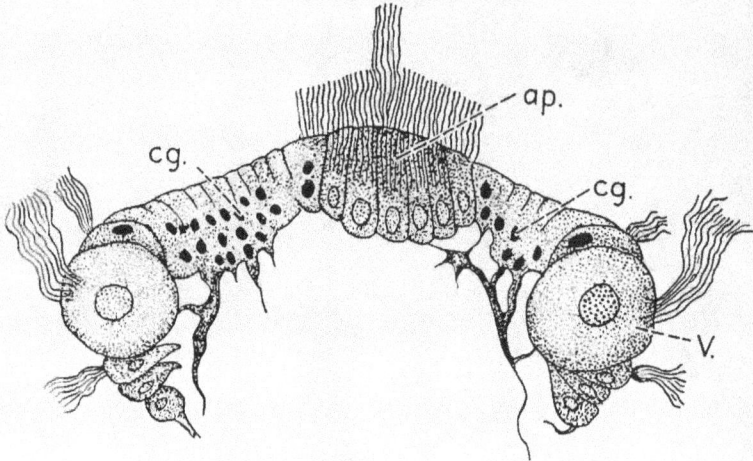

FIG. 108.

Frontal section through the pretrochal region of an old veliger larva of *Patella cærulea*, showing what are regarded as the rudiments of the cerebral ganglia, *cg.*, at the sides of the apical plate, *ap. V. :* velum.

(After Patten, from *Textbook of Embryology*, Vol. 1 : Invertebrata—E. W. MacBride.)

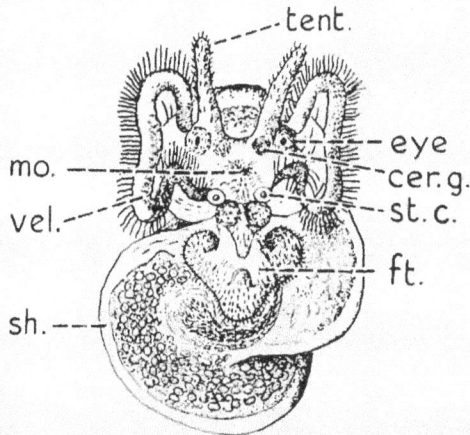

FIG. 109.—VELIGER STAGE OF VERMETUS, A WORM-LIKE GASTEROPOD WHICH IN THE ADULT ANIMAL IS ENCLOSED IN A TUBULAR SHELL. (AFTER LACAZE-DUTHIERS.)

In the veliger the shell is spiral and there are paired eyes and statocysts, the latter being situated in the typical position behind the former.

cer. g. : cerebral ganglion.	*sh. :* spiral shell.
eye : ocellus.	*st. c. :* statocyst.
ft. : foot.	*vel. :* velum.
mo. : mouth.	

form of eye from which the more highly differentiated types of simple ocelli, compound, aggregate, and inverted eyes have been evolved.

When differentiation in any particular line has already taken place and become established, it is probable that—provided the environment remains the same—it will persist, and that the development for instance, of faceted eyes in one class will permanently distinguish that class from another in which inverted eyes have been evolved. The branch of the phylogenetic tree or class of animal which has developed faceted eyes cannot be the parent stock of the branch which has evolved inverted eyes, although both branches spring from a common trunk which includes animals having a simple form of light-perceiving organ, which is capable

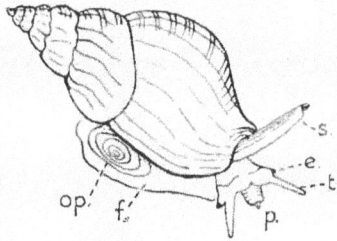

FIG. 110.—SKETCH OF A WHELK (BUCCINUM UNDATUM) IN MOTION.

e. : eye at base of tentacle. *f.* : foot. *op.* : operculum. *p.* : proboscis. *s.* : respiratory siphon or tube by which water is admitted to the gills. (After Nicholson.)

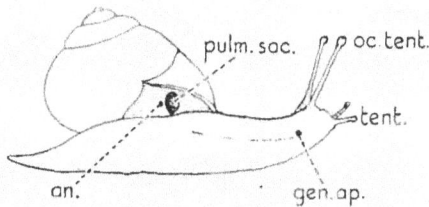

FIG. 111.—HELIX NEMORALIS, SNAIL, SHOWING PAIRED, SIMPLE EYES AT THE FREE ENDS OF THE TENTACLES. (FROM PARKER AND HASWELL.)

an. : anus ; *gen. ap.* : genital aperture ; *oc. tent.* : ocular tentacle ; *pulm. sac* : pulmonary sac ; *tent.* : tentacle.

of evolving in either direction, or may persist in its original form, as seems to have been the case in the limpets, in which the two bilateral cephalic eyes of the fully developed living types have the form of a simple open pit, without lens.

It is noteworthy that the nautiloid group, which was abundant in the Palæozoic era, included during this period a great variety of forms— the shell being straight in Orthoceras—curved in Phragmoceras ; in the form of a flat spiral with the turns not in contact ; or in a close spiral, as in *Nautilus* ; or in the form of a cork-screw helix. *Nautilus* is apparently the only representative of the order living at the present day, although over 1,000 different species of Nautilidæ and Orthoceratidæ were found by Barrande in the Silurian basin of Bohemia alone.   The Ammonites, which are closely allied to the Nautilidæ, were also very varied in type. The condition of the eyes in the extinct Nautilidæ and Ammonites is not certainly known ; it is probable, however, that they were of the same simple type (see Chap. 3, p. 48, and Figs. 112, 113) as in many of the simpler univalve molluscs and their living representative *Nautilus*.

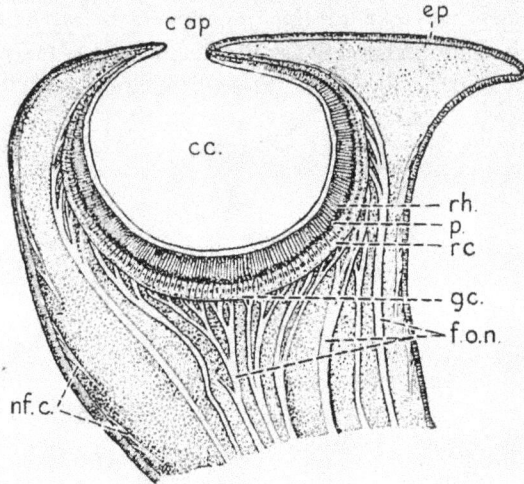

FIG. 112.—SECTION OF EYE OF NAUTILUS, SHOWING 1 : CAVITY OF OPTIC PIT ; 2 : LAYER OF RODS ; 3 : PIGMENT LAYER ; 4 : LAYER OF SENSORY CELLS ; 5 : LAYER OF GANGLION CELLS ; 6 : BRANCHES OF THE OPTIC NERVE ; 7 : EPIDERMIS ; 8 : NERVES OF CUTICLE ; 9 : OPENING BY WHICH THE OPTIC CAVITY COMMUNICATES WITH THE SURROUNDING SEA-WATER. (AFTER HENSEN.)

c. ap. : central aperture.
cc. : central-cavity.
ep. : epithelium.
f.o.n. : fibres of optic nerve.
g. c. : ganglion cells.
nf.c. : nerve-fibres of cuticular epithelium.
p. : pigment.
rc. : sensory retinal cells.
rh. : rods.

Moreover, the habits and the conditions of life of these animals, who lay confined within a rigid shell in which they were carried about by currents in the water, irrespective of any active or purposeful movements on their own part, contrasts markedly with that of the rapid and active movements of the carnivorous octopuses and squids in which highly differentiated eyes have been evolved, and it seems probable that the restriction of move-ment, combined with imperfect vision and almost complete dependence for food on external circumstances, may have had a very considerable influence in bringing about the gradual extinction of these two Orders. The Nautilidæ and Ammonites are a side-branch of the class Mollusca which has almost completely disappeared, but the preservation of the simple type of eye found in *Nautilus*, which has neither lens nor any power of independent movement of the eyeball, well illustrates the way in which an organ which appears to be of subsidiary importance to the life of

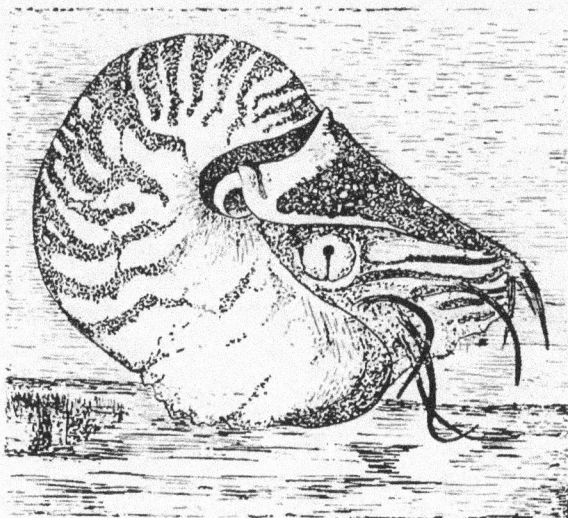

FIG. 113.

Drawing taken from photograph of a living specimen of *Nautilus pompilius*, showing the position of the eye when the animal is in the water. (After A. Willey, *Q. J. Micro. Sc.* **39**.) Note.—The groove which runs vertically downwards from the central aperture to the lower margin of the eye.

the animal as a whole, may be retained as an hereditary structure through millions of years, without—it may be presumed—having undergone any marked change either in the way of evolution or devolution.

A similar preservation of a simple type of eye, adapted to simple needs, has presumably occurred in other types of shellfish belonging to the Class Mollusca and throughout the Invertebrate Kingdom, in all the simpler and less specialized types of animals in which eyes have been evolved ; and it may be inferred from the similarity of the shells of extinct animals and those of the present day that the adult and larval forms of the extinct species correspond with the adult and larval forms of the living, not only in general but also in detail—for example, the structure and relative position of the ocelli and statocysts of the veliger larvæ of the extinct parent stock with those of the living species ; moreover, when we compare the trochophore and veliger larvæ of the Mollusca with those of other classes of invertebrate animals, one cannot fail to be impressed with the essential uni-formity of type, in the general appearance and structure of these larvæ, not-withstanding the wide differences which exist in the adult animals. In illustration of this we need only refer to the trochophore larvæ of the Brachiopods belonging to the phylum Molluscoidea, those of certain of the Annulata and of the Rotifers (see pp. 88, 91, 92, Figs. 56, Chap. 7; 58, 59, Chap. 8). In contrast with the similarity in form of the larvæ of these very different types of animal, it is especially noticeable how changes in the habits and conditions of the adult animal are associated with adaptive changes in special organs, e.g. the development of the highly complicated faceted eyes of some insects, which replace the simple eyes of the larva, e.g. in Dytiscus marginalis (Figs. 78, 79 and 80, Chap. 11, pp. 117, 118). The simple eyes of the larva which were present before metamorphosis had taken place while the larva was living in the water, being followed by an aggregate or composite type of eye, adapted to the special needs of the fully developed animal, which is capable of living on land or flying quickly in the air. These changes occur specially in the higher and more recently evolved types of animal, as compared with the more simple and ancient types of shell-fish which we have been considering previously. More-over, as we have pointed out in a previous chapter (p. 26), along with the specialization of the lateral eyes of these more recent types there has in some cases been a regression of the paired median eyes, accompanied by fusion of these in the median plane and presumably also diminution or loss of function. Moreover, as we shall see later, palæontological evidence indicates that similar regressive changes have taken place in the paired median eyes of vertebrates.

The phylum Mollusca includes bivalved shellfish such as the mussels, cockles, and oysters belonging to the class Lamellibranchiata (Pelycypoda); the Chitons or coat-of-mail shellfish (Amphineura); animals with spiral univalve shells, including whelks, snails, and slugs (Gastropoda); the elephant's-tusk shells (Scaphopoda); and the cuttlefishes, squids, octopods, and Nautili (Cephalopoda).

The eyes, as we have already mentioned, vary markedly both in position and in structure. Thus, they may appear in the usual place on either side of the fore part of the head; on the back, as in *Chiton*; or around the edge of the mantle, as in the scallop or in the thorny-oyster. They may be of the simple, upright type or inverted. The lens may be cuticular or cellular in type. The simple eyes may be open pits without a lens or the pit may be constricted off from the surface and form a vesicle covered by a " secondary cornea " and enclosing a vitreous or a cellular lens. The eyes may be absent in the adult animal, but a pair of ocelli may be present in the trochophore larva or in the veliger stage of development. In the

Cephalopods the eyes may be highly complex, as in *Sepia*, having a retina of the upright type, a vitreous chamber, a biconvex double lens, " ciliary body," " iris," anterior chamber, cornea, sclerotic cartilages, ocular muscles, and palpebral folds, or a simple unclosed vesicular pit, open to the surface and thus containing sea-water as in *Nautilus*. An inverted type of retina is, moreover, present in *Onchidium* (Fig. 39, Chap. 3, p. 54), an aberrant type of snail in which eyes are present on the back of the animal and the nerve fibres lie in front of the retinal cells and rods ; the lens is formed of two (or more) enormous clear cells which fill the whole of the interior of the eye, occupying the space which in a vertebrate eye would be filled by the vitreous humour and lens. The resemblance to a verte-brate eye is further simulated by the way in which the fibres of the optic nerve appear to perforate the retina at the posterior pole of the eyeball.

The Eyes of Bivalved Shellfish (Pelycypoda)

In the freshwater mussels (Anodonta or Unio) and cockles (Cardium) no eyes are present in the adult animal and none have been described in the larval stage, although a typical trochophore larva is developed with an apical plate bearing a vertical tuft of hairs beneath which is a cerebral ganglion, while surrounding the plate is a prototroch or girdle of ciliated cells, as in *Patella* (Fig. 114).

In the scallop, or *Pecten*, Fig. 106, eyes are present round the edge of the mantle. These are peculiar in having an inverted retina and a cellular lens. They probably originate as a special modification of certain tentacles. Each eye forms a dome-shaped projection about the size of a pin's-head. Enclosed within this is an almost spherical vesicle (Fig. 107) the inner half of which is formed by the retina, while the outer includes the cornea and lens. The retina is slightly concave in front where it comes in contact with the lens and is in relation with a circular " blood sinus." It is covered by a basement membrane beneath which is a nerve-fibre layer. The nerve-fibres on one side converge towards a point on the edge of the cup where, joining together, they form one branch of the optic nerve. Other fibres diverge as they pass towards the edge of the cup. On reaching the outer margin of the cup they turn round this, and passing backward on the superficial surface of the sclera converge towards the " posterior " or inner pole of the eye, where they unite to form a second branch of the optic nerve. The two branches join a short distance behind the posterior pole to form a single main optic nerve. Beneath the layer of nerve-fibres is a stratum of large nerve cells which appear to give origin to the optic nerve-fibres, these fibres springing from the superficial end of the cell, namely that nearest the lens. Deep to these large cells is a plexiform layer con-taining small nuclei. This is succeeded by a layer of refractile rods which are separated by a cleft from a tapetum and a pigment layer. The whole is enclosed by a fibrous sheath surrounded by a loose mesenchyme containing blood-vessels. The cellular lens is highly convex on its deep surface, slightly convex superficially, where it is covered by a transparent

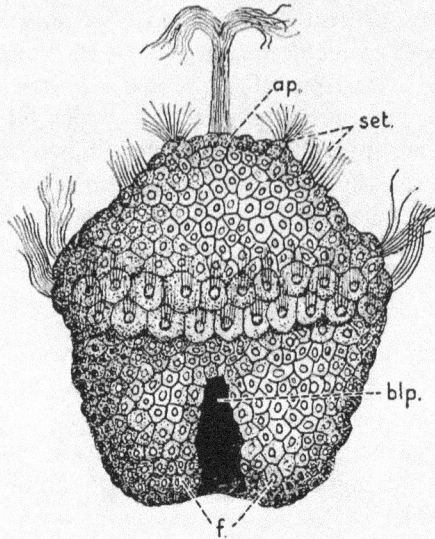

FIG. 114.—TROCHOPHORE LARVA OF PATELLA COERULEA.

Ventral side showing : *ap.*, apical plate ; *blp.*, blastopore ; *f.*, rudiment of foot; *set.*, setæ. Compare with Figs. 58, 108.
(After Patten, redrawn from MacBride.)

cornea. This consists of a thin cuticle covering a layer of hypoderm cells beneath which is a fibrous stratum continuous with and forming part of the fibrous sheath enclosing the eyeball. The clear hypoderm cells of the cornea are continuous circumferentially with the surrounding hypoderm cells which are deeply pigmented and thus function as a fixed iris.

The only cephalic eyes which occur in the class Lamellibranchiata are a pair of ocelli which are found in the bases of the most anterior filament of the inner gill lamina in *Mytilus*, the common sea-water mussel, and some allied genera.

The Eyes of Amphineura

With the exception of the Chitons, or " coat-of-mail shells " (Fig. 115), the Amphineura are a lowly organized class of mollusc in which in the adult animal the region of the head is hardly distinguishable from the body, and it is neither provided with eyes nor tentacles.

The Chitons are characterized by a series of eight overlapping valves, situated one behind another on the back of the animal. These give an appearance of segmentation. This is, however, misleading, as the body itself is not truly segmented. Each plate or valve is developed as a separate scale, the scales later uniting to form a jointed shield or lorica.

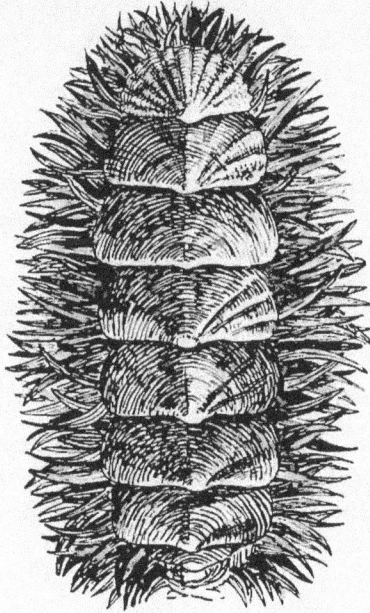

FIG. 115.

Dorsal aspect of *Chiton spinosus*, a mollusc in which the head of the adult animal has no eyes, tentacles, or statocysts. Sensory organs are, however, found in canals which are present in the superficial layer of the shell valves which cover the back. Some of the larger of these organs have the structure of an eye, having a cornea, lens, iris, pigment layer, and retina.

(From *Cambridge Natural History.*)

From beneath the edges of the lorica bristles project, which, diverging from one another in all directions, give a brush-like appearance to the animal. The superficial cuticular layer of the scales is perforated by small vertical canals which lodge sense-organs. These are called " micræsthetes" and " megalæsthetes," and some of the latter are especially differentiated as eyes, having a cornea, lens, sensory retinal cells, a pigment layer, and iris.

Ocelli are also present in the trochophore larva (Fig. 116).

The arrangement and structure of the tubular system and sensory organs of *Chiton* somewhat resemble the sensory organs of the lateral line system of vertebrates, but they differ in certain respects and are considered to have been evolved independently and not to be homologous.

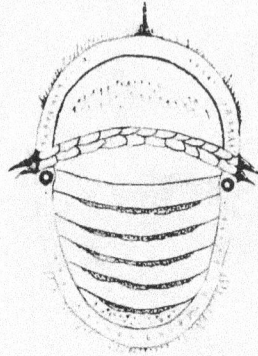

FIG. 116.—TROCHOPHORE LARVA OF A CHITON, SHOWING APICAL TUFT OF HAIRS AND PAIR OF OCELLI. (AFTER KOWALEWSKY.)

The Eyes of Gasteropods

The gasteropods are univalve shellfish and they include such well-known types as the periwinkles, whelks, snails, and slugs. In most cases the eyes, which are of the simple upright type, are situated on tubercles at the bases of the tentacles or appear as slight projections near the middle of the tentacle (Fig. 110), but in the snails and slugs the eyes are borne on the ends of a second pair of tentacles, which are longer than and are placed behind the first pair (Fig. 111). The eyes of all are developed from pit-like depressions of the epidermis, and since the developmental stages of the more complex types are indicated by the adult form of the lower and simpler types, we shall consider the latter first.

1. *Patella, the Common Limpet* (Fig. 33, Chap. 3, p. 48).—Each eye consists of a pit-like depression of the cuticle. The cells lining the pit are elongated and continuous externally with nerve-fibres, which join to form the optic nerve. The inner ends of the cells which are directed towards the hollow of the pit are clear and refractile ; the central part of each cell is pigmented, while the outer part which contains the nucleus is clear.

2. *Trochus.*—The spiral shell of this mollusc is conical in form and since when the outer covering is removed a bright pearly surface is exposed, it is much used for decorative purposes. As in the former type the eyes are formed by a depression of the cuticular epithelium. They

differ, however, in that the mouth of the pit has become constricted by the ingrowth of a circular fold of the cuticular epithelium, which reduces the size of the opening to a small pupillary aperture (Fig. 34, Chap. 3, p. 48). Moreover, the interior of the vesicle is completely filled with a clear, gelatinous material which is apparently secreted by the cells which line the vesicle. This is described as the vitreous humour.

3. *Murex.*—The ornamental spiral shells of this genus have long tapering spines and are commonly known as " venus's combs." In this type the eyes are more highly organized than in the former examples, the mouth of the pit has become closed and the pit is constricted off from the cuticle so as to form a vesicle (Fig. 35, Chap. 3, p. 49). The

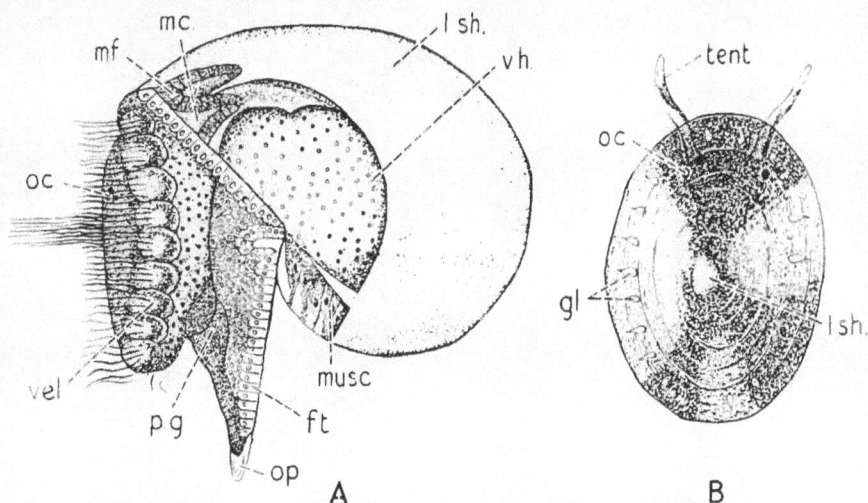

FIG. 117.—A : VELIGER LARVA OF PATELLA CŒRULEA VIEWED FROM THE LEFT SIDE SHOWING OCELLI ON APICAL PLATE. B : DORSAL VIEW OF ACMÆA VIRGINEA, JUST AFTER METAMORPHOSIS, IN WHICH THE OCELLI ARE SEEN TO BE COVERED BY THE MARGIN OF THE SHELL. THE LARVAL SHELL IS RETAINED AS AN APICAL KNOB, WHICH WILL BE CAST OFF LATER. (REDRAWN FROM MACBRIDE : A, AFTER PATTEN ; B, AFTER BOUTAN.)

ft. : foot.	*oc.* : ocellus.
gl. : glands in roof of mantle.	*p.g.* : rudiment of pedal ganglion.
l. sh. : larval shell.	*tent.* : tentacle.
mc. : mantle cavity.	*vel.* : velum.
mf. : mantle fold.	*vh.* : visceral hump.
musc. : muscle.	

outer lamina of the circular cuticular fold joins over the superficial aspect of the vesicle and forms with a layer of ingrowing mesenchyme what is termed the " secondary cornea," whereas the outer part of the epithelial wall of the optic vesicle, which remains thin and transparent, is called the " primary cornea." The remaining inner and larger part of the epithelial wall of the vesicle is differentiated into a retina of the same type as in *Trochus* and *Patella*, consisting of well-defined bacillary, pigment, and nuclear layers. Within the cavity of the optic vesicle the contents have become differentiated into a more solid refractile body, the lens, and a more fluid part which surrounds the lens and, like the vitreous of the vertebrate eye, intervenes between the lens and the retina. Both lens and vitreous are formed by modification of the secretion of the cells lining the vesicle, and a lens of this type is known as a vitreous or non-cellular lens.

The development of gasteropods has been worked out by Patten, Boutan, and others, more especially in *Patella* and *Acmæa*, a nearly allied species. A typical trochophore larva is formed with an apical plate bearing a vertical tuft of cilia, beneath which there is developed from the ectoderm a cerebral ganglion (Fig. 114, p. 156). The ocelli are developed from the same ectodermal layer, just behind and lateral to the bases of the tentacular processes, and are well seen in the veliger larva of *Acmæa virginea* (Fig. 118, A). At a later stage the velum or prototroch is shed and the eyes are covered by the anterior margin of the shell (Fig. 118, B). The relation of the ocelli to tentacles, velum, mouth, statocysts, and foot are well shown in Fig. 109, p. 150), showing the veliger stage of development in *Vermetes*. This is a worm-like gasteropod characterized

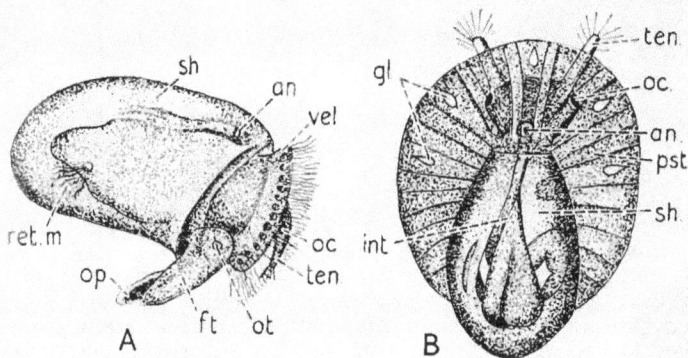

FIG. 118.—ADVANCED STAGES OF DEVELOPMENT OF ACMÆA VIRGINEA. A: LATERAL VIEW OF VELIGER LARVA. B: DORSAL VIEW OF YOUNG ACMÆA, AFTER THE VELUM HAS BEEN CAST

an. : anus.
ft. : foot.
gl. : glands in roof of mantle.
int. : intestine.
oc. : ocellus.
op. : operculum.
ot. : statocyst.
pst. : peristome.
ret. m. : retractor muscle.
sh. : shell.
ten. : tentacle.
vel. : velum.

After the velum has been cast off the young mollusc sinks to the bottom; the periostome enlarges and gives rise to the conical adult shell, the margin of which overlaps the eyes.

(After Boutan—redrawn from MacBride.)

by having a spiral shell in the larva which is replaced in the adult by a straight, tubular shell.

Fossil shells of gasteropods are found in the earliest Palæozoic rocks, and it is probable that the animals contained within them differed little from those living at the present time, and that tentacles, ocelli, and statocysts were developed in them in the same relative positions as in living animals of the same type.

The Scaphopoda

These are worm-like molluscs and include the elephant-tusk shells, or Dentalium. The animal is enclosed in a slightly curved tubular shell which resembles in form an elephant's tusk or tooth. No eyes are found in the adult animal, but statocysts are present in the larva of Dentalium, which passes through typical trochophore and veliger stages.

The Eyes of Cephalopods

These vary from simple optic pits containing sea-water such as are present in *Nautilus*, to the highly organized eyes of the cuttlefish, squids, and octopuses.

We shall commence our description with the simplest form, namely that of *Nautilus*. The eyes are of large size and paired. When the animal is swimming in the water, they appear in a triangular space on each side between the hood above, the bases of the tentacles in front, and the edges of the mantle and opening of the shell below (Fig. 113, p. 153). Each eye has a central opening which leads directly into the cavity of the optic vesicle, which is thus filled with sea-water. From this a shallow groove runs downward to a rim-like fold which surrounds the lower part of the eye. The position of this groove suggests the fœtal or choroidal fissure of a vertebrate eye. There has, however, been no inversion of the outer wall of an optic vesicle, such as occurs in the eyes of vertebrates, and the wall of the optic vesicle in *Nautilus* consists of a single layer, whereas the secondary optic vesicle of the lateral eyes of vertebrates is bilaminar. Although the development of *Nautilus* has not, so far as we are aware, yet been described, it may be assumed that the eye is developed by inversion of the superficial layer of the epidermis, so as to form a simple pit as it does in the initial stage of development in other molluscs.

The microscopic structure of the adult eye of *Nautilus* has been described by Henle. The wall of the cup consists from within outwards (Fig. 112, p. 152) of a bacillary layer formed by the inner ends of the retinal cells, a pigment layer, outside which is a single layer of large nuclei contained in the basal part of the retinal cells, this is succeeded by an

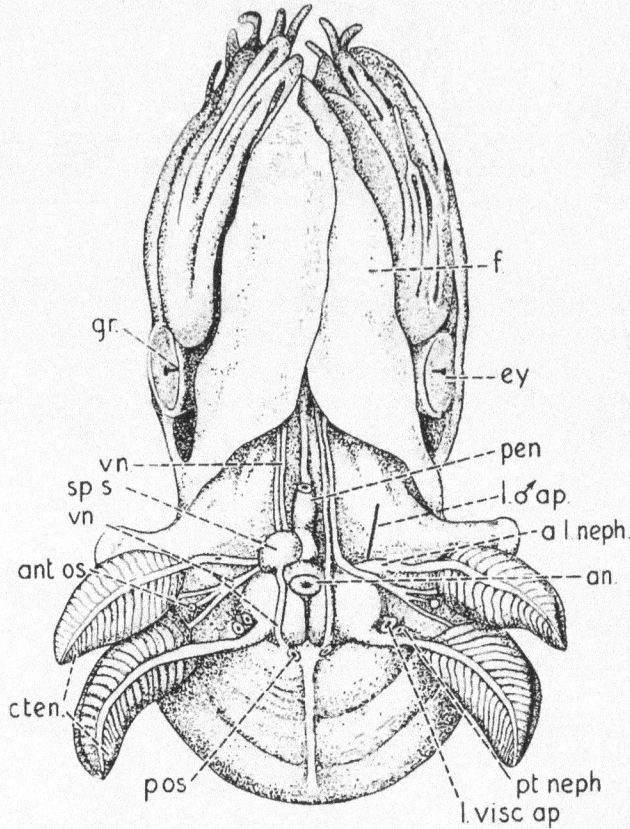

FIG. 119

NAUTILUS POMPILIUS, SHOWING THE CENTRAL APERTURES OF THE EYES. (AFTER
WILLEY, FROM PARKER AND HASWELL'S *Textbook of Zoology*.)

The flattened external surface of the eye is bounded by a slightly raised rim,
which extends round the posterior half of its margin.   From this a narrow
groove extends inwards to the central opening, which has some resemblance
to the choroidal fissure of the lateral vertebrate eye.   The eye of *Nautilus*
is, however, extremely simple, consisting of an open cup, the cavity of which
is filled with sea-water.   It has neither lens, iris, nor vitreous humour.
The rods or inner refractile segments of the cells are directed towards the
light and the nerve fibres originate from the opposite end.   The interior of
the mantle cavity is exposed, the postero-ventral wall having been reflected.

a. l. neph. : oral left renal aperture.
an. : anus.
ant. os. : right oral osphradium
(olfactory organ).
cten. : ctenidia or branchial organs.
ey. : eye.
f. : funnel.
gr. : groove leading to central aperture of eye.

l. ♂. ap. : bristle passed into left re-
productive aperture.
l. visc. ap. : left viscero-pericardial
aperture.
pen. : penis.
pt. neph. : aboral left renal aperture.
p. os. : aboral osphradia.
sp. s. : spermatophoral sac.
v.n. : visceral nerves.

outermost layer of small scattered nuclei and nerve-fibres ; the latter pierce an external limiting membrane and pass inwards through the optic stalk to the cerebral ganglion (anterior part of the œsophageal ring). In the interior of the optic cup there is neither vitreous, lens, nor iris, and as an optical instrument it is comparable to a camera of the simple pill-box type.

Nautilus (Fig. 119) with its simple type of eyes is especially interesting from the phylogenetic standpoint ; it is the only living representative of the extinct Nautiloid tetrabranchiata, which were abundant in the Palæozoic epoch ; the earliest representatives being found in the Cambrian rocks. It also closely resembles the Ammonites, but there are certain differences in the shell, and it is doubtful whether the Ammonites were tetrabranchiate, like *Nautilus,* or dibranchiate. This difference, however, is not so

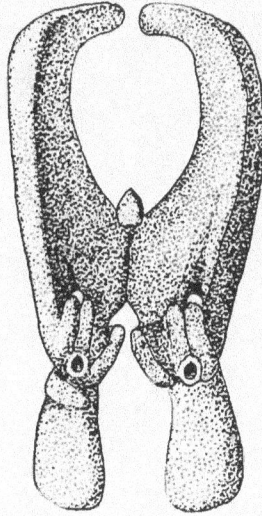

FIG. 120.—CARTILAGINOUS INTERNAL SKELETON OF NAUTILUS POMPILIUS.

fundamental as might be expected from the differences in structure which exist between the branchiæ and eyes of living representatives of these fossils, since there are many points of agreement between dibranchiate and tetrabranchiate cephalopods which outweigh such differences as have occurred in the long geological period which has elapsed since the fossil representatives of the living genera were alive. Incidentally one may mention, as an example of an important structural similarity between these two widely separated orders, the occurrence of a cartilaginous endoskeleton—the " cranial cartilage," Fig. 120—which is present in both *Nautilus* and *Sepia.* It is noteworthy that the cranial cartilages of *Nautilus* and *Sepia* resemble in certain respects the endoskeleton of some chætopods, crustacea, and arachnids, e.g. the entosternite of *Scorpio* and *Limulus.*

On the dorsal aspect of the cranial cartilage of *Sepia*, overlying and protecting the cerebral ganglia is another endoskeletal structure, namely the nuchal cartilage. The hypothetical significance of the existence of these skeletal elements in invertebrates will be discussed later in connection with Gaskell's comparison of the entosternite of *Limulus* with the cartilaginous skeleton of Ammocœtes.

The Eyes of Sepia

The conspicuous large eyes of the cuttlefish have attracted the attention of many zoologists, among the more recent of whom may be mentioned Faussek (1900) and Koeppern (1909). They are much more highly organized than those of *Nautilus* and *Triton* and have a superficial resemblance to the lateral eyes of vertebrates, since they have a lens with a

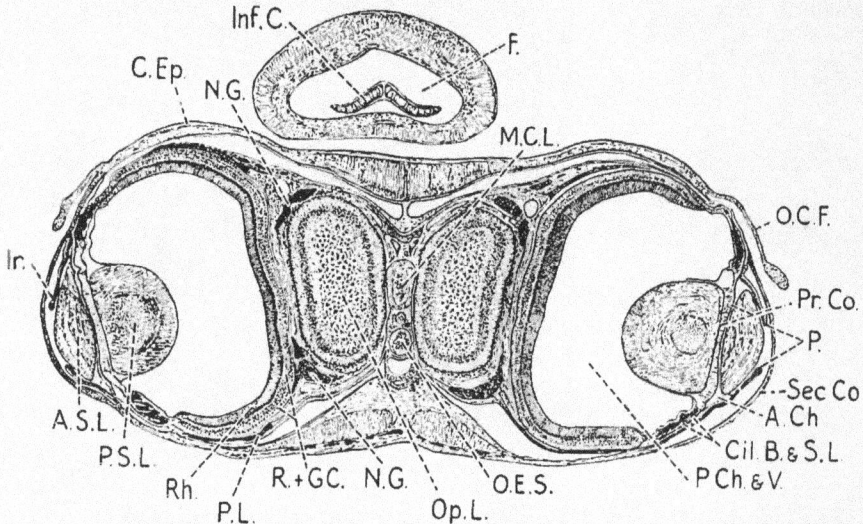

FIG. 121.—TRANSVERSE SECTION THROUGH THE HEAD OF AN OCTOPUS (SEPIOLIA)
(ORIGINAL).

A.Ch. : anterior chamber.
A.S.L. : anterior segment of lens.
C.Ep. : cutaneous epithelium.
Cil. B. & S.L. : ciliary body and suspensory ligament.
F. : cavity of funnel.
Inf. C. : infundibular cartilage.
Ir. : iris.
M.C.L. : middle cerebral lobe.
N.G. : nerve ganglion.
O.C.F. : outer cutaneous fold of eye.

OES. : oesophagus.
Op. L. : optic lobe.
P. : pupil.
P. Ch. & V. : posterior chamber and vitreous body.
P.L. : pigment layer of retina.
Pr. Co. : primary cornea.
P.S.L. : posterior segment of lens.
R + GC. : retinal and ganglion cells.
Rh. : rods.
Sec. Co. : secondary cornea.

The names which are employed to denote the various parts of the invertebrate eye must not be regarded as implying a morphological correspondence with similarly named parts of vertebrate eyes. (R. J. G.)

suspensory mechanism, ciliary body, iris, anterior- and vitreous-chambers, cornea, and a palpebral fold (Fig. 121). They are, however, of the upright type, and are developed as an ingrowth of the epidermis. It must be realized also that the names which have been applied to the various parts do not in most cases denote structures which are strictly homologous with the structures similarly named in the vertebrate eye.

The retina resembles the vertebrate retina in having three principal layers of cell-elements, namely, an inner consisting of the sensory- or visual-cells; an intermediate resembling the bipolar cells of vertebrates; and an outer or ganglionic layer. The retina of the cuttlefish is, however, of the upright type, the rods or receptive ends of the visual cells being directed inward towards the source of light, and the ganglion cells and nerve-fibre layer being peripheral, i.e. nearest the fibrous capsule. The retina of *Sepia* thus agrees with the vertebrate retina in consisting of three principal layers of sensory cells, thus being " compound " in type; but it differs in being upright as contrasted with the inverted retina of the vertebrate eye.

The general structure of the retina will be most easily understood by a reference to its early stages of development, as shown in (Fig. 36, A, B, C, D, E, Chap. 3, p. 50). The eye commences as a simple pit—*optic cup*; this is lined by a single layer of cubical cells, continuous at the mouth of the pit with the epithelium covering the surface of the body. The mouth of the pit then becomes constricted, and later an *optic vesicle* is cut off from the exterior. The deeper cells of the optic vesicle, which will give rise to the *retina*, become columnar and develop thread-like processes which project into the cavity of the vesicle. The cells of the superficial segment of the wall of the vesicle become flattened and form the inner epithelial layer of the future *corpus epitheliale*. Superficial to the optic vesicle is a mesodermal layer covered externally by the epithelium of the body-wall. The latter forms the outer epithelial layer of the future corpus epitheliale and the two epithelial layers with the mesoderm between them form the *primary cornea*. Around this a circular fold rises up and grows inwards over the developing lens; this is known as the *iris fold* (C, D, E). The epithelial body consists of a central portion which is primarily concerned in the secretion of the posterior segment of the lens but later forms a septum between the two segments of the lens and a peripheral portion which is composed of large clear cells, some of which by secretion and also by degeneration give rise to both segments of the non-cellular lens; others which are of small size contribute to the later stages of development of the lens. In the retina, according to Faussek, the primarily tall columnar cells of the inner segment of the optic vesicle, which at first form a single layer resting on the inner surface of the basement membrane, proliferate and give rise to many layers of small round cells, the outer of which pass through the basement membrane and form the intermediate and ganglionic layers of the retina. The inner ends of the receptive cells, however, retain their primary position inside the basement membrane and form the layer of *visual-rods*. Between the visual cells are a certain number of cells which develop pigment. These form a conspicuous band external to the bacillary layer (Fig. 121); outside the *pigment layer* is a narrow, clear zone of nerve-fibres—*inner plexiform layer*; this is succeeded by a wide intermediate band of small, round nuclei—*middle nuclear layer*—another layer of fine nerve-fibres—*outer plexiform layer*—and finally a layer of *ganglion cells*, appearing in the greater part of its extent as a single

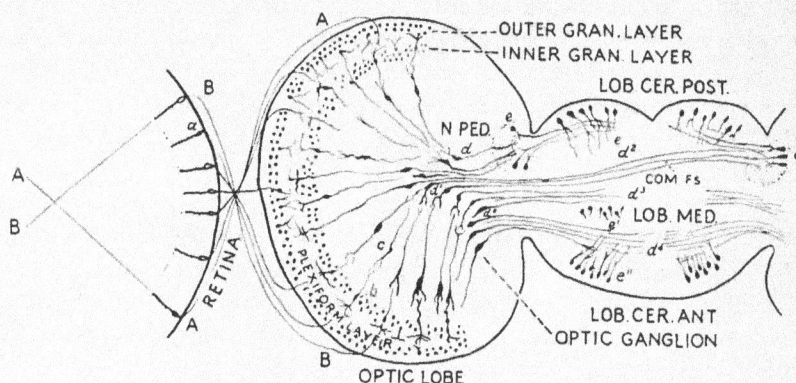

Fig. 122.—Scheme of the Visual Paths and their Central Connections in a Cephalopod, combined from von Lenhossek, Kopsch, and Cajal. According to Cajal most Bipolar Cells (*b*) are located in the Outer Granular Layer. (From C.U. Ariëns Kappers, slightly modified.)

Axons coming from the retinal cells, decussate in the optic nerve, where they form a chiasma. The inverted image on the retina which results from rays passing through the narrow pupil and lens is thus corrected in the cortex of the optic lobe. *a*, *b*, *c*, *d*, d^1, d^2, d^3, d^4, *e*, e^1, e^2, denote relays of neurons.

stratum of large cells, lying in an outer nerve-fibre layer which is limited by an external basement membrane. The nerve-fibres converge towards, the proximal or posterior pole of the eyeball, where, forming a short, thick optic nerve, they pierce the sclera and enter the optic lobe (Fig. 36, F, Chap. 3, p. 50).

The course of the nerve-fibres, according to Cajal, is indicated in Fig. 122, which shows a decussation of axons coming from the retina in the optic nerve; this corrects the reversal of the image formed on the retina. In the optic lobe there are two layers of granule cells placed superficially and separated by a plexiform layer of nerve-fibres; while in the centre is an area consisting of nerve-cells and nerve-fibres, the nerve-cells being chiefly aggregated in a central nucleus and in a peduncular nucleus. .From these nuclei relays of cells carry sensory impulses to the middle-anterior- and posterior-cerebral lobes. The terminal fibres of the axons coming from the retina pass into the plexiform layer of fibres between the two granular layers in the cortical part of the optic lobe ; in this layer they communicate with dendrites of cells in both the superficial and deep granular layers ; while the axons of the granule cells convey the impulse to the central and peduncular nuclei.

Development of Cephalopods

The higher Mollusca differ markedly in their development from the lower types, e.g. the univalve shellfishes (*Patella, Vermetes, Triton*) ; *Chiton ; Dentalium ;* and the bivalve shellfishes such as *Pecten*. In the higher molluscs there is no trochophore or veliger stage of development. The segmentation is partial : meroblastic—a blastoderm or germinal disc being formed on the surface of a large mass of yolk ; moreover, there are many points in the later stages of development which mark a wide diver- gence of the higher cephalopods from the more simple representatives of the class.

The trochophore stage is believed to have been completely eliminated during the descent of the higher from the common ancestors of these and of the simpler types ; and also adult features recently acquired by the higher types have been reflected back or impressed on the early stages of develop- ment of the higher types. The explanation of some of these changes probably lies, as has been suggested by MacBride, in the effect which " the accession of large stores of nourishment " in the eggs has in " almost obliterating the traces of ancestral history in their development, leaving only the most general resemblance in the formation of the layers and the development of the sense-organs as links between them and other Mollusca."

CHAPTER 13

EYES OF INTERMEDIATE TYPES BETWEEN INVERTEBRATES AND VERTEBRATES

THESE, commonly known as Protochordata, are classed in three Sub-phyla:

(1) Hemichorda, including *Balanoglossus*, Fig. 123.

(2) Urochorda, comprising the tunicates (Ascidia or sea-squirts); *Salpa* (Fig. 128, A, Chap. 14, p. 176); Doliolum and allied forms, many of which are fixed and form colonies such as Pyrosoma.

(3) Euchorda (Acrania or Cephalochorda), represented by *Amphioxus* or lancelet (Fig. 129, Chap. 16, p. 179).

All these classes are interesting with respect to the eyes which are present in the larval stages of certain representative types, and from the general standpoint of morphology although they are not in the main line of descent of vertebrates and are to be regarded as side-branches some of which have undergone regressive changes.

There is still considerable difference of opinion with regard to the affinities of each of the three groups enumerated above, which are some-times described together under the general term Protochordata. The disagreement has been specially concerned with the relationships of the Subphylum Enteropneusta, or Hemichorda, which includes such apparently different species, as the free-swimming *Balanoglossus* and the fixed type *Cephalodiscus*. The affinity of these with the vertebrates was at one time definitely denied by many morphologists, although the Urochorda or tunicates have for a long time been recognized as degenerate vertebrates which have undergone adaptational changes, such as a colonial or a fixed condition of life in the adult animal which is similar to that of many protozoa or cœlenterates and aquatic plants.

The very close resemblance of the tornaria larvæ of the Hemichorda (Fig. 125, Chap. 14, p. 172) to the trochophore larvæ of invertebrates, more particularly of the annelids and the echinoderms—a resemblance which includes such likenesses as are found in the apical plate, the cerebral ganglia, the two ocelli ; the disposition of the ciliated bands and apical tuft of hairs (Fig. 124) ; also of the mouth, alimentary canal, and anus—led certain authors such as Spengel to challenge the earlier conclusions of Bateson and others that they were derived from and represented the parent stock, which had given rise to the whole vertebrate kingdom. Later workers, including Ritter and MacBride, have, however, re-affirmed an important item in the original thesis of Bateson, namely that bilateral

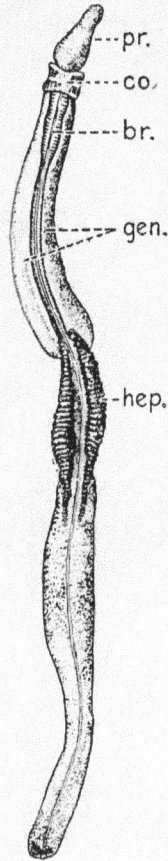

FIG. 123.—BALANOGLOSSUS. (AFTER SPENGEL, FROM PARKER AND HASWELL'S *Textbook of Zoology.*)

br. : branchial regions.
co. : collar.
gen. : genital ridges.
hep. : projections caused by a series of paired hepatic pouches.
pr. : proboscis.

segmented animals have evolved in two directions—one, in which the alimentary canal pierces the nervous system between the supra-œsophageal ganglion and the infra-œsophageal ganglion, leading up to the annelids and arthropods ; and the other, in which the central nervous system is dorsal to the alimentary canal, from which the protochordata and verte-

brates have been evolved.   One important distinguishing character of the
Hemichorda may be noted, which serves to connect them with the vertebrate stock, namely, the presence of a series of paired gill slits behind the
" collar region," which communicate with the pharyngeal region of the
alimentary canal (Fig. 123, p. 169).   Somewhat similar gill slits are also
present in larval tunicates, which combined with a ventral position of
the heart and other definitely vertebral relations of the intestinal organs
indicate that these lowly organized animals, the Protochordata, are side-
branches of the early vertebrate stem ; but it must not be concluded that
they are in the direct line of descent, or, in other words, belong to the true

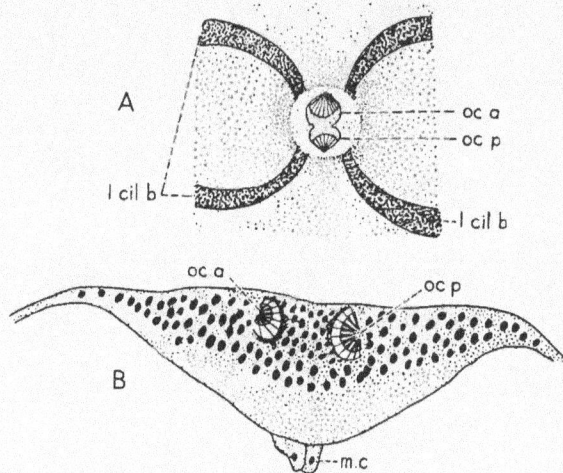

FIG. 124.—THE APICAL PLATE AND EYES OF A FULL-GROWN TORNARIA LARVA
OF BALANOGLOSSUS.   (AFTER MORGAN.)

A. Apical view showing the relation of the plate to the longitudinal ciliated
   band.
B. Antero-posterior, median section through the apical plate and eyes.

                        l. cil. b. : longitudinal ciliated band.
                        m.c : muscle cells belonging to the apical cord.
                        oc. a. : anterior eye.
                        oc. p. : posterior eye.

parental stock of the vertebrates. The intermediate position of *Balanoglossus*
is indicated by the co-existence in it of both dorsal and ventral nerve cords,
as well as the larval characters already mentioned which are common to
both vertebrates and invertebrates, and, as we shall see later, there are
many points which indicate that some of the best known living representatives of the Urochorda and Euchorda, such as the Ascidia and
Amphioxus, have descended from animals which were more highly organized
than their living representatives. This conclusion is partly based on
general considerations and partly on the differences to be observed in the

degree of development of the sense-organs in the larval state as compared with the adult animal ; also the degenerate condition or absence of the same organs in the adult protochordate animal, as compared with those adult vertebrates in which the lateral eyes are certainly functional and also those, such as the cyclostomes and certain reptiles, in which the median eyes show a high degree of structural differentiation, which warrants the assumption that these median eyes also were functional in the ancestral stock from which the cyclostomes and reptiles have descended.

CHAPTER 14

I. *HEMICHORDA*

THIS Class includes *Balanoglossus* (Fig. 123, Chap. 13, p. 169), a burrowing, marine, worm-like animal of which there are several species, varying in length from 2–3 cm. to 2½ metres. No eyes are present in the adult animal, but in the early stages of its development it passes through a stage which is termed the " tornaria " (Fig. 125), which resembles in certain respects the trochophore stage of certain echinoderms, rotifers, annelids,

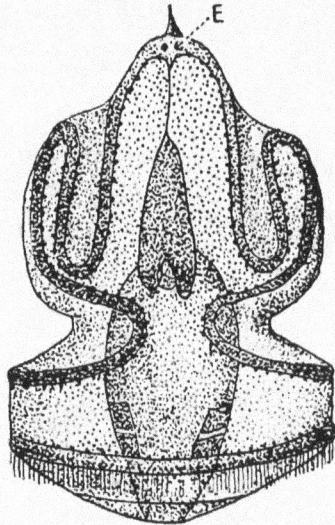

FIG. 125.—LARVAL FORM (TORNARIA) OF BALANOGLOSSUS SHOWING THE EYE-SPOTS ON THE APICAL PLATE. (AFTER SPENGEL.)

Annulata, and Brachiopoda, more especially in the presence of an apical plate, bearing a vertical tuft of cilia and eye-spots. The development of *Balanoglossus* has been described by Spengel, Heider, and Morgan. The last author describes the two eye-cups on the apical plate of the tornaria as being anterior and posterior in position (Fig. 124, A, Chap. 13, p. 170). They consist of a single row of elongated ectodermal cells which are clear and converge towards the centre of the pit ; each is surrounded by a mass of pigment which lies on the outer surface and between the two cups (Fig. 124, B, Chap. 13, p. 170) ; at the base of the plate is a thick layer of nerve-fibres. At a latter stage the apical plate and eyes atrophy and the larva sinks to the bottom and undergoes a metamorphosis whereby it is changed to a worm-like form which leads a burrowing life, like *Amphioxus*, and has no eyes.

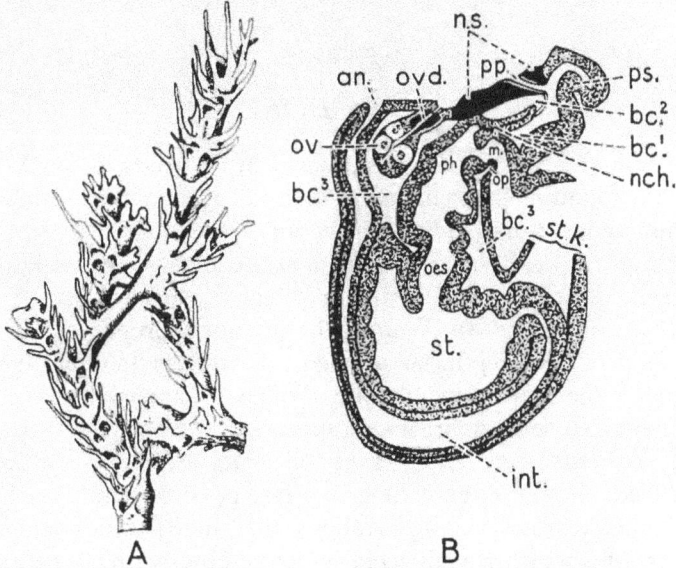

FIG. 126.—CEPHALODISCUS. (AFTER McIntosh and Harmer.)

A : Colony showing gelatinous investment covering separate zooids. B : Diagrammatic representation of longitudinal section of a zooid.

an. : anus.	*op.* : operculum.
bc.[1] : coelom of proboscis.	*œs.* : œsophagus.
bc.[2] : coelom of collar.	*ov.* : ovary.
bc.[3] : coelom of trunk.	*ovd.* : oviduct.
int. : intestine.	*ph.* : pharynx.
m. : mouth.	*pp.* : proboscis pore.
nch. : supposed notochord.	*ps.* : proboscis.
ns. : nerve-strand and ganglion cells.	*stk.* : stalk.

Cephalodiscus is closely related to Balanoglossus, but there is no free-swimming Tornaria, having eye-spots.

Cephalodiscus (Fig. 126) and *Rhabdopleura*, which lead an inactive, fixed life, being associated in colonies, have no eyes in the mature condition, but McIntosh has described eye-spots as being present in the polypides of *Cephalodiscus*.

CHAPTER 15

II. *UROCHORDA*

A GREAT deal of interest has been shown in the study of the " single " eye which is found in the ventricular cavity of the cerebral vesicle of the free-swimming larva of *Ascidia mammillata* or *Phallusia* (Figs. 3, Chap. 1, p. 5, and Fig. 127). Besides the eye, a single statocyst is present in the expanded anterior end of the neural tube, which expansion is usually spoken of as the " sense vesicle." In *Phallusia* the anterior neuropore remains open for a certain period during the larval stage. Later, regressive changes set in which precede the fixed, plant-like life of the adult animal, and the vesicle with its contained sensory organs disappears, the central nervous system becoming reduced to a small ganglion with associated nerve-fibres. The so-called single eye, according to Froriep, corresponds to the right lateral eye of vertebrates, and he has shown that there is a rudiment of a left eye also present, which is connected by nerve fibres with the neural tube. These fibres join the central nervous system at a point corresponding to the termination in the neural tube of the optic nerve of the right eye. The mode of development of this right lateral eye is indicated in Fig. 127, which shows an enlargement and elongation of certain cells forming a part of the right wall of the cerebral vesicle and a deposit of pigment on their inner or ventricular aspect. This placodal thickening of the wall of the cerebral vesicle is later converted into an optic vesicle, which instead of projecting outwards towards the cutaneous ectoderm becomes enclosed in the ventricular cavity. The " lens " and " retina " are formed by the clear cells which originally lay to the outer side of the pigment-mass and formed part of the wall of the cerebral vesicle. The lens is thus formed from neural ectoderm, not cutaneous ectoderm as in the lateral eyes of vertebrates generally, and there is no invagination of the outer wall of the optic vesicle to form an optic cup.[1] Light can only reach the eye-vesicle through the transparent body-wall and the wall of the cerebral- or sense-vesicle.

Owing to the eye of the ascidian larva being single, Salensky and others considered that it could not be homologous with the paired lateral

---

[1] It may be presumed that the absence of a lens developed from the cutaneous ectoderm is probably due to absence of the invagination of the neural ectoderm to form an optic cup. (R. J. G.)

eyes of vertebrates, but was comparable with the parietal eye of verte-brates. Froriep, however, considered that the site of origin of the primary optic plate in the early stages of development of the ascidian larva, namely on the right side of the cerebral vesicle, and the appearance of a similar but more rudimentary optic organ on the left side were presumptive evidence of the organs being homologous with the paired lateral eyes of vertebrates rather than with the " unpaired " median

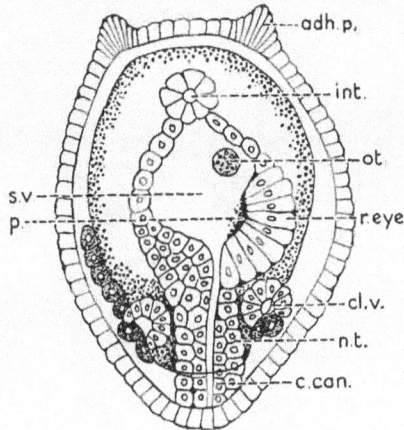

FIG. 127.—HEAD-END OF AN ASCIDIAN EMBRYO, PHALLUSIA MAMMILLATA, SEEN FROM THE DORSAL ASPECT. THE EPITHELIUM OF THE WALL OF THE CEREBRAL VESICLE ON THE RIGHT SIDE IS MODIFIED SO AS TO FORM A RETINAL OR OPTIC PLATE, CONSISTING OF RADIATING COLUMNAR CELLS, THE INNER ENDS OF WHICH ARE PIGMENTED.

adh. p. : adhesive papilla.
c. can. : central canal of medullary tube.
cl. v. : " cloacal vesicle " or atrium.
int. : intestine.
n.t. : wall of medullary tube.
ot. : statocyst.
p. : pigment.
r. eye : right eye.
s.v. : interior of sensory vesicle.

Compare with Fig. 3, which represents an older stage of development.
(From Korschelt and Heider, after Kowalevsky.)

or parietal eye of vertebrate animals. In this connection it is important to note that the statocyst of the ascidian larva is also a single organ, and that in explanation of this it seems likely that the full development of the corresponding area on the opposite side of the head and brain to that on which the existing statocyst has been developed was curtailed or arrested at an early stage. On the other hand, at the time (1906) when Froriep was writing it was not generally appreciated that the " parietal eye " of vertebrates has been derived from paired median organs of

which one has been more or less completely suppressed, while the other
has assumed a median position (*vide* Dendy, Gaskell, Hill, A. S. Woodward, Stensio, and others). The demonstration of the bilateral condition
of the eye in an ascidian larva is thus not in itself conclusive evidence
of the organ not being homologous with the " parietal organ " of verte-

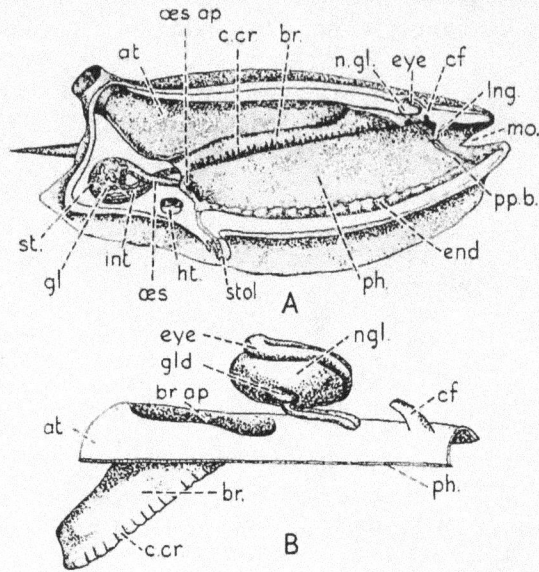

FIG. 128.—SALPA. A. LATERAL VIEW OF SECTION. B. ENLARGED LATERAL VIEW
OF THE EYE AND NEIGHBOURING PARTS (DIAGRAMMATIC).

at. : wall of atrial cavity.
br. : branchia.
c. cr. : ciliated crests on the edge of
the branchia.
cf. : ciliated funnel.
end. : endostyle.
gl. : digestive gland.
gld. : paired " neural gland."
ht. : heart.
int. : intestine.

lng. : languet.
mo. : mouth.
n. gl. : nerve ganglion.
œs. : œsophagus.
œs. ap. : opening of œsophagus.
ph. : pharynx.
pp. b. : peripharyngeal band.
st. : stomach.
stol. : stolon.

In B—*br. ap.* : branchial aperture ; *ph.* : wall of pharynx.
(After Delage and Hérouard, from Parker and Haswell.)

brates. Moreover, the structure of the ascidian eye is more like that
of the parietal organ of vertebrates than that of the lateral eyes, more
especially with regard to the absence of inversion and the formation of
the lens from neural ectoderm ; but as we shall see later, these objections
are not insuperable when we are dealing with degenerate organs, and the
site of origin of the optic plate on the right side of the early ascidian larva
is a point in favour of Froriep's contention.

The Eyes of Salpa and Allied Forms of Tunicata

Salpa, Fig. 128, A, belongs to the sub-order Hemimyaria of the order Thaliacea. It has a single horse-shoe shaped eye placed on the superficial aspect of a large oval nerve-ganglion (Fig. 128, B) and just behind the ciliated funnel which is the expanded opening of the ducts of the right and left " neural gland " (*n. gl.*). The branchial aperture is situated behind the nerve-ganglion. According to von Baer the nerve-ganglion of tunicates is placed upon the ventral surface of the larva, and does not therefore correspond to the cerebrospinal nervous system of vertebrates. More recently, however, the nervous system of the Prochordata has been studied by Bateson, Harmer, and Hill, and according to Kappers in the Enteropneusts (Ptycodera—*Balanoglossus*) both invertebrate and vertebrate types of nervous system are present in the same animal ; the invertebrate type being represented by the œsophageal ring and ventromedian neuroepithelium, and the vertebrate type by the medullary tube in the collar and by the frontal and caudal dorsomedial neuroepithelium. Whereas in tunicates the ventral primordium of the nervous system disappears and the dorsal medullary plate closes throughout the whole length of the body, except at the frontal end, where it remains open at the anterior neuropore, which lies close to the ciliated funnel and communicates secondarily with the pharynx.

The median eye of *Salpa* is sometimes supplemented by accessory eyes. An eye-spot is present in the larva of *Botryllus violacea*, a colonial type of tunicate ; and in one species of *Oikopleura*, a minute tunicate which is enclosed in a transparent envelope, like a glasshouse ; in this is a simple light-perceiving organ without pigment which is incorporated with the statocyst, and it may be noted that in Pyrosoma a single statocyst is placed in close relation to the cerebral ganglion and the ciliated funnel. The significance of the disappearance of one member of a pair of sense-organs, such as the otocysts or eye-vesicles in a degenerate type of animal, will become apparent when we consider the reduction in size or disappearance of one member of a pair of median eyes in vertebrates.

CHAPTER 16

CEPHALOCHORDA—ACRANIATA

THE pigment cells and light-percipient organs found in the lancelet fish, or *Amphioxus*, have been specially studied by Hesse and Joseph; the latter has shown that the pigment spot beneath the unpaired olfactory lobe, which has been described as the eye spot or median eye of the lancelet, consists merely of a cluster of cylindrical cells, filled with pigment granules which occupy the extreme anterior end of the " so-called " cerebral ventricle, and that in his opinion there is no structural resemblance between this group of pigment cells and even the simplest type of vertebrate eye. He also described similar cells in the dorsal region of the anterior part of the spinal cord. Neither the cells of the pigment spot or of the larger group at the anterior end of the spinal cord (cells of Joseph) are in relation with neuro-sensory cells, and it has been proved experimentally that neither are sensitive to light. Moreover, if these regions are removed by decapitation, the body of the animal still reacts to light. The explanation of this lies in the existence of the organs of Hesse (Fig. 129, A and B, p. 179), which consist of a series of single large neuro-sensory cells capped by a crescentic pigment layer which covers over one-half of the organ; a nerve process arises from the sensory cell, either from beneath the edge of the pigment cap, or opposite the centre of the cap. The pigment is arranged in three distinct layers, a thick band in the middle and two thin layers external and internal situated respectively superficial and deep to the middle layer. Between the pigment layers are two unpigmented strata which are believed by Boeke to contain neurofibrillæ in the cell-protoplasm.

The arrangement of the organs of Hesse in the spinal cord is remarkable. They are situated ventral and lateral to the central canal of the spinal cord commencing at the third or fourth segment, where they are most numerous and becoming less frequent towards the tail end. It is said also that on the left side of the cord the " eyes " are directed upward or dorsalward; on the right side, downward or ventralward (Fig. 129, A). Kappers remarks that as the animal usually lies on one side it would in this position perceive light reaching it in a horizontal plane. Beside the organs of Hesse, other neuro-sensory cells are found which lie in the ependyma lining the central canal, the neurites of which pass into the spinal cord (Edinger). This position of neuro-sensory cells is explained by the primary origin of the spinal cord from an open medullary plate lying on the superficial surface of the embryo, in the same morphological situation as the neuro-genetic or neuro-sensory epithelium of invertebrates. Similar cells have also been found in Ptychodera (a species allied to *Balanoglossus*) by van der Horst, in the collar region and extending forward and backward from this situation into the dorsal region.

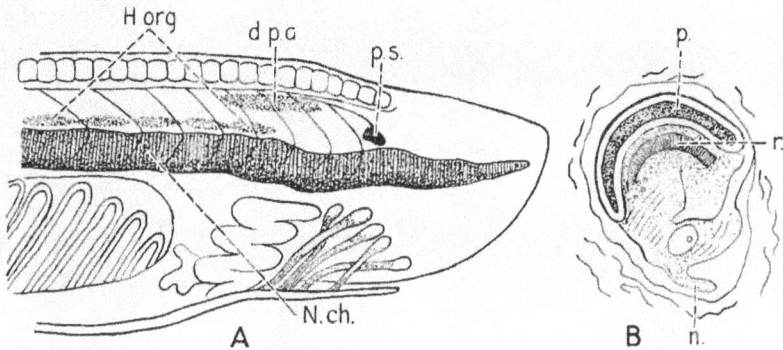

FIG. 129.—A : LATERAL VIEW OF THE HEAD-END OF AMPHIOXUS, SHOWING THE ANTERIOR PIGMENT SPOT, THE DORSAL PIGMENT AREA OF THE SPINAL CORD AND THE ORGANS OF HESSE. B : SECTION THROUGH ONE OF THE ORGANS OF HESSE.

d.p.a. : dorsal pigment area of spinal cord.　　*p.* : pigment.
H. org. : organs of Hesse.　　　　　　　　　*p.s.* : anterior pigment spot (eye).
n. : nerve.　　　　　　　　　　　　　　　　*r.* : rods.
N. ch. : notochord.

With regard to Joseph's statement concerning the histological structure of the pigment-spot of *Amphioxus*, it must be remembered that the cephalic region of this animal, which burrows head-downward in the sand, is degenerate, and that notwithstanding the want of resemblance of the " spot " to either a lateral or median vertebrate eye, the presence of pigment in this situation is significant,[1] as pigment is one of the most persistent of the tissue-elements both from the ontogenetic and phylo-genetic standpoints. It is quite common in aborted and macerated human embryos or fœtuses to find the eyes represented merely by a mass of degenerate pigment cells ; and Klinckowstroem has shown that the position of the pineal organ in sea-gulls and other birds is represented by a mass of irregularly distributed pigment cells in the parietal region (Chap. 3, p. 75).

[1] See p. 215.

CHAPTER 17
THE PINEAL SYSTEM OF VERTEBRATES
THE PARIETAL REGION

BEFORE commencing the description of the pineal system of vertebrates, it will be necessary to define certain terms which are applied
to structures included in the parietal region of the brain, namely, that
part of the roof of the interbrain or thalamencephalon which lies between the paraphysis in front and the posterior commissure of the
midbrain or mesencephalon behind. These structures are seen in their

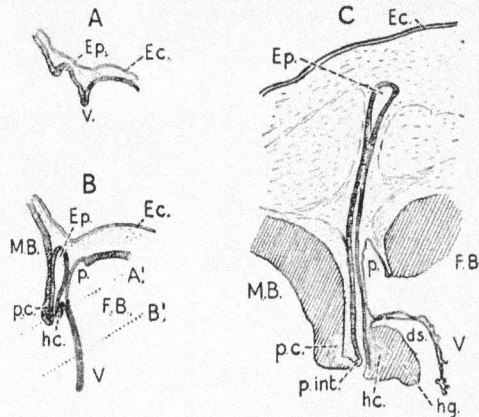

FIG. 130.—SAGITTAL SECTIONS OF ACANTHIAS EMBRYOS, SHOWING STRUCTURES
IN THE ROOF OF THE DIENCEPHALON. (AFTER C. S. MINOT.)

A : 15 mm. embryo ; B : 28 mm. embryo ; C : 70 mm. embryo.
A^1 : Plane of section, Fig. 139, A.
B^1 : Plane of section, Fig. 139, B.

ds. : dorsal sac.	hg. : habenular ganglion.
Ec. : Ectoderm.	p. : paraphysal arch.
Ep. : Epiphysis.	MB. : midbrain.
FB. : forebrain.	pc. : posterior commissure.
hc. : habenular commissure.	p. int. : pars intercalaris.

V. : velum transversum.

simplest form in the embryos of certain Teleostean fishes, e.g. *Acanthias
vulgaris* (Fig. 130), or among reptiles, *Lacerta muralis* (Fig. 173, Chap. 20,
p. 244).

From before backwards these parts include :
    (1) The paraphysis.
    (2) The velum transversum.

(3) The dorsal sac. Tela chorioidea superior.

(4) The habenular commissure (commissura superior).

(5) The pineal organs, including :

    (A) The pineal eye or parietal organ.

    (B) The " parapineal organ."

    (C) The connections of these organs with the central nervous system.

(6) Pars intercalaris (Schaltstück).

(7) The posterior commissure (commissura posterior).

When two pineal organs are present in or near the median plane, the term " Epiphysis I " has been used to denote the more anterior and " Epiphysis II " to denote the more posterior organ. When the term " epiphysis " is used alone it is generally applied to the primary embryonic diverticulum or to the pineal gland as distinct from the pineal eye or parietal organ. Thus the name " epiphysis " is usually applied to the deeply situated solid organ, e.g. that of the mammalian brain as contrasted with the superficial sensory vesicle or pineal eye of the lamprey or *Sphenodon*.

In addition to the above-mentioned structures, which are included in the parietal region of the brain, are accessory parts which comprise :

The fibrous coverings or capsule.

Pigment—(*a*) mesodermal ; (*b*) epidermal.

Pineal vessels and nerves.

The parietal cornea (Studnička).

The parietal plug (Dendy).

The parietal spot (P. fleck).

The parietal scale (P. schuppe).

The parietal plate or pineal plate.

The parietal pit or impression.

The pineal- or parietal-foramen.

The meaning of most of these terms is self-evident. The parietal cornea is, however, defined by Studnička as including all the translucent tissues lying over the parietal organ and between it and the superficial surface of the epidermis, whereas the name " parietal plug " was applied by Dendy to the conical mass of transparent tissue between the lens of the parietal organ and the deep surface of the corium or dermis in *Geotria*. The terms pineal plate or parietal plate are given to the bony plate which sometimes overlies the pineal organ in certain fishes and reptiles. The pineal plate may lie between the frontals, between the frontal and parietal bones, or between the parietal bones. It may or may not be perforated by a parietal foramen. It is perforated in the skull of *Lacerta agilis* ; not perforated in the arthrodiran fish *Dinichthys intermedius* found in the

Upper Devonian of Ohio (Fig. 131) and in that remarkable extinct Elasmo-branch fish *Pleuracanthus* (Fig. 141, B, p. 201). Examples of the latter have been found in the Carboniferous and Permian periods, and it would seem that a complete parietal foramen previously present in this plate had already disappeared at a date which preceded these two periods. The more primitive condition, namely, the presence of a parietal foramen, seen in the two examples cited, is thus exemplified in a living animal, the

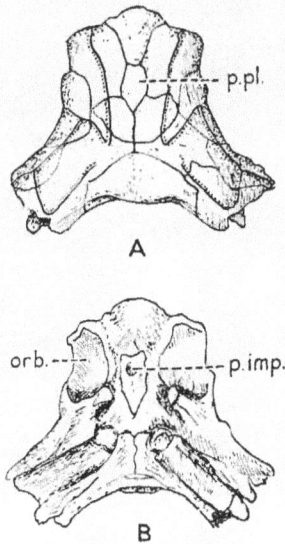

FIG. 131.—HEAD-SHIELD OF DINICHTHYS INTERMEDIUS. (AFTER A. S. WOOD-WARD.)

A—Upper surface.

B—Intracranial surface, the latter showing a well-defined pineal impression, from the upper Devonian of Ohio, U.S.A.

p. imp. : pineal impression.   p. pl. : pineal plate.
orb. : orbit.

lizard ; whereas the closed foramen, indicating a complete loss of visual function and atrophy, is seen in the fossil fish. In the still more ancient fish *Osteolepis*, however, a well-marked pineal foramen is present in a plate formed by the fusion of the two frontals and lying between the orbits (Fig. 132).

Definition of Terms applied to Structures in the Parietal Region of the Brain

1. *Paraphysis* (Fig. 130).—This is a sac-like evagination of the roof of the interbrain, which arises at the junction of the lamina supra-neuroporica and the inwardly projecting transverse fold, the velum transversum. The walls of the paraphysis which at the commencement of

its development are simple are apt to become much folded by the ingrowth of vascular processes of the surrounding mesoderm, so that in the fully developed state the paraphysis has the appearance of a complicated glandular structure and on account of its resemblance to the choroid plexuses of the ventricles was termed by Sorensen the " plexus chorioideus superior."   In some cases, e.g. in *Sphenodon*, it grows backwards

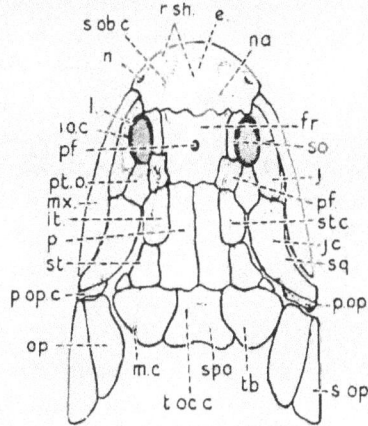

FIG. 132.—DORSAL VIEW OF OSTEOLEPIS MACROLEPIDOTUS, ONE OF THE MOST ANCIENT TYPES OF FOSSIL FISH FOUND IN THE UPPER SILURIAN AND DEVONIAN STRATA, SHOWING A PARIETAL FORAMEN IN THE FRONTAL BONE AND BETWEEN LARGE ORBITAL CAVITIES. (AFTER E. S. GOODRICH.)

e. : ethmoid, included in rostral-shield.
fr. : frontals fused and enclosing pineal foramen.
io.c. : infraorbital canal.
it. : intertemporal.
j. : jugal.
l. : lacrimal.
m.c. : main trunk-canal.
mx. : maxillary.
n. : nostril.
na. : nasal included in rostral-shield.
op. : opercular.
pf. : pineal foramen.
p. op. : pre-opercular.
p. op. c. : preopercular canal.
pt. f. : post frontal.
pt. o. : post-orbital.
r. sh. : rostral-shield.
so. : supra-orbital.
s. ob. c. : supraorbital canal.
s. op. : subopercular.
sp. oc. : dermal supra-occipital.
sq. : squamosal.
st. : supra-temporal or pterotic.
stc. : postorbital and supra temporal canal.
tb. : tabular.
t. oc. c. : transverse occipital canal.

over the dorsal sac between this and the pineal eye (Fig. 252, Chap. 24, p. 369). The paraphysis is frequently absent, e.g. in the adults of many mammals.

2. *Velum Transversum.*—A membranous fold which projects from the roof of the interbrain into the cavity of the ventricle. Its walls are usually smooth and simple, but it may be thrown into folds by the ingrowth of vessels, especially in its lower part. In some cases instead of forming a single transverse fold, it appears as two, paired folds, as in the Dipnoi, or is developed as an unpaired choroid plexus as in tailed amphibia.

3. *The Dorsal Sac.*—Fig. 252, Chap. 24, p. 369, and Fig. 130, p. 180, *ds*. This is an arched membranous fold which lies behind the transverse velum, the posterior layer of which forms the anterior boundary of the lower part of the dorsal sac. It projects towards the roof of the skull, between the pineal stalk and pineal nerve behind and the paraphysis in front. In some cases the dorsal sac grows backward on each side of the stalk of the epiphysis in the form of two blind pouches. The stalk in these cases may be enclosed in a tubular sheath of ependyma, or lie in a groove in the posterior wall of the sac. The wall of the sac is like that of the velum, in some cases smooth and simple, in others thrown into folds which may be vascular and form part of the tela chorioidea superior (Fig. 252).

4. *Commissura Habenularis.*—This, which is also named the superior commissure, appears later and is much smaller than the posterior commissure. It joins the right and left habenular ganglia. In some cases the habenular ganglia are fused in the median plane and the commissure is then enclosed in the centre of the mass, as in *Petromyzon*.

5. *The Pineal Organs.*

A. The *parietal organ*—(parietal eye; pineal eye; sensory-vesicle) (Fig. 133) : the principal or parietal sense-organ which is socketed in the roof of the skull may be derived from either the right (Cyclostomes) or left (*Sphenodon*) member of the primarily paired organ. In Cyclostomes it arises further back than the smaller vesicle which lies below it and to the left. The larger vesicle is therefore sometimes described as Epiphysis II whereas the term Epiphysis I is given to the small vesicle—" parapineal organ " of Studnička—which springs from a point farther forward and is connected with the anterior part of the left habenular ganglion (see Fig. 134, p. 188, and Fig. 22, Chap. 3, p. 28). It must be borne in mind, however, that this attachment in *Petromyzon* is one which has been secondarily displaced forward along with the anterior part of the left habenular ganglion and that the primary outgrowth of the pineal diverticulum was immediately in front of the posterior commissure.

The parietal sense-organ in those animals in which it is best developed, such as in the Cyclostomes and certain lizards, consists of a hollow vesicle, the superficial wall of which is lens-like, while the proximal part is differentiated as a retina of the upright type, having receptive sensory cells, pigment cells, and ganglion cells, with nerve-fibres proceeding from these to form a parietal or pineal nerve which terminates directly in the habenular ganglion of the same side or in either the habenular or posterior commissure, or in both of these and so reaches the habenular ganglia and other nerve centres with which the commissures

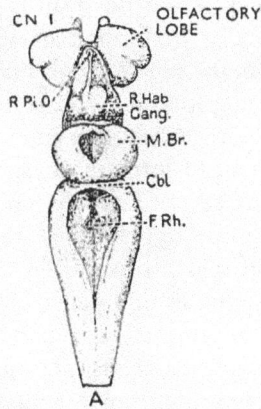

FIG. 133.—DORSAL VIEW OF THE BRAIN OF PETROMYZON MARINUS, SHOWING THE RIGHT PINEAL ORGAN AND LARGE RIGHT HABENULAR GANGLION. (AFTER AHLBORN.)

Cbl. : cerebellum ; *CN. I.* : cranial nerve I. ; *F. Rh.* : fossa rhomboidalis ; *M. Br.* : midbrain ; *R. Pi. O.* : right pineal organ.

are connected. The nerve-fibres may pass by the stalk of the parietal organ as in *Petromyzon*, or they may course independently of the stalk, being formed secondarily as in *Lacerta* (Figs. 172, D, 173, Chap. 20, pp. 243, 244).

The parietal sense-organ may be cut off and separated from the pedicle by the growth of the vault of the skull (Figs. 161, 162, Chap. 19, p. 228). In these cases it may persist throughout life as a functionless organ lying beneath the skin as in the frog, in which animal it remains as the " frontal organ " of Stieda, or it may fail to develop. In both cases the base of the stalk and other parts may persist as the pineal body (pineal organ ; pineal sac ; pineal gland ; conarium ; epiphysis), the detailed structure of which will be considered later.

B. The *parapineal organ :* this is the term which was applied by Studnička to the anterior smaller end-vesicle Epiphysis I of *Petromyzon* in his description of the pineal system of Cyclostomes. In reptiles it is represented according to Studnička by the anterior of the two organs, which in the Reptilia is the more fully developed organ and becomes the parietal eye. The posterior organ (pineal organ or Epiphysis) remains entirely within the cranial cavity, and though as in *Sphenodon* it may develop a terminal vesicle (pineal sac) (Fig. 252, Chap. 24, p. 369) it is cut off from all access of light and cannot function in any way as a visual organ. The same objection to the use of the terms " anterior organ " and " posterior organ " may be raised on developmental and morphological grounds as was made in discussing the terms Epiphysis I and Epiphysis II. The two organs in Sphenodon are developed from a single median diverticulum which afterwards is subdivided into two parts, an anterior vesicle which is separated off as a closed vesicle, the parietal organ or pineal eye and a posterior part which consists of the original stalk and an end-vesicle, the pineal sac. The stalk and pineal sac together form the pineal organ or epiphysis. On both developmental and morphological grounds Dendy regarded the anterior part of the diverticulum which becomes detached, to form the parietal sense-organ in *Sphenodon* as the representative of the primary left pineal eye, and the pineal sac as representing the primary right pineal eye and it would seem that the stalk which is common to both has arisen by approximation and fusion during phylogeny of the bases of a pair of bilaterally placed median eyes. If this interpretation is correct, the parapineal organ does not arise ontogenetically as a separate and distinct outgrowth from the roof of the interbrain, and does not spring from a separate cephalic metamere lying in front of the metamere which gives origin to the pineal organ. The separate anterior diverticulum which arises in front of the pineal diverticulum gives rise to the paraphysis and never develops a terminal sensory vesicle.

    C. The connections of the parietal organ and the parapineal organ with the central nervous system will be described separately with reference to different types of animals.

    6. *The Intercalated Segment* is a part of the roof plate which lies between the base of the pedicle of the pineal body and the posterior commissure. It is characterized by the absence in it of commissural nerve-fibres and it varies greatly in its extent in different types of animal.

    7. *The Posterior Commissure.* This lies immediately above the anterior end of the aqueductus cerebri, and receives some fibres from the pineal organ, in addition to its nuclear connections, and the connections with the median longitudinal bundles. It varies greatly in its size and extent in different animals, Figs. 130 and 208, Chap. 22, p. 303 (rabbit embryo). In some it is spread out in a series of bundles, while in others it is compressed into a rounded cord. The fibres which it receives from the parietal organ in *Petromyzon* are said by Studnička to divide in a T-shaped manner into branches which go to either side, but he was unable to trace their ultimate destination.

The Pineal Eyes of Cyclostome Fishes

The pineal eyes of this primitive class of vertebrates have been specially studied by Ahlborn, Wiedersheim, Studnička, Dendy, Beard and Gaskell. The class comprises the marine and freshwater lampreys (*Petromyzon*) and the Australian form of lamprey (*Geotria*) ; also the slime-eels or hag fishes (*Myxine* and *Bdellostoma*), *Bdellostoma* being so named on account of its leech-like mouth. It is described as being blind, parasitic and degraded in type, and specimens of it have been taken from great depths of the sea. The lampreys, on the other hand, although the median eyes are probably little more than light-percipient organs, have well-developed lateral eyes in the adult animal and are active in their movements. They feed on the flesh of living fishes and are predatory rather than parasitic.

The pineal system of the adult *Petromyzon* is situated close behind the single nasal orifice. It consists of two vesicles : one, the larger, called the *parietal organ*, is situated more superficially ; while the other, which is smaller and less differentiated, lies beneath the former (Fig. 22, Chap. 3, p. 28, and Fig. 134, p. 188). The latter was termed by Studnička the *parapineal organ*. The larger vesicle is connected by a definite tract, the pineal nerve, with the right habenular ganglion (Fig. 14, Chap. 3, p. 19), and also sends fibres into the posterior commissure and right bundle of Meynert (Fig. 134). The smaller vesicle is connected by a few fibres with the left habenular ganglion, posterior commissure, and left bundle of Meynert. Owing to its anterior attachment to the roof of the thalamencephalon or interbrain, the smaller organ is sometimes termed Epiphysis I, while the larger organ, on account of its posterior attachment, is known as Epiphysis II. The right habenular ganglion, in correspondence with the greater size of the superficial vesicle as compared with the smaller deep organ, is proportionally larger than the left habenular ganglion, and the right bundle of Meynert is for the same reason larger than the left bundle (Dendy, A., 1907).

Owing to the connection of the larger vesicle, by means of its pineal nerve, with the large right habenular ganglion, and the similar connection of the smaller vesicle by nerve-fibres with the small left habenular ganglion, and also the position of the smaller organ slightly to the left of the larger, along with other evidence of the bilateral origin of the two organs, Dendy, Gaskell, and others regarded the two vesicles as right and left members of a primarily paired organ, rather than anteriorly and posteriorly arranged unpaired metameric organs arising in the median plane. Professor Dendy also assumed that the smaller vesicle having undergone greater regressive changes than the larger, has been displaced beneath the larger. In this position, where it lies under cover of the superficial vesicle, it is obvious that the smaller, less differentiated organ has become quite functionless as a visual organ and that the small size

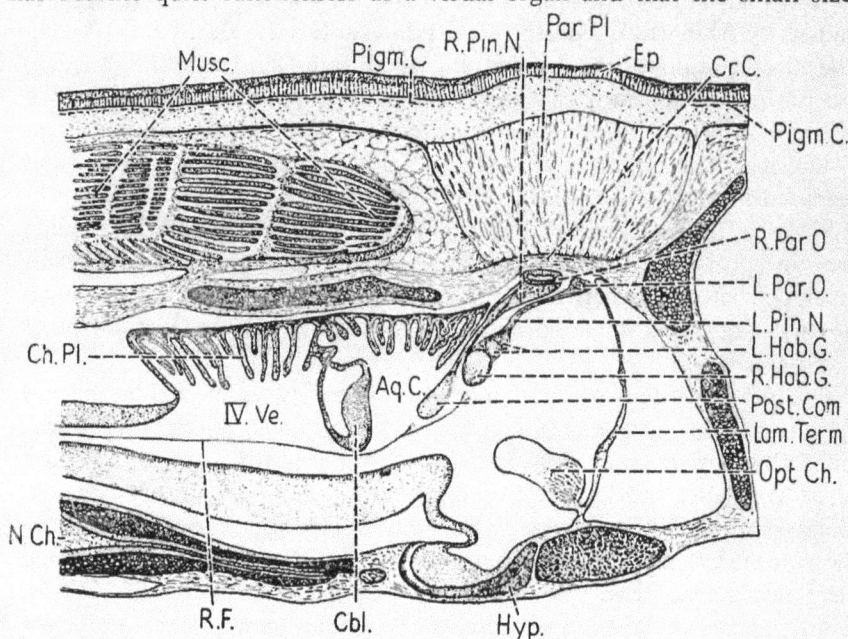

FIG. 134.—SAGITTAL SECTION THROUGH THE HEAD OF THE NEW ZEALAND LAMPREY (*Geotria*), SHOWING THE GENERAL POSITION AND CONNECTIONS OF THE RIGHT AND LEFT PINEAL EYES. (AFTER DENDY.)

Aq. C. : aqueductus cerebri.
Cbl. : cerebellum.
Ch. Pl. : choroid plexus.
Cr. C. : cranial capsule.
Ep. : epidermis.
Hyp. : hypophysis.
Lam. Term. : lamina terminalis.
L. Hab. G. : left habenular ganglion.
L. Par. O. : left parietal organ (parapineal organ).
L. Pin. N. : left pineal nerve.
Musc. : muscle.
N. Ch. : notochord.
Opt. Ch. : optic chiasma.
Par. Pl. : parietal plug.
Pigm. C. : pigment cells.
Post Com. : posterior commissure.
R.F. : Reissner's fibre.
R. Hab. G. : right habenular ganglion.
R. Par. O. : right parietal organ.
IV. Ve. : fourth ventricle.

of the left habenular ganglion as compared with the right, is correlated with this displacement and loss of function. Lying directly over the larger vesicle, is a thick conical plug of translucent mesenchymatous tissue which is especially well developed in *Geotria*, the New Zealand lamprey (Fig. 134).

This fills a gap in the cartilaginous roof of the skull. Above is a layer of loose subcutaneous connective tissue and the epidermis. The hypodermal cells of the latter are peculiar in containing no pigment granules such as are present in this layer elsewhere, neither is there any pigment in the subepidermal tissue. All the tissues between the parietal organ and the superficial surface of the epidermis are translucent and constitute the " parietal cornea " as defined by Studnička. The pineal organ can thus be seen through the cornea and appears as a central white spot (Fig. 48, Chap. 3), as described on p. 71.

Sections of the larger superficial vesicle (Fig. 45, Chap. 3) show that the " eye " is of the ocellar or upright type. It consists of a superficial or distal segment—the " lens "—termed by Studnička the " pellucida " and a deep or proximal segment, the retina. These are continuous with each other at the circumference of the vesicle and they enclose between them a central cavity filled with a loose syncytial tissue which in the living animal is believed to enclose within its meshes a clear semi-fluid material. The whole tissue with the viscous fluid contained in its spaces is termed the vitreous. The cavity is in some specimens funnel-shaped (Fig. 45, Chap. 3, p. 69, and Fig. 14, Chap. 3, p. 19). The distal ends of the columnar cells of the retina converge towards the lumen of the " groove " or " tube " forming the narrow part or stalk of the funnel much in the same way as they do in the cylindrical upright eyes of certain arthropods, e.g. *Acilius sulcatus*, which in the large parietal eyes of young larvæ, about 10–12 mm. long show a central cleft in the retina ; this, as pointed out by Gaskell, is strikingly similar to that in the parietal organ of *Ammocœtes*. The cleft in the *Acilius* larva, moreover, is directly continuous with the virtual cavity which occupies the central axis of the cylindrical " vitreous " segment of the eye of *Acilius sulcatus* (Grenacher). It must be borne in mind, however, that the bottom of the cleft in an *Acilius* or *Dytiscus* larva (Fig. 38, Chap. 3, p. 53) corresponds to the bottom of the optic pit, from which the eye is developed as a downgrowth of the surface epithelium into the sub-epidermal tissue ; whereas in *Ammocœtes* the blind end of the diverticulum from the roof of the interbrain is directed distally away from the stalk, and the cleft or atrium is in the stalk near the proximal end of the vesicle (Fig. 137, B). With reference to the supposed origin of the funnel-shaped prolongation of the cavity of the main vesicle into the distal end of the " optic stalk," it will be convenient to allude here to the position and relations of the atrium, which is a small accessory cavity in the wall of the main parietal organ. The atrium varies considerably in size and shape in different specimens ; it is usually situated behind and below the cavity of the main vesicle with which it communicates in the majority of cases, although it is in some completely cut off and appears as an independent closed vesicle lying between the proximal end of the funnel-shaped cavity and the exit of the pineal nerve. The wall of the atrium is composed of cells which are columnar in type. The free ends of these converge towards the central cavity, while their nuclei are peripheral (Fig. 45). Around these cells is an accumulation of irregularly disposed cells, the nuclei of which resemble those of the surrounding ganglion cells. The atrium therefore has been thought by some writers to represent a nerve ganglion situated in the wall of the vesicle and interposed between the sensory or visual cells and the tract of nerve-fibres which connect it with the habenular ganglion. Others, however, considering the similarity of the columnar cells lining its cavity to the columnar cells of the retina, regard the atrium as a part of the general cavity of the organ which has been either wholly or partially constricted off, and corresponds either to a secondary diverticulum from the main outgrowth or a part of the cavity of its stalk. According to Kuppfer (1894) the primary outgrowth of the diverticulum from the roof of the interbrain is at first directed backward ; later an extension forward takes place, so that in a median sagittal section its cavity including that of the stalk appears T-shaped, and it seems possible that the posterior limb of the cross-bar of the T persists as the atrium whereas the distal part of the vertical bar remains as the stem of the funnel.

The retina (Figs. 45 and 46, Chap. 3, pp. 69, 70) consists of (1) sensory cells ; (2) tall, columnar cells containing the so-called " white pigment " ; (3) ganglion-cells lying in a plexiform layer of nerve-fibres, with a few spindle-shaped neuroglial or connective tissue cells. There are also an internal and an external limiting membrane and a thin fibrous capsule continuous with the pia mater of the brain. The sensory or visual cells end distally in a flask-shaped or bulbar swelling covered over by a cap of clear finely granular material which frequently tapers at its extremity into a fine thread which is continuous with a syncytial fibre of the vitreous. The base of the knob or flask rests on the internal limiting membrane and is continuous through the membrane with the thin rod-like outer end of the body of the cell ; the oval nucleus is situated in a spindle-shaped swelling of the body near the base of the cell. Proximal to the nucleus, the body of the cell tapers into a fine nerve process which subdivides in a plexus of nerve-fibres containing the ganglion cells, the axons of which course in a tangential direction in the latter and join to form the pineal nerve.

The interpretation of specimens prepared by the silver impregnation methods is difficult. Cells which are heavily impregnated are found in the lens, and according to Studnička's description of specimens prepared by Retzius many of the cells which are blackened in the retina are supporting ependymal cells which show typical sole-like thickenings, where their outer or proximal ends are attached to the external limiting membrane, whereas the inner or distal ends of the columnar retinal cells which contain the pigment remain unstained. On the other hand the nerve-fibre layer and the continuity of many of the nerve-fibres with the fibres of the pineal-nerve ; and also of the retinal cells of the parapineal organ and the connections of these with the anterior (left) habenular ganglion and the nerve-fibres of the pineal tract were well brought out by the impregnation process.

The columnar cells containing the " white pigment " (Fig. 45, B) are variously regarded as being : (1) ependymal cells, which function as supporting cells and are comparable to the " fibres of Müller " in the retina of the lateral eyes (Studnička) ; (2) " pigment " cells, which

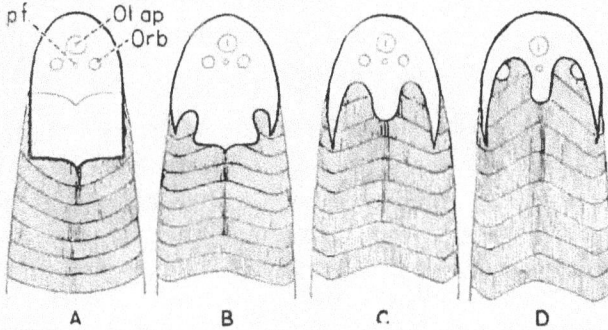

FIG. 135.—DIAGRAM TO SHOW THE DIFFERENT SHAPES OF HEAD-SHIELD, DUE TO THE FORWARD GROWTH OF THE SOMATIC MUSCULATURE. (AFTER GASKELL.)
A : Didymaspis ; B : Auchenaspis ; C : Cephalaspis ; D : Ammocoetes.
Ol. ap. : olfactory aperture ; Orb. : orbital cavity ; p.t. : parietal foramen.

contain a crystalline deposit of calcium phosphate, guanin, and a small quantity only of melanin. The deposit of phosphate of lime was regarded by both Mayer and Gaskell as an indication of degeneration and comparable with the " brain sand " found in the pineal body of mammalia.

The Parietal Foramen of Ammocœtes

The position of the narial and pineal openings in the muco-cartilage which forms the temporary head shield of an *Ammocœte* was studied by Gaskell, who compared the dorsal head-shield of the larval lamprey with the very similar head-shields of certain extinct fishes, belonging to the class Ostracodermata, and more particularly *Didymaspis, Auchenaspis,* and *Cephalaspis* (Fig. 135) ; in all of which the parietal foramen is placed behind the single nasal aperture and between the two orbital cavities for the lateral eyes. He also compared the microscopical structure of the head-shields of the Ostracodermata, as represented by Rohon, with that of the muco-cartilage of *Ammocœtes*, and found a marked similarity, more especially with regard to the disposition of the spaces relative to the matrix. A still further point of agreement which Gaskell emphasized is the relation of the somatic musculature to the head region. The somatic musculature seems to have advanced forward in successive stages of phylogeny and encroached upon the posterior border of the head-shield, causing a gradual absorption of this border on either side of the median hard plate which overlies and protects the brain, thus producing a notch on each side between the tongue-shaped plate which overlies and protects the brain and the lateral cornua. Gaskell further suggested that this plate on account of its position and general relations should receive the same name as the similar plate in the trilobites and be called the " glabella."

Since Gaskell's time the microscopical structure and general architecture of the head-shields of the Ostracodermata has been re-investigated, with the aid of modern methods of technique, by Stensiö and Kiaer, and an account of their work will be found in the section on Geological Evidence of the Existence of Median Eyes in Vertebrates, Chapter 23.

The Pineal Nerve, Chiasma and the Pineal or Habenular Tract.

The nervus pinealis was first described by Ahlborn (1883) as the stalk of the epiphysis. A point of considerable developmental interest is the relation that the delicate pineal nerve of the adult *Petromyzon* has to the original hollow stalk of the pineal diverticulum in the embryo. In other words, does the pineal nerve of the mature lamprey correspond in its mode of development to the optic nerve of the lateral eyes of vertebrates ? Or is it developed independently of the stalk of the primary pineal outgrowth ? Also, is there anything in the pineal system of the lamprey comparable with the optic chiasma, optic tracts, and central connections of the lateral eyes of vertebrates ? These questions are intimately bound up with that of the development of the two pineal vesicles, the nerve-fibres arising from them and the central connections of these with the habenular ganglia and the anterior and posterior commissures. According to Kuppfer (1894) (Fig. 138, A, p. 196) and Johnstone (Fig. 136), two separate pineal diverticula are developed ; a smaller anterior and a large posterior. Studnička (1893) quite independently came to the same conclusion, but Kuppfer's figure shows the anterior diverticulum in front of the anterior commissure, a position which throws a grave doubt on the identity of the small recess which he depicts, with the future parapineal organ (Fig. 22, p. 28). On the other hand, Balfour (4·8 mm. larva of *Petromyzon*), Dohrn (Fig. 138, B, p. 196), and the well-known figures by Dohrn depicting the early developmental stages of the olfactory and pituitary sacs of *Petromyzon*, show only one pineal diverticulum. These authors and others describe only a single diverticulum which spreads forward, backward, and also laterally. In the later stages of development the stalk becomes elongated and its lumen disappears, the two terminal

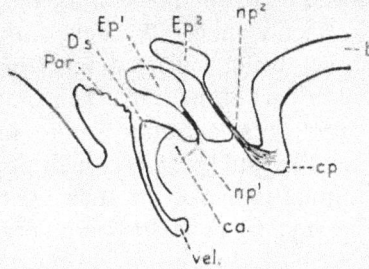

FIG. 136.—SCHEMATIC DIAGRAM DESIGNED TO SHOW THE RELATIONS OF THE TWO EPIPHYSES IN VERTEBRATES. (AFTER J. B. JOHNSTONE.)

ca. : anterior commissure.		np.[1] : nerve of anterior epiphysis.	
cp. : posterior commissure.		np.[2] : nerve of posterior epiphysis.	
D.s. : dorsal sac.		Par. : paraphysis.	
Ep.[1] : anterior epiphysis.		t. : tectum.	
Ep.[2] : posterior epiphysis.		vel. : velum.	

vesicles being carried forward away from the original site of origin of the diverticulum, namely, between the anterior and posterior commissures. On the left side a part of the left habenular ganglion is carried forward with the anterior or ventral terminal vesicle, and forms the " cushion " described by Ahlborn on which the vesicle rests (Fig. 22, Chap. 3, p. 28) ; the remaining part of the ganglion is left in its original position, the two parts of the ganglion being connected by a strand of nerve-fibres called the " pineal or habenular tract." The whole of the larger right habenular ganglion appears to remain in its original position. It is connected with the superficial vesicle or " parietal organ " by the " pineal nerve " and by some commissural or chiasma fibres with the posterior part of the left habenular ganglion ; these fibres constitute the habenular or anterior commissure. The right pineal nerve (Dendy, Studnička) is connected with the posterior commissure and right bundle of Meynert as well as with the right habenular ganglion.

The intermediate stages of development between the adult condition and the embryonic condition have, so far, not been completely filled in. Studnička, however, showed that the pineal nerve of a 35-mm. *Ammocœtes* (Fig. 137, *a*) extended backward from the parietal organ to the posterior-commissure, and that the nerve-fibres at this stage were enclosed throughout the whole length of the nerve in a nucleated sheath which was continuous anteriorly with the wall of the parietal organ. In transverse sections of the pineal nerve, obtained from an *Ammocœtes* of similar age, the proximal end of the nerve (Fig. 137, *d*) consisted almost exclusively of

13

nerve-fibres, while at the distal end near the atrium (Fig. 137, *b*) the
greater part of the section was occupied by epithelial cells; the nerve-
fibres here being confined to the lower and lateral parts in the periphery
of the section.   In the middle of the nerve (Fig. 137, *c*) the nerves were
in the lower part of the section, the cells above; the nerve-fibres were
evenly distributed, not yet being collected together in cords.   In the
adult *Petromyzon* in the last part of the stalk, the nerve-fibres are arranged
in definite layers; moreover, outside the nerve-fibres in the fully developed
pineal nerve, separate cells are still present which Studnička regarded as
being vestiges of the original tissue of the stalk.   These cells are found
either in the centre (Fig. 137, *e*) or at the periphery.   The special pia-

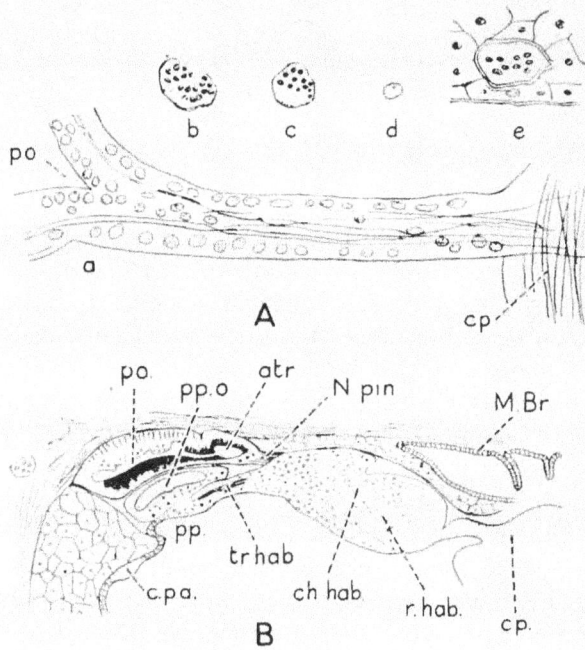

FIG. 137.

A—*a.* : Longitudinal section of the pineal nerve of a 35-mm. *Ammocœtes*;
   b, c, d : Transverse sections through different parts of the pineal nerve from
   a similar specimen; *b* : near the atrium; *c* : about the middle of the
   nerve; *d* : through the proximal part; *e* : transverse section through the
   pineal nerve of an older Ammocœtes.   (After Studnička.)

B—Sagittal section through the parietal region of the brain of an older *Ammocœtes*.
   The atrium of the parietal organ is exceptionally large, and is situated at
   the same level as the lumen of the parietal organ.

   atr. : atrium.   *po.* : parietal organ.
   cp. : commissura posterior.   *pp.* : paraphysis.
   c.p.a. : commissura pallii anterior.   *pp. o.* : parapineal organ.
   ch. hab. : chiasma habenularis.   *r. hab.* : right habenular ganglion.
   M. Br. : midbrain.   *tr. hab.* : tractus habenularis.
   N. pin : nervus pinealis.

matral sheath of the stalk which is continuous with that of the parietal organ, and covers a limiting neuroglial membrane is also considered by Studnička as evidence of the pineal nerve being formed from and representing the stalk of the primary diverticulum. The pineal nerve of *Petromyzon* thus appears to differ from that of *Lacerta* (see p. 243), in which the nerve-fibres are developed separately and independently of the original stalk (Figs. 172, 173, Chap. 20). The explanation of this difference probably lies in the circumstance that while in Cyclostomes the stalk remains for a sufficiently long period to form a ready made pathway for the nerve-fibres to take, in their growth from the retina to the habenular ganglion; in amphibia and in reptiles the parietal organ is cut off from the stalk before the growth of the nerve-fibres commences.

On the left side the statement that true nerve-fibres pass from the left terminal vesicle to the anterior part of the left habenular ganglion is said by Studnička not to have been confirmed, but whether the fibres joining the two parts are true nerve-fibres or not, the connection between the vesicle and the ganglion obviously represents the stalk of the left pineal organ, in which, if the vesicle should retain any sensibility to light, the nerve-fibres would be developed.

With regard to the term " pineal tract " which is rightly applied to the strand of nerve-fibres connecting the two parts of the left habenular ganglion (Fig. 137, B, and Fig. 22, Chap. 3); if the ganglion cells of the right parietal organ of *Petromyzon* are regarded in the same light as those in the retina of a lateral vertebrate eye, namely as retinal, then the right pineal nerve of the lamprey, like the " optic nerve " of the human eye, is strictly speaking a " nerve tract," similar to inter-ganglionic nerve-tracts in the central nervous system generally, and the distinction implied between the terms " pineal nerve " and " pineal tract " is misleading. From the morphological standpoint the ganglion-cells around the atrium and elsewhere in the retina of the right parietal organ of *Petromyzon* probably correspond to those of the anterior part of the left habenular ganglion and the pineal nerve of the right pineal organ represents and corresponds to the pineal tract of the left organ. On the right side the anterior ganglion cells appear to have been incorporated in the retina; on the left side they have remained as a separate ganglion outside the vesicle, but connected with it by a wide stalk of neuroglial tissue, which is surrounded by a constricting fold of pia mater.

The Development of the Parietal Organ of Petromyzon

According to Studnička's description of the development of the two parietal organs, the " pineal organ " is the first to develop (Fig. 138). It appears at the posterior part of the roof of the interbrain in the form of a small, caudally directed diverticulum, the wall of which is formed by a single layer of cells. This soon becomes bent forward, and after having considerably increased in size two parts may be distinguished, a proximal

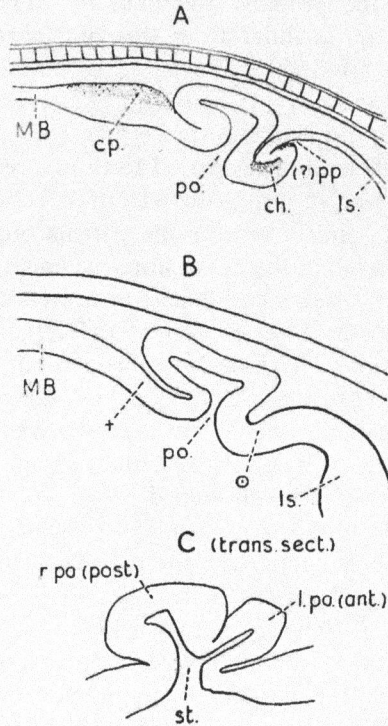

FIG. 138.

A and B : Median sagittal sections of the parietal region of the brain, showing early stages in the development of the pineal organs of *Petromyzon*. (A after Kuppfer ; B after Dohrn.)

C—Transverse section of the rudiments of the pineal organs of a 37-day-old embryo of *Salmo fontinalis*. (After Hill.)

> *ch. :* habenular commissure.
> *cp. :* posterior commissure.
> *l. po. :* left pineal organ (anterior).
> *ls. :* lamina supraneuroporica.
> *MB. :* roof of midbrain.
> *po. :* pineal organ.
> *pp. :* parapineal organ (Kuppfer and Studnička).
> *r. po. :* right pineal organ (posterior).
> *st. :* common stalk of right and left pineal diverticula.

hollow stalk immediately in front of the posterior commissure, which has meanwhile been developed, and a dorsoventrally flattened vesicular end-part which lies over the stalk, namely the " terminal vesicle " (Fig. 139). The terminal vesicle at this stage of development lies directly over the ganglia habenulæ, which are already present, and it raises the skin over it so as to form a slight prominence. The whole organ at this period is, relatively to the brain, exceptionally large ; its transverse diameter being little less than that of the interbrain. The terminal vesicle which at first had a large lumen becomes transformed into a " loaf-like " structure. Its upper wall remains thin and single layered, whilst its lower wall becomes thickened, its superficial surface being arched upwards so that the floor and roof of the vesicle are in close contact with each other, and in transverse section the lumen appears as a crescentic cleft, convex superficially (Fig. 139). After a time, however, the lumen again enlarges and the two walls of the vesicle become separated again. Still later (Fig. 137, B), the lumen of the stalk disappears, except below where a small part persists as the recessus pinealis, which lies in front of the posterior commissure, and

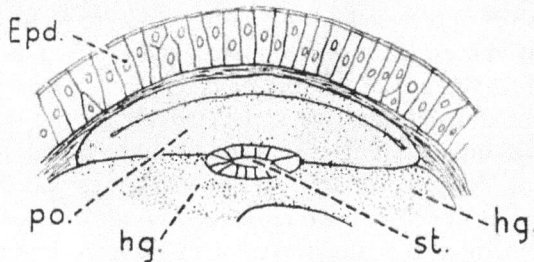

FIG. 139.—TRANSVERSE SECTION THROUGH THE PINEAL ORGAN OF A 6-mm. EMBRYO OF PETROMYZON PLANERI. (AFTER STUDNIČKA.)

Epd. : epidermis.   po. : pineal organ.
hg. : habenular ganglion.   st. : stalk.

above in the situation where the stalk becomes continuous with the terminal vesicle. From the lower wall or retina of the terminal vesicle nerve-fibres grow into the stalk, the cells of the latter being pushed aside or penetrated in the same way as in the development of optic nerves of the paired [lateral] eyes, and it is in this way that the nervus pinealis is developed. At the upper end of the stalk, there is formed at a later stage a fairly large hollow cavity, the " atrium," the walls of which " remind one " of the structure of the retina, and as a rule the atrium opens into the cavity of the end vesicle near the centre of the retina, where there is a funnel-shaped recess. Subsequently the parietal organ is shifted forward from its point of origin in the region of the ganglia habenulæ to a position, in the fully developed brain, in the region of the hemispheres.

Studnička's description of the development of the parapineal organ is not so explicit and it is probable that the recess which is shown in Kuppfer's diagram in front of the anterior commissure does not give origin to the parapineal organ, but that this arises as a subdivision of the primary pineal diverticulum.

From the foregoing description it will be evident that the pineal system of the Cyclostomes may be considered as a vestigial apparatus, which consists of an imperfectly developed pair of median eyes of the upright type, of which one, the left, is more degenerate than the other, and has been displaced beneath the other less degenerate right organ. Since the latter is placed immediately beneath a transparent " cornea " and has a retina provided with sensory cells, the inner ends of which are connected with the dendrites of ganglion cells, and by nerve-fibres arising from these with the habenular ganglia and posterior commissure ; the right organ may be regarded as capable of receiving impressions of light and transmitting these to the central nervous system. But owing to the imperfect development of the dioptric system no distinct image of an object on the retina is possible. It may be conjectured, however, that in the ancestors of the Cyclostomes both eyes were equally developed, were structurally more highly differentiated and reached to the surface of the body. The absence of a cuticular or epidermal lens in the living representatives of the class may be accounted for by the withdrawal of the eyes from the surface. This supposition being granted, the structure of the pineal eye does not differ very greatly or essentially from the upright median eyes of certain invertebrates.

The development of the lateral eyes of *Petromyzon* is similar to that of vertebrates in general ; an optic cup being formed by inversion of the distal part of the primary optic vesicle to form the sensitive part of the retina, while the proximal segment gives rise to the outer or ensheathing layer of the cup and becomes pigmented. The lens also is derived from the cutaneous ectoderm in the usual manner, a hollow vesicle becoming separated from the superficial epithelium by an ingrowth of mesoderm (Fig. 252, Chap. 24, p. 369).

Variations of the Pineal System in the Different Orders of the Class Cyclostomata

It is unnecessary to give a detailed description of the variations which occur among the different species of *Petromyzon*. It is of interest, however, to note that in *Mordacia mordax*, the pineal organ of which was described by Spencer in 1890, he found no trace of a parapineal organ. Also in the hag-fishes, belonging to the Order Myxinoidei, although several authors have described a single vestigial diverticulum without any thickening of the lens, or pigment in the retina, there seems some doubt as to whether these outgrowths were true pineal diverticula, and according to Kuppfer, who carefully examined a series of specimens in 1900, the parietal region behind the velum is quite smooth and he found no trace of an epiphysis. Both *Myxine* and *Bdellostoma* are said to be blind, to a large extent parasitic and of degraded type. Like the lampreys, they feed on the flesh of fishes, but instead of clinging on to the surface of the body, they actually bore their way into the flesh.

The description of the pineal system of the extinct Ostracoderms, which have been shown by Stensiö and Kiaer to be very closely related to the living representatives of the Cyclostomata, will be referred to in Chapter 23, on the Geological Evidence of Median Eyes in Vertebrates and Invertebrates.

CHAPTER 18

THE PINEAL SYSTEM OF THE CLASS PISCES

THIS class includes the cartilaginous and bony fishes, the Holocephali and Dipnoi. Besides the living representatives of the class, there are many extinct forms (for example, Fig. 140) the consideration of which is of the greatest importance with respect to the history and nature of the pineal system as a whole.

The study of the pineal organs in the various types of living fishes

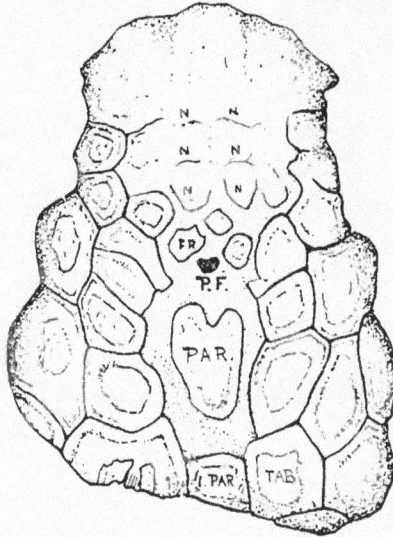

FIG. 140.—DORSAL VIEW OF THE HEAD OF DIPNORHYNCHUS, A PRIMITIVE FOSSIL FISH FROM THE MIDDLE DEVONIAN ROCKS OF NEW SOUTH WALES. (REDUCED ¼.)

A median spine subdivides the anterior border of the parietal foramen, there being a crescentic notch on each side of it. This is considered to be an indication of the bilateral origin of the parietal organ.

P.F. : parietal foramen.	*FR.* : frontal.
PAR. : parietal.	*N.* : nasal.
I. PAR. : interparietal.	*TAB.* : tabular.

(After E. S. Hills.)

at first sight appears as if it would be somewhat barren. There is no well differentiated sense-organ such as that in Cyclostomes and certain reptiles ; nor is there any special development of the proximal part, as in the pineal gland or epiphysis of birds and mammals. The general impression is that of a vestigial structure, any variations of which, such as are present in different types of living fish, being chiefly accountable on

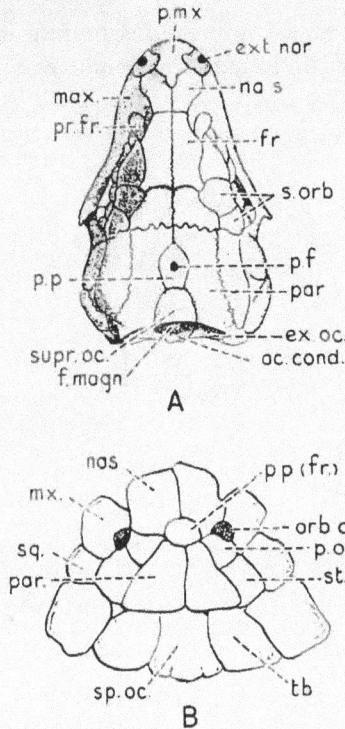

FIG. 141.—THE PARIETAL OR PINEAL PLATE OF LACERTA AGILIS AND OF PLEURA-
CANTHUS, A PRIMITIVE TYPE OF FOSSIL FISH BELONGING TO THE CARBONI-
FEROUS AND PERMIAN ERA. IN LACERTA A PARIETAL FORAMEN AND PARIETAL
SENSE-ORGAN ARE STILL PRESENT. IN THE EXTINCT PLEURACANTHUS THE
PARIETAL FORAMEN HAD ALREADY DISAPPEARED.

A : *Lacerta agilis.* (After W. K. Parker.)

ex. oc. : exoccipital.	*par. :* parietal.
ext. nar. : external nares.	*p. mx. :* præmaxilla.
f. magn. : foramen magnum.	*p.f. :* parietal foramen.
fr. : frontal.	*pp. :* pineal plate.
max. : maxilla.	*pr. fr. :* praefrontal.
nas. : nasal.	*s. orb. :* supraorbitals.
oc. cond. : occipital condyle.	*supr. oc. :* supraoccipital.

B : *Pleuracanthus.* Dermal bones of the head seen from above. (After Davies.)

mx. : maxilla.	*pp. (fr.):* pineal plate, probably repre-
nas. : nasal.	senting fused frontals.
orb. c. : orbital cavity.	*sp. oc. :* supra-occipital.
par. : parietal.	*sq. :* squamosal.
po. : postorbital.	*st. :* supratemporal.
	tb. : tabular.

the hypothesis of there being a greater or less degree of retrogressive change from a more highly evolved system which existed in the extinct ancestors of the living species to the relics of that system which are left in the fishes of to-day.

A comparison of the pineal impressions present in fossil types of fish with the conditions found in living representatives of the class (Fig. 132, Chap. 17, p. 182, Fig. 231, Chap. 23, p. 330, and Fig. 49, Chap. 3, p. 73) reveals different stages in the devolution of a system in which paired and

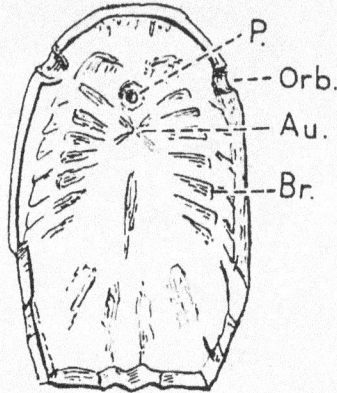

FIG. 142.—UNDER SURFACE OF THE HEAD SHIELD OF CYATHASPIS (JAEKEL), UPPER SILURIAN.

P. : Impression which is believed to have been produced by median eye (epiphysis).
Orb. : Orbital notch for lateral eye.
Br. : Impressions supposed to be for branchial sacs.
Au. : Impressions thought to have been caused by the auditory organs.

presumably sensory end-organs existed outside the skull immediately beneath the skin, to the vestigial condition which is found in many of the living adult forms of fish, in which all traces of the bilateral nature seem to have disappeared and nothing but a simple tubular stalk and the proximal part or base persist. There are, however, a few cases in which a double or partially subdivided parietal foramen has been recorded in living types of fish (Cattie), and indications of the bilateral nature of the pineal diverticulum have been recorded in the embryos of several species of fish belonging to different orders (Figs. 149, 150, 151, 152).

Some interesting observations were made by Locy on the earliest stages of the development of the pineal system in dog-fish embryos. He stated that in the neural plate of an embryo 3 mm. long of *Squalus acanthias,* before the closure of the plate to form the neural tube, there are three pairs of depressions : namely, an anterior, which gives rise to the optic vesicles of the lateral eyes, and two pairs of accessory depressions (Fig. 143), of which the anterior pair, placed immediately behind the optic grooves, gives rise to the walls of the thalamencephalon and the principal outgrowth from it, the epiphysis. When the neural tube is closed the two members of the pair unite to form the epiphysis which in his opinion is therefore double in origin, being formed from a united pair of accessory optic vesicles. He also considered it highly probable that the enlarged distal end of the epiphysis in *Squalus* is homologous with the pineal eye of those forms in which it is differentiated as a median eye.

With reference to these observations it would be interesting to obtain further observations on these early stages in other animals. The majority

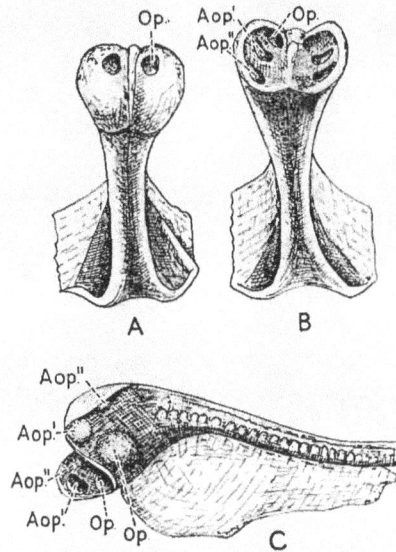

FIG. 143.

A : Embryo of *Squalus acanthias* 3 mm. long; three somites; showing the first appearance of the optic vesicle, *Op*.
B : Slightly older embryo showing in addition to the primary pair of optic vesicles two pairs of accessory vesicles, *Aop.'*, *Aop."*
C : Embryo with open neural groove placed in such a position as to give an external view of the vesicles on one side and an internal view on the opposite side of the neural folds. Locy believed that the accessory vesicles were homologous with the optic vesicles and that the pineal outgrowth was formed in *Squalus acanthias* by the union of the anterior pair of accessory optic vesicles.

(Redrawn from Locy's figures : *Anat. Anz.*, 1893, Bd. IX.)

of writers describe the pineal outgrowth as being primarily single and first appearing after the neural tube has become closed, the subdivision of the primarily single diverticulum into parietal sense-organ (when this is developed) and epiphysis taking place later. As far as we are aware, the development of two separate diverticula, arising independently of each other in the median plane, has not been described, although such have sometimes been shown in a diagram, such as Fig. 136, p. 193, and Fig. 138, Chap. 17, p. 196, which is intended to represent in a simple, schematic form the relations which exist either in the embryonic condition or the adult animal in certain types, such as *Petromyzon*.

The Pineal Organ of Elasmobranchs

It will be convenient to describe first the development of the parietal region of the brain of a typical cartilaginous fish, e.g. *Squalus acanthias*, the spiny dog-fish. The different stages of development of this fish were especially investigated by C. Sedgwick Minot in embryos ranging from 11·5 mm. to 86 mm. in length (Figs. 130, A, B, C, Chap. 17, p. 180). All the component parts of the roof of the diencephalon are present in *Acanthias*, namely the paraphysal arch, including the paraphysis ; the velum transversum ; the post-velar arch or dorsal sac ; the habenular commissure ; the epiphysis, pars intercalaris, and posterior commissure. Associated with the habenular commissure are, on each side, the habenular ganglia, which as compared with the corresponding ganglia in higher types are of relatively large size in *Acanthias* (Fig. 130, C).

In the early stages, e.g. a 15-mm. embryo, the paraphysal arch (Fig. 130, B) is a simple, rounded elevation projecting from the roof of the diencephalon immediately in front of the pineal diverticulum. In a sagittal section it might readily be mistaken for an anterior pineal diverticulum. Its walls are, however, thin, and at a later stage of development it gives rise to the paraphysis. The latter appears at the summit of the arch in a 34-mm. embryo, and at the 70-mm. stage is a simple but slightly folded sac which projects vertically upward immediately in front of the stalk of the pineal diverticulum. The velum transversum hangs downwards in the ventricular cavity, where it forms a transverse fold the lateral edges of which are continued forward as the choroid plexuses of the ventricle. The dorsal sac is inconspicuous, whereas the epiphysis in the 70-mm. embryo is a long, tubular process reaching from the interval between the habenular and posterior commissures to the level of the cranial vault, which in an 86-mm. specimen shows a definite gap, representing the parietal foramen. The distal end of the tube shows a club-shaped expansion, but there is no special differentiation of this part to form a retina and lens corresponding in structure to that of the parietal sense-organ of the lamprey. The growth in length of the epiphyseal tube is in a downward direction relative to the roof of the skull, for the slightly expanded distal end of the tube retains its primary close relation to the ectoderm, while the proximal part is gradually separated from the superficial structures by an increase in depth of the area between the cranial vault and the base of the pedicle—compare A, B, C, Fig. 130. This extension of the epiphyseal tube is largely due to the increase in size of the midbrain and hemispheres; though in some types, e.g. *Spinax* (Fig. 49, Chap. 3, p. 73), there is a displacement forward, relative to the brain, of the parietal pit in the roof of the skull; and there is a horizontal portion of the tube the lengthening of which is produced as a result of this displacement. In *Spinax* also there is a thickened and slightly expanded proximal part of the tube which lies between the pineal recess and the upper margin of the habenular ganglion. This corresponds in position to the epiphysis of mammals, but beyond a slight increase in the thickness and folding of its walls, there is no structural change in this segment and in most species the proximal part passes insensibly into

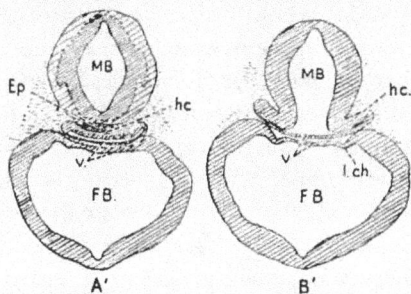

FIG. 144.—TRANSVERSE SECTIONS OF THE 28-MM. ACANTHIAS EMBRYO IN THE PLANES A, B, WHICH ARE INDICATED IN FIG. 130, B, p. 180.

Ep. : epiphysis.
FB. : forebrain.
hc. : habenular commissure.

l. ch. : lamina choroidea.
MB. : midbrain.
v. : velum.

the stalk, without any abrupt change to mark the transition of the one into the other. The relation of the habenular commissure to the habenular ganglia and the walls of the midbrain is shown in the transverse sections A and B, Fig. 144. The earliest stages of the development of the pineal region of *Acanthias* were studied by Locy (1893–5). He described (see p. 203) three paired hemispherical depressions arranged serially one behind the other near the outer edge of the unclosed medullary plate. The first pair give rise to the optic vesicles. The second and the third pair he described as " accessory optic vesicles." With regard to the second pair of primary depressions or anterior pair of " accessory optic vesicles," Locy states :[1] " I have been able to follow the anterior pair step by step through a graded series of embryos without having once lost trace of them, and to see that they enter the thalamencephalon, and give rise to the pineal outgrowth. The posterior pair, which are smaller, are not to be followed in this definite way; they become fainter and I believe they fade away." Later he states that " the bulging of the walls to form the midbrain vesicle

[1] W. A. Locy, 1893, *Anat. Anz.*, Bd. IX.

has come on insidiously, and has taken up a position behind the vesicles of the paired eyes, in apparently the same position previously occupied by the accessory vesicles. These transpositions are confusing, as they resemble the accessory optic vesicles grown larger." It will be unnecessary to enter into details of the discussion which followed the publication of Locy's work. This was chiefly concerned with the position of the accessory vesicles relative to the lateral optic vesicles and the supposed homology between the accessory optic vesicles and the median paired eyes of arthropods ; and if Locy's conception that " there are preserved on the cephalic plate of certain Elasmobranch embryos three pairs of optic vesicles "—the lateral and two accessory pairs—were true, a condition would be present in the embryo of these fishes which is well known in certain invertebrates, and it would provide a basis for the supposition that the ancestors of the vertebrates possessed two or more pairs of eyes arranged serially and that one pair, the lateral eyes, have evolved to form the highly differentiated and inverted lateral pair of eyes of living vertebrates ; whereas the other accessory pair (or pairs) have degenerated, or possibly have evolved along a different structural plan and functional direction, and have persisted as the pineal organ. Locy's conception of the ultimate fate of the depressions *A.op.'* ; *A.op.''*, and their connection with the pineal diverticulum, has however not been generally accepted by later authors.

Structure of the Pineal Organ of Selachia [1]

The walls of the end-vesicle and stalk are throughout their whole extent built up on a foundation of ependymal cells which extend between the inner and outer limiting membranes. The oval nuclei of these cells are situated at varying distances from the internal limiting membrane. The ends of the cells where they are attached to the membrane are often expanded, as is the case in the supporting radial fibres of Müller in the retina of the lateral eyes of vertebrates. These conical expansions are most noticeable at the outer ends of the cells. At the inner end some of the cells terminate flush with the membrane with which they are blended. Others send small club-shaped or irregularly tapering processes through the membrane, which project into the lumen of the tube. These processes are seen both in the terminal vesicle and in the stalk. No definite ciliated epithelium is, however, present. In many cases the lining membrane is quite smooth, though in others thread-like protoplasmic processes project inwards which end in a nucleated syncytial network, like the " vitreous " of the end-vesicles in *Petromyzon*. In some cases there is a coagulum resembling an inspissated secretion, such as is frequently seen in the ventricular cavities and central canal of the

[1] Cartilaginous fishes belonging to the sub-order of Elasmobranchii which includes the Sharks and Dog-fishes.

spinal cord. At later stages in development a certain degree of differentiation takes place, into neuroglia cells and cells which resemble ganglion cells. Neuroglial fibres and nerve-fibres also may be distinguished, the latter being most abundant near the base of the stalk, where they become collected together in bundles. A definite pineal tract is present in the posterior part of the stalk near its base, which according to Studnička is traceable into the posterior commissure ; other fibres have occasionally been traced into the habenular commissure and ganglia, e.g. in *Acipenser*. The structure of the proximal part of the pineal organ is essentially the same as that of the stalk. In some specimens, however, e.g. *Spinax*, the wall may be considerably thickened and thrown into folds. Folding of the wall is also frequent in the end vesicle, but this is not so common as in the bony fishes, in some species of which it is so pronounced that the organ somewhat resembles a racemose tubular gland, more especially as the spaces between the folds are occupied by vascular connective tissue (Fig. 155, p. 220). In the cartilaginous fishes the wall is usually only slightly folded or is smooth. It is covered by a thin sheath of pia mater and accompanied by vessels which form a plexus around the terminal vesicle. Pigment is frequently present in the connective tissue around these blood-vessels, but not in the walls of the vesicle itself.

The General Form and Position of the End-vesicle of Cartilaginous Fishes

The end vesicle of these fishes, as compared with that of Cyclostomes and certain reptiles, is relatively small, and in some cases it is probable that it simply represents the slightly dilated distal extremity or blind end of the stalk—the true sensory vesicle not having been developed, or if developed in early embryonic life having been cut off from the stalk and subsequently degenerated, as appears to be the case in some amphibians. There are, however, certain points with regard to its shape, structure, and situation that seem to favour the view that it does in reality represent the sensory vesicle, in the majority of cases. In no instance, however, does it reach its full development, but remains small and imperfectly differentiated. With reference to its shape, certain cases occur in which the end-organ shows evidence of bilaterality : it may be heart-shaped, having a distinct notch on its anterior border, e.g. *Raja clavata* and *Acanthias vulgaris* (Cattie) ; or it may be mallet-shaped, forming with the distal extremity of the stalk a T-shaped junction which projects beyond the hemispheres, e.g. *Centrophorus granulosus*. Moreover, the stalk is frequently accompanied by two principal arteries which spring from the right and left sides of the arterial anastomosis which surrounds its base. In many cases, however, the end vesicle has been described as conical, club-shaped, round, oval, or disc-shaped, and the shape appears to vary within the same species. It is quite likely that some cases in which the end vesicle is in reality heart-shaped have been erroneously described as oval or club-shaped owing to the difficulty of forming a true estimate of its shape when it is seen only in sagittal sections. Unless a reconstruction of the organ is made from a complete series of such sections, an actually heart-shaped organ might easily be regarded as conical. The specimens described by Cattie were drawn from actual dissections of the region, and he gives detailed accounts of their size, relations to membranes, and vascular supply. He also describes in one specimen of *Acanthias vulgaris* two bilaterally placed parietal foramina separated by a median antero-posterior bridge. Bilateral parietal foramina or impressions are also occasionally found in ancient fossil fishes, e.g. *Pholidosteus, Rhinosteus,* and *Titanichthys* (Figs. 225, 226, Chap. 23, p. 325), a circumstance which considerably adds to the significance of their occurrence in living species—which although infrequent should, we think, be regarded as an indication of an inherited trait which is of distinct historical value.

The end vesicle in cartilaginous fishes is often flattened dorso-ventrally and in some cases the proximal or under surface is thicker than the upper, as in the Cyclostomes. The reverse condition has, however, sometimes been observed, but the similarity in structure of the end vesicle of the fishes generally to that of Cyclostomes may be taken as an indication that in some cases the proximal segment of the end vesicle in fishes, corresponds to the proximal or retinal segment of the " pineal eyes " of the lamprey and the convex distal segment to the " pellucida " or lens.

Relations of the Pineal Organ to the Roof of the Skull in Selachians

The end vesicle may lie in a foramen in the anterior part of the carti-laginous roof of the skull and be situated in the median plane between the orbits. Although this foramen is often called the parietal foramen, it must be borne in mind that this region in fishes generally corresponds to the frontal or prefrontal region of the cranial vault (Fig. 132, Chap. 17, p. 182, and Fig. 141, B, p. 201). The term " parietal," signifying wall, is, strickly speaking, correct, but the opening is not necessarily in the region of the parietal bone or bones, as in amphibia and reptiles (Fig. 170, Chap. 19, p. 237, and Fig. 171, A, p. 237). The foramen may be closed superficially by a membrane which is continuous at the margins of the opening with the perichondrium and the dura-mater lining the canal. The end vesicle is usually attached to the walls of the canal by a loose connective tissue, containing vessels, as in *Acanthias*. In other cases the cartilaginous roof is not completely perforated, the canal being closed externally by cartilage and thus ending blindly, as in *Spinax* (Fig. 49, Chap. 3, p. 73) and the curious spoon-bill or paddle-fish (*Polyodon*) (Fig. 50, Chap. 3, and Fig. 229, Chap. 23, p. 329). The end vesicle may reach the surface in front of the cartilage at the prefrontal foramen, as in the thornback

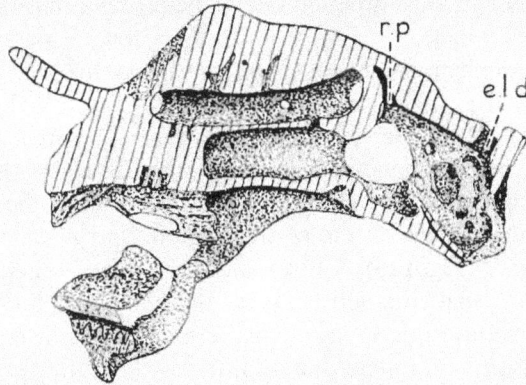

FIG. 145.—SAGITTAL SECTION THROUGH THE SKULL OF CALLORHYNCHUS ANTARCTICUS, A PRIMITIVE FORM OF FISH ALLIED TO CHIMÆRA. (AFTER PARKER AND HASWELL.)

The pineal organ has been withdrawn from the surface and lies wholly within the skull, its terminal vesicle lying at the apex of a recess—*r.p.*; while the endolymphatic duct of the vestibule, *e.l.d.*, perforates the skull.

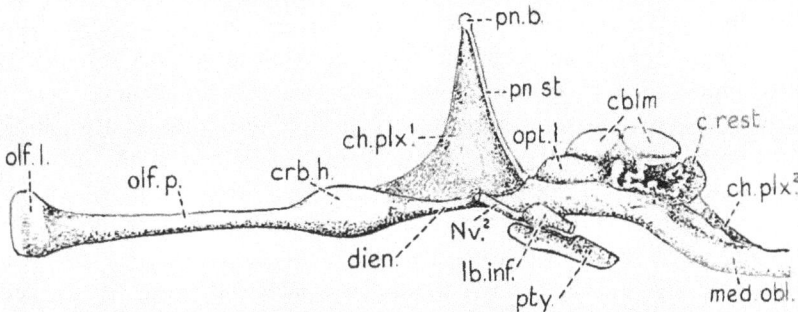

FIG. 146.—LATERAL VIEW OF THE BRAIN OF CALLORHYNCHUS ANTARCTICUS, SHOWING THE PINEAL BODY AND MEMBRANES IN PLACE.

cblm. : cerebellum.
ch. plx.[1], *ch. plx.*[2] : membranous roof and choroid plexus of the third and fourth ventricles.
c. rest. : corpus restiforme.
crb. h. : cerebral hemisphere.
dien. : diencephalon.
lb. inf. : lobus inferior.

med. obl. : medulla oblongata.
Nv.[2] : optic nerve.
olf. l. : olfactory bulb.
olf. p. : olfactory stalk.
opt. l. : optic lobe.
pn. b. : pineal body.
pn. st. : pineal stalk.
pty. : pituitary body.

skate, *Raja clavata* and the eagle-ray or devil-fish (*Myliobatis*). In the latter and in *Ophidium barbatum* (Fig. 153, p. 219) the pedicle of the pineal organ is exceptionally long, the end vesicle reaching to a point considerably in front of the hemispheres of the brain. It is enclosed in a connective tissue capsule which is loosely attached to the membrane which forms the roof of the skull in this situation, there being no groove or pit for the reception of the vesicle.

In the Holocephali, namely in *Chimæra monstrosa* and in *Callorhynchus*, there is a conical recess in the cartilaginous roof of the skull (Fig. 145). This is lined by dura mater which is continuous at the margins of the foramen with the perichondrium on the outer surface of the skull. The recess is filled by a tent-like prolongation of the roof of the diencephalon, which represents the dorsal sac of this region, and is called the " membranous pallium " (Fig. 146). The stalk of the pineal organ is attached to the brain in the usual situation between the habenular and the posterior commissures and ascends in front of the midbrain and on the posterior aspect of the dorsal sac to end in a minute vesicle at the apex of the recess in the cranial vault.

Structure of the Pineal Organ of a Fully Developed Sturgeon (Acipenser)

As compared with the simple ependymal structure of the pineal diverticulum in the early stage of its development (Fig. 147) sections through the fully developed organ show that a differentiation has taken place into two principal types of cell, namely, supporting cells which retain their ependymal character and cells of a sensory type. Two other types of cells are also found, but are less frequent ; these are large ganglion cells and neuroglia cells. Nerve-fibres and neuroglia fibres are also present. The same structure is met with throughout the whole extent of the organ, including the proximal part, the stalk, and end vesicle. Fig. 148 represents a part of the walls of the proximal part of the stalk, stained with iron-hæmatoxylin and highly magnified. The outer ends of the ependymal cells are attached by a slightly expanded foot to the external limiting membrane ; the inner end of each cell is slightly notched and lacks any special character (e.g. cilia). The cell bodies are palely stained and the cytoplasm has a loose reticular structure ; the nucleus also is feebly stained and has a fine nuclear reticulum. The cells of the sensory type on the other hand are deeply stained with hæmatoxylin, both as regards the denser cytoplasm and the nucleus ; the outer end of the cell is often prolonged into a process which resembles a nerve-fibre and runs in a direction parallel to the surface forming a right angle with the long axis of the body of the cell. The inner ends of these

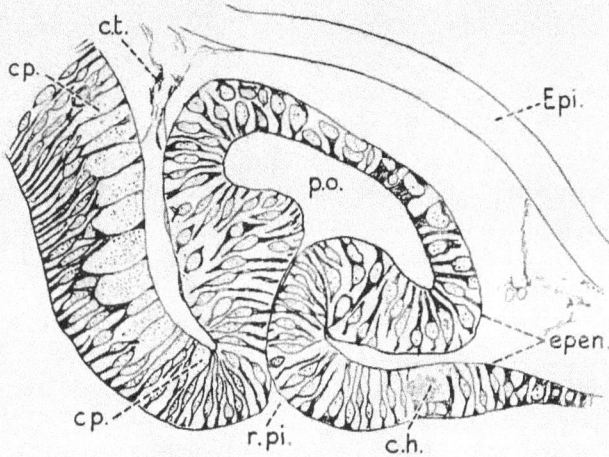

FIG. 147.—LONGITUDINAL MEDIAN SECTION THROUGH THE PINEAL DIVERTICULUM OF AN EMBRYO OF A STURGEON (ACIPENSER), SHOWING THE CONTINUITY AND SIMILARITY OF STRUCTURE OF THE WALL OF THE DIVERTICULUM WITH THE EPENDYMAL ROOF OF THE INTERBRAIN, AND THE POSITION AND EXTENT OF THE POSTERIOR AND HABENULAR COMMISSURES. (AFTER STUDNIČKA.)

c.h. : habenular commissure.
c.p. : posterior commissure.
c.t. : connective tissue.
epen. : ependyma.

Epi. : epidermis.
p.o. : pineal organ.
r. pi. : recessus pinealis.

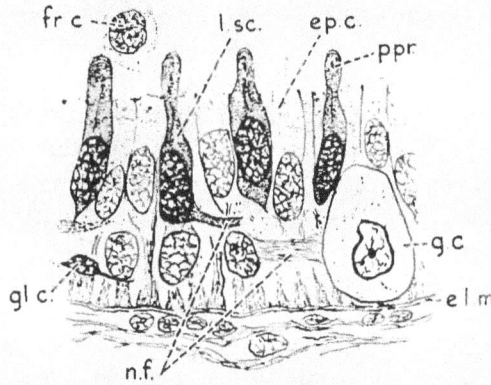

FIG. 148.—SECTION THROUGH THE PROXIMAL PART OF THE STALK OF THE PINEAL ORGAN OF A STURGEON (ACIPENSER STURIO), HIGHLY MAGNIFIED. (AFTER STUDNIČKA.)

e.l.m. : external limiting membrane.
ep. c. : clear ependymal cell without cilia.
fr. c. : free cell in lumen of stalk.
g.c. : ganglion cell.
gl. c. : neuroglial cell.
n.f. : nerve-fibres.
p. pr. : protoplasmic process.
l. sc. : deeply stained cell resembling the sensory cells of the retina in the lamprey.

cells often protrude into the lumen of the tube between the inner ends of the ependymal cells ; here they form cylindrical or club-shaped swellings, with rounded free extremities and sometimes show a constriction at the level of the free ends of the ependymal cells. They frequently contain fine granules and threads, which are probably mitochondrial in nature. A few large ganglion cells are found, chiefly in the vicinity of the external limiting membrane ; they are feebly stained, the cell-body being clear or finely granular. The nucleus is also palely stained, but shows a well-defined nucleolus. The neuroglial cells are small, mostly spindle-shaped, with tapering processes ; the amount of cytoplasm relative to the size of the nucleus is very small, and the nucleus is deeply stained. Nerve-fibres are seen singly or in bundles, mostly lying parallel to the surface, and fine neuroglial fibres are also present.

The proximal part of the pineal organ of the sturgeon, as well as the stalk and end-organ, thus appears to have a structure, which is comparable with that of the parietal sense-organ of the Cyclostomes and reptiles rather than with that of a secreting gland.

With regard to the destination of the nerve-fibres ; these were studied by J. B. Johnston in *Acipenser*. He described a nerve-fibre layer which passes from the dorsal surface of the pineal sac to the roof of the brain, where the fibres passed across from one side to the other, dorsal to the habenular commissure, in what he called the " epiphyseal commissure." He was able to follow the fibres on into the region of the nucleus anterior, and he considered that these fibres at least in part had the value of neurites of the cells of the epiphyseal sac. Other fibres of the " decussatio epiphysis " were seen to end freely between and in contact with the cells forming the wall of the stalk. In the decussatio epiphysis a third type of cell was demonstrated, namely, cells, the fibres of which simply decussated and could be followed into the region of the nucleus anterior in front of the ganglion habenulæ.

Other fibres were traced by Johnston from the proximal end of the stalk which turned laterally over the upper side of the epiphyseal sac to the upper border of the decussatio epiphysis ; some of these fibres then crossed forward and passed into the ganglia habenulæ, about an equal number being distributed to each side.

This bundle of commissural fibres is probably the same as that described by Eycleshymer and Davis in the epiphyseal region of *Amia calva* (p. 213, Fig. 149, E).

The pineal organs of some special types of fish may now be alluded to with the view of drawing attention to certain points which are of value in the study of the pineal system as a whole. Among these is the primitive Ganoid fish *Amia calva*, which is commonly known as the American bow-fin. Its pineal organs were specially investigated by Hill (1894), Eycleshymer and Davis (1897), and Kingsbury (1897). Hill found that in the early embryonic stages both parietal organs were present, there being

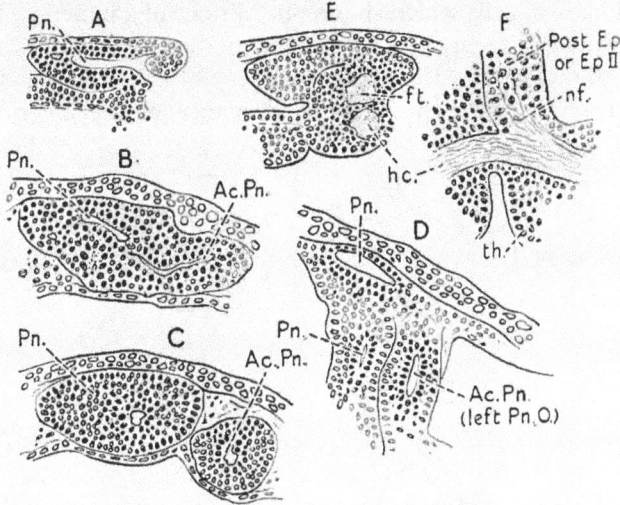

FIG. 149.—DRAWINGS OF SECTIONS SHOWING THE EARLY DEVELOPMENT OF THE EPIPHYSES IN AMIA. (AFTER EYCLESHYMER AND DAVIS.)

A—Sagittal section of primary vesicle of a larva 8–9 days old ; 5–6 mm. ;   160.

B—Transverse section through the epiphysis of a larva 10 days old ; 7–8 mm., showing the bifid cavity.

C—Transverse section through a larva at the same stage of development as B, and Fig. 150, C ; showing the right and left pineal organs, lying side by side.

D—Transverse section through a larva, 14–15 days old ; 9–10 mm. at the same stage as Fig. 150, D, showing the right and left pineal organs.

E—Sagittal section of epiphysial region of larva 12–13 mm., showing fibre tract *ft.* lying in ventral portion of primary vesicle.

F—Section showing nerve-fibres passing to the posterior epiphysis from the superior or habenular commissure.

a larger posterior organ—which probably corresponds to the posterior or right pineal organ of *Petromyzon*—and a smaller organ which lay in front and to the left, which appears to be homologous with the anterior or left parietal organ of *Petromyzon* or the " parapineal organ " of Studnička. In 10-mm. embryos the larger posterior pineal organ has developed into an ovoid vesicle with a pointed anterior extremity. Its upper or distal wall is convex and consists of a single layer of cells, while the lower wall has three or four layers of nuclei. The vesicle is joined to the roof of the diencephalon by a tubular stalk, which arises in the usual situation between the habenular and posterior commissures. In older embryos the organ rises perpendicularly from the brain and comes in contact with the skin. The anterior parietal organ is situated close in front of and to the left of the posterior organ. Its distal end is directed forward and encloses a small cavity which communicates with the ventricle. In 15-mm. embryos this communication is found to be closed ; anteriorly it ends in a solid ovoid mass of cells which shows only a trace of a lumen. According to Eycleshymer (Figs. 149 and 150) a lumen appears first in 5 to 6-mm. embryos. He also describes nerve-fibres which, coming from the habenular commissure, penetrate the substance of the anterior organ ;

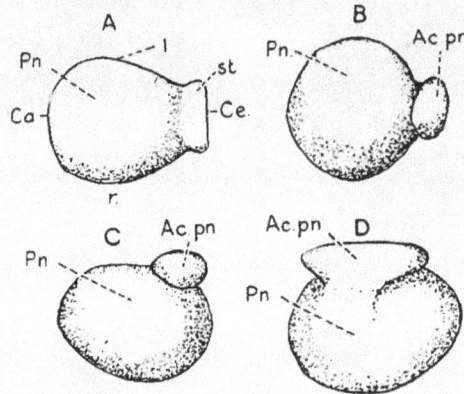

FIG. 150.—DRAWINGS OF MODELS OF THE EPIPHYSES OF AMIA, RECONSTRUCTED FROM SERIAL SECTIONS ; SEEN FROM ABOVE. (AFTER EYCLESHYMER AND DAVIS.)

A—Larva 6-7 days old ; 4-5 mm. ;   100.
B—Larva 9 days old ; 6-7 mm. ;   100.
C—Larva 10 days old ; 7-8 mm. ;   100.
D—Larva 14-15 days old ; 9-10 mm. ;   100.

Ac. pn. : accessory epiphysis, or left pineal organ.
Ca. : caudal end.   *Pn.* : pineal organ (Epiphysis II or
Ce. : cephalic end.   posterior epiphysis).
l. : left side.   *r.* : right side.
                                       st. : stalk.

and, in an earlier stage—12 to 13-mm. embryos—similar nerve-fibres which enter the posterior organ (Fig. 149, F). Later the anterior organ was found by Hill to have disappeared ; but Kingsbury has described an adult specimen of *Amia calva* (Fig. 151) in which the left pineal organ was still present although less developed than the right organ. It consisted of a hollow vesicle which was connected by a thick nerve-cord with the left habenular ganglion. The left habenular ganglion, in correspondence with the small size of the left pineal organ as compared with the right pineal organ, was smaller than the right habenular ganglion (Fig. 151). The two organs were enclosed in a membranous septum formed by two opposed layers of the dorsal sac. This sac is very large in *Amia*, and is prolonged backwards in the pineal region where in the section shown in the figure, four posterior diverticula have been cut across. From the above descriptions it will be seen that the pineal system of *Amia* shows definite evidence of bilaterality, and also indications of degenerative or devolutionary changes in both organs, but more especially of the left, which in some cases exists only in the early embryonic stages of development.

Eycleshymer and Davis, commenting on the question of the bilateral origin of the pineal organ, remark that : " The embryologist who con-

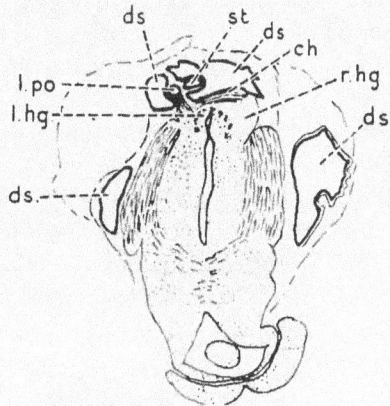

FIG. 151.—TRANSVERSE SECTION THROUGH THE DIENCEPHALON OF AMIA CALVA, SHOWING THE STALK OF THE RIGHT PINEAL ORGAN, AND THE LEFT PINEAL ORGAN IN A MEMBRANOUS SEPTUM BETWEEN TWO DIVERTICULA OF THE DORSAL SAC. (AFTER KINGSBURY.)

The left pineal organ is connected by nerve-fibres with the habenular commissure ; the left habenular ganglion is smaller than the right habenular ganglion.

ch. : chiasma.	*l. po.* : left pineal organ.
ds. : dorsal sac.	*r. hg.* : right habenular ganglion.
l. hg. : left habenular ganglion.	*st.* : stalk of right pineal organ.

templates the study of the pineal organ recalls the syllogistic statement : ' The pineal organ is probably a sense-organ. The sense-organs are paired structures ; ergo, the pineal organ should be a paired structure.' " They also quote from an article by Dr. Ayers (*J. Morph.*, 4, 1890, p. 228): " After a careful study of the *Amphioxus* eye-spot and related structures, I have become convinced that the animal presents us with the earliest stage in the phylogenetic development of the vertebrate eye." Although this pigment presents a variety of forms the author finds " the most usual form that of a slightly bilobed mass, the lobes being placed to the right and left of the median line, so as to cover the roots of the first pair of cranial nerves. . . . For greater functional power, the central median portion of the pigment spot has grown upwards (dorsal) and carrying with it a portion of the ventricular wall, has produced the median eye. . . . The parietal pineal eye of the Cyclostomata and other vertebrates has been

developed from a median portion of the pigmented eye of *Amphioxus*. . . .
The rudiments of the eye were developed from (segmental) sense-organs,
but the eye itself is never developed from two right and left halves, in so
far as the closure of the medullary folds would necessitate this."

We have quoted these extracts in full because they illustrate, besides
the important observation with regard to the bilateral disposition of the
pigment of the eye-spot in *Amphioxus*, several errors of interpretation
which were common at the time, more especially with regard to the position
of *Amphioxus* in the vertebrate phylum, namely—not as an offshoot from
a branch of the main stem, but as a living representative of the parent
stock from which the various higher types of vertebrates, including the
Cyclostomes, have descended ; secondly, the assumed visual function of the
pigment spot of *Amphioxus* which has been disproved (see pp. 178, 179) ;
thirdly, the denial of the possibility of two laterally situated sense-organs,
right and left, becoming united in a single organ : this we now know occurs
normally in the formation of the triple median eye of arthropods which is
produced by the fusion of the right and left members of one of two pairs
of ocelli, the other pair coming into contact but not being completely
fused ; fourthly, the failure to recognize the degenerate condition of the
anterior end of *Amphioxus*, the whole animal being regarded as having
reached only a very simple stage of evolution, whereas it is in many respects
highly evolved, and it is probable that the head-region was in the less
remote ancestors of *Amphioxus* much more highly developed than it is in
the living representatives of the species.   It seems more probable that the
pigment-spot of *Amphioxus* instead of " representing the earliest stage in
the phylogenetic development of the vertebrate eye " is merely a vestige of
a more highly developed organ, or possibly a *pair* of light-percipient sense-
organs which were present in the head of the remote ancestors of the
present stock, before the latter took to burrowing head downwards in the
sand at the bottom of the sea.

Polypterus Bichir [1]

Another example of enormous development of the dorsal sac and special
modification of the pineal organ is found in the primitive Crossopterygian
ganoid fish *Polypterus*, found in the Congo and Upper Nile.   In this
fish the dorsal sac arises by a relatively narrow stalk and expands as
it extends upwards towards the cranial vault.   It thus appears triangular
in a sagittal median section, the apex of the ▽ being directed downwards.
The posterior wall of the sac is folded by vascular ingrowths, but elsewhere it is smooth and membranous.   The pineal organ consists of a

[1] J. Waldschmidt, 1887, "Beitrag zur Anatomie des Zentralnervensystems und des
Geruchsorganes von Polypterus bichir," *Anat. Anzeiger.*, Jahrg. 11.

hollow, tubular stalk which arises immediately behind the habenular commissure. It extends upwards and backwards, in close relation with the posterior wall of the dorsal sac, to its posterior angle, where it bends sharply forwards and becomes continuous, without any abrupt change in diameter, with an elongated tubular end vesicle. This extends forwards, in a slight groove on the superficial aspect of the dorsal sac, as far as the level of the posterior ends of the hemispheres, where it terminates in a pointed extremity. In the posterior part of this remarkable end vesicle, the wall is slightly folded, while in the anterior part the walls are smooth and the lumen somewhat larger. The wall of the vesicle shows the usual ependymal structure, containing certain cells which resemble sensory-cells. The lumen contains a few free cells, but no special syncytial formation. No parietal impression or foramen was found in the roof of the skull.

Teleostean Fishes

In adult bony fishes, as a rule, only one pineal organ has been found in the adult animal, although definite indications of two organs have been described by Hill in early embryos of several types of fish belonging to this class, namely : *Salmo* (Fig. 138, C, Chap. 17, p. 196) ; *Catostomus teres* (sucking-carp) ; *Corregonus albus* (Fig. 152) ; *Stizostedion* (perch) ; and *Lepomis*. Of the two organs, one, the smaller, is placed in front and to the left ; the other, the larger, is behind and to the right. These observations are of considerable value, as they tend to confirm the view held by Locy with respect to the bilateral origin of the pineal organ, which was based on his observations of paired hemispherical evaginations near the outer edge of the unclosed neural-plate of dog-fish embryos, and also the observations recorded by Eycleshymer and Davis on the early developmental stages of *Amia*, and that of Kingsbury on an adult example of *Amia calva*.

The pineal organ of the teleostean fishes is much more variable, both in structure and in form, than it is in the Selachii and ganoids. It may consist of a minute end vesicle at the end of a thin, elongated stalk, as in *Ophidium* (Fig. 153), or a small solid nodule without a definite stalk. In other cases the end vesicle is expanded and has the shape of a flat, toad-stool fungus ; its structure is also complicated by the intergrowth of vascular folds of the surrounding mesoderm and outgrowing buds or folds of the neuro-epithelial wall. A good example of such is found in the pineal organ of the gar-pike (*Belone acus*) (Fig. 155). In bony fishes there is, in general, a tendency for the stalk of the pineal organ to be short and the end vesicle large, as compared with the cartilaginous fishes and ganoids, in which the stalk is usually long and the end vesicle small.

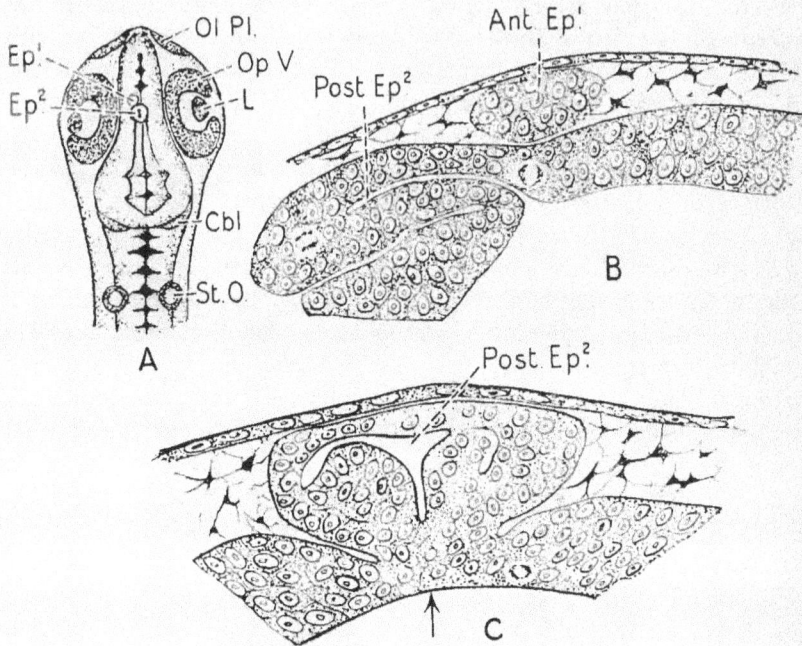

FIG. 152.—THE PINEAL ORGANS OF CORREGONUS ALBUS. (AFTER CHARLES HILL.)

A. : Dorsal view of embryo of *Corregonus albus*, showing the position of the rudimentary epiphysis to the left of the median plane.
B. : Longitudinal section through the anterior and posterior epiphysis of a 7-mm. embryo of *C. albus*.
C. : Transverse section through the posterior epiphysis of an embryo of *C. albus*; the arrow marks the median plane.

Ant. Ep.[1] : Epiphysis I.	*Ol. Pl.* : olfactory placode.
Cbl. : cerebellum.	*Op. V.* : optic vesicle.
Ep.[1] : anterior epiphysis.	*Post. Ep.*[2] : Epiphysis II.
Ep.[2] : posterior epiphysis.	*St. O.* : static organ.
L. : lens.	

Hill considered that the posterior epiphyseal vesicle of teleosts and *Amia* is homologous with the " epiphysis " of *Lacertilia*, and that the anterior vesicle is homologous with the parietal eye of *Lacertilia*.

The general structure of the pineal organ of the bony fishes is very similar to that of the cartilaginous fishes, namely, a neuro-epithelium of ependymal character, containing a few glial cells and cells resembling nerve-cells, enclosed between two limiting membranes (Fig. 154). Cytoplasmic processes frequently project through the internal limiting membrane into the lumen of the organ. The vessels surrounding the pineal organ form a rich anastomotic plexus, but they do not appear to enter the epithelial walls. The end vesicle is never differentiated into an eye-like structure, such as that of *Petromyzon*, although cells resembling sensory-cells, unipolar nerve-cells, and ganglion-cells ending in nerve-fibres have been described; also in some cases there is a definite nerve-tract ending in the posterior commissure, and in embryos of *Clupea* Holt has demonstrated nerve-fibres entering the habenular commissure.

According to Galeotti some of the cells in the pineal organ of the so-called white fish *Leuciscus* show indications of a secretory function, some of the nuclei containing special fuchsinophile granules and secretory products being found by him in the lumen of the organ. According to Holt, however, the lumen of the organ contains only plasmatic strands connecting the opposite sides of the walls, or a delicate syncytium (Clupea).

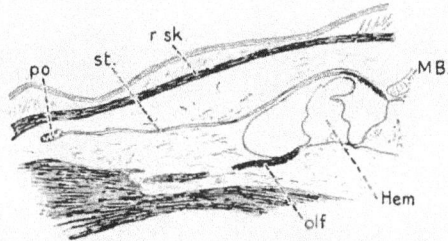

FIG. 153.—THE PINEAL ORGAN OF OPHIDIUM BARBATUM, ALLIED TO THE BLIND DEEP-SEA FISH TYPHLONUS. IT IS REMARKABLE FOR THE GREAT LENGTH OF THE STALK AND INSIGNIFICANT SIZE OF THE END VESICLE. (AFTER STUDNIČKA.)

Hem. : hemisphere.	*po.* : pineal organ.
MB. : midbrain.	*r. sk.* : roof of skull.
olf. : olfactory nerve.	*st.* : stalk.

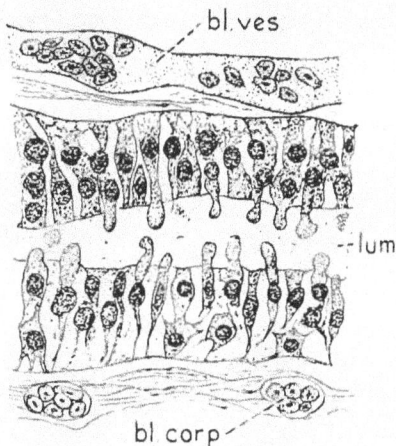

FIG. 154.—LONGITUDINAL SECTION THROUGH A SINGLE TUBE OF THE PINEAL ORGAN OF A GAR-PIKE (BELONE ACUS), SHOWING KNOB-SHAPED PROJECTIONS INTO THE LUMEN OF THE TUBE. THESE RESEMBLE THE REFRACTILE-KNOBS WHICH ARE PRESENT IN THE SENSORY VESICLE OF PETROMYZON, AND WERE CONSIDERED BY STUDNIČKA NOT TO BE SECRETORY. THE CELLS ARE EPENDYMAL IN ORIGIN, AND THE LARGE MULTIPOLAR CELLS BENEATH THE EXTERNAL LIMITING MEMBRANE RESEMBLE GANGLION CELLS. (AFTER STUDNIČKA.)

bl. corp. : blood corpuscles ; *bl. ves.* : blood vessel ; *lum.* : lumen.

Relation of the Pineal Organ to the Roof of the Skull in Teleostean Fishes

The tip of the end vesicle of the pineal organ may either simply come in contact with the roof of the skull, or the whole superficial area of an expanded vesicle may be in relation with the roof as in the gar-pike (Fig. 155). Sometimes the stalk is so short that the end vesicle does not reach the vault. It is only occasionally that the under surface

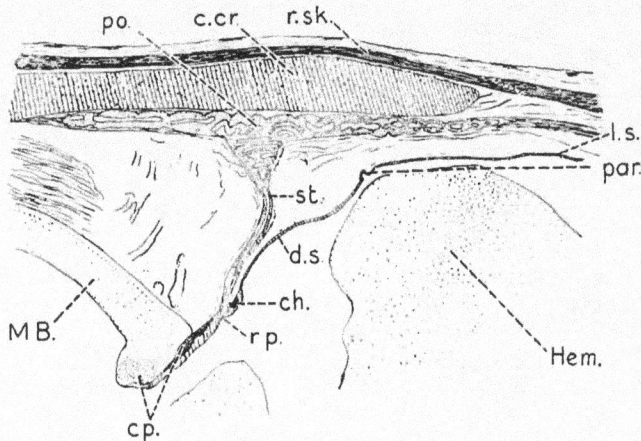

FIG. 155.—THE PARIETAL REGION OF THE BRAIN AND PINEAL ORGAN OF A GAR-
PIKE (BELONE ACUS). LONGITUDINAL SECTION. ADULT SPECIMEN, EN-
LARGED. (AFTER REICHERT.)

c. cr. : cartilaginous roof of cranium.   MB. : midbrain.
ch. : habenular commissure.   par. : paraphysis.
cp. : posterior commissure.   po. : pineal organ.
d.s. : dorsal sac.   r.p. : recessus pinealis.
Hem. : hemisphere.   r. sk. : roof of skull.
l.s. : lamina supraneuroporica.   st. : stalk.

of the skull shows any depression for the reception of the end vesicle, or a part of this; such has, however, been observed by Cattie in the common pike (*Esox lucius*) and in the Salmon (*S. salar*); also by Rabl Rückhard (*S. fario*) and Hill (*S. purpuratus*). Cases in which a parietal foramen closed superficially by fibrous membrane, is present either in the cartilaginous or bony skull are exceptional. Handrick has, however, published figures of such in *Argyropelecus hemigymnus*, a species of fish allied to the salmonoids and the herrings; and Klinckostroem has shown a true parietal foramen in the bony vault of the skull in *Callichthys asper*, belonging to the cat-fish family. It is noteworthy, however, that in this case, although a parietal foramen is present, the pineal organ is not well developed.

The Pineal Region of the Dipnoi

The primitive nature of this sub-class, the three genera of which are collectively known as lung-fishes, might lead one to expect a specially instructive condition of the pineal system. This anticipation is, however, hardly realized, for although from many standpoints these fishes— *Ceratodus*, *Protopterus*, and *Lepidosiren*—are of prime importance in the study of comparative anatomy, the parts of the brain included in the pineal system do not show a high grade of organization. No pineal eye is present. The pineal organ shows signs of degeneration and all trace of a parietal foramen has disappeared. Incidentally, it may be mentioned that the lateral eyes of *Lepidosiren* are relatively small and show a peculiarity in development which was described by Graham Kerr (1919), namely, instead of the optic vesicle being formed as a hollow outgrowth it is developed as a solid bud from the forebrain, which at the time when the optic rudiment first appears is itself solid ; later a cavity appears as a secondary formation in the primarily solid optic outgrowth, and the subsequent development of the eye follows the usual course. Another peculiarity which the lateral eyes of the Dipnoi share with Elasmobranchs and Cyclostomes is the absence of a processus falciformis. The origin of the lateral eyes as solid buds is probably a devolutionary rather than an evolutionary change. Moreover, with regard to the structure of the end vesicle of the pineal organ of *Polypterus*, Studnička found the walls markedly folded, the lumen thus being almost obliterated. He also found that some of the epithelial cells contained a brown pigment, both of which conditions indicate a degenerate state of an organ previously more highly developed. It would seem, therefore, that we are not only dealing with a class of animals which is primitive in the evolutionary sense, the Dipnoi having persisted up to the present age from the early Mesozoic period without having undergone much further developmental organization—that is to say, have remained in a more or less stationary condition—but that during or even before this period retrogressive changes have taken place both in the development of the lateral eyes and in the pineal organ.

Ceratodus Fosteri

Huxley (1876) described the pineal organ as consisting of a cylindrical stalk ending anteriorly in a heart-shaped expansion, the latter lying in a depression in the cartilaginous roof of the skull. He also gave an admirable illustration of the bones on the dorsal surface of this remarkable skull (Fig. 156), which closely resembles Krefft's figure. In neither of these is there any indication of a parietal foramen on the superficial aspect of the skull. A more detailed description of the pineal region of *Ceratodus* is given by Studnička (1905), more especially with regard to the relation of the pineal organ to the posterior wall of the dorsal sac, and of the end vesicle which extends forward to and overlaps the paraphysis as in *Protopterus*.

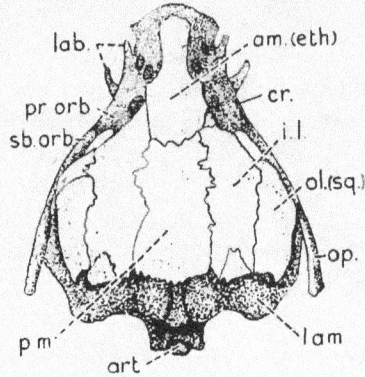

FIG. 156.—DORSAL VIEW OF SKULL OF CERATODUS FOSTERI. (AFTER HUXLEY.) Investing bones, lightly stippled. Cartilage, dark stipple.

am. : anterior median bone.
art. : articular surface for 2nd fin ray.
cr. : cartilaginous cranium.
i.l. : inner lateral bone.
lab. : labial cartilages.
lam. : process covering lungs.
ol. : outer lateral bone.
op. : operculum.
p.m. : posterior median bone.
pr. orb. : preorbital.
sb. orb. : suborbital.

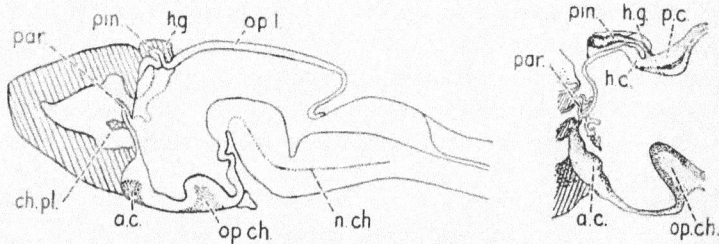

FIG. 157.—SAGITTAL SECTIONS THROUGH BRAIN OF LEPIDOSIREN. *Left :* EARLY STAGE. *Right :* DETAIL OF LATER STAGE OF DEVELOPMENT. (AFTER J. GRAHAM KERR.)

a.c. : anterior commissure.
ch. pl. : choroid plexus of lateral ventricle.
h.c. : habenular commissure.
h.g. : habenular ganglion.
n. ch. : notochord.

par. : paraphysis.
p.c. : posterior commissure.
pin. : pineal diverticulum.
op. ch. : optic chiasma.
op. l. : optic lobe.

Lepidosiren

The development of the South American lung- or mud-fish was specially studied by Graham Kerr (1919). The pineal organ arises in the usual situation between the habenular and posterior commissures and extends forwards on the roof of the diencephalon as a tubular, " carrot-shaped " diverticulum, which reaches a point just behind the hemispheres and well above the paraphysis (Fig. 157). On either side of it are the well-developed habenular ganglia, which as they enlarge become connected by a transverse bridge of nerve fibres, the habenular commissure. The roof of the mesencephalon, which lies close behind the pineal organ, becomes slightly thickened on each side of the mesial plane, forming the arched tectum opticum, but " correlated with the small size of the eyes in *Lepidosiren* the thickening never becomes so great as to produce projecting optic lobes such as are formed in most vertebrates."

Protopterus

The pineal organ of the South African lung-fish was described by Burckhardt in 1892 and another specimen was described by Studnička in 1905. In both these specimens the organ was divisible into three parts, a club-shaped end vesicle which was subdivided into several compartments by folds of its wall ; an elongated stalk which in Studnička's case was hollow throughout, whereas in Burckhardt's specimen the central part was solid, only the third or proximal part having a lumen. The lumen, however, was closed at its base, there being no communication with the ventricle. This proximal part probably corresponds to the " pineal gland " or epiphysis of mammals ; the stalk and end vesicle may fail to develop as in the higher vertebrates, or the latter may be cut off by the growth of the skull from the proximal part, the end vesicle persisting as Stieda's organ, e.g. in the frog, while the proximal part differentiates as the epiphysis.

CHAPTER 19

THE EYES OF AMPHIBIANS

THIS class includes the tailed amphibia—Urodela ; the tailless amphibia
—Anura ; the degraded blind and limbless amphibia—Apoda ; and the
extinct labyrinthodonts—Stegocephala.

The pineal system of amphibians is particularly interesting on account
of the light that it sheds on intermediate stages between the more highly
evolved types of the parietal sense organ or pineal eye, such as is found
in the lampreys and lizards, and those types in which the end-organ fails
to develop and in which it appears that the proximal end only, grows and
becomes modified to form the epiphysis or pineal organ as in birds and
mammals.

The Pineal System of the Urodela

In this primitive order, which comprises the Tritons ; salamanders ;
the common British newts ; *Amblystoma* (Axolotyl) ; *Amphiuma ;*

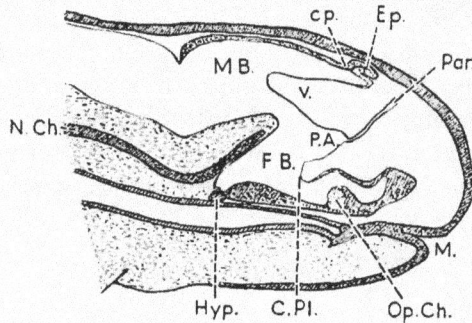

FIG. 158.—MEDIAN SAGITTAL SECTION THROUGH THE HEAD OF AN 18-MM. LARVA
OF NECTURUS MACALATUS, SHOWING THE STRUCTURES IN THE PARIETAL REGION
OF THE BRAIN. (AFTER C. S. MINOT.)

cp. : posterior commissure.	*M.* : mouth.
C. Pl. : choroid plexus.	*MB.* : midbrain.
Ep. : epiphysis.	*Op. Ch.* : optic chiasma.
FB. : forebrain.	*P.A.* : paraphysal arch.
Hyp. : hypophysis.	*Par.* : paraphysis.

Necturus (Fig. 158) ; and *Proteus*, the pineal organ is very rudimentary
and in the adult lies entirely within the cranial cavity. The whole organ
consists at first of a flattened hollow vesicle, connected by a short

stalk with the roof of the diencephalon, to which it is attached in the usual situation between the habenular and posterior commissures. The superficial or distal wall of the end vesicle is formed by a single layer of epithelium, whereas the deep or proximal wall shows two or three layers of nuclei ; the inner ends of these cells in some specimens, e.g.

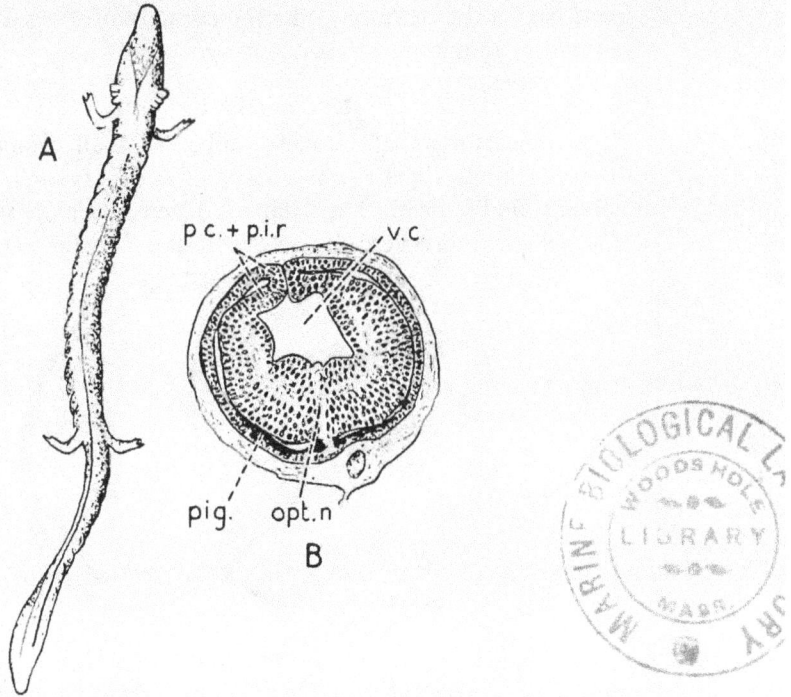

FIG. 159.

A—*Proteus*—Adelsberg grotto, reduced. The lateral eyes are invisible externally. There is a small pear-shaped pineal organ within the cranial cavity.
B—Vertical section, through one of the rudimentary lateral eyes.

opt. n. : optic nerve ; *p.c.+p.i.r.* : pars ciliaris+pars iridica retinæ. The lips of the optic cup meet in front owing to the absence of the lens. *p.g.* : pigment ; *v.c.* : vitreous cavity. Arrest of development has taken place at an early stage, and the retina is unusually thick.

(After Semper.)

Salamander maculosa and *Proteus anguineus*, contain pigment granules ; and in a specimen of *Necturus* described by Kingsbury (1895), two or three medullated nerve-fibres on each side were seen by him to pass from the brain into the epiphysis. Whether these nerve-fibres were efferent fibres passing from the brain to the epiphysis or afferent fibres passing from a vestigial sensory vesicle to the brain is a problem regarding the solution of which we have no direct evidence which will help us to come to a decision. The presence, however, of nerve-fibres passing between

15

the parietal sense organ and the brain in lampreys and reptiles, and the homologous nerve connecting the vestigial sense organ with the roof of the brain in the common frog do afford indirect evidence which justifies the assumption that these fibres are primarily afferent in nature, although their original function of transmitting impulses from the terminal sense organ to the brain has, like the capacity of the sense organ itself to receive these sensations, ceased long ago.

1. Urodela Caudata

The pineal organ of Urodeles appears in all examples which have hitherto been examined to show signs of degeneration. Thus in *Triton*, de Graaf found indications of " fatty " degeneration (probably vacuolation of the cells) ; moreover, the cavity of the vesicle was irregularly sub-

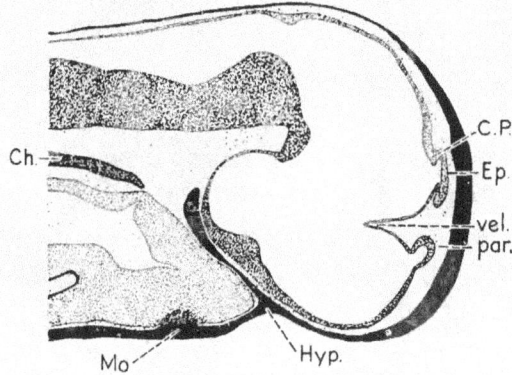

FIG. 160.

A median sagittal section of the head of an embryo of *Amblystoma punctatum* (Axolotl), showing the relations of the paraphysis, *par.* ; velum, *vel.* ; and epiphysis, *Ep.* ; *Ch.* : notochord ; *c.p.* : commissura posterior ; *hyp.* : hypophysis ; *mo.* : mouth. The dorsal sac will be formed between the velum and epiphysis, and the anterior or habenular commissure in front of the epiphysis.

(After J. B. Johnstone.)

divided by partitions into loculi, the septa being produced by folding of its walls. The vesicle is often dorsoventrally compressed, being flattened out between the cranial wall and roof of the brain, and the lumen is thus reduced to a mere slit. In *Desmognathus*, according to Fish (1895), no trace of a lumen is to be found in the pineal organ of the adult animal. In *Typhlotriton* and *Proteus anguineus*, both of which are cave-dwellers and blind, the lateral eyes are also degenerate and buried beneath the skin of the head. In *Proteus* (Fig. 159) Galeotti found that the epiphysis was a small, pear-shaped structure showing no evidence of secretory function, but he observed that in certain cells near the nucleus pigment granules were present—this being the only place in which pigment was found to be present in the brain of *Proteus*. This snake-like amphibian, which lives in the subterranean waters of Carniola and Dalmatia, is in its natural state described as being of " fleshy whiteness and transparency." The absence of pigment in the skin and its presence in the epithelium of the pineal organ appear to indicate a more feebly inherited tendency towards the formation of pigment in the skin and a marked tenacity of the inherited character with respect to the deposit of pigment in the epithelium of the end vesicle of the pineal organ. On the other hand, it may be argued that the pigment in the epithelium of the pineal organ is simply due to chemical changes occurring in a degenerate tissue ; but since the pigment is strictly limited to the epithelium of the pineal organ and is not found in the surrounding mesodermal tissue and other parts of the brain, nor in the body generally, this interpretation does not seem to be the correct explanation of its presence in the pineal organ.

A paraphysis (Fig. 160) is usually well developed in the Urodela, and may appear as a simple tubular diverticulum or it may be branched and glandular in appearance.

The parietal foramen which is present in the skull of certain extinct Urodeles has disappeared in living forms, e.g. in the newt (*Molge cristata*), W. K. Parker, and *Typhlototriton*, H. Riese. In these, paired frontal and parietal bones are separated by a cruciate suture.

2. Apoda (Cæcilia)

The best-known example of this order is the slimy eel-like creature *Ichthyophis glutinosa*, in which the lateral eyes are very small and are imbedded in the skin. The adult animal has no limbs, but vestiges of the hind limbs have been recognized in the embryo. The pineal organ described in 1891 by Burckhardt is a small, pear-shaped hollow vesicle the walls of which are infolded and the stalk attached to the roof of the diencephalon just behind the habenular commissure. The paraphysis is well developed and viewed in profile has the shape of a geological hammer, the posterior limb of which overlaps and conceals the pineal organ. Some fibres passed between the pineal organ and the roof of the diencephalon. Burckhardt was uncertain, however, whether these were nervous or supporting in nature. The skull described by Sarasin, like that of other living orders of Amphibia, shows no parietal foramen.

In the genera *Gymnopis* and *Herpele* the lateral eyes have not only sunk beneath the skin as in some other forms but they actually lie beneath the bones of the skull.

3. Anura (Acaudata)

The development of the pineal organ in tailless amphibia is more pronounced than in Urodela and Apoda, and in many at one period in their development an end vesicle—stalk and proximal part—are distinguishable

(Fig. 161). The end vesicle, however, soon becomes cut off from the stalk by the ingrowth of the roof of the skull (Fig. 162), and the stalk disappears leaving only the proximal part or epiphysis in connection with the roof of the diencephalon.

The end vesicle, or parietal organ (Fig. 167, p. 233), is situated beneath the epidermis, being imbedded in the corium and lying completely outside the roof of the skull. Its position in the living animal is indicated by a small, pale area, the parietal spot where the pigment in the sub-epithelial

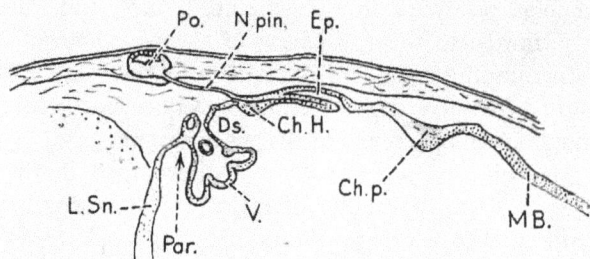

FIG. 161.—THE PARIETAL REGION AND PINEAL ORGAN OF A TADPOLE (RANA TEMPORARIA)—INTERNAL GILLS AND HIND LIMBS APPEARING AS STUMPS. (AFTER BRAEM, 1898.)

Ch. H. : chiasma habenularis.
Ch. p. : chiasma posterior.
Ds. : dorsal sac.
Ep. : epiphysis.
L. Sn. : lamina supra-neuroporica.
MB. : midbrain.

N. pin. : nervus pinealis or stalk of pineal organ.
Par. : paraphysis.
Po. : pineal organ.
V. : velum.

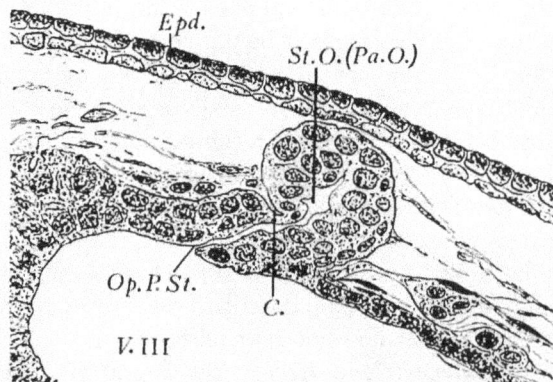

FIG. 162.

Median longitudinal section of the pineal diverticulum of a frog tadpole, showing a constriction in the plane of the cranial capsule, which indicates the future line of separation of the parietal organ (Stieda) from the epiphysis or pineal sac. The apex of the organ is directed forward, and is to the right in the figure.

(Original R. J. G.)

C. : constriction ; Epd. : epidermis ; Op. P.St. : opening of pineal stalk ; St. O. (Pa. O.) : parietal organ (Stieda) ; V. III. : third ventricle.

layer of the skin is absent or scanty, and the cutaneous glands are also either absent or are reduced in size and number. The spot is variable in size and degree of distinctness in different species and in some is absent altogether. It is well seen in the common frog, *Rana temporaria* (Fig. 163), and also in *R. subsaltans*, of which a drawing clearly showing the " fleck " was published by Gravenhorst in 1829, although its significance was not appreciated at the time ; and later, when Stieda discovered the vesicle beneath it, he considered it to be glandular in nature, and it

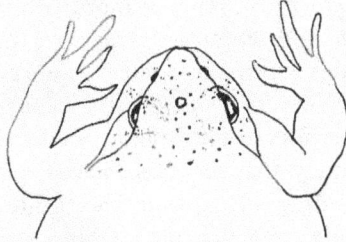

FIG. 163.—HEAD OF FROG (RANA TEMPORARIA), SHOWING THE PARIETAL SPOT WHICH LIES OVER STIEDA'S ORGAN AND BETWEEN THE LATERAL EYES. (FROM STUDNIČKA.)

became known as the " frontal gland " (" Stirndrüse "). Goette (1873–75), who first recognized the existence of the proximal part or epiphysis in the early stages of development of *Bombinator igneus,* was also the first to establish the connection of this with the end vesicle and homologize these parts with the pineal organ of other classes of vertebrates, although he was in error with regard to the connection which he believed to exist between the pineal organ and the anterior neuropore (see p. 5).

Development.—The pineal diverticulum in *Rana* is at first elliptical in form, but soon becomes tubular, the expanded blind-end growing forward while the attached end remains at its site of origin, between the habenular and posterior commissures. A constriction then appears marking off the end vesicle from the proximal part, and as the head enlarges and the end vesicle, which is attached to the skin, is carried forward, a narrow neck appears which becomes elongated and forms the stalk. Later the lumen in the stalk disappears and finally the epithelial wall becomes interrupted, and in the fully developed animal the end vesicle or parietal organ is completely separated from the epiphysis by the roof of the skull, which in living representatives of the order has no parietal foramen. The proximal part, or epiphysis, retains its lumen for a considerable period, and this may persist even in the fully grown animal, as in the example shown in Fig. 166, which shows the hollow tubular organ lying on the roof of the diencephalon and extending forward as far as the habenular commissure. The pineal recess lies immediately in front of the posterior commissure and the pineal tract passes backwards on the dorsal aspect of the epiphysis to end in the ventral part of the posterior commissure.

The end vesicle or parietal organ is usually a round, hollow, epithelial cyst, but is sometimes solid. In the former the superficial or distal wall of the cyst is formed of a single layer of epithelium, while the proximal wall shows two or three layers of nuclei, which in *Bufo*, according to Studnička, are radially arranged, and may contain pigment granules. The end vesicle of *Bufo* thus shows a more primitive (less degenerate) condition than in *Rana*, and resembles somewhat the end vesicle of *Petromyzon*, but is not so highly differentiated. The cavity of the end vesicle varies considerably in size and shape. In some cases it is irregularly constricted and has the form of the figure eight placed horizontally ∞ (*R. esculenta*); or kidney-shaped (*Bombinator igneus*) (de Graaf); or horse-shoe shaped (Leydig). It is sometimes quite irregular in form and crossed by protoplasmic strands. The whole vesicle is enclosed in a loose connective tissue capsule composed of flattened cells, between which and the vesicle is a space which Leydig (1891) has shown in *Bombinator* is traversed by nerve-fibres and capillary vessels. The superficial surface of the vesicle is formed by a layer of flattened neuro-epithelium (external limiting membrane), which constitutes the inner boundary of the space. As a rule the epithelial cells forming the walls of the end vesicle remain undifferentiated, but in some specimens of adult animals Studnička has observed at least two layers of cells in the proximal or retinal section and a differentiation of an inner layer of high cylindrical ependymal cells and beneath these (more superficially) rounded cells. Among the former Studnička describes in *Bufo*, cells of a distinctly rod-like character, and Galeotti has seen rounded protoplasmic masses projecting into the lumen, like those in *Petromyzon*. The structure of the vesicle thus resembles a degenerate sense organ rather than a gland, and its cells differ markedly from those of the surrounding cutaneous glands.

Nerves of the Parietal Organ and Epiphysis in Anura

The fine strand of fibres which sometimes connects the " Stirndrüse " or " frontal gland " with the roof of the skull was first described by Stieda in 1865. This slender band may contain nerve-fibres, or be composed simply of connective tissue, or it may be absent. It is generally considered to originate as the stalk of the pineal organ which in the course of development has become thinned out and elongated, as represented in Fig. 161 (p. 228) by Braem, of the parietal region of a tadpole of *Rana temporaria*. Nerve-fibres may appear in the stalk at a later stage and it was thought at the time that the stalk was transformed into

the " pineal nerve." Whether the nerve-fibres are actually formed in
the stalk or grow into the stalk from neuro-sensory or ganglion cells in
the end vesicle is a problem which it is difficult to decide ; for, according
to the later publications of Leydig (1891), the nerve-fibres do not actually
enter the vesicle as they appear to do in Fig. 164, but both nerves and
vessels pass beneath or around the vesicle and join a plexus of nerve-
fibres and capillary vessels in the surrounding connective tissue (Fig. 165).

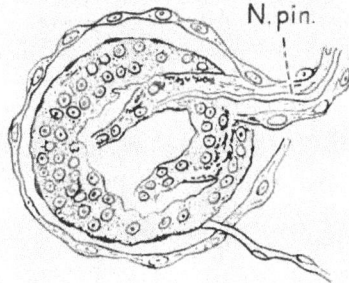

FIG. 164.

Another drawing of the same specimen as Fig. 165, showing pigment granules in
the epithelium of the wall of the frontal organ (Stieda) and the pineal nerve.
(After Leydig.)   *N. pin.* : nervus pinealus.

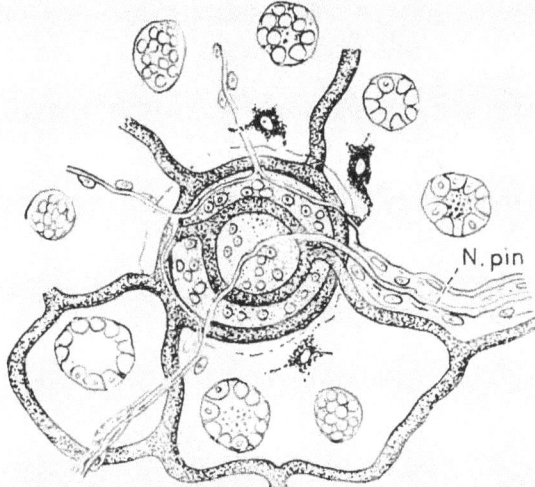

FIG. 165.—THE FRONTAL ORGAN OF BOMBINATOR IGNEUS (STAGE OF TWO-LEGGED
LARVA), SEEN FROM BELOW.

Surrounding the organ are blood-vessels and nerves. Three-branched pigment
cells of the connective tissue type are present, and sections of cutaneous
glands. *N. pin.* : nervus pinealis.

(From a drawing by Leydig, 1891.)

Moreover, neither fully differentiated neuro-sensory cells nor ganglion
cells have been described in the end vesicle, but on the contrary in most
cases the epithelium shows signs of degeneration and the nerve-fibres

or even the whole stalk are frequently found to be absent in adult specimens, a circumstance which suggests that the development of nerve-
fibres when it occurs is merely a transitory phase in the existence of a
degenerate organ which is variable in the degree of differentiation to
which it attains in different examples of the order or even in individuals
of the same species. The occasional presence of nerve-fibres in the stalk
of the end vesicle, although not constant, is of morphological importance,
and the following detailed description by Braem (1898) of both the extracranial and intracranial course of the pineal nerve is especially interesting.
He distinguishes between the " nervus pinealis " of the parietal organ and
the " tractus pinealis " of the epiphysis (Fig. 166).

Dealing first with the pineal nerve of *Rana*, Braem states that it consists
of thick medullated fibres accompanied by blood-vessels. These fibres
enter the organ from below, either at the middle or near the hinder pole.
Having entered the vesicle they gradually become imperceptible and are
lost. Connective tissue elements enter slightly into the composition
of the nerve, and Studnička mentions that he has found pigment cells on
the surface of the nerve and, further, that he considers the elongated
nuclei seen in the course of the nerve to be connective tissue in nature.
In any case, there is at least a fine endothelial sheath, which separates

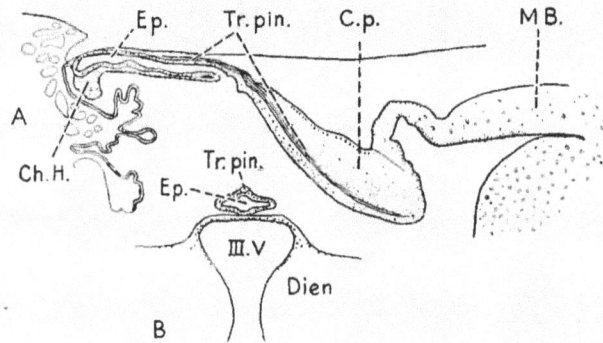

FIG. 166.

A—Sagittal section through the Epiphysis (proximal part of the pineal organ)
    showing the pineal tract, from an adult example of *Rana temporaria*.
B—Transverse section through the epiphysis and roof of the diencephalon.

Ch. H. : Chiasma habenularis.	*MB.* : midbrain.
C.p. : commissura posterior.	*Tr. pin.* : tractus pinealis.
Dien. : diencephalon.	*III. V.* : third ventricle.
Ep. : epiphysis.	

(After Braem, 1898.)

the nerve and the accompanying blood-vessels from the cranio-dorsal
lymph space in which the greater part of the nerve lies. Braem further
describes the nerve as passing through the lymph sac and sooner or later
piercing the skull in an oblique direction between the two frontal (fronto-

parietal) bones, close behind the ethmoid and thus just above the olfactory lobe.   Having entered the cranial cavity, it courses backwards on the superficial aspect of the dura mater, to which it is closely applied, to the paraphysis.   It then passes over the latter to the epiphysis.   In its course thither the nerve is pushed for a short distance away from the median line by a dense plexus of blood-vessels.   Braem saw the commence-ment of the nerve near the apex of the epiphysis, but he was unable to see any connection of its fibres with those of the " tractus pinealis," although he considered such a connection was more than probable. Studnicka also mentions that he was unable to trace any connection between the pineal nerve and pineal tract in his specimens of quite young tadpoles of *Rana*.   Braem saw no indications of degeneration ; nevertheless, he considered it possible that the nerve in some cases might be absent, an opinion which is supported by the observations of de Graaf and Leydig, and by a young specimen of a frog tadpole, of our own (Fig. 167).

The course of the pineal tract in an adult specimen of *Rana temporaria*

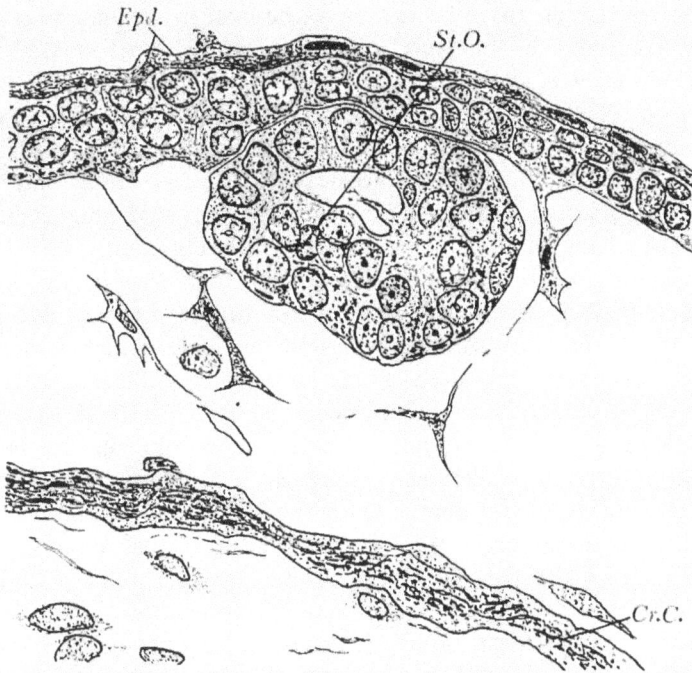

FIG. 167.—SECTION THROUGH STIEDA'S ORGAN OF A FROG TADPOLE, AT A LATER
STAGE OF DEVELOPMENT THAN THAT SHOWN IN FIG. 164.

The terminal vesicle (parietal organ) is completely cut off from the epiphysis,
    and careful search through sections behind the vesicle failed to reveal any
    nerve tract or remnant of the original connection between it and the epiphysis,
    or brain.   (Original, R. J. G.)
    Cr. C. : cranial capsule ; *Epd.* : epidermis ; *St. O.* : Parietal organ (Stieda).

is shown in Fig. 166—A, in sagittal section ; and B, in transverse section. It commences on the dorsal aspect of the epiphysis near its apex and courses backwards either on or in the substance of its dorsal wall, and finally enters the ventral part of the posterior commissure. According to Braem the fibres composing the tract arise from ganglion cells in the posterior commissure, while Haller states that the tract arises by two roots from the part of the thalamus which lies medio-ventral to the posterior commissure.

Gaupp[1] also describes a bundle of nerve-fibres which he saw in one specimen on the ventral side of the stalk of the epiphysis.

The Epiphysis or Proximal Part of the Pineal Organ of Anura

The epiphysis (Fig. 166, p. 232) usually has the form of a hollow tube ending blindly in front and opening posteriorly in the third ventricle, just behind the habenular commissure. Occasionally in the adult animal the lumen has disappeared in its basal part, which thus forms a solid stalk. In transverse section the tube is seen to be oval in outline, as if dorso-ventrally compressed, the lower wall being thicker than the upper. On each side a row of short lateral diverticula are present, which according to Braem in *Rana* are eight in number, the more anterior diverticula being larger than the posterior. The epiphysis thus has a glandular appearance like that in certain teleostean fishes, e.g. *Salmo purpuratus*. This condition we shall see occurs also in reptiles, birds, and mammals, but in these attains a much higher degree of differentiation.

The Character of the Epithelial Cells forming the Walls of the Epiphysis.— Those next to the lumen tend to become columnar in type, and sometimes bear cilia or cylindrical protoplasmic processes which project into the lumen, as in the stalk of certain teleostean fishes. These have been regarded by Galeotti as secretion processes, but Studnička states that their rod-like form in the adult animal is more like that of sensory-epithelial cells, such as are seen in the parietal organ of *Petromyzon*. These cells are especially abundant in the lower wall of the epiphysis, where there is an outer layer of rounded cells in the situation of the ganglion cells of the parietal organ of the lamprey. The cells in the dorsal wall of the epiphysis are, like those of the ventral wall, ependymal in character, but are mostly round. In its distal part the pineal tract is found imbedded in the wall of the tube, but near the base it becomes superficial and lies in a groove on its dorsal aspect. The general impression which is given by examination of the structure of the epiphysis is that of an aborted neuro-epithelial tissue, the attempted differentiation of which has become arrested.

[1] E. Gaupp. Zirbel, Parietalorgan und Paraphysis. *Ergebnisse der Anat. und Entwicklungsgeschichte,* von Merkel und Bonnet.

The Parietal Foramen of the Labyrinthodonts

The extinct Stegocephala or labyrinthodonts were very variable in size and in shape. Thus, the length of the skull, only, of *Mastodonsaurus* was 1·25 metres, while the total length of some of the smaller examples of *Melanerpeton* is only 2·5 cm. They were mostly tailed amphibians with two pairs of short limbs, the anterior, the smaller, having four or five toes ; the posterior, the larger, having five toes. Illustrations of the imprints of these feet are familiar to all who are in the least interested in the study of palæontology. They occur in stratified deposits of fossilized mud, which often shows irregular cracks, and have been found in North America, Thuringia, Saxony, and Bohemia ; and also in the Karoo formation of South Africa. The hand-like form of the footprints of *Cheirotherium barthi*, figured by Owen, are especially remarkable. Another notable characteristic of these amphibia, which has given rise to the name " labyrinthodont," is the remarkable radial arrangement and folding of the dentine which is seen in the larger and geologically later types of Stegocephala. The skull was characterized by a series of dermal plates, firmly fixed to the chondrocranium and grooved by canals of the lateral-line system. Some types resembled the more primitive types of fossil fish, such as *Lepidosteus*, but lack the opercula ; others are reptilian in type. In some the skull is wide, with elongated posterolateral horns, e.g. *Diplocaulus magnicornis* (Fig. 168), in which the orbital cavities are

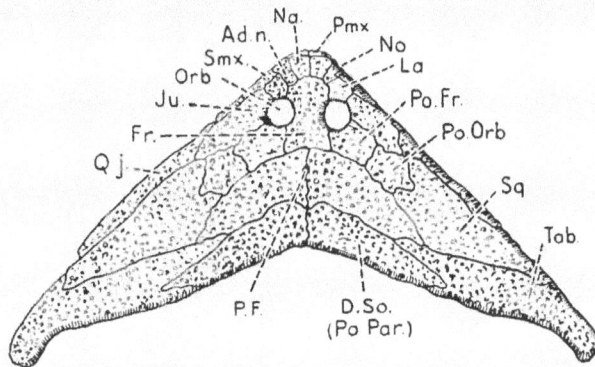

FIG. 168.—DORSAL VIEW OF SKULL OF DIPLOCAULUS MAGNICORNIS. PERMIAN OF TEXAS. (AFTER O. ABEL.)

Ad. n. : lacrimal (adnasal).
D.So. : posterior parietal.
Fr. : frontal.
Ju. : jugular.
La. : prefrontal or lacrimal.
Na. : nasal.
No. : external nostril.
Orb. : orbit.

PF. : parietal foramen.
Pmx. : premaxilla.
Po. Fr : postfrontal.
Po. Orb. : postorbital.
Qj. : quadratojugal.
Smx. : maxillary.
Sq. : squamosal.
Tab. : tabular.

(From E. S. Goodrich.)

close together on the top of the head, and a relatively small parietal foramen lies some distance behind them. In other cases (Fig. 169) the skull is narrow, as in *Dolichosoma longissimum*, found in the lower Permian, Bohemia. In this the parietal foramen is of moderate size and the frontal and parietal bones are fused in the median plane, and are partially fused with each other, so as to form a fronto-parietal plate, as in living types. In the primitive type *Branchiosaurus amblystomus* and in *Protriton* (Fig. 170) the parietal foramen is relatively very large, and the parietal and frontal bones are separate. This is the case also in *Eryops megacephalus* and *Capitosaurus* (Fig. 171, B). A special feature of some of the primitive types such as *Protriton* (Fig. 170) is the presence of circumorbital bones excluding the frontal bone from participation in the formation of the orbit and a ring of sclerotic plates for the protection of the eye within the orbit.

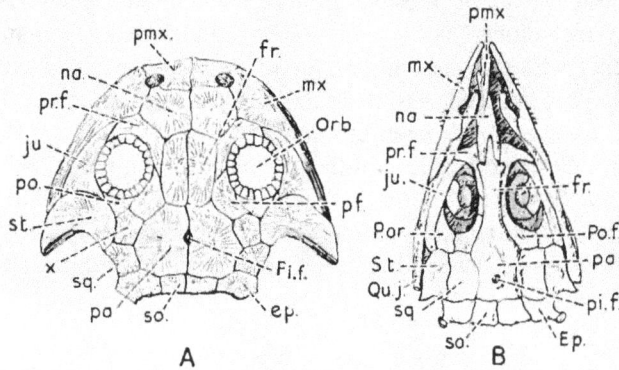

FIG. 169.

A—Dorsal aspect of skull of *Metanerpeton pulcherrimum*, showing the broad type of head with separate parietal and frontal bones. (Fritsch 1 1, after Credner.)
B—*Dolichosoma longissimum*, showing narrow type of skull with fused parietal and frontal bones. Lower Permian, Bohemia. 3 1. (After Fritsch.)

ep. : epiotic.	*po.* : postorbital.
fr. : frontal.	*Po. f.* : postfrontal.
ju. : jugular.	*pr. f.* : prefrontal.
mx. : maxilla.	*Qu. j.* : quadratojugal.
na. : nasal.	*so.* : supraoccipital.
Orb. : orbit.	*sq.* : squamosal.
pa. : parietal.	*st.* : supratemporal.
pi. f. : pineal foramen.	*x.* : anterior.
pmx. : premaxilla.	

A general consideration of the skull of labyrinthodonts in all six orders of which a conspicuous parietal foramen is present, while it appears to be generally absent as a recognizable feature in macerated skulls of modern amphibians corroborates the impression gained by the study of the parietal foramen in fishes, namely, that its presence as a relatively or actually large foramen in the skulls of the more ancient types of fossils and the tendency for it to lessen in size or disappear in the more recent types and living species indicate that the pineal organ itself was more highly evolved

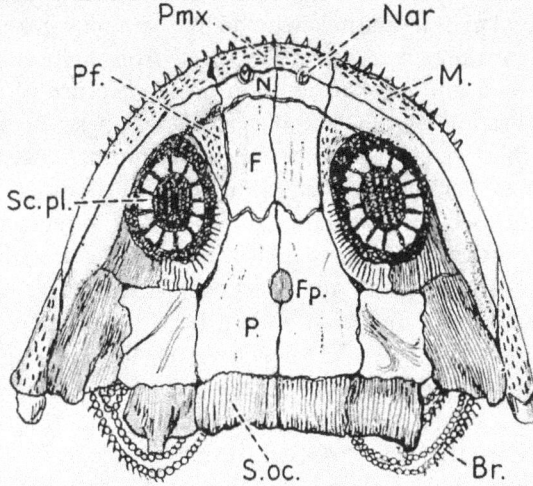

FIG. 170.—DORSAL VIEW OF SKULL OF PROTRITON, ONE OF THE SMALLER STEGO-
CEPHALA, MAGNIFIED.

Br. : branchial arches.	*Nar.* : nostril.
F. : frontal.	*P.* : parietal.
Fp. : parietal foramen.	*Pf.* : prefrontal.
M. : maxilla.	*Sc. pl.* : sclerotic plates.
N. : nasal.	*S. oc.* : supraoccipital.

(From Wiedersheim, after Fritsch.)

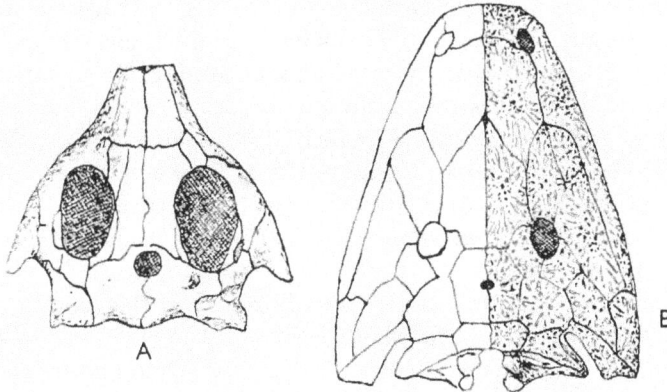

FIG. 171.

A—Dorsal aspect of skull of *Procolophon* (Seeley), a primitive reptile showing a large parietal foramen.

B—Cranium of *Capitosaurus* (Zittel), an extinct tailed amphibian belonging to the order Stegocephala, or labyrinthodonts, showing a parietal foramen.

in the more ancient and primitive types, and has become vestigial in the living representatives of these types, both in fishes and Amphibia.

Before passing on to the description of the pineal system of Reptilia it will be worth while to recall some of the effects which ensue from the disuse of the lateral eyes in animals which have for many generations lived in situations where they are completely cut off from light and are unable to use the eyes as a guide to locomotion or the capture of food. The structural degeneration of the lateral eyes under these circumstances is very similar to that which has occurred in the pineal sense organs. In both cases there is a withdrawal of the unused sense organ beneath the superficial structures, a disappearance of the refractile mechanism and of the sensory or optic nerve-fibres which connect the eye with the central nervous system. Examples of these degenerative changes are found in widely different classes of animals and in both vertebrates and invertebrates. They are well known in such cave-dwelling animals as *Proteus anguineus*; burrowing animals such as the mole or common earth worm, or as we have previously mentioned *Balanoglossus* and *Amphioxus* which bury themselves in the sand. Other instances occur in the deep-sea fishes which live in total darkness, 2,000 to 3,000 fathoms beneath the surface of the ocean, and there are also the parasitic worms and other animals which live imbedded in the flesh, tissues or organs of their hosts, and those which in their adult state become fixed like the barnacles to rocks or other objects, and which though possessing motile processes or cilia are incapable of locomotion and become blind.

One of the most interesting examples of such structural degeneration is the olm, or *Proteus anguineus* (Fig. 159, p. 225). It lives in the subterranean streams and pools of Carniolia, Carinthia, and Dalmatia, and resembles a lizard, but has external gills uncovered by an operculum; these may be removed without causing the death of the animal, which has lungs like those of other amphibia. The colour of the animal has been described as being of a " fleshy whiteness and transparency," and in this respect as well as in the retention of its external gills it resembles the Mexican axolotls (*Amblystoma tigrinum*) which also retain the larval condition of their gills.

The general appearance of *Proteus anguineus* and the condition of the eyes have been well described by Karl Semper (1883). The eye is completely buried beneath the superficial structures, being entirely covered by the skin. It has with the exception of the lens and the adjoining ciliary apparatus and iris all the characteristic parts of the eye. The development of these parts has, however, been arrested at an early embryonic stage. Inversion of the retina has taken place, and there is a deposit of pigment in its outer layer. Notwithstanding the imperfect development of the eyes, Semper was able to prove from observations he made on a family of *Proteus* that he kept for four years that the creatures were " highly sensitive to diffused light," and he remarked that " as this light contains no heat rays the eye of the *Proteus* can receive no impression but that of light."

Semper also writes of the mole, this animal " has true eyes from which none of the essential parts of the eyes of vertebrates are absent, although these parts are all of the simplest embryonic structure. The whole eye is very small, deeply imbedded in muscles, and quite covered by the skin, so that it is quite invisible externally. The lens consists of a number of minute and little altered embryonic cells. The retina, in the same way, is much simpler than in the eyes of other vertebrates. True degeneration, then, such as makes the eye incapable of seeing, has not taken place ; nevertheless the eye of the mole is reduced to almost total inefficiency, even when by chance it has an opportunity for using it. This almost total blindness of the mole is the result of complete degeneration of the optic nerve, so that the images which are probably formed in the eye itself can never be transmitted to the animal's consciousness. Occasionally the mole can see a little, for it has been found that both optic nerves are not always degenerated in the same individual, so that one eye may remain in communication with the brain, while the other has no connection with it. In the embryo of the mole, and without exception, both eyes are originally connected with the brain by well-developed optic nerves, and so theoretically (are capable of becoming) efficient. This may be regarded as a perfectly conclusive proof that the blind mole is descended from progenitors that could see."

CHAPTER 20

REPTILES

It is in the class Reptilia that the greatest insight into the nature of the pineal system has been obtained, and more especially with reference to the pineal eye of that archaic lizard, the Tuatara of New Zealand, or *Sphenodon*, which has sometimes been alluded to as a " living fossil."

Most valuable information has also been gained by the study of the parietal foramen in the various orders of fossil reptiles, which, like that in Pisces and Amphibia, not only indicates the antiquity and universality of distribution of the median eye in the widely separated orders of the class, but that, judging from the large size of the foramen in some of the more primitive examples as compared with their living representatives, the pineal eye itself is, both actually and relatively to the size of the animal, smaller in living species than it was in their remote ancestors.

As in fishes and amphibians, there is indubitable evidence of two organs being included in the pineal system of reptiles ; there is a difference of opinion, however, as to whether the two components are essentially separate and independent median structures or whether they are derived from a primarily bilateral pair of sense organs which are homologous with each other and have been secondarily shifted into the median plane.

There is in reptiles the same subdivision of the whole pineal organ into proximal part, stalk, and end vesicle, as in fishes and amphibians, and there are the same connections with the roof of the diencephalon. There is, however, much variability in the degree of differentiation of the pineal system in different orders of the class and in individual species.

Valuable information has also been gleaned from the study of accessory parietal organs in reptiles and of the degenerative changes which have been observed in some cases, e.g. the presence of pigment in the lens ; absence or inconspicuous appearance of the parietal spot ; and degenerative or pathological changes in the neuro-epithelial tissue.

In Crocodilia neither parietal organ nor epiphysis is present in the adult animal, although the habenular and posterior commissures are well-developed and distinct, being separated by a small part of the roof of the diencephalon ; the dorsal sac and paraphysis are also present— alligator (Sorensen, 1894) ; *Crocodilus madagascarensis* and *Caiman niger* (Voeltzkow, 1903).

Development of the Pineal System in Reptiles

In addition to the pioneer work of Leydig, Strahl and Martin, Béraneck and others, the early stages of development of the pineal outgrowth have been studied by Nowikoff (1910) in *Lacerta muralis* and *L. vivipara*, and by Dendy (1899-1911) in *Sphenodon*. According to Nowikoff, the first indication of the pineal outgrowth occurs as a thickening of the neural-epithelium forming the roof of the diencephalon. It is situated in the median plane and indicates the junction of the diencephalon with the midbrain. A transverse groove divides it into an anterior segment which will become the parietal eye, and a posterior segment (Fig. 172, A). At the 4-mm. stage (Fig. 172, B) the apex of the evagination is seen to be directed forward, and the groove now forms a constriction which completely surrounds the tubular evagination. In a 6-mm. example of *L. muralis* (Fig. 172, C) the anterior segment has become detached from the posterior or proximal part, and now forms a closed vesicle lying between the epidermis and the brain. Later in a 9-mm. embryo of *L. vivipara* (Fig. 172, D) the parietal vesicle is seen to be separated from the roof of the diencephalon by an ingrowth of mesoderm containing blood-vessels. Traversing the mesoderm is a bundle of nerve-fibres which connect the parietal eye with the right habenular ganglion. This lies in front of the posterior segment or pineal sac and it was considered by Graham Kerr (1919) to have arisen by the development of nerve-fibres in the primary bridge which connected the wall of the vesicle with the roof of the brain, when these were in contact, as shown in Fig. 172, C. The connection of the nerve with the right habenular ganglion through the habenular commissure agrees with the description by Klinckowstroem (1894) of the connection of the " pineal " or parietal nerve in *Iguana tuberculata*, but differs from that in *Sphenodon* which was described by Dendy (1899), in which the connection is with the left habenular ganglion. A thickening of the superficial or distal wall of the parietal organ in *Lacerta* which was first noticeable in the 6-mm. stage becomes marked off later as the lens (Fig. 172, C), while the remaining portion of the vesicle becomes differentiated into the sensory or receptive part—the retina—the structure of which will be described later (p. 253). At the 25-mm. stage (Fig. 173) the parietal organ becomes further separated from the pineal sac by the interposition of the paraphysis and dorsal sac, around which the greatly elongated pineal nerve courses in its passage from the parietal organ to the habenular commissure.

Several views have been expressed in explanation of the appearances seen in the early stages of development of the pineal system ; briefly stated, these are :

16

(1) There is a single median evagination, the tip of which being cut off, forms the pineal eye, while the basal part retaining its connection with the brain, forms the epiphysis, a pineal stalk, sometimes represented by the pineal nerve, persisting between the two parts—Strahl (1884), *Lacerta* ; Spencer (1886), *Anolis ; Moloch horridus.*

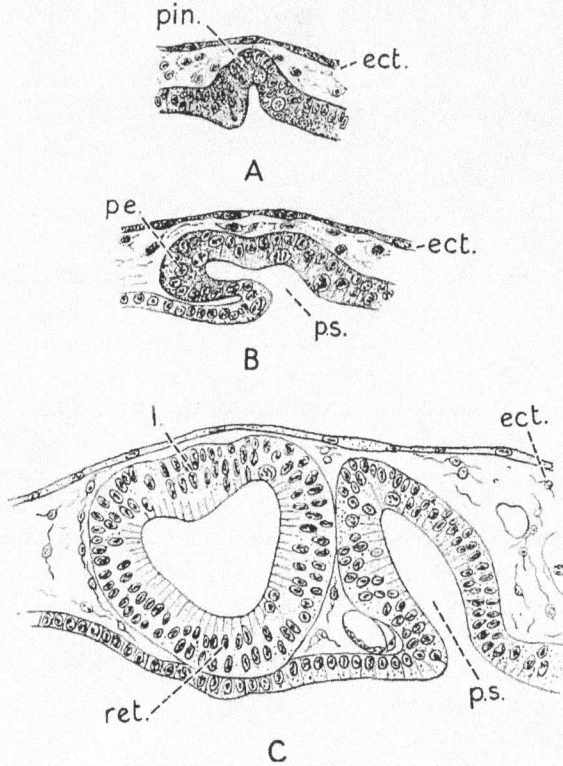

FIG. 172, A, B, C.—SAGITTAL SECTIONS THROUGH THE PINEAL ORGAN OF EMBRYOS OF *Lacerta*. (AFTER NOWIKOFF.)

A : *Lacerta vivipara*, 3 mm.
B : *Lacerta vivipara*, 4 mm.
C : *Lacerta muralis*, 6 mm.

ect. : cutaneous ectoderm.　　*pin.* : pineal nerve.
l. : lens.　　*p.s.* : pineal stalk.
p.e. : pineal eye.　　*ret.* : retina.

(2) There are two separate and morphologically distinct evaginations, situated in the median plane one behind the other, of which the anterior gives rise to the parietal eye and the posterior to the epiphysis—Leydig (1891) ; Studnička (1893).

(3) A single median evagination, which is subsequently divided into two : (*a*) an anterior vesicle, the parietal eye, having an independent

nerve, the nervus parietalis, not connected to the epiphysis, but joining the habenular commissure ; (b) a posterior part, the epiphysis—Hoffmann, *Lacerta agilis* (1886) ; Strahl and Martin, *Anguis, L. vivipara* (1886).

(4) A single diverticulum, the distal part of which becomes divided by an incomplete transverse septum into an anterior and posterior part, in such a way that the lumina of the two end vesicles communicate with the lumen of a common stalk—Béraneck, *Lacerta* (1894).

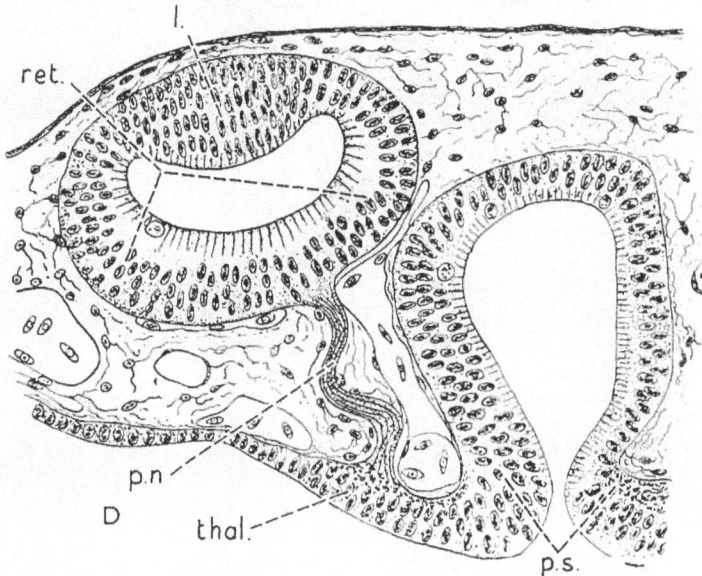

FIG. 172, D.—SAGITTAL SECTION THROUGH THE PINEAL ORGAN OF AN EMBRYO OF LACERTA VIVIPARA, 9 MM. (AFTER NOWIKOFF.)

The nerve-fibres were traced through the habenular commissure into the right habenular ganglion. According to Graham Kerr, they are formed at the time when the vesicle is in contact with the roof of the thalamencephalon and afterwards elongate as the vesicle becomes gradually separated from the brain (see Fig. 173).

l. : lens; pn. : parietal nerve; p.s. : pineal stalk and pineal sac. ; ret. : retina; thal. : roof of thalamencephalon.

(5) The parietal eye arises not as an independent structure but as an outgrowth from the anterior wall of the primary diverticulum—Klinckowstroem, *Iguana* (1894) ; McKay, *Grammatophora muricata* (1888) ; and Schauinsland, *Sphenodon* (1899).

(6) Two completely independent outgrowths soon unite with each other—Francotte, *L. vivipara* (1894).

(7) The rudiments of two pairs of serially arranged sense organs become fused in the median plane, the anterior giving rise to the parietal organ, the posterior to the epiphysis, and when present an accessory parietal or pineal organ.

(8) The parietal eye is phylogenetically bilateral. In ontogeny, indications of this condition are present in reptiles, e.g. *Sphenodon*, and also in other classes of vertebrates, e.g. *Geotria*. Thus in *Sphenodon*

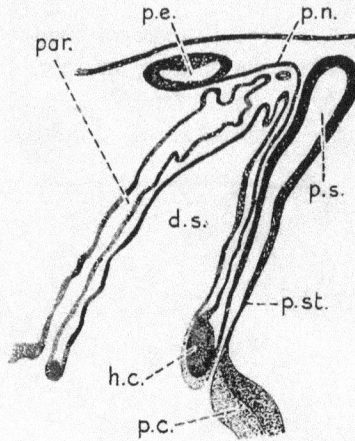

FIG. 173.—LONGITUDINAL VERTICAL SECTION THROUGH PINEAL ORGAN OF LACERTA MURALIS (25 MM.) SHOWING TERMINAL VESICLE. (NOWIKOFF.)

d.s. : dorsal sac.	*p.e.* : parietal eye.
h.c. : habenular or anterior commissure.	*p.n.* : parietal nerve.
par. : paraphysis.	*p. st.* : pineal stalk.
p.c. : posterior commissure.	*p.s.* : pineal sac.

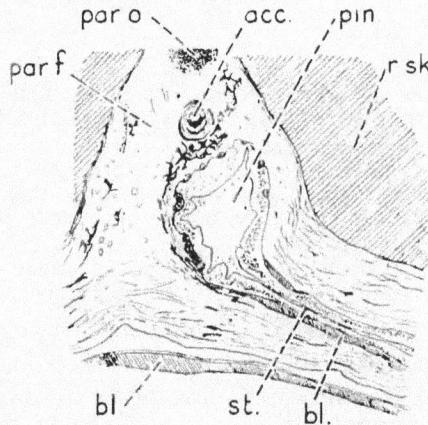

FIG. 174.—THE END VESICLE AND THE DISTAL PART OF THE STALK OF THE PINEAL ORGAN, AND A PART OF THE PARIETAL EYE OF PSEUDOPUS PALLASII. (AFTER STUDNIČKA.)

acc. : accessory pineal organ.	*pin.* : end vesicle of pineal organ.
bl. : blood-vessel.	*r. sk.* : roof of skull.
par. f. : parietal foramen.	*st.* : stalk.
par. o. : part of the parietal organ.	

the anterior diverticulum is at first situated to the left of the posterior part, and the nerve which arises from the retina of the parietal eye, at a later stage of development is connected with the left habenular ganglion— Dendy, *Sphenodon*, 1899 ; Gaskell, 1908 ; Patten, 1890 ; and others.

Dendy's view of the bilateral origin of the parietal sense organ, which was also held by Hill, Gaskell and others, is supported by the geological evidence of the existence in certain extinct fishes of two parietal impressions or foramina, placed side by side in the roof of the skull, as seen in Figs. 140, 229, 230 (Chap. 18, p. 200, and Chap. 23, pp. 329, 330), of *Dipnorhynchus*, *Pholidosteus*, *Rhinosteus*, and *Titanichthys*. It also receives strong support from the occasional development of an accessory parietal

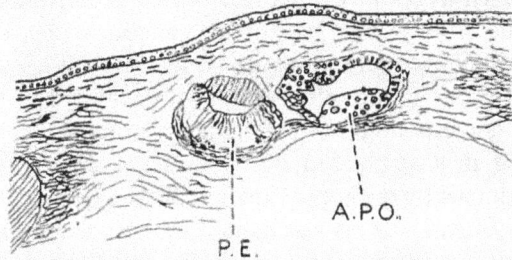

FIG. 175.—SAGITTAL SECTION THROUGH THE PARIETAL FORAMEN OF A HORNED LIZARD (PHRYNOSOMA CORONATUM).

Lying in the foramen are a parietal eye and an accessory parietal organ. (After Ritter, from *Die Parietal-organe Studnička*.)

P.E : parietal eye. A.P.O. : accessory parietal organ.

sense organ which lies close to or is in continuity with the tip of the pineal organ, as in Pseudopus palassii, described by Studnička in 1905 (Figs. 174, 177), and *Phrynosoma coronatum* (Fig. 175) (after Ritter).

The nerves and nerve Ganglia of the Pineal System of Reptilia.

A detailed study of the nerves of (1) the parietal sense organ and (2) the pineal organ, including the pineal sac or end vesicle with the stalk and the basal or proximal part, is instructive from several standpoints, more particularly (A) as an aid to the solution of the question as to its origin— namely, whether from two serially homologous parts placed one behind the other or from vestiges of primarily bilateral sense organs ; (B) ascertaining whether the pineal system shows signs, both phylogenetically and onto-genetically, of degeneration, or of the evolution of an endocrine organ.

An important point to bear in mind is that no nerve-fibres are found in connection with the rudiment of the parietal sense organ until after the vesicle has been completely separated from the basal part of the evagination, as indicated in the drawings of Strahl and Martin (1888), *Anguis fragilis, Lacerta vivipara* ; Béraneck (1892) in *Anguis* and *Lacerta*, and Nowikoff (1910), *L. agilis, L. vivipara*, and *A. fragilis*. The earlier observations made on the embryos of *Lacerta* and *Anguis* were later confirmed by Studnička, and additional observations were made by Klinckostroem, Spencer, Dendy, and others on different species of reptiles, e.g. *Iguana, Varanus*, and *Sphenodon*. The general result of these researches may be briefly stated as follows. The parietal nerve originates from ganglion cells in the retina of the parietal sense organ ; it courses backwards over the dorsal sac and then turns downwards towards the brain in front of the epiphysis and between this and the posterior wall of the dorsal sac, and finally terminates in the roof of the diencephalon, where it has been traced into : the right habenular ganglion—*Iguana tuberculata* (Strahl and Martin) ; the left habenular ganglion—*Sphenodon* (Dendy) ; two parietal nerves, right and left, each of which ended in the habenular ganglion of the corresponding side—Iguana (Klinckostroem) ; a single nerve terminating in a nucleus in the roof of the diencephalon (formed according to Studnička by the approximation of the right and left habenular ganglia)—*Anguis fragilis*. This was named by Béraneck *le noyau pariétal*. Spencer described a case of longitudinal splitting of the parietal nerve in *Varanus* giganteus (Fig. 176), and he also described nerve-fibres passing in the remnants of the original stalk of the pineal eye to the epiphysis. Ritter in *Phrynosoma coronatum* describes the parietal nerve as extending between the posterior commissure and the parietal eye ; and cases have been described in which a nerve is absent. The failure to find a nerve in adult or later larval stages is explained by the degeneration of a nerve which, although developed as a transitory structure in embryonic life, has either disappeared altogether or is represented only by its fibrous sheath. The nerve-fibres when the whole nerve is at the height of its development are provided with medullary sheaths and there is an outer covering of neurilemma, the trunk being invested by a fibrous sheath which is continuous with the capsule of the parietal eye and with the pia mater.

The pineal nerve,[1] or tractus pinealis, or nerve of the epiphysis differs from the parietal nerve, or nerve of the parietal sense organ, in its position relative to the epiphysis and its termination ; arising from cells in the wall of the pineal sac or end vesicle, it passes towards the brain on the posterior aspect of the proximal part of the organ and ends in the posterior commissure (Figs. 166, 187, pp. 232, 264). The earlier description of nerve-fibres

---

[1] The name " pineal nerve " is still frequently used to denote the nerve of the " parietal sense organ," or " pineal eye." The distal connection of the nerve with the parietal organ should, however, prevent confusion when the term " pineal " is used in this sense.

which were seen by Leydig in *Platydactylus* lying in the stalk of the epiphysis was considered by Melchers to be incorrect, the appearance of fibrillation being due to the persistence of connective tissue fibres in the degenerated stalk of the epiphysis. According to Klinckowstroem the tractus pinealis in an 18-day embryo of *Iguana tuberculata* sinks into the posterior wall of the epiphysis at the junction of its proximal two-thirds with the distal

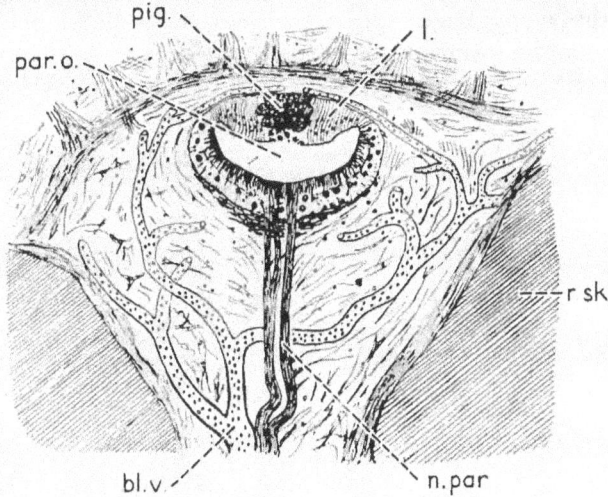

FIG. 176.—SAGITTAL SECTION THROUGH THE PARIETAL EYE, AND PARIETAL FORAMEN OF VARANUS GIGANTEUS, SHOWING DEPOSIT OF PIGMENT IN THE CENTRAL PART OF THE LENS AND A DIVISION OF THE PARIETAL NERVE INTO TWO MAIN BRANCHES. (AFTER SPENCER.)

bl. v. : blood-vessel. *par. o.* : parietal organ.
l. : lens. *pig.* : pigment.
n. par. : parietal nerve. *r. sk.* : roof of skull.

third, and from this point to its termination in the posterior commissure the tract lies free in the surrounding connective tissue. It is thus comparable with the pineal tract observed by Braem in *Rana temporaria* (Fig. 166, Chap. 19, p. 232). Whether there is also a connection with the habenular commissure or ganglia and the exact destination of the fibres which enter the posterior commissure are questions which seem to be unsettled. It seems probable, however, that degenerative changes similar to those which occur in the parietal nerve take place and that the tract disappears in late larval stages or during adult life.

The Pineal Organ of Reptiles

It is only in rare cases that the pineal organ of reptiles is seen to consist of all three parts—end vesicle, stalk, and expanded proximal or basal part, the latter of which represents the epiphysis or pineal gland of birds and mammals. The end vesicle is in most cases absent, but its existence in a rudimentary form and the presence in it of pigment in some species such as *Pseudopus Palasii* (Studnička) (Figs. 174, 177) and the occasional occurrence of a fibrous connection between the tip of the pineal organ and the parietal eye such as occurs in the early developmental stages of certain Amphibia, e.g. *Rana temporaria*, Braem (Fig. 161, Chap. 19, p. 228), is of the greatest significance. It affords additional support to the hypothesis based on the ontogenetic development of the pineal organ and on geological evidence that the proximal part and stalk of the end vesicle represent the common stalk of a primarily bilateral sense

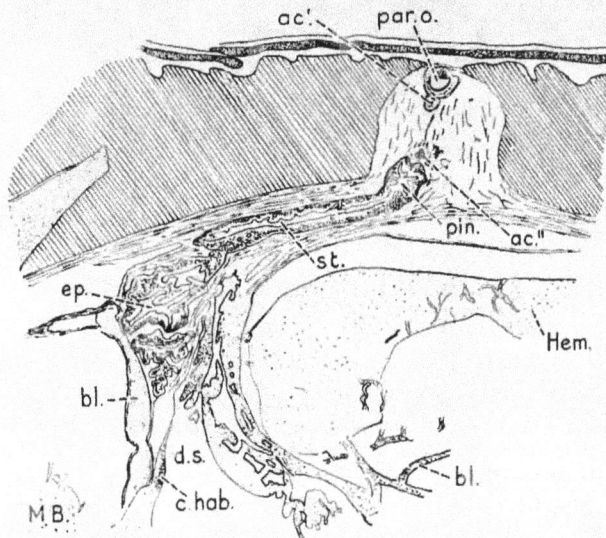

Fig. 177.—Sagittal Section through the Parietal Region showing a Large Parietal Foramen, containing a Parietal Organ, the End Vesicle of the Pineal Organ and Two Accessory Organs, from an Adult Example of Pseudopus Pallasii. (After Studnička.)

ac.', *ac."* : accessory organs.	*Hem.* : hemisphere.
bl. : blood vessel.	*MB.* : midbrain.
c. hab. : habenular commissure.	*par. o.* : parietal organ.
d.s. : dorsal sac.	*pin.* : end vesicle of pineal organ.
ep. : epiphysis.	*st.* : primary stalk of pineal organ.

organ, the end vesicles of which in some types are completely absent; in others, one of the sense organs has become more highly evolved, and retaining its connection with the superficial structures becomes separated from the parent stem; while the other, the growth of which early becomes arrested, either retains its original connection with the common stalk or, like the parietal sense organ, becomes separated off as an accessory pineal organ. Such an accessory organ may lie close to the parietal sense organ; between this and the pineal organ (Fig. 177); or in continuity with the tip of the pineal organ. The frequent presence of pigment in the epithelium of the accessory organ and its location in the proximal segment of the accessory vesicle, or when continuity with the end vesicle of the pineal organ is preserved, its attachment to the distal extremity of this, form in our opinion, important evidence in favour of the accessory organ being the vestige of a light-percipient organ and of its homology with the parietal sense organ.

Structure of the Pineal Organ of Reptiles

The microscopic structure of the wall of the pineal sac of an adult *Sphenodon* is shown in Fig. 178, after Dendy. The appearances are very

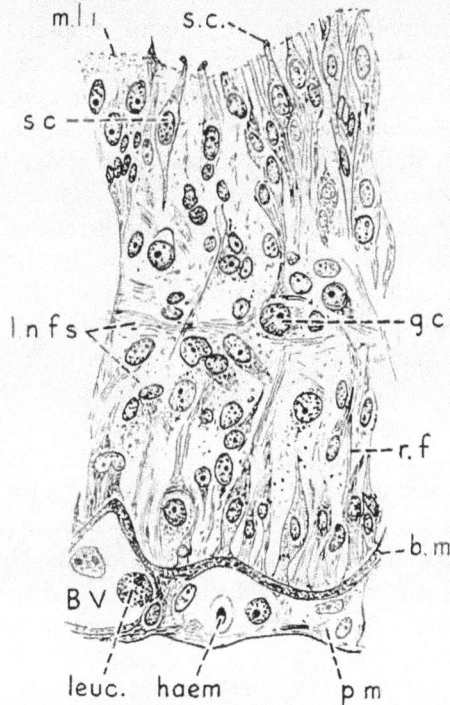

FIG. 178.—PART OF A LONGITUDINAL VERTICAL SECTION THROUGH THE WALL OF THE PINEAL SAC OF AN ADULT MALE SPHENODON (AFTER DENDY), SHOWING DETAILS OF MICROSCOPIC STRUCTURE, WHICH CLOSELY RESEMBLE THOSE OF THE PINEAL EYE (Fig. 181).

b.m. : basement membrane.
B.V. : blood-vessel.
g.c. : ganglion cell.
hæm. : hæmatid.
leuc. : leucocyte.

l.n.f.s. : layer of nerve-fibres of pineal sac.
m.l.i. : membrana limitans interna.
p.m. : pia mater.
r.f. : radial fibres.
s.c. : sensory cells.

similar to those seen in the retina of the parietal organ, but there is in most specimens a lack of pigment in the inner epithelial layer and of large ganglionic nerve cells such as are present in the retina of the parietal sense organ. The pineal sac is invested by an outer fibrous sheath, continuous with the pia mater and containing blood-vessels. Beneath this is a basement membrane or membrana limitans externa, while internally next to the lumen is a less defined membrane, pierced by the inner ends of cells forming the internal epithelial layer. Between these two membranes is a supporting basis of ependymal glial tissue, the cell-elements and fibres of which are arranged for the most part in a radial manner. In addition to the supporting glial element, nerve-fibres are present which form a definite layer running parallel to the surface and about midway between the two limiting membranes. Some of these fibres appear to be continuous with the tapering deep-ends of the sensory cells of the inner epithelial layer, and others with processes of cells, which resemble nerve-cells, belonging to the outer epithelial layer. In young specimens of *Sphenodon* the wall of the pineal sac is less differentiated and its structure resembles that of the stalk and proximal part. In all three parts of the organ, the wall consists of a single or double layer of ependymal cells, the oval nuclei of which are arranged radially to the axis of the tube, and there is a tendency where the tube is narrow, as in the stalk for the cells to form a single layer and become cubical in form, whereas in the expanded segments of the tube, two or more layers of nuclei are present and the cells become elongated. In adult specimens of some species of reptiles, e.g. *Sphenodon* (Spencer), *Anguis* (Leydig), and *Pseudopus* (Studnička) in which the proximal or " epiphyseal segment " becomes expanded, the walls of this part become thickened and in-folded ; the spaces between the folds being filled with vascular con-nective tissue, so that sections of it have a glandular appearance, which closely resembles that of the paraphysis and of the choroid plexuses. In older specimens there is a tendency towards degeneration in all segments of the pineal organ. This is also attended by folding of the walls and ingrowth of vessels. The degenerative processes are still more marked in the epiphysis of *Ophidia* and *Chelonia*, there being an early arrest of development and lack of differentiation which sometimes results in the disappearance of the cavity of the epiphysis or that of its constricted " neck " called by Studnicka the secondary stalk. In late stages the vessels may disappear and intracellular and intercellular spaces appear in a solid mass of degenerated glial tissue, as in *Tropinodotus* (Fig. 179) (Leydig).

There is the same difference of opinion with regard to the nature of the processes projecting through the internal limiting membrane of the distal part of the epiphysis that we mentioned in the case of teleostean fishes (Figs. 148, 154, Chap. 18, pp. 211, 219), namely, as to whether these represent secretory threads, cilia, or protoplasmic processes of the cells, similar to those present in the pineal eye of *Geotria* or *Petromyzon*.

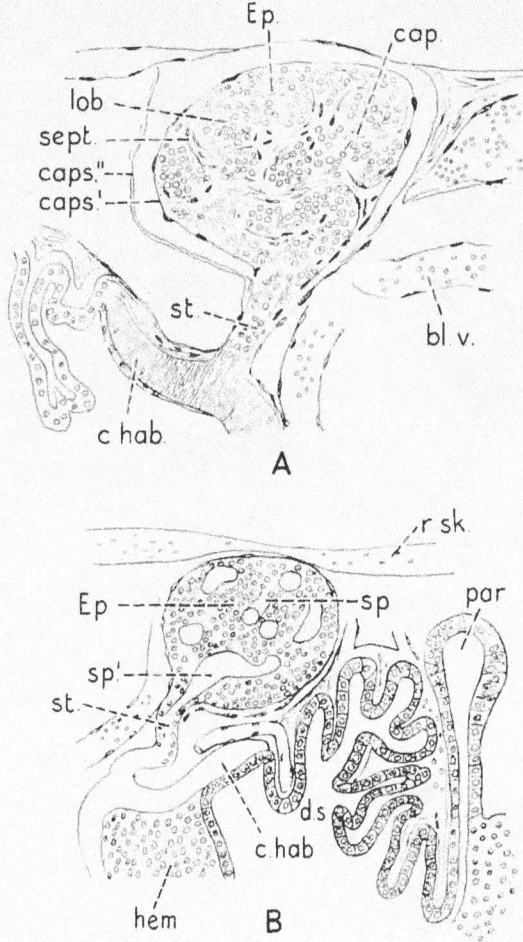

FIG. 179.

A—The epiphysis of a young embryo of a water snake, *Tropidonotus*. The ependymal tissue is penetrated by ingrowing septa of connective tissue, containing capillary blood-vessels, and is subdivided into rounded lobules.

B—The epiphysis of an older specimen of *Tropidonotus*; the organ now appears as a solid mass of tissue; all traces of lobulation and plexus of capillary vessels having disappeared; degeneration being indicated by the formation of spaces which are not lined by endothelium. (After Leydig.)

bl. v. : blood-vessel.	*hem.* : hemisphere.
c. hab. : habenular commissure.	*lob.* : lobule.
cap. : capillary.	*par.* : paraphysis.
caps', caps" : internal and external capsule	*r. sk.* : roof of skull.
	sp. : space
d.s. : dorsal sac.	*sp'.* : remnant of primary cavity.
Ep. : epiphysis.	*st.* : secondary stalk.

They lack the regularity of shape and size which characterizes the smooth club-shaped ends of the sensory-cells of the pineal eye of *Geotria* (Fig. 45, Chap. 3, p. 69), but they give the impression of being degenerated processes of the epithelium rather than a secretion product or cilia.

The Parietal Organ of Reptiles

No parietal eye is developed in many of the lizards ; thus it is absent in *Cyclodus gigas* and in the tegu, a large lizard which frequents the forests of the Amazon ; there is also no parietal eye in certain geckos, e.g. *Hemidactylus, Gehyra, Platydactylus* ; nor in some Agamidæ, namely *Draco, Ceratophora, Lyriocephalus*. A definite parietal eye is also absent in the snakes, tortoises, turtles, crocodiles, and alligators.

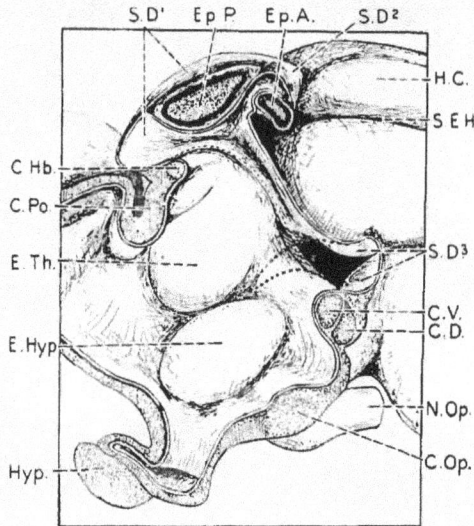

FIG. 180.—RECONSTRUCTION OF THE STRUCTURES ON THE MEDIAL ASPECT OF THE DIENCEPHALIC REGION OF THE BRAIN OF TESTUDO GEOMETRICA (40); SHOWING THE RELATIONS OF THE ANTERIOR EPIPHYSIS AND POSTERIOR EPIPHYSIS TO THE DORSAL SAC. (REDRAWN FROM G. W. H. SCHEPERS.)

C.D. : dorsal commissure.	*Ep. A.* : anterior epiphysis.
C. Hb. : habenular commissure.	*Ep. P.* : posterior epiphysis.
C. Op. : optic chiasma.	*H.C.* : cerebral hemisphere.
C. Po. : posterior commissure.	*Hyp.* : hypophysis.
C.V. : ventral commissure.	*N. Op.* : optic nerve.
E. Hyp. : hypothalamic eminence.	*S.D.* [1], [2], [3] : dorsal sac.
E. Th. : thalamic eminence.	*S.EH.* : sulcus endohippocampi.

In some of the above-mentioned examples in which a parietal eye is stated to be absent, there is a subdivision of the primary pineal evagination into two parts, an upper and a lower. Thus in the tegu, there is a difference of opinion as to whether " the upper division of the embryonic evagination represents the rudiment of a parietal eye which at a later stage of development becomes incorporated with the end vesicle of the pineal outgrowth, and thus fails to form an independent parietal organ " (Klinckowstroem) ; or whether, as Studnička believed to be more probable, the upper subdivision from the first represents the end vesicle of the pineal outgrowth, the parietal organ being absent.

Quite recently an interesting paper by G. W. H. Schepers has been published in the *J. of Anatomy* (Vol. 72, 1938), in which he describes two epiphyseal vesicles in the brain of a South African land tortoise, *Testudo geometrica*. In this animal the epiphyses were situated in the usual position between the cerebral hemispheres and midbrain ; the smaller vesicle was antero-inferior in position, whereas the large vesicle was postero-superior. They were enveloped in a large dorsal sac or parencephalon (Fig. 180), and were situated between the ependyma and pia mater. No stalk or nerve-fibres were found connecting the vesicles with the central nervous system. The larger, superficial vesicle lay in a depression in the roof of the dorsal sac, in close relation with the vessels of the choroid plexus ; while the smaller, anterior vesicle lay in relation with the anterior wall of the sac, below and between two anterior horns of the sac. The walls of both cysts, but more especially the anterior, showed signs of cellular degeneration. Schepers concludes that the vesicles are neural derivatives and that the larger structure is comparable with the pineal body ; the smaller with the " parapineal body."

Structure of the Parietal Organ of Sphenodon

A. The Retina

Beneath the thin inner fibrous capsule (Fig. 181), there is a well-defined external limiting membrane ; while next to the lumen is an internal limiting membrane pierced by the projecting inner ends of the sensory cells. Between the two limiting membranes is a supporting tissue formed by the elongated bodies of the ependymal cells, the outer ends of which are expanded and continuous with the external limiting membrane. The neurosensory elements consist of an inner layer of sensory cells, the cylindrical bodies of which extend from the internal basal membrane towards a middle layer of nerve-fibres. These course parallel to the surface and midway between the two limiting membranes ; as the cell bodies pass towards the middle stratum of nerve-fibres they taper into fine processes which appear to end in this layer. External to the nerve-fibre layer is found a stratum of nerve-cells, some of which are large and contain a clear vesicular nucleus with a well-defined nucleolus. These are the ganglion cells, processes of which join the nerve-fibre layer. Besides the nerve elements just described there are in the internal layer cells containing pigment granules, which are mostly arranged in a radial manner parallel to and between the sensory cells; pigment granules are also found in and between the sensory cells and in the outer layer, where they are often deposited in large round cells called " pigment balls "; small neuroglial cells with branched processes are also present. Moreover, a considerable amount of pigment is contained in the connective tissue around the parietal organ, namely, between the inner and outer layers of the fibrous capsule and in the loose areolar tissue beyond the capsule.

B. The Lens

The lens varies markedly in form both in different species and in different examples of the same species. It is usually biconvex, but one side may be more convex than the other or it may be approximately plano-convex. In the latter case the flatter surface may be directed superficially, or it may be directed towards the cavity of the parietal organ. Other lenses are irregular in form; in some cases sections of the lens may show what appears to be a central notch, lying beneath a clump of rounded pigment cells as in Fig. 176, showing the parietal eye of a specimen of *Varanus giganteus*, described by Spencer. In a similar case in which pigment was present in the centre of the lens in a specimen of *Anguis fragilis*, described by Béraneck (Fig. 182), there was a peculiar seam on the superficial surface of the lens, which suggests that the lens was formed by the growth in contact with each other of the rudiments of two lenses. In some cases the lens may be flattened and very wide, more especially in those cases in which the whole parietal organ is wide and appears to be dorso-ventrally compressed. It is especially in this flattened, wide type of lens that central pigment cells have most frequently been observed. An exception to the above statement, however, occurs in an example of a very narrow, almost cylindrical parietal organ in *Anolis*, an American type of Iguana described by Spencer. In this specimen the vertical or axial diameter of the lens is little less than the transverse diameter, pigment cells were nevertheless present in the middle of the inner half of the lens. The growth of the whole organ appears to have been arrested at an early stage of development, and the retina to have been composed simply of elongated ependymal cells separated by wide intercellular spaces. It may be noted also that the parietal foramen in this specimen was especially narrow, being little wider than the parietal organ. With reference to these conditions it may be mentioned that in a nearly related type of *Anolis* Spencer found a dorso-ventrally flattened form of parietal eye, and that the occurrence of such opposite extremes in the shape of the parietal organ and its lens in the same genus merely exemplifies the tendency to variation which exists in degenerating organs, and does not contradict

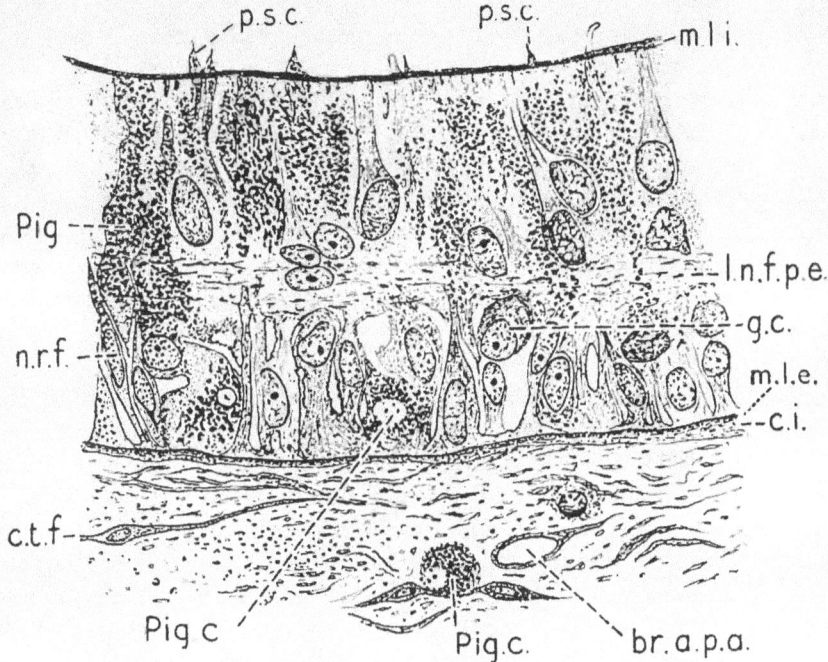

FIG. 181.—SECTION OF THE RETINA OF THE PINEAL EYE OF SPHENODON PUNCTATA.
(AFTER DENDY.)

br. a.p.a. : branch of anterior
   pineal artery.
c.i. : capsula interna.
c.t.f. : connective tissue fibre.
g.c. : ganglion cell.
l.n.f.p.e. : layer of nerve-fibres
   of pineal eye.

m.l.e. : membrana limitans externa.
m.l.i. : membrana limitans interna.
n.r.f. : nucleus of radial fibre.
pig. : pigment.
pig. c. : pigment cell.
p.s.c. : processes of sensory cells.

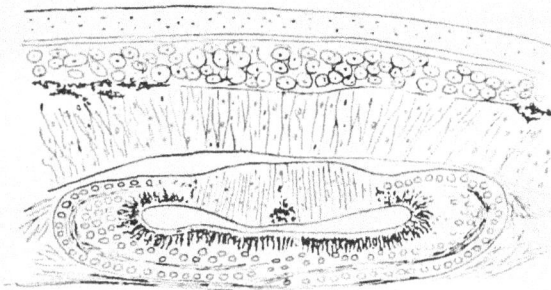

FIG. 182.—PARIETAL EYE OF A 7·6-MM. EMBRYO OF ANGUIS FRAGILIS. (AFTER
(BERANECK.)

Pigment is present in the central and deep part of the lens.   The lens is very wide,
   and is continuous at its periphery with the retina.   The nerve-fibre layer of
   the retina is interrupted below the central mass of pigment in the lens.
   Pigment is absent in the corium and epidermis of the tissues lying superficial
   to the eye.

the general statement with regard to the frequency of pigment cells in the centre of the wide type of lens.

Besides variations in the form of the lens in the parietal eye of reptiles, cases occur in which the lens is absent, its place being simply marked by a thin part of the wall of the vesicle which is destitute of pigment, and although not an homologous structure, it resembles the cornea of the lateral eyes ; a good example of absence of the lens was described by Spencer in a specimen of *Moloch horridus*. This was, however, a very exceptional case in which the parietal eye was almost completely filled with pigmented tissue, leaving only a small space in front, like the anterior chamber of a lateral eye. The parietal organ lay in the parietal foramen, and was connected by a solid stalk with the distal end of the epiphysis. The specimen appears to be a case of arrested development in which the parietal organ has failed to separate from the parent stem, and has failed to differentiate into lens and typical retina. If this interpretation is correct the end vesicle of the epiphysis has also failed to develop. It is possible, however, that the structure described by Spencer as the parietal organ, since it was directly connected by a stalk with the epiphysis, was itself the end vesicle of the pineal organ and it was the parietal organ which was lacking—a view which was first suggested by Studnička.

The frequent appearance of pigment in the centre of the lens of the parietal organ, and the occasional presence in such cases of a notch on the under surface of the lens or of a seam on the superficial surface, may be of significance with reference to the theory of a dual origin of the parietal organ. A parallel condition is met with in cases of cyclopia, whether this anomaly occurs in single individuals or in double monsters, more particularly in certain cases of Cephalothoracopagus monosymmetros or Diprosopus triophthalmos. In these cases varying degrees of blending of the two eyes occur in the development of the cyclops eye, namely, between simple approximation of two eyes lying in a single orbital cavity and an apparently single eye in which a compound lens is found which is formed by the fusion of two halves. Thus, according to the classification of the various degrees in the development of cyclopia by Bock, with reference to the fusion of the paired lateral eyes, cases occur in which :

1. The two bulbs are united only by the sclera.

2. The optic nerves are approximated ; the common scleral tissue between the bulbs has become thinner ; the cornea, iris, lens, vitreous, and retina are double.

3. The cornea is single ; the iris, lens, vitreous, and retina double, the optic nerves separated merely by a narrow space filled with connective tissue.

4. One cornea ; two lenses united in the median plane of the compound eye ; sclera, chorioidea, retina, and optic nerve single.

5. An eye without visible doubling of any part may lack an optic nerve.

6. An apparently single eye, in which the lens is found to be compounded of two halves.

The possibility of the apparently single median or " third " eye of certain fishes and reptiles being compounded of elements of parts of two eyes growing in contact with each other is thus evident, and appearances such as those shown in Fig. 176, p. 247, and Fig. 182, p. 255, are readily explained. It is quite possible that the rounded pigment cells in the centre of the lens represent a vestige of interposed median parts of retinæ which have become included between the two halves of the compound lens ; and the presence of a median notch on the under surface of the lens or a seam on the superficial surface affords additional evidence of the fusion, moreover, the deep brownish-black colour of the pigment and its deposit in large, rounded cells are typical of retinal pigment rather than a mere degeneration product ; although the element of degeneration is undoubtedly present, the localization of the pigment in the centre of the proximal half of the lens is strongly in favour of the cells in which it is deposited being retinal in origin.   A reference to Fig. 175, p. 245, in which a " parietal organ " and an " accessory organ " are seen lying close together, in a sagittal section through the parietal foramen of *Phrynosoma coronatum* will show how if these two vesicles were fused, the opposed portions of the retinæ between the two lenses would almost certainly be included in the centre of the compound lens.   It may also be noted that the two vesicles are surrounded by a common fibrous capsule, and that pigment is less in the more degenerate accessory organ than in the more highly differentiated parietal organ.

Structure of the Lens.—The lens of the parietal organ is formed of transparent elongated cells lying parallel to each other, and extending from its superficial to its deep surface. The cells are longer in the centre of the lens than at its periphery.   Their form and general arrangement resembles that of the cells forming the posterior wall of the embryonic lenses of the lateral eyes ; there is, however, at no period of development any cavity or thin anterior lamina, as in the lateral eye, the lens of the parietal eye being solid from the first—it having been developed from a segment of the superficial wall of the vesicle, which was primarily directly continuous with the retinal segment, the two parts passing insensibly into each other, and a definite limiting membrane only being formed at a later stage.

The lenticular cells are cylindrical or prismatic in type, and show no special thickening in the situation of the nucleus. The nuclei are sometimes arranged in an approximately single plane, but in young embryonic specimens four or five nuclei may be present between the two surfaces,

17

and they are irregularly disposed. There is a tendency towards degeneration seen in some of the older specimens, this being evidenced by the appearance of spaces between the cells and disappearance of the cell outlines. Leydig and others have described the presence of granules in the cells, producing an appearance of longitudinal striation. Leydig also described a radially striated layer on the surface of the lens in one specimen of *Anguis fragilis*, which somewhat resembled the layer of cuticular rods seen in some invertebrate eyes. The nature of these is obscure and the case seems to have been quite exceptional. On the other hand protoplasmic cilium-like processes on the inner surface of the lens, and projecting into the cavity of the vesicle are more common. In some cases these are continuous with syncytial strands of the vitreous tissue filling the cavity of the vesicle.

C. The Vitreous Body

In well-fixed preparations there is present in the cavity of the parietal organ a delicate syncytium which consists of an irregular network of fine protoplasmic strands showing a few oval nuclei imbedded in the thickened nodes of the reticulum. Peripherally it is continuous with the rod- or club-shaped processes of the inner layer of sensory and pigmented cells of the retina and sometimes with similar tapering protoplasmic processes which project inwards from the inner surface of the lens. In one case a thickened band of protoplasm containing closely packed nuclei extended inwards from the retina with which it appeared to be continuous. It is probable that during life the meshes of the reticulum contain a clear albuminous fluid. In imperfectly preserved specimens this tissue may be condensed and form an almost uniform layer lining the inner surface of the retina, and appearing as a coagulum. In other cases it may be thrown down as a flocculent precipitate which occupies the whole cavity. The few cases in which a true syncytium has been demonstrated indicate that in the living animal there is normally a definite syncytium, enclosing spaces filled with clear fluid, and similar to that described in the median eyes of *Petromyzon* and *Geotria* and in the lateral eyes of vertebrates generally.

Nerve Supply of the Pineal System of Sphenodon

The nervous system of adult specimens of *Sphenodon* was minutely studied by Dendy in 1911, who employed serial transverse and longitudinal sections stained with picro-indigo-carmine. He described (1) a left pineal nerve (n. parietalis) and (2) a right pineal nerve (tractus pinealis).

(1) The left pineal nerve commences in the nerve-fibre layer of the retina, passes from the proximal pole of the eye through the space which is enclosed by the outer fibrous capsule of the eye, being covered here by a sheath continuous with the inner fibrous capsule (Figs. 183 and 184).

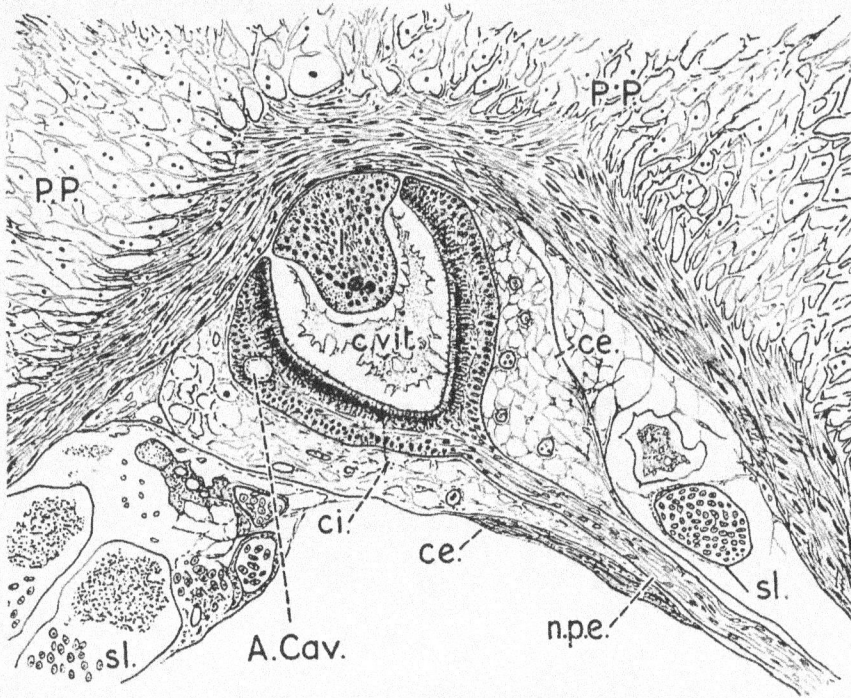

FIG. 183.—SAGITTAL SECTION OF THE PINEAL EYE OF SPHENODON, SHOWING THE PINEAL NERVE, LENS, VITREOUS BODY, ACCESSORY CAVITY, CAPSULA INTERNA, CAPSULA EXTERNA, PARIETAL PLUG, AND VESSELS INCLUDING BRANCHES OF THE LONGITUDINAL SINUS. (AFTER DENDY.)

A. Cav. : accessory cavity.
ce. : capsula externa.
ci. : capsula interna.
c. vit. : vitreous body.

l. : lens.
n.p.e. : pineal nerve.
P.P. : pineal plug.
sl. : longitudinal sinus.

It then passes into and through the dura mater, where it comes into relation with branches of the anterior pineal artery. Here it divides into two and then three branches and lies between two vessels formed by a loop of the sinus longitudinalis. It lies above the paraphysis. Hitherto the nerve has been approximately in the median plane just beneath the dense connective tissue of the cranial wall and in the dura mater. It now passes once more as a single strand to the left of the pineal artery, and, having left the dura mater, it reaches the anterior extremity of the pineal sac and passes beneath its ventral wall to the left of the median plane. The nerve accompanied by the artery is enveloped for some distance in folds of the pineal sac. Near the lower end of the sac its histological structure undergoes an abrupt change, the small oval nuclei

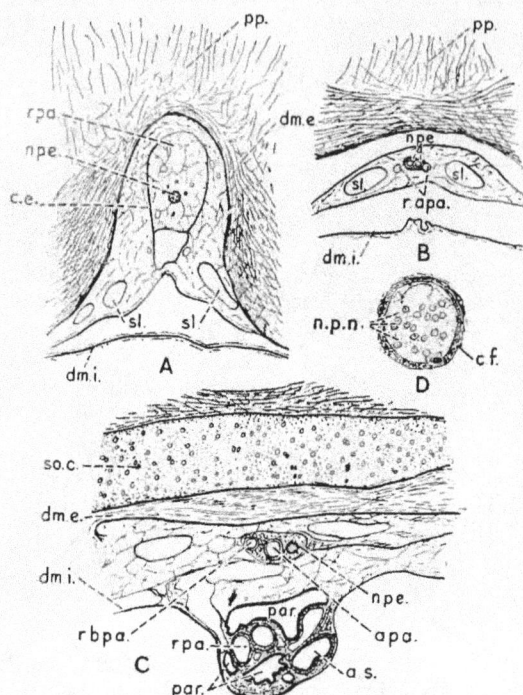

FIG. 184.—A, B, C.—TRANSVERSE SECTIONS SHOWING SOME OF THE RELATIONS OF THE NERVE OF THE PINEAL EYE (N. PARIETALIS), OF AN ADULT SPHENODON. THE SECTIONS PASS FROM BEFORE BACKWARDS. (AFTER DENDY, 1911.)

A—Nerve enclosed in capsule of eye. B—Nerve divided into two strands. C—The subdivisions of the nerve have reunited to form a single nerve, which lies above the distal end of the paraphysis. D—Transverse section through the nerve of the pineal eye, showing its fibrous sheath, and nuclei of the non-medullated fibres. These disappear in the proximal part of its course.

a.p.a. : anterior pineal artery.
a.s. : saccular artery.
c.e. : external capsule.
c.f. : fibrous sheath.
d.m.e., and d.m.i. : external and internal layers of dura mater.
n.p.e. : nerve of pineal eye.
n.p.n. : nuclei of pineal nerve-fibres.
par. : paraphysis.

p.p. : parietal plug.
r.a.p.a. : branch of anterior pineal artery.
r.b.p.a : recurrent branch of anterior pineal artery.
r.p.a. : anastomosing branch of pineal artery.
sl. : superior longitudinal sinus.
so. c. : suboccipital cartilage.

which are present in the course of the nerve-fibres throughout the first part of its course cease and the single nerve breaks up into a number of separate non-nucleated fibres, which spread out in the narrow interval between the pineal sac and the posterior wall of the dorsal sac. Dendy was unable to follow individual fibres continuously to the habenular region,

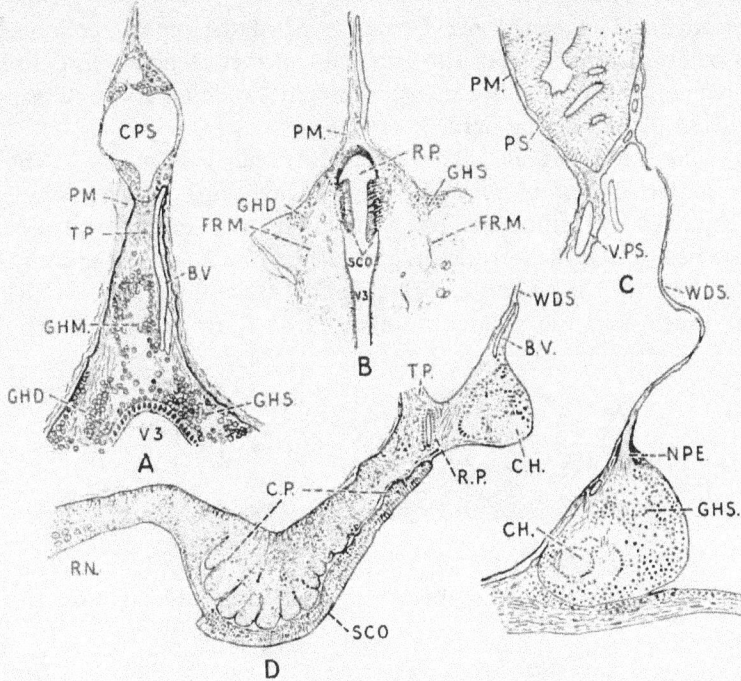

FIG. 185.
(AFTER DENDY, 1911.)

A—Transverse section through the lower part of the tractus pinealis, and the habenular ganglia of an adult *Sphenodon*; note the cavity in the pineal sac, with an ependymal groove in its floor. B—Transverse section through the same specimen as A at the junction of the tractus pinealis with the brain, showing the recessus pinealis, the subcommissural organ, and the fasciculus retroflexus of Meynert. C—Longitudinal vertical section through the pineal region of an adult *Sphenodon*, showing a bundle of nerve-fibres N.P.E. entering it from the posterior wall of the dorsal sac. D—Combined drawing from several sections of the same series as the preceding, showing the lower end of the tractus pinealis, the posterior, and the habenular commissures and the subcommissural organ.

B.V. : blood-vessel.
C.H. : habenular commissure.
C.P. : posterior commissure.
C.P.S. : cavity of pineal sac.
FR.M. : fasciculus-retroflexus of Meynert.
G.H.M., G.H.D., G.H.S., ganglion habenulæ medius—dexter—sinistræ.
N.P.E. : nerve of parietal eye.
P.M. : pia mater.

P.S. : pineal sac.
R.N. : cells of roof nuclei.
R.P. : recessus pinealis ("infra-pineal recess").
SC.O. : subcommissural organ.
T.P. : tractus pinealis.
V.P.S. : vessel of pineal sac.
V.3. : third ventricle.
W.D.S. : wall of dorsal sac.

but he found that numerous fibres entered the left habenular ganglion from the wall of the dorsal sac. Fibres from the same area were also traced to the median habenular ganglion and the right habenular ganglion, but the bulk of the fibres joined the left ganglion, and although some non-nucleated fibres from the nerve-fibre layer of the pineal sac joined the series of fibres coming from the left pineal nerve, Dendy considered that the greater number of fibres which entered the left habenular ganglion came from the left pineal nerve.

(2) The right pineal nerve (tractus pinealis) (Fig. 185). Dendy, using the term " tractus pinealis " in the wide sense in which this name was employed at the time, namely, as including the " entire band or cord of tissue which unites the lower extremity of the pineal sac to the roof of the brain," describes it as commencing in the nerve-fibre layer of the wall of the pineal sac, the greater number of its fibres leaving at its lower

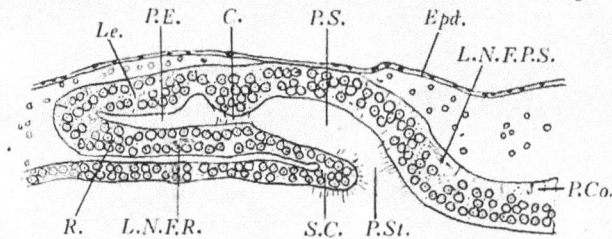

FIG. 186.—SEMI-DIAGRAMMATIC REPRESENTATION OF A MEDIAL LONGITUDINAL SECTION OF AN EMBRYO *Sphenodon*, SHOWING A CONSTRICTION MARKING OFF THE ANTERIOR (LEFT) LOBE, OR PARIETAL ORGAN, FROM THE POSTERIOR (RIGHT) LOBE, OR PINEAL SAC. THE ANTERIOR END OF THE ORGAN IS DIRECTED FORWARD AND IS TO THE LEFT IN THE FIGURE. (AFTER A. DENDY.)

C. : Constriction.	*L.N.F.R.* : Layer of nerve-fibres in retina.
Epd. : Epidermis.	*P. Co.* : Posterior commissure.
Le. : Lens.	*P.E.* : Pineal eye.
L.N.F.P.S. : Layer of nerve-fibres in pineal sac.	*P.S.* : Pineal sac.
	P. St. : Pineal stalk.

S.C. : Superior or habenular commissure.

pole and passing downwards in the stalk to the roof of the brain ; here, between the habenular commissure in front and the posterior commissure behind, some fibres pass to the right and others to the left of the infra-pineal recess and, passing towards the posterior extremities of the habenular ganglia, some fibres appear to terminate in these ganglia, while others appear to end in the median habenular ganglion. Dendy also stated that some fibres passed backwards towards the posterior commissure and subcommissural organ and that possibly some fibres were continued directly into the bundles of Meynert.

The Early Development of the Pineal Nerves in Sphenodon

Dendy also studied the early stages of development in the parietal organ of *Sphenodon*. The earliest indication of the development of nerve-fibres was in embryos, of approximately Stage O when the visceral clefts have begun to close.[1]   (Fig. 186).

[1] Dendy, A., 1899. *Q. J. Micr. Sc.*, **42**, N.S.

In one case he was able to recognize nerve-fibres even before the two pineal vesicles had separated from one another. Both the habenular and the posterior commissures were recognizable. The nuclei in the ventral or future retinal wall of the pineal eye were just beginning to show an arrangement into principal layers separated by a nerve-fibre layer. These fibres were limited to the retinal part of the eye-vesicle, and he concluded that as, now, fibres were visible in the adjacent wall of the brain, the fibres appear first in the retina and from thence grow into the brain wall, as in the case of the ordinary paired eyes. As the pineal eye becomes separated from the roof of the brain by the development of intervening mesoderm, the left pineal nerve, which has now grown out from the retina, grows longer and longer, being attached at its ventral extremity to the brain roof. It is absolutely independent of the pineal sac and its stalk.

In two series of transverse sections at a later stage of development, Dendy was able to trace the nerve continuously from the eye to the left side of the habenular commissure, and he also traced the nerve into the left habenular ganglion in a longitudinal series of sections, belonging to the same developmental stage. He never found it joining the brain roof in the middle or on the right side (see p. 261).

Development of the Right Pineal Nerve.—When the first nerve-fibres have become recognizable in the retinal wall of the pineal eye, a similar band of fibres is visible in the posterior wall of the pineal sac, close to where it joins the roof of the diencephalon in the region of the posterior commissure (Fig. 186). These fibres appear in the outermost zone of the wall, external to all the nuclei. From this point the nerve-fibres extend at a later stage of development upwards into the wall of the pineal sac and downwards into the posterior commissure. When later the nuclei in the wall of the pineal sac assume their characteristic arrangement in two principal layers, the nerve-fibres are found between the two layers of nuclei, as in the retina of the pineal eye. Also when the cavity of the proximal portion of the pineal sac becomes obliterated the nerve-fibres form the most important constituent of the stalk or " pineal tract." The nerve-fibres are associated here with the remains of epithelial cells, connective tissue, and blood-vessels, as in the adult.

Dendy believed that there was no doubt about the connection of the right pineal nerve with the posterior commissure, but that the right pineal organ (pineal sac) was also primarily associated with the right habenular ganglion ; and he considered also that the connection of the pineal sac with the posterior commissure was secondary and " possibly correlated with change of function which the pineal sac has evidently undergone." Several points of interest arise from this description.

First, the primary position of the nerve-fibres in the outermost zone of the wall of the pineal sac recalls the conditions found by Braem and Studnička in *Rana temporaria*. In *Rana* the nerve-fibres commence deeply in the wall of the distal part of the pineal organ, but as they approach the stalk they converge and form a definite tract, which lies upon its dorsal

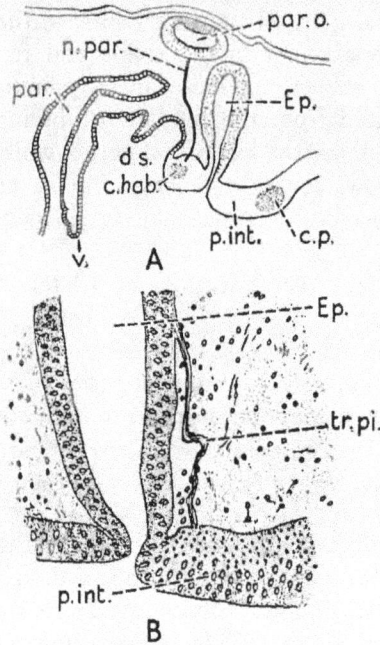

FIG. 187.

A—The parietal region of a 26-mm. embryo of *Anguis fragilis*, showing the position of the parietal nerve in front of the epiphysis and passing towards the habenular commissure. Diagram constructed from three sections. (After Béraneck.)

B—The proximal part of the epiphysis from an 18-day embryo of *Iguana tuberculata*, showing the position of the pineal tract, which, emerging from the posterior wall of the epiphysis, passes to the posterior commissure. (After Klinckostroem.)

c. hab. : habenular commissure.	*p. int.* : pars intercalaris.
c.p. : posterior commissure.	*par.* : paraphysis.
d.s. : dorsal sac.	*par. o.* : parietal organ.
Ep. : epiphysis.	*tr. pi.* : tractus pinealis.
n. par. : nervus parietalis.	*v.* : velum

aspect and finally leaves this to join the posterior commissure (Fig. 166, p. 232); while in *Iguana tuberculata* (Fig. 187), as shown by Klinckow-stroem, the nerve quits the posterior wall of the pineal organ high up and runs an independent course through the connective tissue to the posterior commissure. Although a striking contrast is afforded between these cases and those in which the nerve-fibres pass to the posterior commissure within the stalk, it is probable that the difference in the route which is taken by the nerve-fibres in the two cases is not of morphological importance. Finally, it is probable that if Dendy had been in possession of the large amount of negative evidence with regard to the supposed function of the pineal gland which we possess at the present time, he would not have used the word " evident " with reference to the presumed change of function which at that time the pineal organ was thought to have undergone.

The Connections of the Pineal Organs with the Central Nervous System

The nerves of the pineal system in *Sphenodon* appear to end (Fig. 185) in the habenular and posterior commissures and in the habenular ganglia, and to be continued from the latter by means of the bundles of Meynert to the base of the brain (fasciculi retroflexi, v. tractus habenulo-peduncularis). Each of the fasciculi passes obliquely downwards and backwards in front of the recessus geniculi to the interpeduncular ganglion. The habenular and posterior commissures are recognized at a very early stage of development. The former, being much the smaller of the two, connects the right and left habenular ganglia and lies beneath the median habenular ganglion ; where it forms with the latter a projection into the third ventricle just above the pineal recess. The posterior commissure is closely connected from the first with the tractus pinealis, as well as with other structures outside the pineal complex. It grows rapidly in size and soon becomes folded transversely ; at the same time, the epithelium beneath it becomes converted into the subcommissural organ, which in its turn is connected with the anterior end of Reissner's fibre, that remarkable elastic filament which extends in *Sphenodon*, as in *Geotria* (Fig. 134, Chap. 17, p. 188), along the whole length of the central canal of the spinal cord.

The right and left habenular ganglia are situated above the postero-median and dorsal part of the optic thalami and are prolonged upward on each side into the wall of the dorsal sac ; the prolongation is greater on the left than on the right side, the difference being associated with the termination on this side of the left pineal nerve (n. parietalis) in the apex of the habenular ganglion. Beyond this extension, however, there is no obvious difference in the size of the right and left habenular ganglia, as is the case in *Geotria* (p. 188), and there is no appreciable difference in the size of the bundles of Meynert as in *Geotria*. The lack of any marked difference in the size of a right and left habenular ganglia in *Sphenodon*, notwithstanding the absence of a right parietal nerve, is probably largely due to the presence of other connections of the habenular ganglia besides those with the pineal system, and the very small size of the pineal nerve.

The Vascular Supply of the Pineal System of Sphenodon

According to Dendy (Fig. 188), there is much individual variation among different specimens of *Sphenodon*, but the arteries concerned in the supply of the system appear to be always derived from the posterior

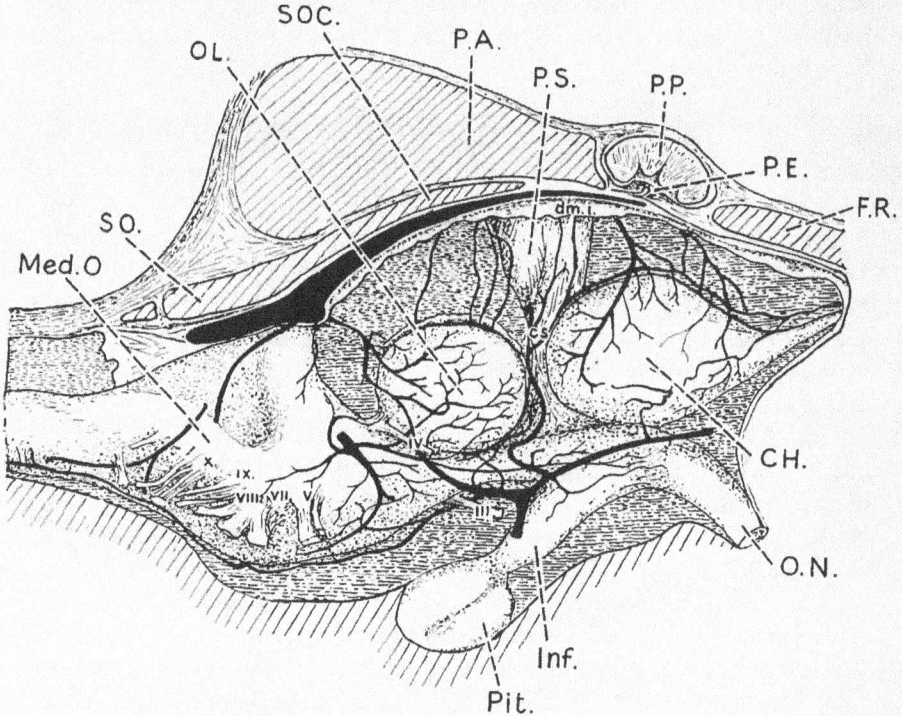

FIG. 188.—THE BRAIN AND PINEAL SYSTEM OF SPHENODON PUNCTATUS.
The right side of the skull has been removed, showing the brain and large sub-dural space. The latter is traversed by blood-vessels. The minute pineal eye (0·53 mm.) is seen in the parietal foramen, lying beneath the parietal plug, which is formed of translucent connective tissue. (After Dendy.)

CH. : cerebral hemisphere.	P.E. : pineal eye.
cs. : connecting stalk.	Pit. : pituitary gland.
dm. i. : dura mater interna.	P.P. : parietal plug.
F.R. : frontal bone.	P.S. : pineal sac.
Inf. : infundibulum.	SO. : supraoccipital bone.
Med. O. : medulla oblongata.	SOC. : supraoccipital cartilage.
O.L. : optic lobe.	iii., iv., v.,
O.N. : optic nerve.	vii., viii., cranial nerves.
P.A. : parietal bone.	ix., x.,

cerebral artery and all the venous blood is returned via the sinus longitudinalis. The posterior cerebral artery divides on each side into an artery to the dorsal sac—saccular artery, and the superior cerebral artery. The superior cerebral artery gives off numerous branches to the hemisphere and the anterior choroidal artery. The saccular artery gives off, on either the left or the right side : (1) the anterior pineal artery, which goes to the pineal eye ; and (2) the posterior pineal artery which supplies the hinder part of the pineal sac. The anterior pineal artery in one case described by Dendy arose directly from the posterior cerebral artery of the left side. It was unpaired ; it passed upwards on the left side of the pineal sac, where it was hidden in folds of its walls and gave off branches to the sac ; it gave off a recurrent branch which passed to the right and finally accompanied by the left pineal nerve it entered the space between the inner and outer fibrous capsules of the pineal eye, where it broke up into capillary vessels which ramified in the connective tissue, but did not enter the eye itself. This fact is of considerable importance, as it is unlikely that an organ which has no demonstrable blood supply could be actively functional, and it indicates impending degeneration.

The Parietal Foramen of Reptiles

The parietal foramen is not present in all orders of the class Reptilia. When present it is usually situated in the anterior part of the interparietal suture. It is found in this position in *Sphenodon* (Fig. 189), which is the

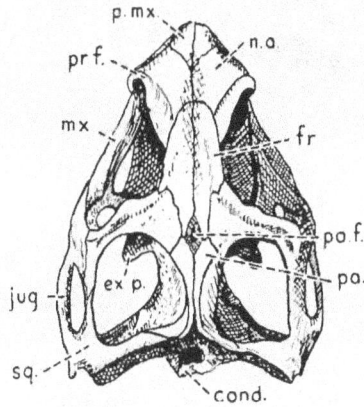

FIG. 189.—DORSAL VIEW OF SKULL OF SPHENODON, SHOWING THE PARIETAL FORAMEN.

cond. : condyle.	*p. mx.* : premaxilla.
ex. p. : external pterygoid.	*pa* : parietal.
fr. : frontal.	*pa. f.* : parietal foramen.
jug. : jugular.	*pr. f.* : prefrontal.
mx. : maxilla.	*sq.* : squamosal.
na. : nasal.	

(From the *Cambridge Natural History*.)

only living example of the Prosauria ; and it is present in the same situation in *Palæohatteria* and in *Conodectes*, one of the most primitive of the Permian reptiles. It is found also in the same site in the less primitive mammal-like reptiles, the Therocephalia and in the Plesiosauria.

In some extinct reptiles the foramen is farther forward, as in the Ichthyosauri, being situated at the junction of the two frontal bones with the two parietal bones (Fig. 190) ; or it may be far back near the exoccipitals as in *Nothosaurus mirabilis*.

In cases in which the lateral or supratemporal fossæ are large, these may be separated by a median antero-posterior bony ridge. This is formed chiefly by the inner borders of the parietal bones, but the frontals may participate in its formation, as in *Mesosuchus* and *Mixosaurus atavus* (Fig. 191). In some types this ridge is reduced to a relatively slender sagittal crest, as in *Trachyodon mirabilis* and *Iguanodon*. In these cases the parietal bones become fused and the interparietal suture and the

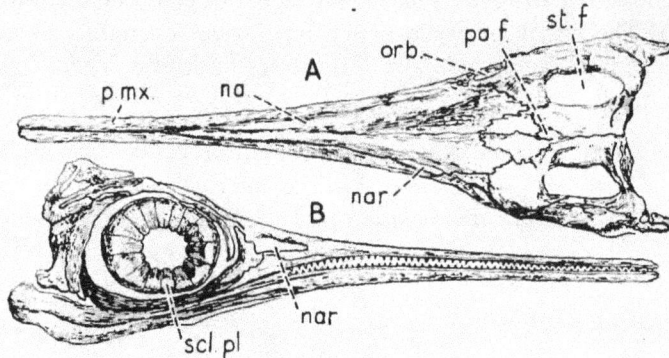

FIG. 190.—ICHTHYOSAURUS ACUTIROSTRIS, OWEN. UPPER LIAS. CURCY, CALVADOS.
          A—Dorsal view of skull.   B—Lateral view of skull.

na. : nasal bone.   *p. mx.* : premaxilla.
nar. : external nares.   *scl. pl.* : sclerotic plates.
orb. : orbit.   *st. f.* : supratemporal fossa.
pa. f. : parietal foramen.

(After E. Deslongchamps, from Zittel.)

parietal foramen disappear. These animals were of enormous size ; they walked on their hind legs, using the tail also as a support for the body. Thus the fore-limbs were free and could be used as arms, as in the kangaroos and wallabies. Their temporal muscles were strongly developed, and encroaching on the sides of the skull they obtained an additional origin from the lateral aspects of the crest, which was formed between them, as is the case in the gorilla. A long median crest is also conspicuously developed in certain Ophidia (*Python*) and Chelonia (*Trionyx gangeticus*), in neither of which a parietal foramen is present. The formation of the crest will not only tend to reduce the width of the parietal canal, but it will increase the thickness of the skull in this situation and the distance of the cranial cavity from the superficial surface of the skull. Thus, although not the prime cause of the atrophy of the parietal organ and of its vascular and nerve-supply, the evolution of the crest when this is present would have probably acted as a contributory factor in the final obliteration of the parietal foramen and its contents.

In some cases in which a " parietal eye " is absent, a parietal foramen is nevertheless present in the cartilaginous roof of the embryonic skull.

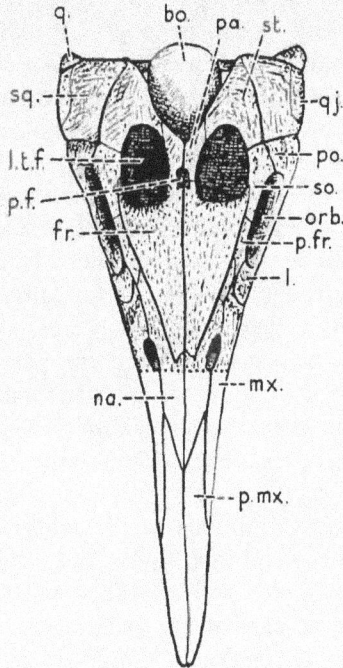

FIG. 191.—DORSAL VIEW OF SKULL OF MIXOSAURUS ATAVUS, FROM THE TRIAS, GERMANY, SHOWING THE PARIETAL FORAMEN, LYING BETWEEN THE TEMPORAL FOSSÆ AND AT THE JUNCTION OF THE PARIETAL WITH THE FRONTAL BONES. (AFTER F. V. HEUNE.)

bo. : basi-occipital.	*pf.* : prefrontal.
fr : frontal	*p. mx.* : premaxilla.
l. : lacrimal.	*po.* : postorbital.
l.t.f. : lateral temporal fossa.	*q.* : quadrate.
mx. : maxilla.	*qj.* : quadratojugal.
na. : nasal.	*so.* : supraorbital.
orb. : orbital cavity.	*sq.* : squamosal.
pa. : parietal.	*st.* : supratemporal.

(Redrawn from E. S. Goodrich.)

Immediately beneath and partially occupying the foramen are the distal ends of the paraphysis, dorsal sac, and the end vesicle of the pineal organ, as shown in an example of a 33-mm. embryo of *Platydactylus muralis*, described and figured by Melchers (1899). The foramen is, however, usually absent, at any rate in the adult animal in those cases in which no parietal eye is developed, e.g. *Gecko verus*.

The size and shape of the parietal foramen differ considerably in different types. Apart from variations in the actual diameter of the foramen which accompany variations in the size of the animal, there is a wide difference in the proportional size of the foramen relative to the size of the skull. Thus in *Procopholon* (Fig. 171, A, Chap. 19, p. 237), in which the skull is only 5 cm. in length, the diameter of the circular parietal foramen is 3·3 mm. ; whereas in *Ichthyosaurus*, which has a skull 50 cm. long, the parietal foramen is 16 mm. long and 8 mm. wide. The foramen is thus actually much larger in *Ichthyosaurus* than in *Procopholon*, although it is relatively smaller. In both animals the orbits are very large relative to the size of the head, but they are exceptionally large in *Procopholon*. The shape of the foramen also varies, the superficial opening usually being either oval or circular in outline. In *Mixosaurus* the anterior margin of the opening is slightly concave forward, but it is not definitely heart-shaped. In section the parietal canal may be tubular with straight sides, or the edges may be bevelled, the central part being narrow (*Lacerta agilis*). In other cases it is funnel-shaped, the narrow end of the funnel being either superficial, as in *Pseudopus Pallasii* (Fig. 177, p. 248), or the smaller opening may be below and the larger above, as in *Varanus giganteus* (Fig. 176, p. 247). The opening is usually closed superficially by a fibrous membrane continuous at the margin of the foramen with the periosteum and the membrane lining the canal. The membrane is destitute of pigment, as are the structures which lie superficial to it ; moreover, the superficial part of the parietal eye is firmly adherent to the membrane, so that if traction is employed in removal of the organ from the foramen the eye is liable to be damaged. Exceptionally, the lower aperture may be closed by membrane continuous with the dura mater, so that the parietal organ is, strictly speaking, outside the cranial cavity, as in certain amphibia (Fig. 161, Chap. 19, p. 228). This condition is found in chameleons. The foramen in the adult animal is in bone ; in the embryo it is in cartilage, as in the Selachia. Its contents vary ; as a rule the parietal organ is situated superficially in contact with the external closing membrane and its diameter is about one-third the diameter of the foramen. It is surrounded by a loose, fibrous connective tissue, often containing pigment and sometimes fat. In *Sphenodon* there is a special inner and outer fibrous capsule containing blood-vessels and traversed by the parietal nerve. In addition to these structures, the parietal recess may contain a part of the end vesicle of the pineal organ and one or more accessory organs (Fig. 177). In some instances it has been noted that in the embryo the parietal organ does not lie in the foramen, but below this, and it is only at a later period that it is found actually in the foramen, e.g. *Lacerta vivipara* (Owsjannikow, 1888), and

Iguana (Klinckostroem, 1894). In one instance in *Sphenodon* (Spencer) the central axis of the parietal organ was directed obliquely forward, so that rays of light entering through the foramen could only fall directly on one part of the retina. This condition is, however, exceptional and does not appear to have been described in other adult specimens. Dendy's figures show a less pronounced degree of obliquity in two embryos of *Sphenodon*, but it is probable that this condition would have been rectified by the time the animal had reached maturity.

More important from the standpoint of interference with function is the occurrence of pigment in the substance of the lens—*Anolis* (Spencer), *Anguis fragilis* (Béraneck), *Varanus* (Spencer) ; and the encroachment from the surrounding tissue of black pigment, which may grow inward over the area occupied by the subjacent lens, as in a case described by Leydig of *Lacerta muralis* (1891) ; also, irregularity in form and structural degenerative changes, previously alluded to as occurring in the lens of a specimen of an adult *Iguana* described by Klinckowstroem (1894). Calcareous concretions have also been found in the parietal foramen, which, although in relation with the end vesicle of the pineal organ rather than the parietal organ, indicate localized degenerative processes occurring within the area of the pineal system. These concretions have been noted by Leydig (1891), who described four rounded, calcareous nodules lying over the tip of the epiphysis, and by Studnička, in *Varanus nebulosus*, who found similar structures in the neighbourhood of the pineal bud. In this case there was one large and several small calcareous balls, the latter being arranged in a semicircle around the pineal outgrowth. These conditions indicate not only interference with function and degenerative changes in the living animals in which they have been observed, but loss of function of the parietal eyes and accompanying degeneration of structure, which must have commenced in quite remote ancestors of the living generations of reptiles. The parietal cornea, corneal scale, and parietal spot of reptiles have already been alluded to in the general description of these structures.

Notes on the Pineal System of Special Examples of Living Saurian Reptiles

Further reference to the significance of the parietal foramen of extinct Saurian reptiles will be made in the chapter on the morphology of the skull in so far as it is concerned in the geological evidence of the antiquity of the median and lateral eyes of vertebrates. The following notes will deal chiefly with the pineal system of embryonic and mature examples of different types of lizard.

Geckonidæ.

In the geckos no parietal organ is developed and the pineal organ consists of a long, tubular outgrowth springing from the usual site between the habenular and posterior commissures and passing upwards to the roof of the skull behind a well-developed dorsal sac and paraphysis. In a 31-mm. embryo of *Gehyra oceanica*, described by Stemmler, the base of the outgrowth is constricted so as to form a secondary stalk in which the lumen has become obliterated and the distal end is slightly expanded into an end vesicle, the tip of which is prolonged forward as a beak-like process ; this is connected to the dura mater of the skull roof by a fibrous cord. The lumen of the end vesicle is smooth, there being no folds or lobulation. The conditions are, therefore, very similar to those which are found in the tubular type of pineal system present in the Selachia. In older specimens, e.g. *Hemidactylus verruculatus*, brown pigment has been observed in the epithelium of the distal end of the epiphysis (Leydig). The same author described in *Platydactylus muralis* fine striated strands in the stalk of the epiphysis near the posterior commissure, which he was inclined to believe were nerve-fibres passing from the posterior commissure into the epiphysis. The existence of a true pineal nerve in geckos, however, appears to be very doubtful, and in certain specimens, e.g. *Hemidactylus mabouia*, it has been definitely stated that it could not be demonstrated.

The epiphysis in older embryonic specimens may show a certain degree of differentiation with thickening of its wall ; in late stages of development and in mature animals kinking and irregularity of the wall has been present, accompanied by penetration of vessels. The epiphysis has, moreover, been found separated from the roof of the brain, presumably by constriction of its stalk, attended by loss of its lumen and final rupture, as in the case published by Melchers in 1899.

The changes which have been observed in the late stages of development of the epiphysis of geckos include : elongation of the cells ; disappearance of cell contours ; vacuolation of cellular bands ; penetration of blood-vessels ; deposit of pigment in and around the capsule and the separation of the whole organ from its connection with the roof of the brain. Taken together, and more particularly the complete severance of the epiphysis from the central nervous system, these changes indicate that the epiphysis in the mature animal shows indubitable signs of retrogression.

Agamidæ.

This family includes lizards of widely varying types. One of the most remarkable is the little flying dragon *Draco volans*, in which the hinder ribs are expanded and covered by a thin membrane ; this forms a kind of parachute or gliding apparatus by which the animal is enabled to pass by long leaps from tree to tree. There is also the frilled lizard, *Chlamydosaurus*, which has a whig-like expansion growing out around the head, neck, and shoulders. It is found in sandy deserts, has a long tail, and walks with long strides on its hind legs. The family includes the horned-lizard, *Ceratophorus aspera ; Calotes versicolor*, which, like the chamæleon, is capable of changing its colour ; the thorny-tailed lizard, *Uromastix* ; and the Australian lizard, *Moloch horridus*, which is covered all over with large conical spines.

In this family a parietal foramen, parietal scale, and parietal spot are described as being present in most of the species that have been examined, though these differ in their degree of development. Thus, in *Ceratophorus* the foramen is only indicated by vessels traversing the bone, while in *Calotes ophiomachus* all three are specially well developed.

In Agamidæ a parietal organ and end vesicle are not as a rule both present in the same individual ; hence it is often difficult to determine whether the organ found lying in the parietal foramen is the parietal sense organ or the end vesicle of the pineal organ, more especially as the " eye " is in most cases not separated from the stalk of the epiphysis ; moreover, in some cases there is no distinct differentiation into lens and retina, and no pigment. A differentiated eye is, however, definitely present in *Calotes, Agama, Phrynocephalus*, and *Grammatophora*. Moreover, in an adult specimen of the latter described by McKay (1888) the parietal eye was separated from the epiphysis, as in *Lacerta vivipara* or *Sphenodon*. It showed a biconvex lens and a well-differentiated retina, in which McKay distinguished rod-like cells, round cells, a molecular layer, a layer of spindle-formed elements, and special triangular cells (? multipolar nerve cells) ; pigment was deposited in horizontal layers in the rod-like cells, and a corneal scale was present. Speaking generally, in those cases in which a well-developed parietal foramen, parietal scale, and parietal spot are present, the parietal eye is well developed. In cases such as *Ceratophora*, in which the existence of a parietal foramen is only indicated, it is doubtful whether the imperfectly developed organ beneath it really represents a parietal sense organ or is a modified end vesicle, the parietal organ being absent.

Draco volans.

Spencer described a parietal organ having the form of an ovoid vesicle, the longest diameter of which lay in the median plane. There was no differentiation into lens and retina. Pigment was absent in the vesicle itself, but was present in the connective tissue membranes behind the vesicle. It lay in a parietal foramen, the position of which was in most

18

cases indicated by a modified scale and a transparent parietal spot. According to Studnička's observations on one specimen of *Draco*, there is no parietal eye, but the pineal organ ends in a dorso-ventrally compressed end vesicle which lay beneath a parietal pit closed superficially by a lamella of cartilage. The end vesicle was not pigmented.

Calotes ophiomachus.

In a specimen described by Spencer (1886) there was a pentagonal corneal scale (Fig. 192, B) with the broad end anterior ; a little behind the centre of this was the parietal spot which was slightly convex superficially

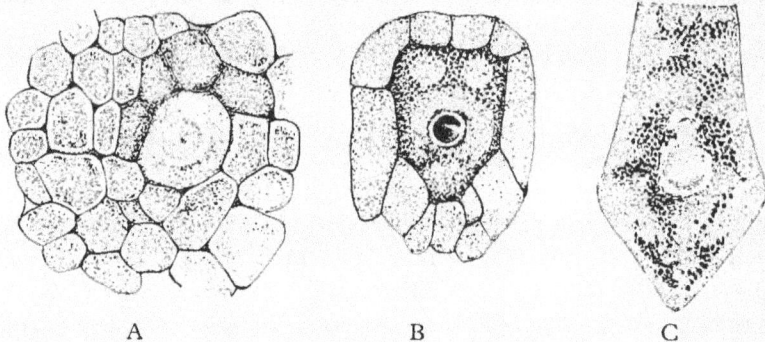

A   B   C

FIG. 192.—THE PARIETAL OR CORNEAL SCALE AND ITS SURROUNDINGS IN THREE FORMS OF REPTILES.

A : *Varanus giganteus* (after Spencer) ; B : *Calotes versicolor*, a tree lizard so named on account of its power or changing its colour (after Spencer) ; C : *Lacerta muralis*, var. *cærulea* (after Leydig). In the centre of the parietal plate is seen the parietal eye spot ; through this is seen in *Calotes*, in which this part is definitely transparent, the parietal eye. In *Lacerta muralis* pigment granules encroach on this area.

and bounded by a circular rim. The parietal eye was a dorso-ventrally flattened vesicle having its longest axis in the median plane. Some of the cells of the lens contained pigment at their inner or central ends. The parietal organ was separated from the epiphysis. The latter consisted of two parts, a vertical basal segment and a horizontal terminal part which was directed forward, its tip ending at the posterior border of the parietal foramen near the parietal eye.

Agama hispida. Spencer (1886).

The parietal eye lay in a parietal foramen, beneath a pigmentless parietal cornea and modified scale, through which could be seen a remarkable hour-glass-shaped parietal spot. The retina of the parietal eye was so deeply pigmented that its structure was obscured, and pigment was also present in the lens.

Agama caucasica (Owsjannikow, 1888).

The parietal eye, which was exceptionally large, lay in a parietal foramen surrounded by connective tissue containing numerous pigment cells. Both lens and retina showed cells the inner ends of which terminated in pencil-like refractile processes which projected into a vestigial vitreous body.

Grammatophora (Spencer, 1886 ; McKay, 1888).

In Spencer's specimen the parietal eye was spherical and strongly pigmented in its lower segment. Externally it was covered by a white substance. Superficial to it the tissues contained no pigment and there was a conspicuous corneal scale. McKay's case has already been alluded to (p. 273).

Moloch horridus (Spencer, 1886).

The parietal spot was visible in the middle of a small area surrounded by horny processes, which cover the skin in this region ; it appeared as a black dot surrounded by a dark circular rim. The parietal organ lay in a parietal foramen and was continuous, by means of a slender cylindrical stalk, with the epiphysis. This widened out insensibly into a conical epiphysis. The stalk was solid throughout. The interior of the parietal organ was almost completely filled with pigmented tissue, and the lens was absent.

Iguanidæ.

This family, which closely resembles the preceding, comprises very various species, which are mostly found in America and in neighbouring islands such as the Galapagos. Some, such as *Anolis*, are arboreal ; others, such as the snub-nosed *Amblyrhynchus cristatus*, live to a great extent in the sea and feed on seaweed. The Californian toad *Phrynosoma*, which is found in the United States of America and in Mexico, lives in sandy deserts and preys on small beetles and other insects. The girdled lizards Zonuridæ are remarkable for the primitive character of their skulls, the hinder and lateral parts of which are completely roofed over by dermal bones.

In contrast to the Geckonidæ, the parietal organ is usually present and well developed, and the Iguanidæ in this respect resemble the Agamidæ and the remaining families of Lacertilia which we shall describe in the following pages. The parietal organ is usually well developed and lies beneath a transparent scale, near the centre of which is a circular dark spot surrounded by a pale rim. The epiphysis is usually subdivided into a proximal thick-walled part, a stalk, a flattened vesicle, and frequently a fibrous cord which connects the tip of the epiphysis with the parietal organ. The latter is generally regarded as the fibrous sheath of the nerve of the parietal organ, the fibres of which have disappeared. It must be remembered, however, that in *Lacerta vivipara* and other species the parietal nerve has been shown by Nowikoff to be developed independently and in front of the epiphyseal evagination, after the parietal organ has been separated from the epiphyseal part of the primary diverticulum.

Anolis.

One specimen described by Spencer (1886) differs from the typical in that the long axis of the parietal organ is vertical, and that it lies in an exceptionally narrow parietal foramen which is almost completely filled by the parietal eye. It was connected with the epiphysis by a fibrous cord, which was regarded by Spencer as its nerve; but, as pointed out by Studnicka, the cord as shown in Spencer's figure is clearly continuous with the fibrous sheath of the parietal organ, and no fibres are seen entering the retina. In another specimen of *Anolis* described by Spencer, the parietal organ was dorso-ventrally flattened. It is probable, therefore, that the cylindrical parietal organ of the first specimen was exceptional, and does not represent a peculiarity of this particular family. The central cells of the lens in its deepest part contained pigment in the first specimen.

Leiolæmus nitidus (Spencer, 1886).

The parietal organ (Fig. 193) is dorso-ventrally flattened; the central part of the retina is slightly arched upwards towards the lens, so that the

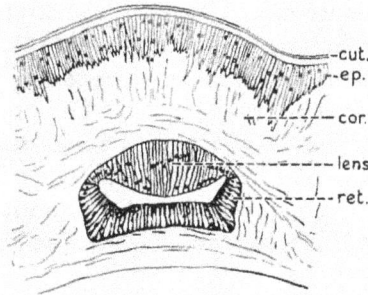

Fig. 193.—Sagittal Section through the Parietal Eye of Leiolæmus nitidus, showing a Flattened, Undifferentiated Retina of Ependymal Type, Biconvex Lens, and a Corium with Exceptionally Tall Papillæ. (After Spencer, 1886.)

cor. : corium.
cut. : cuticle.
ep. : epidermis.

lens : lens.
ret. : retina.

cavity of the organ is much reduced in its vertical diameter; the lateral walls formed by the peripheral part of the retina are almost vertical, but slope slightly outward as they ascend to the margin of the lens. The retina is composed of a single layer of cells containing pigment in their rod-like inner extremities, while the outer ends terminate in conical expansions the bases of which are continuous with the external limiting membrane ; oval nuclei were present in the bodies of the cells near the centre. The lens was biconvex and consisted of elongated cells, the oval nuclei of which lay for the most part in a single plane. A thick layer of corium lay between the parietal organ and the epidermis. This and the epidermis with the overlying corneal scale were destitute of pigment. The corium was remarkable with regard to the exceptionally large size of the papillæ which entered the epidermis. The corneal scale was slightly arched upwards, like the glass of an old type of watch. No nerve was described, and it is worth while noting that the absence of a nerve in association with such a simple structural type of retina is what might be expected, the differentiation of the cells from the primary single layer of ependymal elements having advanced very little beyond the stage of deposit of pigment in the inner ends of these cells.

A nearly allied species, *Leiolæmus tenuis*, also described by Spencer, showed very similar conditions to those described above.

Plica umbra (Spencer).

The pineal system of this animal is remarkable for the extraordinary length of the epiphysis, which, arising from the roof of the diencephalon in the usual situation, is seen to consist of a proximal nearly vertical part and a horizontal segment which comprises the greatly elongated stalk, at the distal end of which is a small pigmented vesicle of doubtful nature, which has been regarded by different authors as the end vesicle of the pineal organ ; as a part of, or offshoot of the parietal organ ; or an accessory organ. Both the upper and lower walls are pigmented. The true parietal organ is a small flattened vesicle lying far forward and in an exceptionally large parietal foramen. The superficial wall, corresponding to the lens in other specimens, is unpigmented ; the lower or retinal segment is deeply pigmented. There was a specially large corneal scale in the middle of which was a small, slightly arched parietal speck.

Iguana tuberculata.

The pineal system of *Iguana* has been specially studied by Spencer (1886), Leydig (1896), and Klinckowstroem (1895). The latter author also followed out in detail the developmental history of *Iguana*. His conclusions from the general standpoint are so important that we shall give them in full, in place of detailed descriptions of individual specimens.

I. The Parietal Eye.

1. The parietal eye of *Iguana*, arising from the constriction at the distal part of the primary epiphyseal evagination, appears on the 9th day as an oval vesicle which is more or less constricted off from the proximal epiphysis.

2. The originally markedly biconvex lens in the course of development takes on a flat, slightly biconvex form or even a plano-convex form.

3. From the 14th to 18th days the entire inner side of the eye cavity is covered with cilia. A strong nerve unites the under side of the eye vesicle with the roof of the diencephalon. The retina shows two zones, one inner without cells and an outer cellular zone. Black pigment begins to appear on the retinal cells, and from the surrounding mesoderm a connective tissue capsule is formed which envelops the nerve and eye.

4. In 24 to 26 days the parietal nerve has reached its highest degree of development. Through the inward growth of the nerve-fibres the retina is divided into an outer and inner cell layer, between which the subdivisions of the nerve can be seen as a nerve-fibre layer. In the inner zone an abundance of pigment has been formed.

5. In 35 to 40 days the nerve and nerve-fibre layer shows significant signs of degeneration. The amount of pigment has greatly increased.

6. In the adult *Iguana* the pineal eye shows the varied features which are characteristic of rudimentary organs.

7. The nervous elements seem to have entirely disappeared in the retina, and the formation of pigment has become so excessive that a recognition of the structural relations is often impossible.

II. The Parietal Nerve.

1. The nerve which enters the pineal eye is dissimilar in its development to that of the optic nerves of the paired eyes.

2. At the end of the 9th day there is still no trace of a nerve to be seen entering the vesicle, which has already separated from the pineal.

3. By the 14th day the nerve is formed, and passes from the floor of the eye vesicle to a cell accumulation lying in the roof of the diencephalon, called the centrum parietale.

4. The parietal centre lies asymmetrically to the right of the middle line, immediately in front of the pineal evagination.

5. In 24 to 27 days the nerve is surrounded by a connective-tissue sheath (perineurium), and the parietal centre now lies in a direct line with the right ganglion habenulæ.

6. In 35 to 40 days the nerve shows undoubted signs of degeneration that already appear to have produced atrophy of its central part.

7. In adults the nerve elements are completely atrophied and only the thickened perineurium remains.

8. In one embryo of *Iguana* there are two parietal nerves, one from each ganglion habenulæ.

III. The Proximal Pineal.

1. At the end of the 9th day the pineal has the form of a vesicle communicating with the third ventricle ; this shows a structure comparable with the parietal eye vesicle.

2. In the course of development the pineal becomes covered with cilia internally and is gradually transformed into a long funnel.

3. The proximal part of the pineal retains a structure which is suggestive of that of the medullary tube ; the development of the distal part resembles that of the retina of the parietal eye.

4. The conical pineal of adult animals retains at its distal end the funnel-shaped form of the embryo, while its proximal part undergoes a follicular transformation during the growth of its wall.

5. The epiphyseal evagination in the tegu shows in the early stages of development, just as in *Iguana*, a constriction causing a division into a distal part (pineal eye vesicle) and a proximal part (pineal).

6. Later this constriction disappears and the entire primary epiphyseal evagination is developed into a pineal.

7. The pineal of the tegu, in a stage corresponding to 24–26 days of *Iguana*, shows traces of pigmentation that appear to vanish afterwards.

8. In an embryo of *Iguana* nerve bundles from the diencephalic roof, entirely similar to the parietal nerve, enter the posterior part of the pineal (Fig. 187, B, p. 264).

9. On the end of the proximal pineal of one *Iguana* embryo and in an adult a secondary pigmented pineal eye was developed.

Among the special points which Klinckowstroem emphasizes in the summary of his observations on *Iguana* one may note : (1) the separation of the parietal vesicle, by means of a constriction from the anterior part of the primary evagination ; (2) the independent formation of the parietal nerve, which takes place after the separation of the eye vesicle from the epiphysis ; (3) the connection of the parietal nerve with the right habenular ganglion in some cases, and the demonstration in one embryo of *Iguana* of two parietal nerves, one ending in the right habenular ganglion and the other in the left habenular ganglion ; (4) the degenerative changes in the retina and parietal nerve which occur in the late stages of development, which eventually lead to a total disappearance of the nerve-fibres ; (5) the distinction between (a) the proximal part of the epiphysis, which undergoes a follicular transformation and an accompanying thickening of its wall, and (*b*) a distal part, the structure of which resembles and suggests that of the retina of the parietal eye.

Lacertidæ.

The different species of *Lacerta* have been studied by Spencer, Owsjannikow, Strahl and Martin, Leydig and Nowikoff. All the typical parts of the pineal system are represented in the ordinary lizards, and the variations in form and structure which are met with are largely due to age and the concomitant degeneration found in old specimens. The different stages of development were described by Nowikoff in 1910, and have already been alluded to (p. 242). They confirm Klinckowstroem's observations on *Iguana* with respect to the separation of the parietal vesicle by constriction and the independent origin of the parietal nerve subsequent to the separation of the parietal vesicle.

The pineal system of the adult lizard comprises the following parts, which, passing from the superficial surface of the head towards the brain, are :

A pentagonal parietal scale, near the centre of which is a slightly raised dark spot, the " parietal spot " (Fig. 192, C, p. 274).

A pigment-free, transparent parietal area, which is formed of a mucoid connective tissue, lying between the superficial closing membrane of the parietal foramen and the epidermis.

The parietal eye and parietal nerve.

The terminal or habenular ganglion.

A membranous fibrous capsule which encloses the retinal segment of the parietal eye, and the parietal nerve ; in old specimens in which the nerve-fibres have degenerated the fibrous sheath of the nerve may persist as a cord uniting the parietal eye with the brain roof or with the tip of the epiphysis.

A pineal organ which consists of : a proximal part, springing from the diencephalic roof between the habenular and posterior commissures ; a tubular body or stalk : an end vesicle, which is sometimes prolonged forward as a fibrous cord which ends in the vicinity of the parietal organ or is united with its fibrous sheath.

The end vesicle of the pineal organ is surrounded by blood-vessels which are contained in a fibrous connective tissue which is sometimes deeply pigmented. This is continuous with a similar vascular and pigment-bearing connective tissue around the parietal organ.

Striations have been observed in the peduncle of the proximal part of the pineal organ, which Leydig considered were nerve-fibres, but no separate pineal tract, such as that figured by Klinckowstroem in *Iguana tuberculata*, appears to have been described.

In some cases the walls of the epiphysis may be folded ; thus Studnička describes in a specimen of *L. agilis* a series of lateral buds, right and left, on each side of an elongated sac-like epiphysis ; and Leydig found a similar condition in *L. ocellata*. In this specimen the epithelial cells at the distal end of the epiphysis were pigmented, as in a case of *Anguis fragilis* also described by Leydig.

Scincidæ.

The skink family comprises a number of different species, mostly found in sandy deserts and often showing retrogressive features, such as the union of the premaxillæ and diminution in the size and number of the limbs, the fore-limbs or both fore and hind-limbs being absent in some species. In *Chalcis flavescens*, a long, worm-like animal, both pairs of limbs are present, but are less than 2 mm. in length. One interesting adaptation to a dust-blown sandy environment is the existence in certain skinks of a transparent window in the lower eyelid of each lateral eye, which allows the eye to be used when closed, while at the same time it serves as a protective covering for the eye.

Cyclodus gigas.

A description of the pineal system of this animal was given by Spencer in 1886. A corneal scale, parietal fleck, and parietal foramen were all present. The pineal organ took origin from the roof of the diencephalon in the usual situation, and coursing forward with an arch-like bend, ended in a vesicular expansion above the anterior part of the hemispheres and in the region of the parietal foramen, which it partly filled. Spencer regarded this expansion as a parietal eye which had remained in an undeveloped and rudimentary condition. Studnička, however, states that there can be no doubt that the structure described by Spencer as a parietal eye was in reality the well-developed end vesicle of a completely formed pineal organ, and that the parietal organ had not been developed. Both the upper and the lower wall of the end vesicle was composed of long, cylindrical cells from which cilium-like processes projected into the lumen of the vesicle.

Gongylus ocellatus.

Legge (1897) described the pineal diverticulum of an embryo 10 mm. long, which was divided into a distal part, which he considered to be the rudiment of the parietal eye, and a proximal part, the epiphysis. The distal segment, namely, the parietal eye (or possibly the end vesicle of the epiphysis), had disappeared in those specimens which had passed the embryonal period, and there remained only the true epiphysis which had become greatly enlarged. This consisted of a proximal vertical segment and a horizontal part which was directed forward ; it showed saccular outgrowths and ended in a pointed extremity, the walls of which were of equal thickness.

The parietal eye, which is only present in the embryonic stage of development, has a distinctly biconvex lens consisting of elongated cells and a retina containing brown pigment. The retinal cells ended in long rod-like processes, which projected into the lumen of the vesicle ; and between the bases of these small round cells could be distinguished. Neither nerve-fibres nor parietal nerve could be recognized. No parietal foramen was present, nor was there any specially modified corneal scale, the scales in the pineal and the surrounding region being small and of approximately equal size.

The published description of other species of the Skink family, such as *Scincus officinalis, Hinulia,* and *Chalcides tridactylus,* do not differ essentially from that of *Cyclodus* and *Gongylus,* and it will be unnecessary to give a special account of each of these. It will suffice to give a general idea of the structure of the pineal organ by the drawing (Fig. 194) reproduced, with the kind permission of the author, from a photograph of a section through the parietal eye of *Scincus officinalis* and published by Jean Calvet in his work *L'Épiphyse,* 1934. This shows the lens, retina, and parietal nerve, with the general relations of the organ. Calvet also gives photographs showing the position of the parietal scale in *Varanus* and *Iguana.*

Rhipidoglossa.

This family, which is represented by the chamæleons, is from the standpoint of the pineal system as remarkable as it is in other respects. The pineal system in general resembles that of *Lacerta,* but although all parts of the complete system are represented in the embryonic condition, the parietal organ in some examples has disappeared in the adult animal. A detailed account of the pineal system of chamæleons was given by Spencer in 1886 and one two years later by Owsjannikow. In both of these examples and in another mentioned by Studnička, which was examined by himself, there is substantial agreement with reference to the presence of a parietal foramen. In Studnička's case the contained parietal organ was surrounded on all sides by a dense plexus of anastomosing vessels, and in all, the tissue overlying the organ was devoid of pigment and its position on the head was indicated by a small, slightly raised transparent scale or nodule. According to Spencer's description, the pineal organ (epiphysis) was a hollow, tubular structure, which was directed at first dorsally and was then bent sharply forward. In its distal part the wall was folded, and from the extremity of this portion a cord, which he regarded as the nerve, coursed forward to the parietal eye.   Owsjannikow, however, considered that this cord consisted of connective tissue rather than of nerve-fibres.   The parietal organ in Spencer's specimen was a slightly flattened hollow vesicle which was elongated in the antero-posterior direction.   No distinction in the structure of different parts of its wall could be recognized, neither lens nor retina being distin-

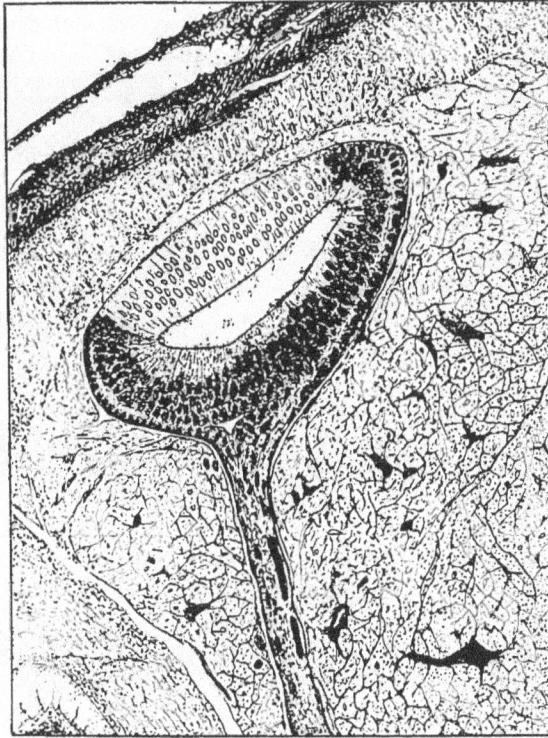

FIG. 194.—VERTICAL SECTION THROUGH THE PINEAL EYE OF A SKINK, SHOWING THE LENS, RETINA, NERVE, AND PIGMENT CELLS.

It will be noted that there is a considerable amount of pigment in the epidermis and subepidermal tissue lying over the pineal organ.
(Drawn from a photograph—J. Calvet.)

guishable.   The walls throughout were composed of cells of approximately equal length, and the inner ends of these cells bore long cilia which projected into the cavity of the vesicle.   No pigment was present.   The lower wall of the vesicle, moreover, showed on its inner aspect a small invagination which Spencer took to be a remnant of the primary connection of the lumen of the parietal organ with that of the epiphysis.

Owsjannikow's specimen differed from Spencer's in the more complete differentiation of the parietal eye, a definite lens and retina being distinguishable. He described two layers in the retina : an inner composed of deeply pigmented, long, rod-like cells bearing cilia, and an outer layer which was devoid of pigment and contained fibres and cells with round nuclei. The lens was biconvex, contained no pigment and was formed of elongated cells. In the cavity of the vesicle there was a fine granular mass, which represented a vestige of the vitreous body. The conclusion to be drawn from these two widely different examples is that a variable degree of differentiation of the parietal organ may occur in different specimens, the development proceeding farther in some cases than in others, in which it becomes arrested at an early stage—the arrest being followed by degenerative changes. Another interpretation of the differences between these two specimens is the possibility of the hollow structure devoid of pigment, which was described by Spencer as the parietal eye, being the end vesicle of the pineal organ, the parietal eye having failed to develop or having been present only for a short period during embryonic development, as in the examples of disappearance of the organ described by Legge in *Gongylus* (p. 281).

The Pineal System of Ophidia.

The pineal system of the snakes is represented only by the epiphysis, the parietal eye being absent. In one case, however, published by Hanitsch in an embryo of the common viper (*Pelias berus*) a well-differentiated parietal organ with a lens, which contained much pigment in its interior, was described. The epiphysis had the usual form, and had the appearance of twisted tubes between which connective tissue was interposed, giving it a glandular appearance. The case seems, however, to have been exceptional and the parietal organ has not been seen in other species. In view of the temporary embryonic existence of a parietal organ in *Gongylus* (described by Legge, p. 281), the correctness of this single observation cannot be denied, and the very occasional occurrence of a parietal eye in snakes must be regarded as awaiting further confirmation.

The skull in living species of snake has no parietal foramen, and in the python the parietal bones are fused in the median plane so as to form a prominent keel-like ridge in which it is unlikely that any remnant of a parietal canal would persist. A foramen is, however, present in the skull of the extinct Pythonomorpha, in which the parietal bones, although united, are not produced upwards as an intermuscular ridge, but form a flat, triangular plate with the parietal foramen near or at its anterior border. Examples are met with in *Clidastes propython* (Cope), Upper Cretaceous, Alabama ; and *Platecarpus coryphæus* (Cope), Upper Cretaceous, Kansas. These were marine, lizard-like animals of large size (5 metres), having anterior and posterior paddles adapted for swimming. The parietal foramen of *Platecarpus* was oval in outline, the longest diameter being about 2 cm., it was in the median plane and situated at the anterior border of the triangular parietal bone, immediately behind the frontal bone. Although possessing certain characters which differentiate them from the Lacertilia, the Pythonomorpha or Mosasauridæ are more nearly allied to lizards than the snakes, and fossil skulls of the true Ophidia which are of comparatively recent date do not appear to differ markedly from the skulls of living species.

The pineal system of living examples of Ophidia has been studied by Sorensen, 1894; Leydig, 1897; Studnička, 1893; and Rabl-Rückhard, 1894. The epiphysis of the common ringed snake, *Tropidonotus*, a non-poisonous British species, is developed as a simple hollow evagination from the roof of the diencephalon in the usual situation between the habenular and posterior commissures, and there is usually a well-developed paraphysis and dorsal sac. Later it becomes pear-shaped, and eventually the cavity disappears in the distal part, which becomes a solid rounded mass, and at the base, where the neck becomes constricted and cord-like. What appears to be a remnant of the original cavity may, however, persist at the junction of the stalk with the body of the organ (Fig. 179, Chap. 20, p. 251).

In the adult the body is surrounded by blood-vessels which penetrate into its substance and produce a lobulated appearance. The whole is enclosed in a sheath consisting of an inner and outer layer of connective tissue, which is continuous with the pia mater and encloses a space. Leydig described a striated appearance in the pedicle, which he thought was produced by nerve-fibres connecting the organ with the posterior commissure. In one case the distal end of the organ was surrounded by deeply pigmented cells. Studnička considered that the lobulation and penetration of the organ by connective tissue septa containing capillary blood-vessels might be an indication of its transformation into a gland of internal secretion. It is quite common, however, to find degenerating nervous or neuroglial tissue invaded by blood-vessels, and the appearance is very different from that of a typical endocrine gland.

The Pineal System of the Chelonia.

The parietal organ and parietal foramen are lacking and the pineal organ is represented merely by a rudimentary epiphysis.

The development of the parietal region of the brain has been studied by Voeltzkow (1903) in *Chelone*, and in *Chelydra serpentina*, the snapping turtle, by Humphrey (1894). Voeltzkow found that in the early embryonal stages the epiphysis had the form of a simple tubular evagination of the roof of the thalamencephalon, which in later stages, becoming thinner at its basal or proximal part, developed a secondary stalk. Still later, by a further attenuation of the stalk, the epiphysis became completely separated from the roof of the brain. A detailed description of the parietal region in an embryo of *Chelydra* (Fig. 195) shows that this region of the roof of the brain differs little from that of other reptiles. The tubular epiphysis springs from the roof of the third ventricle in the usual situation in front of the posterior commissure and passes upwards on the posterior wall of the dorsal sac, and then forwards over its superficial surface as far as the velum and tip of the paraphysis. Its lumen widens

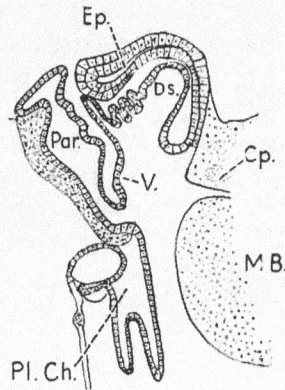

FIG. 195.—PARIETAL REGION OF THE BRAIN OF AN EMBRYO OF A SNAPPING TURTLE (CHELYDRA SERPENTINA), SHOWING THE RELATION OF THE EPIPHYSIS TO THE DORSAL SAC AND PARAPHYSIS. (AFTER HUMPHREY, 1894.)

Cp. : posterior commissure.   MB. : midbrain.
Ds. : dorsal sac.   Par. : paraphysis.
Ep. : epiphysis.   Pl. Ch. : plexus choroideus.
                    V. : velum.

as it passes forwards and the wall of the epiphysis, which in the basal part consists of a single layer of epithelial cells, shows two layers of nuclei at its rounded distal end.

In the adult animal the lumen in some cases is found to have disappeared, in the stalk and also in the body of the epiphysis; in other cases it may persist, and in one specimen of *Cistudo europæa* described by Faivre it contained small granules of calcium phosphate. The shape of the organ varies, being described as ovoid, conical, or tuberous; it is surrounded by blood-vessels and ingrowths of fibrous tissue may penetrate the wall, giving a lobulated appearance to its surface, but there is no outgrowth of epithelial buds or true lobulation. The structure of the epiphysial wall of an adult specimen of *Cistudo europæa* was described by Studnička (1905); the wall was thick and penetrated here and there by connective tissue bundles derived from the capsule. The lumen was lined by a single layer of cylindrical ependymal cells, which were everywhere of the same size and ended at the same level on the inner surface of the wall. The wall was composed of elongated ependymal cells which were attached by their outer ends to the external limiting membrane. The ependymal fibres tended to unite in bundles, which gained attachment to the ingrowing fibres from the connective tissue capsule. The tissue consists of peculiar stellate cells which send out slender protoplasmic processes and probably correspond to neuroglia cells, although no true neuroglial fibres are present. The cells are widely separated from each other and the tissue thus has a somewhat spongy appearance. There are no true ganglion cells, nor are any nerve-fibres present. In many places the inner surface of the wall shows pits which are due to small diverticula of the single central lumen; external to these are small closed cavities lying in the substance of the wall. Sometimes the diverticula and cavities are lined by cylindrical ependymal cells, similar to those bounding the main cavity; at others by the ordinary cells of the surrounding tissue. There were no indications of a secretory process in the walls of the epiphysis. In the central cavity some isolated cells were found, the protoplasm of which seems to have been slightly changed, and in the diverticula and spaces a few separate cells or small amœba-like syncytia were present. The stalk of the epiphysis had no lumen, but small cavities similar to those in the body of the epiphysis were present, and also spaces lying between the stellate cells which form the bulk of the tissue of the stalk. No nervous cord could be seen in the interior of the stalk. The epiphysis of the Chelonia thus appears to occupy an intermediate position between that of the saurian reptiles and that of birds.

The pineal system of Crocodilia has already been alluded to (p. 47), and it will only be necessary to note that the absence of the parietal organ in all species examined is contrary to expectation in these animals which live in tropical climates, should the theory of the function of the parietal eye being an organ for the estimation of heat be correct.

CHAPTER 21

THE PINEAL SYSTEM OF BIRDS

IN birds there is no parietal eye and no parietal foramen. Also there is usually no indication of a parietal spot. The pineal organ, moreover, is only represented by the proximal part, or epiphysis. The epiphysis, however, in many forms undergoes an important and characteristic transformation, which although foreshadowed in lower classes of vertebrates is not definitely evolved. This change consists in the outgrowth from the primary embryonic diverticulum of hollow epithelial buds the cavities of which are at first continuous with the lumen of the primary diverticulum (Fig. 196). At a later stage of development these often become cut off from the main stem and form independent vesicles lined by columnar epithelium. The vesicles or follicles are at first separated by a considerable amount of interfollicular connective tissue containing blood-vessels, and on section the organ has a glandular appearance resembling in some respects the thyroid gland. The epithelium lining the follicles in the pineal organ of birds is, however, ependymal in type and composed of tall, columnar cells as contrasted with the low, cubical cells of the thyroid gland ; and the content of the follicles of the pineal organ of adult animals seems to correspond to that of the ventricles of the brain, with a small amount of cell detritus, there being no colloid material. The whole organ is at first pear-shaped and the hollow epithelial buds at first communicate with the central lumen or one of its branches. Later, however, when the follicles are separated, the stalk becomes elongated and eventually its lumen disappears. The stalk may persist as a fibro-vascular cord connecting the main organ with the roof of the brain or it may become ruptured and the organ freed from its primary connection with the diencephalon. Thus all escape of secretion into the cavity of the third ventricle is prevented. Up to this period the epithelium lining the follicles is in a sound, healthy condition, the cell outlines being well defined and the alignment of the cells being quite even (Fig. 197). Later, however, degenerative changes take place in the cytoplasm and nuclei, and cell detritus accumulates in the cavities of the follicles (Fig. 198). The follicles also diminish in size and come nearer together, the whole organ forming a dense mass of closely packed small vesicles in many of which the lumen has become greatly reduced in size, or has completely disappeared.

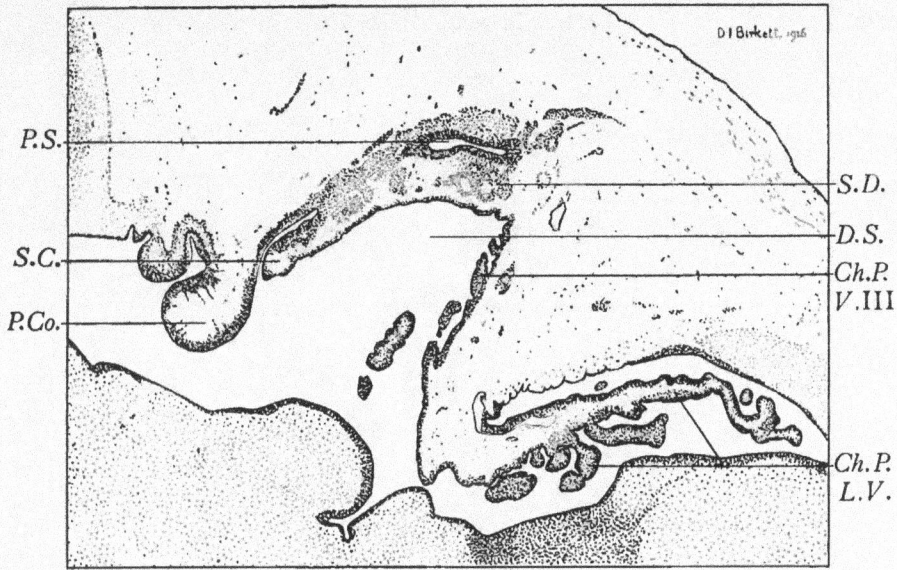

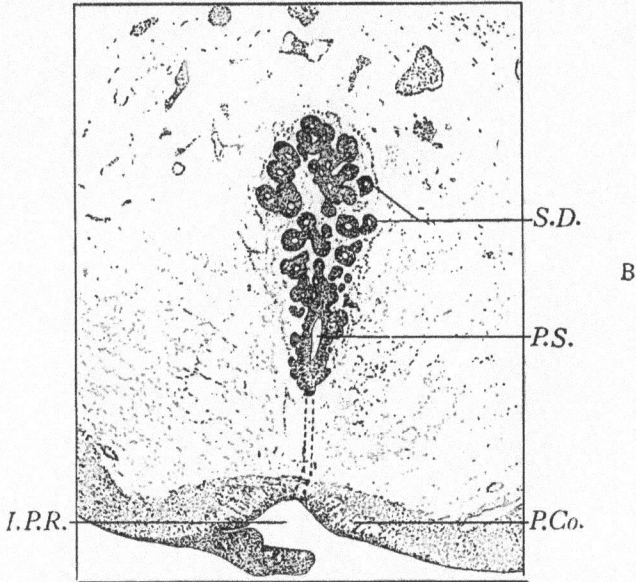

Fig. 196.—*Upper :* Medial longitudinal section of a chick embryo (8 days), showing the main pineal diverticulum and secondary diverticula, which have arisen as hollow outgrowths of the former ; also the relation of the superior and posterior commissures to the stalk of the main diverticulum, and the dorsal sac.

Lower : Oblique coronal section of pineal organ of a chick embryo, of the same age as A, showing the primary and secondary diverticula and some fibres of the posterior commissure.

Ch.P. V.III. : choroid plexus of third ventricle.
Ch.P. LV. : choroid plexus of lateral ventricle. *D.S. :* dorsal sac.
I.P.R. : infrapineal recess.

P. Co. : posterior commissure.
P.S. : pineal sac.
S.C. : superior commissure.
S.D. : secondary diverticula.

19

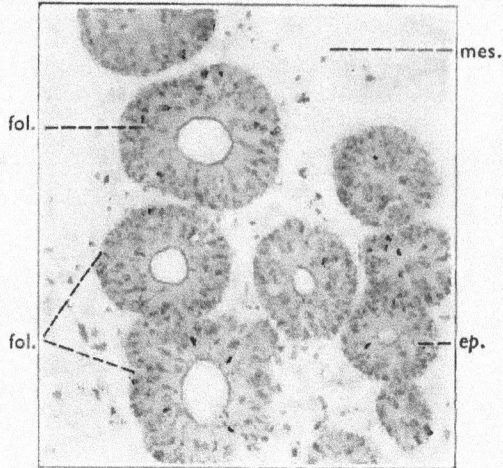

FIG. 197.—TRANSVERSE SECTION OF THE PINEAL ORGAN OF A CHICK EMBRYO,
INCUBATED 8 DAYS, SHOWING HOLLOW FOLLICLES, *fol.*; LINED BY EPENDYMA,
ep.; AND THE SURROUNDING MESENCHYME, *mes.* (R. J. G.)

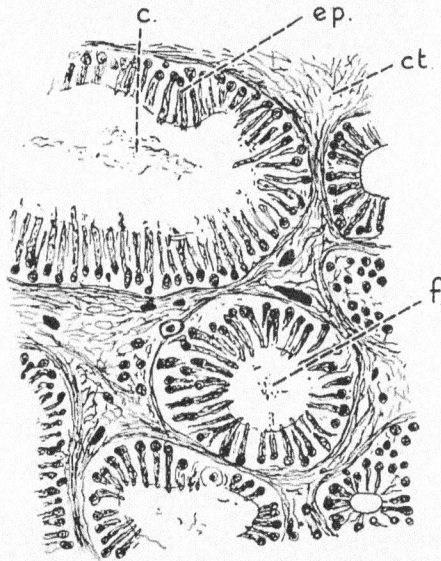

FIG. 198.—SECTION OF EPIPHYSIS OF ADULT MELEAGRIS, SHOWING FOLLICLES
LINED BY EPENDYMAL CELLS, AND CONTAINING A COAGULATED MATERIAL.

c. : coagulum.
ct. : interfollicular connective tissue.
ep. : ependymal cells.
f. : lumen of follicle.
(After Mihalkowics—highly magnified.)

No nerve-fibres connecting the pineal organ with the brain are present either within or near the stalk ; the nerve-fibres of the habenular and the posterior commissures are, therefore, derived from sources entirely outside the pineal system, and in those cases in which the pedicle has been ruptured it is obvious that all nervous connections with the brain by means of it, should they have existed in embryonic life, will have disappeared in the adult.

The pineal organ of birds, however, does not always conform to the type described above ; it is often a simple elongated tube, arising in the usual situation between the habenular and posterior commissures and extending upwards towards the vault of the skull, beneath which it ends in a slightly lobulated expansion (Fig. 199). This is, however, not regarded

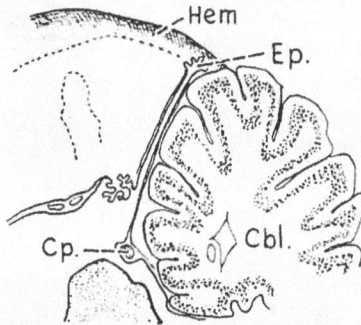

FIG. 199.—PARIETAL REGION AND CEREBELLUM OF A SPARROW. (AFTER GAZE.)
Cbl. : cerebellum.   Ep. : epiphysis.
Cp. : posterior commissure.   Hem. : hemisphere.

as an end vesicle. The tube is hollow and communicates in young specimens with the cavity of the third ventricle. It occupies the narrow interval between the cerebellum, which lies behind, and the two hemi-spheres, which are in front and lateral. Owing to the large size of the hemispheres and cerebellum in birds, the tube is of considerable length. It is invested by a fibrovascular sheath continuous with the pia mater at its attachment to the brain.

The Development of the Pineal System of Birds

This has been studied chiefly in the chick, and since the early stages of development in the chick do not differ essentially from those of other types of bird, we shall confine our description to that of the chick, and only refer to special points in the development of the system in other birds when these have some bearing on the general problem we are considering.

The first indication of the development of the pineal organ in the chick is a thickening of the epithelium forming the roof of the third ventricle, which soon grows forward in the form of a hollow diverticulum. It rises a short distance in front of the posterior commissure and is approximately mesial in position. Rarely two epiphysial outgrowths have been observed. Thus in 1897 Saint Remy found on each side of the neural tube, before this had become closed, a small evagination of the epithelium in the pineal region. Hill in 1900 observed two small diverticula close to each other in the same region of a chick embryo in which the brain was already closed. Cameron in 1903 saw similar outgrowths in chick embryos, which he considered to be an indication of the primary bilateral origin of the pineal organ. It is possible that some of these cases may be explained on the assumption that they are simply due to an abnormal development, but their occurrence in birds, considered along with the evidence of similar indications of the bilateral development of the pineal organs in other classes of vertebrates, does lead one to think that the pineal, like other sense-organs, is a bilateral structure. Thus important evidence of its bilateral origin has been found in cyclostomes, Dendy; in Selachian and Teleostean fishes (Locy, Hill); in *Amia* (Kingsbury); besides important embryological and geological evidence in Amphibia and reptiles.

The pineal diverticulum at the fourth day in the chick embryo is a conspicuous hollow, club-shaped organ (Fig. 200). Its wall consists of an, as yet, undifferentiated ependymal layer, which is continuous at its base with the ependyma forming the roof of the brain. Capillary vessels lie in the receding angle between it and the roof of the brain. The superior commissure has not yet appeared. The posterior commissure, on the other hand, is well-developed and forms a broad band some distance behind the pineal outgrowth. A low post-velar arch and velum are already recognisable. There is no evidence of any connection with the cutaneous ectoderm, a fairly thick stratum of loose mesenchyme lying between the diverticulum and the epidermis. Its distal end already shows a slight indication or lobulation, which increases as age advances and is most marked on its anterior surface and sides.

In an 8-day chick embryo, Fig. 196, A and B, the pineal organ, which is still directed forward over the superficial aspect of the dorsal sac, is seen to have budded out a number of hollow vesicles, lined by ependyma (Fig. 197), and separated from each other by a loose mesenchyme. The cavities of the vesicles are at first continuous with the central lumen or with branches which are given off from this, but already some are constricted off and form closed, independent vesicles which are surrounded on all sides by mesoderm. The mesoderm at this stage has condensed on the surface of the organ into a thin, fibrous capsule outside which are a number of dilated capillary vessels and small venous sinuses. A secondary stalk has developed at its base and its lumen has already become constricted, but still remains in communication with the third ventricle. At the eighth day the superior commissure has made its appearance and is connected on each side with the habenular ganglion. The posterior commissure has now become folded and forms a rounded cord immediately behind the pineal recess.

The development of the superior commissure in birds was specially studied by Cameron in 1904. Owing to its late appearance, the com-

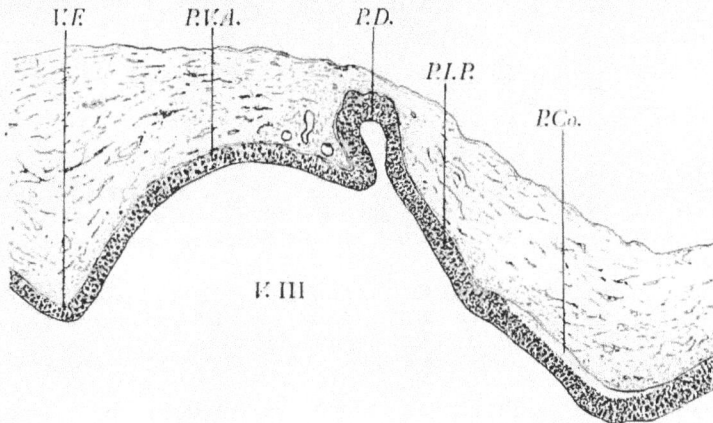

FIG. 200.—MEDIAN LONGITUDINAL SECTION OF THE PINEAL DIVERTICULUM OF A CHICK EMBRYO (FOURTH DAY). THE APEX IS DIRECTED FORWARD. (R. J. G.)

P. Co. : posterior commissure.   P.V.A. : post-velar arch.
P.D. : pineal diverticulum.   V.F. : velar fold.
P.I.P. : posterior intercalary plate.   V. III. : third ventricle.

missure was thought by authors writing previous to this date to have been absent in Aves. Cameron, however, demonstrated its presence in a 9-day chick embryo. He states that " the nerve-fibres are found to emerge from the ganglion habenulæ—from the cells of which they take origin. They pass backwards for a considerable distance (histologically speaking) in the lateral wall of the thalamencephalon, and then cross the mesial plane immediately in front of the epiphysial opening, and pass to the ganglion habenulæ of the opposite side, in which they appear to end. Therefore, although both the ganglia and nerve-fibres appear early (by the 5th day), it takes the latter some time to grow backwards in order to cross the median plane. It is thus obvious that they will appear last of all at the latter position. This explains why it is not until the 8th or 9th day that they are seen in vertical mesial sections of the same region."

Cameron was unable to find distinct evidence of fibres passing from the superior commissure to the epiphysis in chick embryos, and concluded that if they do exist they must be very scanty, but in the blenny, *Zoarces vivipara*, he described and figured a bundle of nerve-fibres passing from the upper part of the superior commissure some of which ended in the epiphysial segment of the same side, while others, decussating, crossed to the epiphysial segment of the opposite side (Fig. 201). He also published photographs of sagittal and horizontal sections through the superior

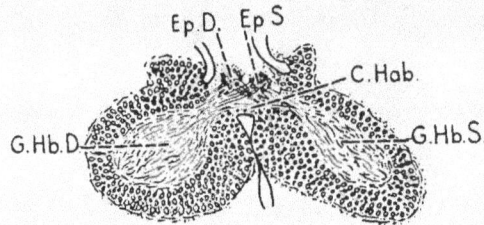

FIG. 201.—TRANSVERSE SECTION THROUGH THE GANGLIA HABENULÆ AND EPIPHYSEAL ELEMENTS OF AN EMBRYO BLENNY (ZOARCES VIVIPARA) SHOWING DECUSSATION OF THE UPPER FIBRES OF THE SUPERIOR COMMISSURE. (AFTER CAMERON, 1904.)

C. Hab. : commissura habenularis.   *G. Hb. D.* : right ganglion habenulæ.
Ep. D. : right epiphyseal element.   *G. Hb. S.* : left ganglion habenulæ.
                        Ep. S. : left epiphyseal element.

commissure in the adult human subject, prepared by the Weigert-Pal method, and showing the same division of the habenular commissure into an upper and lower segment, the former sending decussating fibres into the pineal body, the lower and posterior segment being composed of commissural fibres between the two habenular ganglia and of fibres joining the striæ medullares.

Structure and Contents of the Adult Pineal Organ of Birds

Three different types of pineal organ were described by Studnička :
1. Simple tubular.
2. Follicular.
3. Solid lobular.
1. The simple tubular type is further subdivided into :
   (a) Epiphyses with thin walls.
   (b) Epiphyses with thick walls.
The first (Fig. 199) is exemplified by the pineal organ of the sparrow, which has an elongated tubular epiphysis ending in a small lobulated vesicle. It lies immediately in front of the cerebellum, between the

hemispheres ; and in young birds the cavity, which is lined by columnar ependymal cells, communicates with the third ventricle. No nerve-fibres are present either in the stalk or external to it.

The second type of tubular epiphysis with thick walls (Fig. 202) occurs in the grosbeak, which is allied to the finches. The organ is a thick-walled tube ending blindly beneath the roof of the skull. It is somewhat lobu-lated, and in the adult animal is frequently separated from its original connection with the roof of the brain, its narrow stalk having been rup-tured. Its lumen is lined by ependymal epithelium and sends tubular diverticula into the substance of the wall, but there is no true formation of follicles.

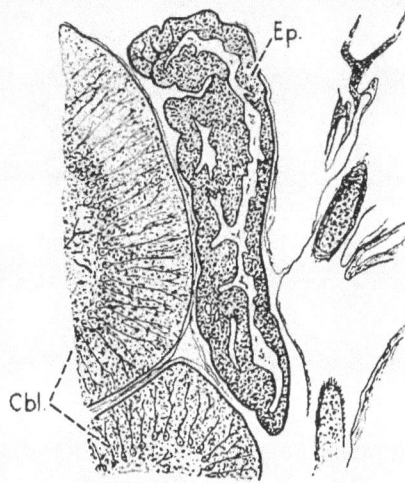

FIG. 202.—SAGITTAL SECTION THROUGH THE CEREBELLUM AND EPIPHYSIS OF A GROSBEAK, COCCOTHRAUSTIS VULGARIS. (AFTER REICHERT.)
Cbl. : cerebellum.   *Ep.* : epiphysis.

2. The follicular type of epiphysis is the most common. It consists of a mass of completely separated hollow follicles and short tubes which have originated as outgrowths from the original embryonic diverticulum from which they have subsequently been cut off as independent vesicles. Even in the adult some follicles may still retain their primary connection with the central lumen or one of its branches. A vascular connective tissue is interposed between the follicles, which is continuous externally with a thin fibrous capsule. There is a rich vascular supply, but, as in the other types, no nerves connecting the epiphysis with the central nervous system are present.

3. The solid lobular type (Fig. 203). The organ consists of a con-glomeration of solid lobules held together by thin fibrous septa. The cavities of the lobules are either partially or completely obliterated, and

it is possible that in some cases the lobules may have arisen as solid out-growths. In the adult the main body of the organ is often separated from the roof of the brain by rupture of the thinned-out stalk. It lies in the narrow triangular space between the cerebellum and the two hemispheres. This relation in the adult bird contrasts markedly with the embryonic condition in which there is a wide interval between the cerebellum and the pineal outgrowth, which space is occupied by the prominent optic lobes. The space is reduced in the later stages of embryonic development by the straightening out of the cephalic flexure of the brain and the relatively greater growth of the hemispheres and cerebellum as com-pared with the optic lobes.

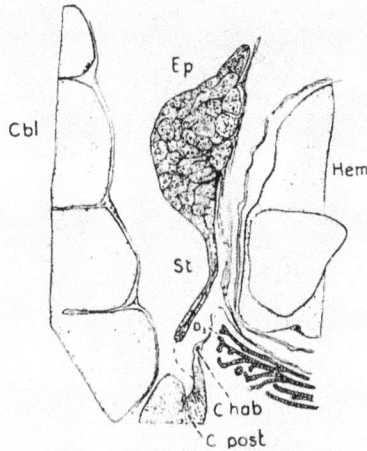

FIG. 203.—THE PARIETAL REGION OF THE THALAMENCEPHALON AND THE EPIPHYSIS OF AN ADULT FOWL (GALLUS DOMESTICUS), SHOWING THE ALMOST SOLID CONDITION OF THE FOLLICLES AND INGROWTH OF CONNECTIVE TISSUE. (AFTER STUDNIČKA, 1905.)

Cbl. : cerebellum.	Ep. : epiphysis.
C. hab. : habenular commissure.	Hem. : hemisphere.
C. post. : posterior commissure.	St. : stalk.
Ds. : dorsal sac.	

The shape of the epiphysis in the adult is usually either spindle-shaped or clavate, and it is directed almost vertically upward towards the roof of the skull. The solid type of epiphysis may be seen in the adult fowl, but different grades exist between the embryonic follicular form (Figs. 196, 197) and the almost solid form sometimes seen in adult examples.

Between these three principal types of epiphysis there are all degrees of intermediate forms, and different parts of the organ in a single individual may conform to the character of any of the three types. In some examples there are evident signs of degeneration, such as the disappearance of the external limiting membrane and mingling of the outer ends of the ependymal cells with the fibres of the surrounding vascular connective tissue, as is shown in Fig. 204, of a part of the wall of one of the follicles in the epiphysis of an owl. This observation, which we owe to Studnička, is of great importance in the comparative study of the structure of the pineal body in man and mammals, as it represents a stage in the late fœtal development which is paralleled in the development of the mammalian organ, and explains certain difficult points in the interpretation of the appearances seen in the late fœtal and post-natal stages of its growth in the human subject.

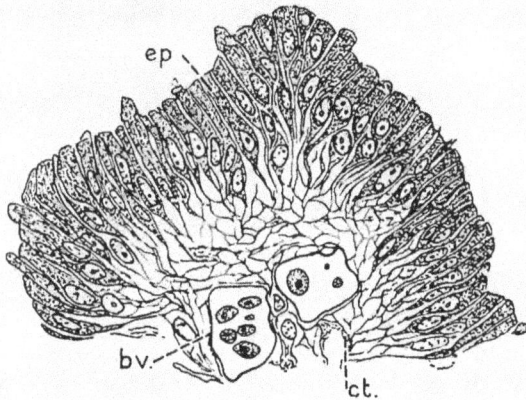

FIG. 204.—SECTION THROUGH A PART OF THE WALL OF THE EPIPHYSIS OF AN OWL, STRIX FLAMMEA, SHOWING ABSENCE OF AN EXTERNAL LIMITING MEMBRANE, AND APPARENT CONTINUITY OF THE TAPERING PROCESSES OF THE OUTER ENDS OF THE EPENDYMAL CELLS, WITH THE FIBRES OF THE SUPPORTING TISSUE. (AFTER STUDNIČKA.)

bv. : blood-vessel. *ct.* : connective tissue.
ep. : ependyma.

The inner ends of the ependymal cells in this specimen, Fig. 204, show the same rounded projections of protoplasmic material and thread-like processes that are seen in the epiphyses of some fishes, Figs. 148, 154; amphibia, p. 230; and reptiles, Fig. 178, p. 249; and there is the same difference of opinion as to whether these projections are evidence of a definite secretion or are simply due to degenerative changes in the cytoplasm and extrusion of effete material from the cell into the lumen of the follicle. The contents of the follicles are very similar to those found in the cavity of the epiphysis in fishes and reptiles, namely, a few detached groups of cells either fused in a syncytium or separate, and thin coagula containing cell-detritus such as are sometimes seen in the ventricles of the brain.

The structure of the adult epiphysis of birds, in spite of the resemblance which the developing organ has to a compound racemose gland with a secretory duct opening into the ventricular system, does not bear out the expectation which might be anticipated from its embryonic history. Degenerative changes seem to occur soon after the obliteration of the lumen of the duct, and it thus neither resembles an ordinary racemose gland nor does it truly resemble a ductless gland such as the thyroid, which gland continues to develop and shows signs of secretory activity after the follicles have been cut off from the parent stem.

CHAPTER 22

THE PINEAL ORGAN OF MAMMALS

ONLY the basal segment of the organ, the epiphysis or conarium, is recognizable in man and mammals generally ; the terminal parts, namely, the parietal sense-organ, the end-vesicle or pineal sac, and the stalk, are seldom present in the adult animal, and in many cases it is doubtful whether any vestige of these parts, even in a rudimentary condition, is found in the embryo. It is possible, however, that the occasional occurrence of bifid pineal diverticula and accessory organs and the development in the fœtus of an anterior lobe may be attributed to an inherited trait, which has not yet been completely exhausted or suppressed, and which serves as an indication of its primary dual origin. The sagittal or parietal fontanelle of the human skull and the parietal foramina which are formed at its lateral angles, each of which transmits a small vein and artery, may also be regarded as possible vestiges of the parietal foramen which in certain reptiles and fishes lodges the parietal sense-organ. Although in the adult human skull the roof is separated from the pineal organ by the whole depth of the falx cerebri and the splenium of the corpus callosum, in the human fœtus at the 7th week, when the rudiment of the pineal is first recognizable, the roof of the diencephalon is quite near the condensation of mesenchyme which represents the future membranous capsule of the brain, and there is a special development of endothelial lined vascular spaces in this situation. Further, the occasional appearance of pigment in the skin of the head of the pineal region in certain swimming birds (Klinckowstroem), mentioned on p. 75, and the occasional occurrence of a parietal foramen in the skull of the goose (Mrázek), more especially in those examples which possess a tufted crest, indicate that remnants of a parietal fleck and a parietal foramen may persist in the higher classes of vertebrates long after all remnants of the parietal eye have disappeared ; and that, if this is true, the validity of the supposed morphological significance of the parietal foramen in the human subject is not so difficult to accept as was formerly thought. The hypothesis that the parietal fontanelle and the parietal foramina of the human skull are homologous with the parietal foramen of reptiles, amphibia, and fishes has, moreover, received a considerable amount of support from recent geological evidence of the foramen in fossil skulls of the Therapsids or mammal-like reptiles discovered in America and South Africa (Broom). Thus in the middle or upper Permian period a group of higher Synapsids * were evolved which are allied to the Theromorphs of America. These were the large Dinocephalia, some of which were 16 to 18 ft. in length ; also small rat-like animals and others with grotesquely shaped broad skulls. Changes in the skull of these types, and more especially in the parietal region, show transitions between reptilian and mammalian forms. They not only show transitional stages in the gradual obliteration of the parietal canal, but they also suggest how in certain orders of mammals the canal may have been retained, or if not quite obliterated may have reappeared in association with the widening of the skull which is correlated with an increase in the size of the brain.

Dicynodon (Fig. 205), although not directly in the line of mammalian

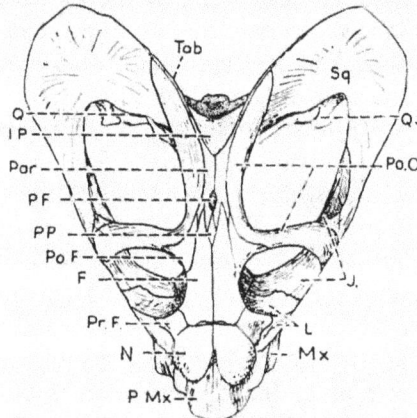

FIG. 205.—SKULL OF AN ANOMODONT REPTILE, DICYNODON KOLBEI, BROOM, VIEWED FROM ABOVE.

It shows an oval pineal foramen and narrow parietal bones, separated from the temporal fossa by a backward prolongation of the post-orbital bone. Although greatly specialized, Broom regards the skull as essentially similar to the mammalian type.

F. : frontal.	*Po. F.* : post-frontal.
IP. : interparietal.	*Po. O.* : post-orbital.
J. : jugular.	*P.P.* : pre-parietal
L. : lacrimal.	*P. Mx.* : pre-maxilla.
Mx. : maxilla.	*Pr. F.* : pre-frontal.
N. : nasal.	*Q.* : quadrate.
Par. : parietal.	*QJ.* : quadratojugal.
P.F. : pineal foramen.	*Sq.* : squamosal.
Tab. : tabular.	

descent, is very instructive with respect to reduction of width of the parietal bones, and the diminution in the transverse diameter of the

---

¹ Synapsida : ἀψίς, arch or recess—the type of cranial roof of Tetrapods in which there is a single temporal fossa.

parietal foramen, which becomes still further reduced in the Cynodont reptile *Glochinodontoides gracilis* (Haughton) (Fig. 206). In this the two parietals are fused and the antero-posterior ridge between the temporal fossæ, mentioned on p. 268, is already prominent. In the skull of the small Ictidosaurian [1] reptile (Fig. 228) found in beds of a later period (Rhœtic or Lower Jurassic) the development of this longitudinal ridge is still more pronounced, the parietal bones being fused throughout their whole length and the parietal canal having disappeared

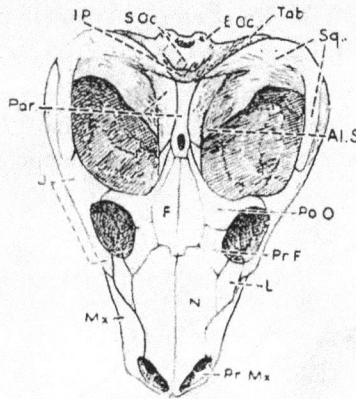

FIG. 206.—VIEW FROM ABOVE THE SKULL OF A PRIMITIVE CYNODONT REPTILE, GLOCHINODONTOIDES GRACILIS, HAUGHTON. NATURAL SIZE. (AFTER BROOM.)

The two parietal bones have fused to form a median longitudinal crest. The pineal foramen is still present and is oval in form. The parietal bones share in the formation of the temporal fossa.

Al. S. : ala of sphenoid.	*Par.* : parietal.
E. Oc. : ex-occipital.	*Po. O.* : post-orbital & post-frontal.
F. : frontal.	*Pr. F.* : pre-frontal.
I.P. : inter-parietal.	*Pr. Mx.* : pre-maxilla.
J. : jugular.	*S. Oc.* : supra-occipital.
L. : lacrimal.	*Sq.* : squamosal.
Mx. : maxilla.	*Tab.* : tabular.
N. : nasal.	

completely. In this animal, besides the keel-like interparietal crest, there are two occipital condyles and the articulation of the lower jaw with the base of the skull is still more mammalian in type than it is in the preceding forms, for although the joint between the articular and quadrate is still present, the dentary almost reaches the squamosal. For these and other reasons the Suborder Ictidosauria is regarded as forming one of the connecting links between the cynodonts (dog-toothed reptiles) and the Mammalia.

A more human type of the parietal region of the skull-roof is met with in the Gorgonopsian reptile *Scylacops capensis* (Broom). This, although

---

[1] Ἰκτίδες, weasel-like.

in other respects it is much more reptilian in character, serves as an example of the earlier type of fossil reptile-skull, in which the parietal foramen lies in the suture between two horizontally placed parietal bones, which are separated from the single temporal fossæ merely by a backward prolongation of the postorbital. This bone is reduced in Glochinodontoides, and the parietal bone shares in the formation of the temporal fossa, as it does in the human subject and other living orders of mammals.

Development of the Pineal Organ of Mammals

Despite the wide differences in the general form and structure of adult types of mammalia, the early stages of development of the pineal organ appear to be very similar in all. We shall therefore give a short description, in the first place, of the development of the human pineal

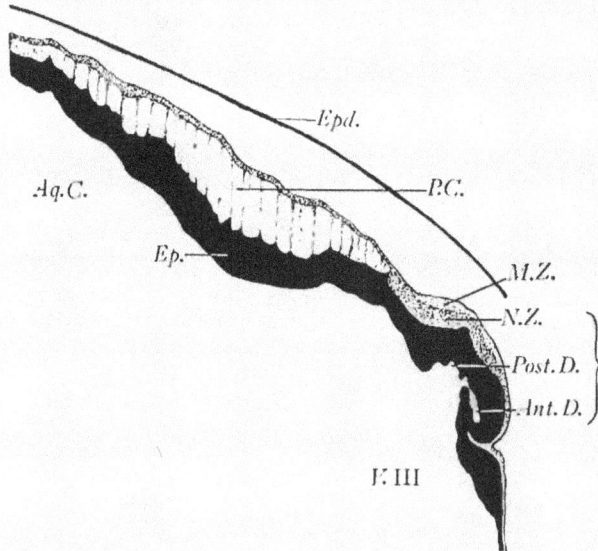

FIG. 207.—MEDIAN LINEAR RECONSTRUCTION OF THE PINEAL REGION AND POSTERIOR COMMISSURE OF A 20-MM. HUMAN EMBRYO. THE APEX OF THE PINEAL DIVERTICULUM IS DIRECTED FORWARD. (R. J. G.)

Ant. D. : anterior diverticulum.	*N.Z.* : nuclear zone.
Aq. C. : aqueductus cerebri.	*M.Z.* : marginal zone.
Ep. : ependyma.	*P.C.* : posterior commissure.
Epd. : epidermis.	*Post. D.* : posterior diverticulum.

V. III. : third ventricle.

organ, of which we have a more complete knowledge than of other types, and will only refer to the development of the pineal system in lower mammals with respect to any corroborative evidence or peculiarity of structure which may be of general interest.

One of the first indications of the development of the pineal system

in man is a thickening of the ependyma in the posterior part of the roof
of the diencephalon and the adjacent parts of the alar laminæ. This
thickening has the form of a longitudinal band which is slightly raised
above the general surface and is grooved on its under surface. It lies in
front of the posterior commissure, which commissure has already appeared
and extends backwards for a considerable distance above the ventricle
of the midbrain, which becomes the future aqueduct of Sylvius. Soon,

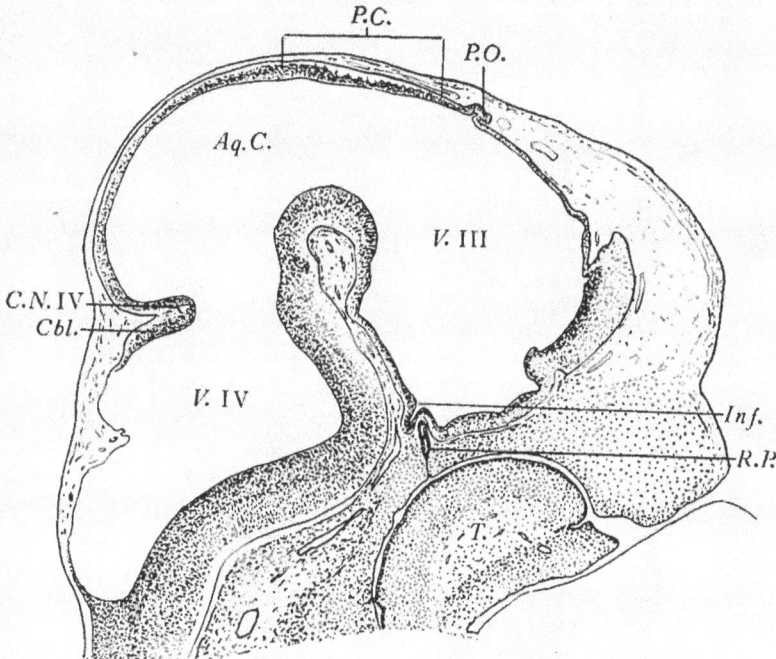

FIG. 208.—MEDIAN LONGITUDINAL SECTION OF A RABBIT EMBRYO (16 DAYS,
11 MM.). THE APEX OF THE PINEAL BODY IS DIRECTED FORWARD, AND THE
DIVERTICULUM SHOWS A CENTRAL CONSTRICTION. (R. J. G.)

Aq. C. : aqueductus cerebri.	P.O. : pineal organ.
Cbl. : cerebellum.	R.P. : pouch of Rathke.
C.N. IV. : Cranial nerve IV.	T. : tongue.
Inf. : infundibulum.	V. III. : third ventricle.
P.C. : posterior commissure.	V. IV. : fourth ventricle.

by a forward growth of the anterior end of the thickened band and a
deepening of the groove, the rudiment assumes the typical form of the
primary diverticulum in lower classes of vertebrates : namely, a rounded
anterior segment with a small lumen which is separated by a slight constriction from the lumen of the basal segment, which opens freely into
the cavity of the third ventricle (Figs. 207, 208, 209.)

In a 20-mm. human embryo the wall of the diverticulum shows a
division into the three typical zones of the neural tube, namely, an inner,

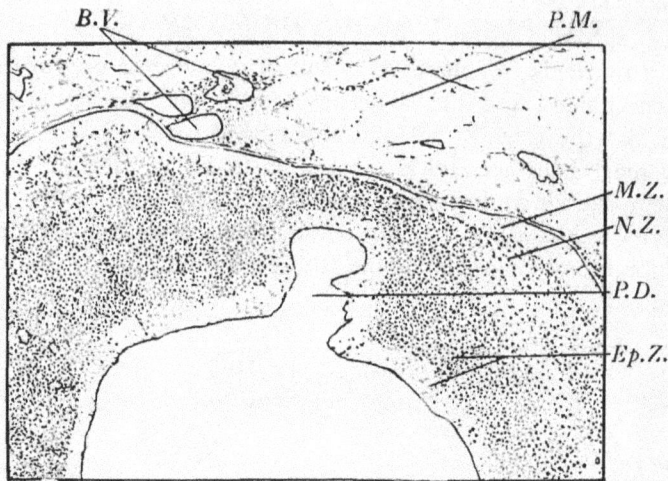

FIG. 209.—PINEAL EVAGINATION, 20-MM. HUMAN EMBYRO. THE SECTION
PASSES TRANSVERSELY THROUGH THE POSTERIOR PART OF THE DIVERTICULUM,
WHERE ITS LUMEN IS CONTINUOUS WITH THE CAVITY OF THE THIRD VENTRICLE.

B.V. : blood-vessels.   N.Z. : nuclear zone.
Ep. Z. : ependymal zone.   M.Z. : marginal zone.
                    P.M. : pia mater.

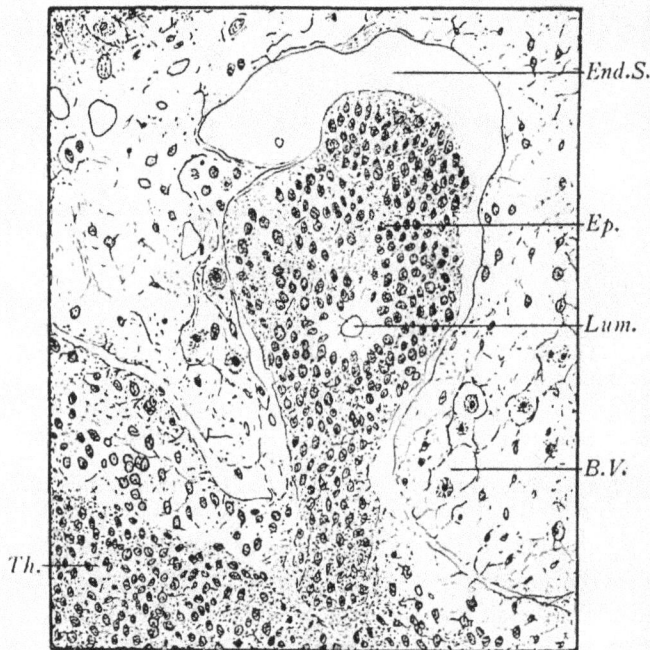

FIG. 210.—PINEAL ORGAN OF THE SAME EMBRYO AS FIG. 209. THE SECTION
PASSES TRANSVERSELY THROUGH THE ANTERIOR PART OF THE ORGAN, AND
SHOWS THE CENTRAL LUMEN SURROUNDED BY RADIALLY ARRANGED EPENDYMAL
CELLS. (R. J. G.)

B.V. : blood-vessel. Ep. : ependyma. End. S. : endothelium-lined space.
        Lum. : lumen.   Th. : thalamencephalon.

thick ependymal layer (*Ep.Z.*), a thin middle layer or nuclear zone (*N.Z.*), and an outer reticular or marginal zone (*M.Z.*). The inner ends of the ependymal cells which immediately surround the lumen are clear and destitute of nuclei ; they show a radial arrangement and are bounded by an internal limiting membrane (Figs. 209, 210). The outer zone is limited by a less defined external membrane and pia mater, and it is in relation with large endothelium-lined spaces and capillary vessels which

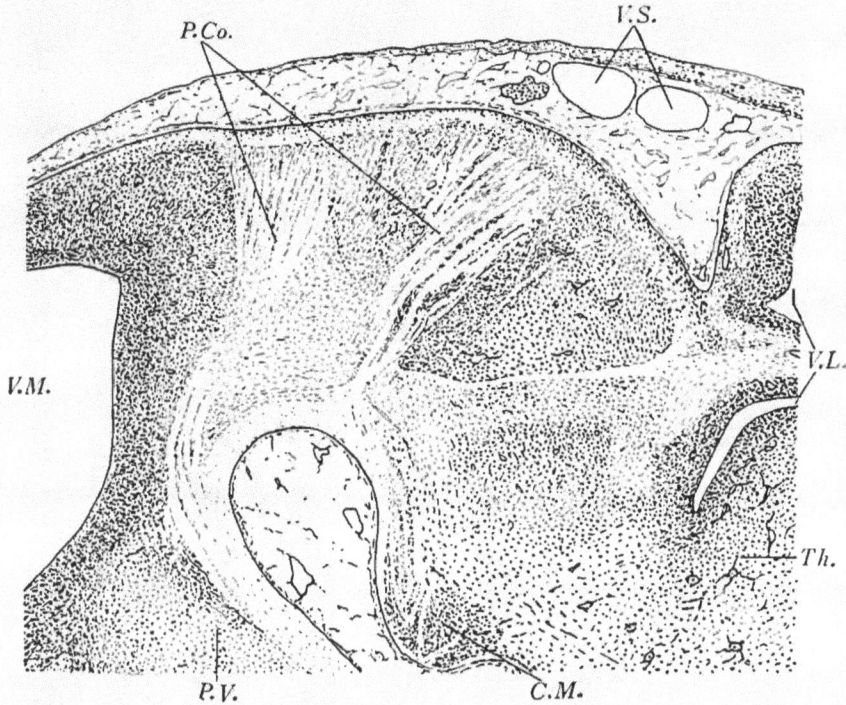

FIG. 211.—PARAMEDIAN SECTION THROUGH THE MID-BRAIN OF A RABBIT EMBRYO (18 DAYS), SHOWING THE DIRECTION OF THE FIBRES OF THE POSTERIOR COMMISSURE AND THEIR CONNECTIONS WITH THE PONS VAROLII AND INTERPEDUNCULAR REGION. (R. J. G.)

C.M. : corpus mammillaris.   *V.M.* : ventriculus mesencephali.
P. Co. : posterior commissure.   *V.S.* : venous sinuses.
P.V. : pons Varolii   *V.L.* : ventriculus lateralis.
Th. : thalamus.

lie in the surrounding loose mesenchymal tissue. The extent and thickness of the posterior commissure at this stage of development are well seen in Figs. 207, 208, which represent the region in a human embryo and in a rabbit embryo at a corresponding stage of development (16 days, 11 mm.). Fig. 211, of a slightly older rabbit embryo (18 days), shows the direction of the fibres of the posterior commissure as seen in a paramedian sagittal section.

20

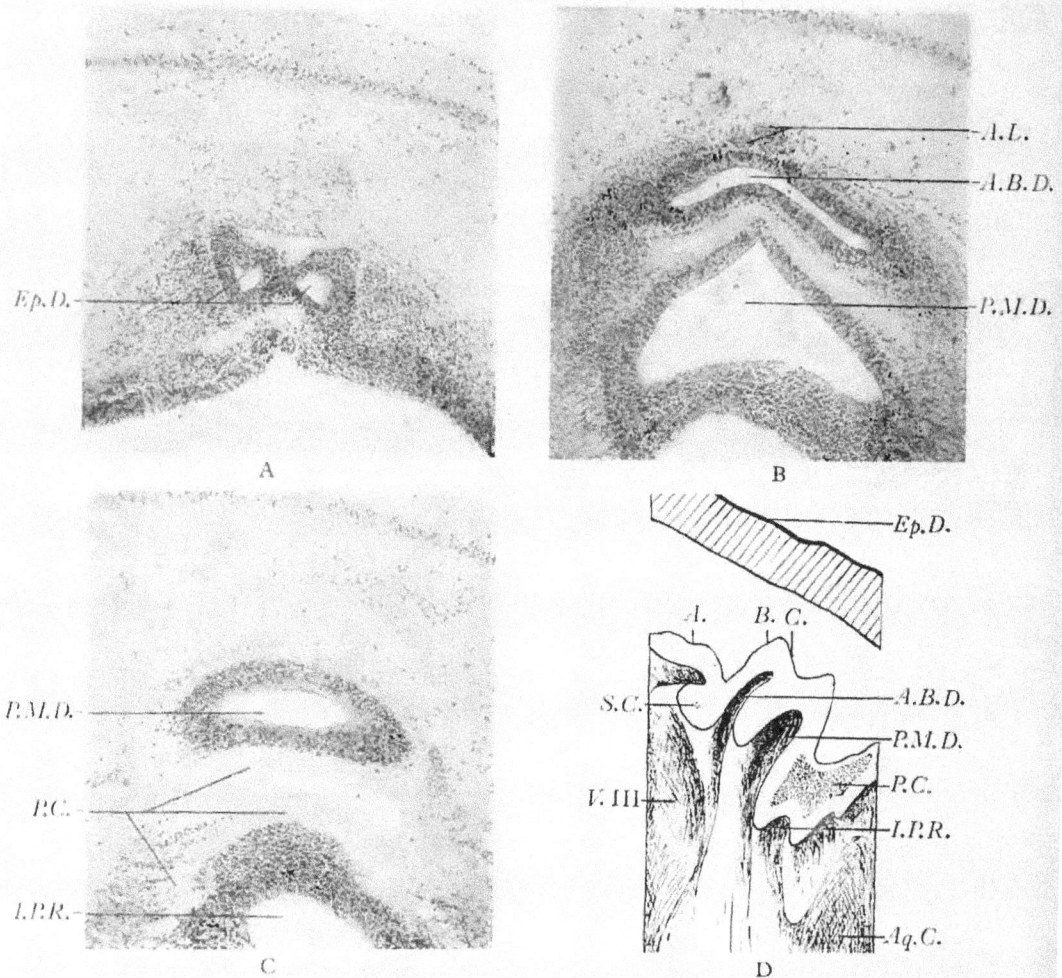

FIG. 212.—TRANSVERSE SECTIONS OF PINEAL REGION OF A 22-MM. HUMAN EMBRYO AND MEDIAN ASPECT OF THE RIGHT HALF OF A MODEL RECONSTRUCTED FROM THE CORRESPONDING SERIES OF SECTIONS. (R. J. G.)

A—Section through the posterior bifurcated end of the anterior ependymal diverticulum in the plane A of the model.

B—Section through the anterior bilobed diverticulum and posterior median diverticulum in the plane B of the model.

C—Section through the posterior median diverticulum and posterior commissure in the plane C of the model.

D—Drawing of the median aspect of the right half of the model showing the relations of the superior and posterior commissures to the pineal diverticula.

A. B. C., in D indicate the planes of the sections in A, B, and C.

A.B.D. : anterior bilobed diverticulum.   Epd. in D : epidermis.
A.L. : epithelial buds forming rudi-   I.P.R. : infrapineal recess.
   ment of anterior lobe.   P.C. : posterior commissure.
Aq. C. : aqueductus cerebri.   P.M.D. : posterior median diverticulum.
Ep. D. in A : ependymal diverticulum.   S.C. : superior commissure.
           V. III. : third ventricle.

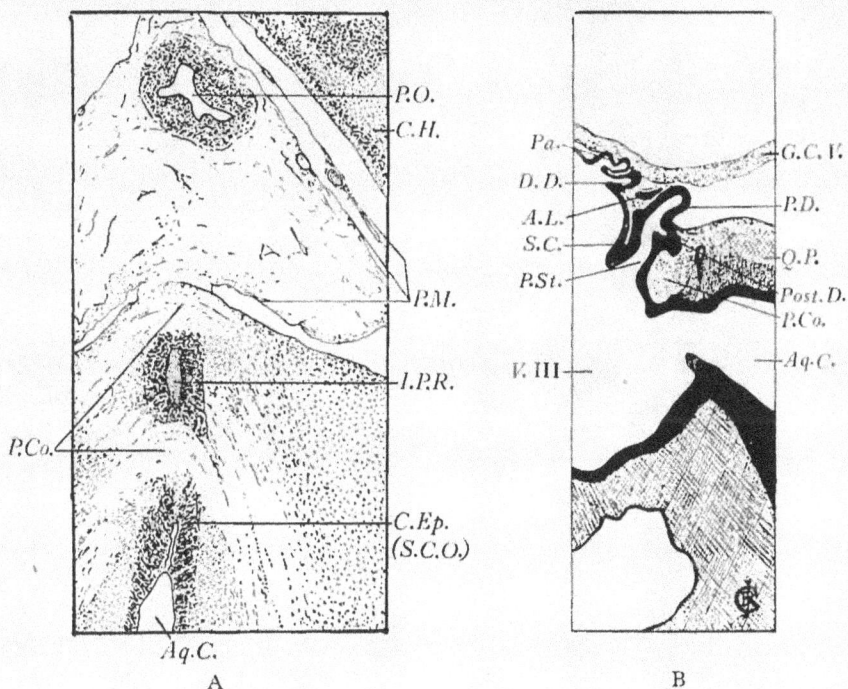

FIG. 213.

A—Transverse section through the pineal organ of a human embryo (6 cm.) showing its relations to the membranes, posterior commissure, and subcommissural organ.

B—A median linear reconstruction of the pineal region of a human embryo (6 cm.) showing the main diverticulum, infrapineal recess, anterior lobe, superior and posterior commissures, the dorsal sac, and an anterior diverticulum possibly representing a vestige of the paraphysis; also the great cerebral vein and opening of the aqueductus cerebri. (R. J. G.)

A.L. : anterior lobe.	P.D. : pineal diverticulum.
Aq. C. : aqueductus cerebri.	P.M. : pia mater.
C. Ep. : columnar epithelium.	P.O. : pineal organ.
C.H. : cerebral hemisphere.	Post. D. : posterior diverticulum.
D.D. : dorsal diverticulum or supra- pineal recess.	P. St. : pineal stalk.
	Q.P. : quadrigeminal plate.
G.C.V. : great cerebral vein.	S.C. : superior commissure.
I.P.R. : infrapineal recess.	S.C.O. : subcommissural organ.
Pa. : ? paraphysis.	V.III. : third ventricle.
P. Co. : posterior commissure.	

In a 22-mm. human embryo, Figs. 212, A, B, C, D, the simple primary diverticulum is subdivided by a transverse fold into a hollow, bilobed anterior segment, B, *A.B.D.*, and a single median posterior segment, B, *P.M.D.* The superior or habenular commissure has also appeared and two diverticula from the dorsal sac have commenced to grow back-

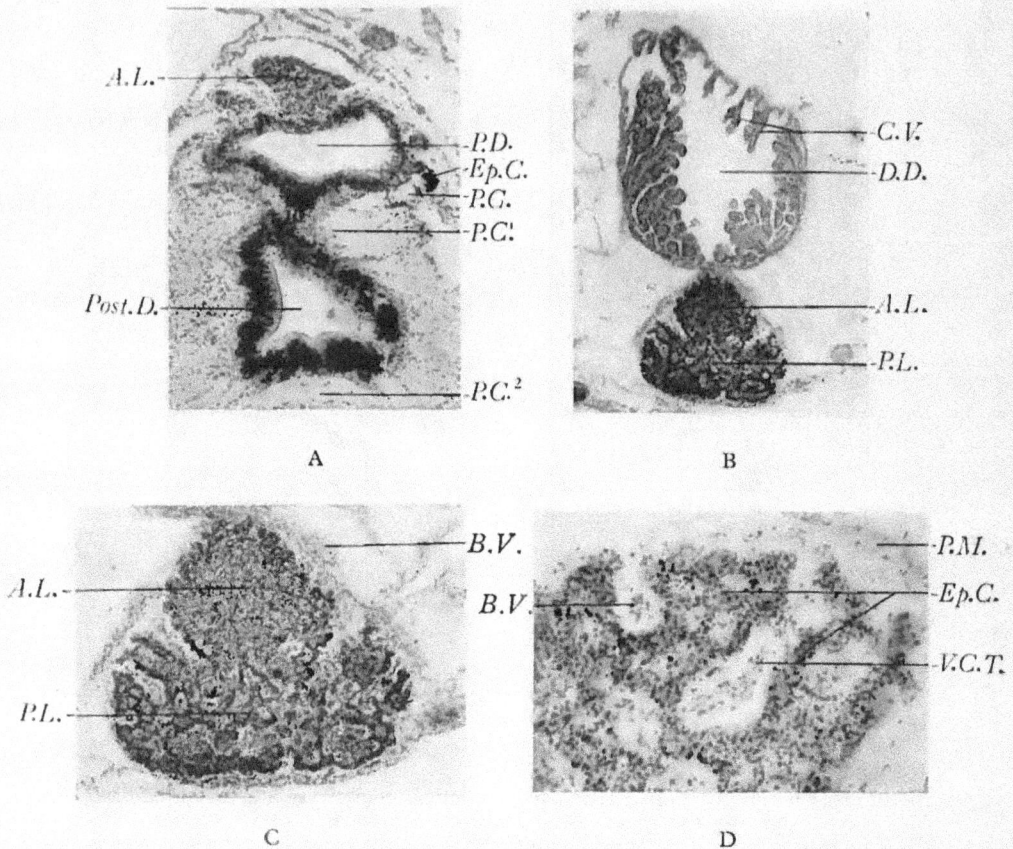

FIG. 214.—TRANSVERSE SECTIONS OF THE PINEAL REGION OF A 6-CM. HUMAN
EMBRYO, AND OF A 4½-MONTH FŒTUS. (R. J. G.)

A—Section through the basal part of the main pineal diverticulum of a 6-cm.
human embryo showing, in the upper part of the photograph, the solid
anterior lobe. Below this is the main pineal diverticulum, the wall of which
shows proliferating cords of ependymal cells growing outward, into the
surrounding tissue. Below the pineal evagination is a section through the
infrapineal recess, the epithelial lining of which is assuming a columnar
type. Fibres of the posterior commissure are seen at the sides and below
the pineal region.

B—Coronal section through the pineal region of a 4½-month human fœtus showing
the relation of the dorsal diverticulum (suprapineal recess) to the pineal
gland. Clusters of elongated choroidal villi project into the lumen of the
diverticulum. The pineal gland shows partial subdivision into an anterior
and posterior lobe.

C—The pineal gland more highly magnified, showing the ingrowths of vascular
processes of the pia mater between the outgrowing neuro-epithelial cords.

D—Peripheral portion of the gland ×55 D., showing pale areas containing a
central core of vascular pia mater, alternating with dark zones composed of
neuro-epithelial cords.

[Continued at foot of next page

ward on each side of the main pineal diverticulum, A, *Ep. D.* There is also a slight indication of the development of the anterior lobe, which appears as two solid epithelial buds from the anterior wall of the pineal diverticulum, B, *A.L.* An infrapineal recess was also present in this specimen, D, *I P.R.*, which probably represents a temporary fold and would have disappeared at a later stage of development, when the apex of the pineal organ becomes rotated backward and comes to lie on the dorsal aspect of the quadrigeminal plate.

In a 6-cm. human embryo, the anterior lobe has considerably increased in size and a secondary pineal stalk has developed and forms rather more than one half of the total outgrowth, the distal end of which consists of the main pineal diverticulum (Fig. 213, A, *P.O.*, and B, *P.D.*) and a smaller posterior diverticulum (Fig. 213, B, *Post. D.*), which lies immediately above the posterior commissure. The anterior lobe consists of a number of irregularly branched processes of epithelium, which grow into the vascular mesenchyme in front of the main pineal diverticulum and above the habenular commissure. Similar proliferating outgrowths of ependymal cells from the sides of the main diverticulum are seen invading the mantle zone ; these, however, lie beneath the external limiting membrane Fig. 214, A, *A.L.*, *Ep. C.*, and have not, as yet, come into contact with the blood-vessels of the surrounding mesenchyme. Two diverticula were present in front of the pineal organ ; the more posterior of these probably represents the diverticulum from the dorsal sac, which will become the suprapineal recess (Fig. 213, B, *D.D.*) ; the more anterior is possibly a rudiment of the paraphysis (*Pa.*). The close relation of the great cerebral vein to the epiphysis is indicated in the lineal reconstruction (Fig. 213, B, *G.C.V.*) and also the position of the epidermis, which at this stage is raised a considerable distance above the pineal organ. The exact position relative to the membranes of the brain is shown in Fig. 213, A, *P.O.* The organ lies in a triangular space bounded below by the roof plate of the neural tube and the layer of pia mater which invests the brain stem, and laterally by right and left membranous laminæ, which are attached above to the lower border of the interhemispheric septum or primary falx cerebri. Along the line of junction of the lateral laminæ with the interhemispheric septum is a membranous channel which encloses the great cerebral vein (Fig. 215, *G.C.V.*). At a later stage of development, when the corpus callosum and fornix grow backward over the

A.L. : anterior lobe.	*P.C.*[1], *P.C.*[2] : posterior commissure.
B.V. : blood-vessel.	*P.L.* : posterior lobe.
C.V. : choroidal villi.	*P.M.* : pia mater.
D.D. : dorsal diverticulum.	*Post. D.* : posterior diverticulum.
Ep. C. : epithelial cords.	*V.C.T.* : vascular connective tissue.

diencephalon and midbrain, the thin lower part of the interhemispheric septum disappears (Fig. 215, S.), while the thick upper part persists as

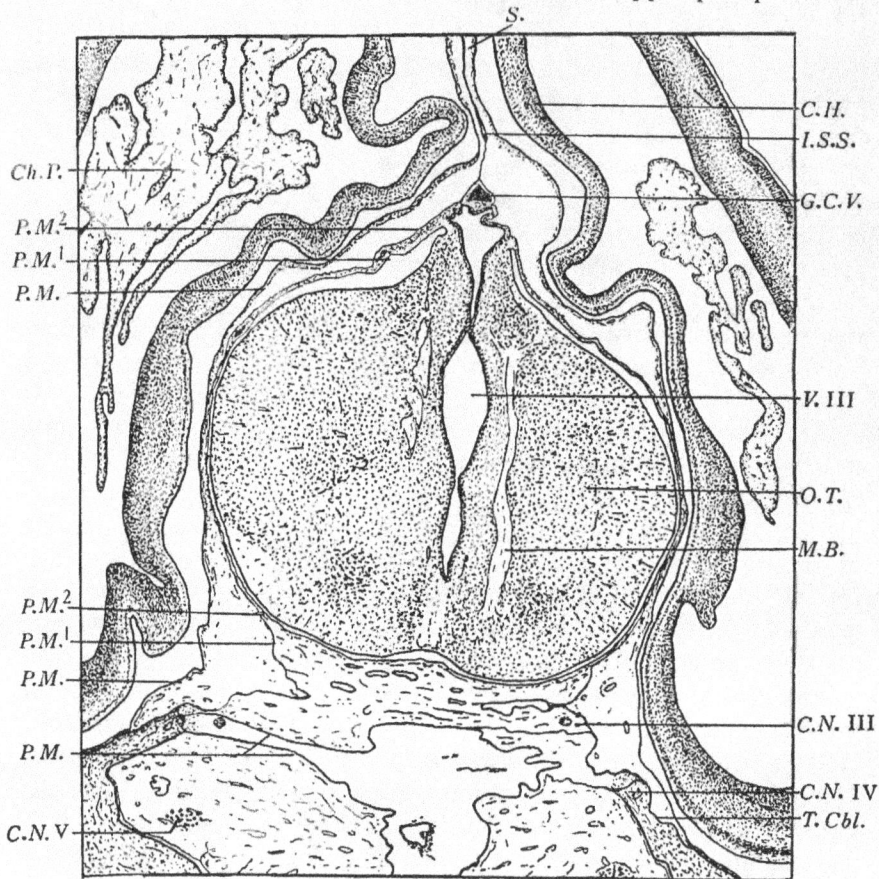

FIG. 215.—TRANSVERSE SECTION THROUGH THE POSTERIOR THALAMIC REGION OF A 6-CM. HUMAN EMBRYO IN FRONT OF THE PINEAL ORGAN, SHOWING THE RELATION OF THE CEREBRAL MEMBRANES TO THE GREAT CEREBRAL VEIN AND NEURAL TUBE AT THE JUNCTION OF THE LATERAL PLATE WITH THE DORSAL LAMINA, AND THE EXTREME THINNESS OF THE MEMBRANE (LOWER PART OF INTERHEMISPHERIC SEPTUM) WHICH JOINS THE SHEATH OF THE GREAT CEREBRAL VEIN TO THE LOWER MARGIN OF THE FALX CEREBRI. (R. J. G.)

C.H. : cerebral hemisphere.
Ch. P. : choroid plexus.
C.N., III., IV., V. : cranial nerves.
I.S.S. : inferior sagittal sinus.
G.C.V. : great cerebral vein.
M.B. : bundle of Meynert.

O.T. : optic thalamus.
P.M., P.M.^{1}, P.M.^{2} : pia mater.
S. : septum interhemisphericum (falx cerebri).
T. Cbl. : tentorium cerebelli.

the definitive falx cerebri, the inferior sagittal sinus (Fig. 215, I.S.S.) being developed in its lower border. The septum in the earlier stages of development is very much thicker than at the stage described, and is formed by a median condensation of the loose mesenchyme which occupies the space between the developing hemispheres. It is not formed by the

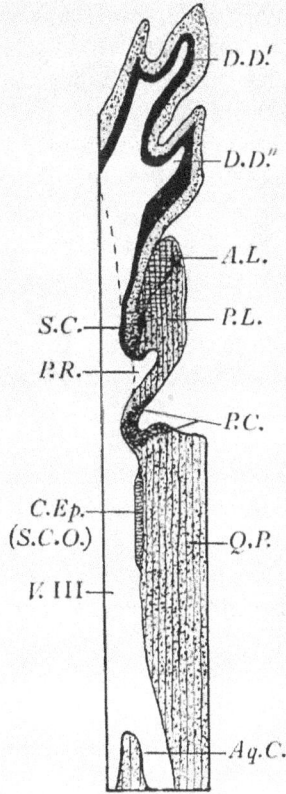

FIG. 216.—MEDIAN LINEAR RECONSTRUCTION OF THE PINEAL REGION OF A 4½-MONTH HUMAN FŒTUS SHOWING ANTERIOR OPENING OF AQUEDUCTUS CEREBRI; THE COLUMNAR EPITHELIUM OF THE SUBCOMMISSURAL ORGAN BETWEEN THIS AND THE POSTERIOR COMMISSURE, ABOVE WHICH IS THE PINEAL ORGAN, CONSISTING OF A MAIN POSTERIOR LOBE WHICH IN THE GREATER PART OF ITS EXTENT IS SOLID AND A SMALL ANTERIOR LOBE. ABOVE AND IN FRONT OF THE PINEAL RECESS IS THE SUPERIOR COMMISSURE AND ABOVE THIS THE BIFID DORSAL DIVERTICULUM. (R. J. G.)

A.L. : anterior lobe.	P.L. : posterior lobe.
Aq. C. : aqueductus cerebri.	P.R. : pineal recess.
C. Ep. : columnar epithelium.	Q.P. : quadrigeminal plate.
D.D.', D.D." : dorsal diverticulum.	S.C. : superior commissure.
P.C. : posterior commissure.	S.C.O. : subcommissural organ.

union of the two layers of a fold, and the same remark applies to the formation of the tentorium and the falx cerebelli.

The recess (Fig. 213, B, *Post. D.*) which projects backward from the posterior wall of the main diverticulum probably corresponds to the posterior pineal diverticulum described in the preceding specimen

(22-mm. human embryo). This pocket, which has been described as the infrapineal recess, disappears at a later stage of development, probably by opening out into the cavity of the third ventricle ; and it seems probable that the cavity of the secondary pineal stalk (Fig. 213, B, *P. St.*) also becomes absorbed into the ventricle in the same way, leaving only its apical part, which persists in the adult as the definitive pineal recess. The central cavity of the body of the main pineal diverticulum, which according to Krabbe becomes closed by constriction at the neck, persists for a variable time ; thus the cavity has usually disappeared at birth, but the pineal body may be solid, with the exception of the pineal recess at its base, at a much earlier stage, e.g. in a 4½-month human fœtus, which we shall describe next (Fig. 216, and Fig. 214, B and C).

The mid-fœtal stage of development of the pineal organ in the human subject is very instructive. The anterior lobe, which is medial in position, is seen in a coronal section to be partially separated from the main part of the organ by two fibro-vascular septa, which pass obliquely downwards and medially towards the centre of the organ, each traversing about one-third of its total width, the remaining median third corresponds to a zone where the anterior lobe is continuous with the substance of the main posterior lobe. The structure of the two lobes is similar, but that of the anterior lobe, especially its central part, is more homogenous. Each lobe consists of a lobulated mass of small epithelial cells with deeply stained oval nuclei. The most active growth is at the periphery, where irregularly branched epithelial processes are growing out into the sur-rounding vascular connective tissue. The epithelial cells appear to be mostly directly derived from the inner ependymal zone of the diverticulum, but there are also a certain number of cells which have the character of the nuclear or mantle zone, which may be distinguished by their position and by their nuclei being vesicular and pale in colour, as contrasted with the deeply stained nuclei of the undifferentiated ependymal cells. At the surface branched finger-shaped or club-shaped processes interdigitate with vascular processes, which appear to grow inward between the epithelial cords (Fig. 214, B, C, D). Further, if cross-sections of the interdigitating processes are observed, it will be seen that the vascular processes of pial tissue appear paler than the surrounding zones of densely packed small epithelial cells. The vascular mesenchymal areas are at first separated from contact with the neural epithelium by the external limiting membrane, between which and the deeply stained ependymal cells are a few sparsely scattered cells, with pale vesicular nuclei belonging to the mantle zone. The general arrangement of the epithelial tubes or cords and their relation to the ingrowing vascular processes, are seen with diagrammatic clearness in Fig. 217, B and D, photographed from a section of the wall of the pineal sac of an adult Sphenodon.[1] In the illustration, Fig. 217, it will be observed that the wall of the pineal sac is folded, and that between the hollow epithelial outward projections of the wall there are ingrowths of vascular connective tissue. Such an ingrowth is seen in the centre of Fig. 217, D, and it will be noted that the vascular core, *B.V.*, which lies in the middle of the lobule is surrounded on all sides by neuroepithelium. Should a cross-section of such an *apparent* lobule be examined, it will be seen to consist of a core of sinusoidal blood-vessels surrounded by a perivascular sheath of pial tissue, which is in contact peripherally with the external limiting membrane of outgrowing neuroepithelial processes. Proceeding farther outward from the central pale area formed by the vessels and their loose mesenchymatous sheath, there will be found beyond the limiting membrane the reticular and nuclear zones, the latter containing pale cells with large vesicular nuclei. Finally, there is a peripheral zone of deeply stained ependymal cells and the internal limiting membrane.

The deeply stained cells surrounding the clear vascular areas have the appearance of epithelial cords cut in various directions. When the section is transverse (Fig. 217, F) the cords appear as rings of cells, " rosettes," with deeply stained oval nuclei arranged radially round a small palely stained central zone, which is formed by the inner ends of the cells coming into contact in the central axis of the cord. If the section of the cord is longitudinal, two parallel rows of nuclei are seen, which are separated by a palely stained axial zone, where the inner, palely stained ends of the cells come into contact in the situation of a virtual lumen. These cords of proliferating ependymal cells are usually grouped in lobules (Fig. 214, D), which grow outward between the vascular ingrowths of the pia mater.

In the later stages of development neither the internal nor external limiting membrane is visible, and it appears that the lumen of the outgrowing epithelial lobules, seen in Fig. 217, A and B, is replaced by a virtual lumen, which forms the central axis of the solid cords which are seen in cross-section in Fig. 214, D, and Fig. 217, F. The external limiting membrane also disappears, as it has been shown to do in birds, and the ependymal tissue mingles with the connective tissue, as was clearly demonstrated by Studnička to be the case in *Strix* (Fig. 204, p. 297).

[1] This specimen is from one of a series of microscopical sections illustrating the development and the structure of the adult pineal region of *Sphenodon* and *Geotria* which were prepared by the late Professor Dendy of the University of London, King's College, and we take this opportunity of thanking Professor D. Mackinnon for permission to make use of this most valuable collection in our recent investigation.

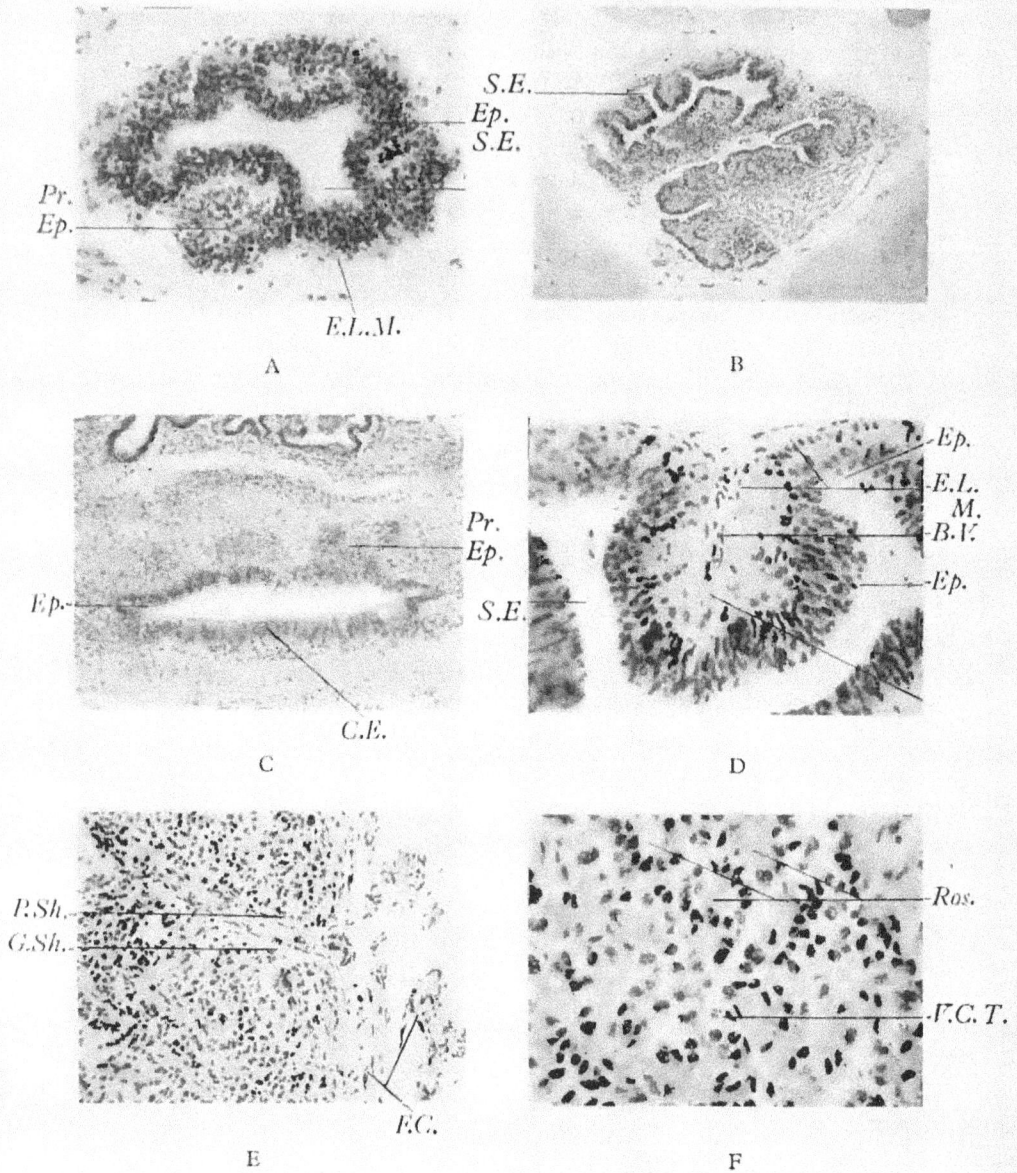

FIG. 217.

A—Transverse section through the distal end of the pineal evagination of a
6-cm. human embryo. It shows folding of the wall of the diverticulum and
outgrowth of the proliferating ependymal cells into the mantle zone.

B—Section through the pineal region of an adult *Sphenodon* (Dendy collection),
showing in the upper part of the photograph the pineal evagination, the wall
of which is folded in a manner similar to the human, but the extension of

[Continued at foot of next page

There is thus an appearance produced, by cross-sections of the cords, of groups of deeply stained epithelial cells arranged in ring-like zones or " rosettes." These surround the vascular ingrowths, which appear pale. This arrangement of alternating series of branched epithelial and vascular cords is the key to the mosaic appearance which is described by Globus and Silbert as characteristic of the later stages of fœtal and early postnatal life. The " streams" of deeply stained epithelial cells described by these authors are longitudinal sections of the epithelial cords. The central parts of the large clear areas of the mosaic pattern are transverse or oblique sections through the ingrowing vascular processes surrounded by pale cells with vesicular nuclei. Owing to the radial disposition of the epithelial cells around a central axis, which is destitute of nuclei, the general appearance of a group of epithelial cords cut transversely is similar to that of an acinar gland, but with the important difference that in the human subject the acini usually have no lumen and no ducts are present.

The later fœtal and early post-natal stages of development of the human pineal organ have been specially studied by Globus and Silbert, 1931, and Krabbe, 1915 ; the former have published an excellent series of photographs of the pineal body, illustrating the structure of the organ

the lumen of the diverticulum into the outgrowing processes is much more pronounced. Below and to the right of the photograph are seen sections of portions of the paraphysis and dorsal sac.

C—Transverse section through the basal part of the pineal evagination of the 4½-month human fœtus, seen in Fig. 214, B, C, and D, showing outgrowth of neuro-epithelial cords, more especially from the anterior aspect and sides of the tube ; on the posterior aspect (below in photograph) the epithelium is differentiating into the columnar type characteristic of the subcommissural organ.

D—Detail of B, × 139 D., showing in the centre a pseudo-lobule, with its central core of vascular pia mater, between two hollow neuro-epithelial outgrowths.

E—Section through the subcapsular part of a pineal gland of an infant (1 year 4 months), showing the fibrous capsule and the penetration of a blood-vessel into the substance of the gland. The vessel is surrounded by a perivascular sheath of fibrous connective tissue, outside which is a glial sheath the cellular and fibrous components of which are continuous with the neuro-spongium which forms the supporting tissue of the lobules and contains the parenchyma cells.

F—Portion of the same specimen × 261 D., showing the predominance at this stage of the cells with small dark nuclei and the arrangement of the cells in cords, which when cut in cross-section are seen to be disposed radially round a central core which is destitute of nuclei, giving the acinar appearance sometimes described as " rosettes." (R. J. G.)

B.V. : blood-vessel.	M.Z. : marginal zone.
C.E. : columnar epithelium.	P. Sh. : pial sheath.
E.L.M. : external limiting membrane.	Pr. Ep. : epithelial processes.
Ep. : ependyma.	Ros. : " rosette."
F.C. : vessels in fibrous capsule.	S.E. : secondary evagination.
G. Sh. : glial sheath.	V.C.T. : vascular connective tissue.

in human fœtuses from $5\frac{1}{2}$ months to the time of birth, and of 18 infants in the first month of post-natal life, during which critical period considerable changes in structure occur which have been described by these authors and also by Krabbe. Globus and Silbert have also described the pineal organ of children varying in age from 2 months to $5\frac{1}{2}$ years and of older persons up to the age of 72 years. They distinguish two principal types of cell-elements, namely, small cells with deeply stained oval nuclei and larger cells with more abundant protoplasm and pale vesicular nuclei. The latter, more especially during the first two months of post-natal life, occupy the central zones of lobular areas, which are bounded externally by the small dark cells. These rounded or polygonal areas appear to form structural units of a system which on section has a mosaic-like appearance. About the beginning of the 2nd month of post-natal life the mosaic appearance becomes less pronounced, and from this time up to the 10th month these authors believe that a transformation takes place of the small dark cells into fibroblasts. Krabbe, on the other hand, holds the view that the small, darkly staining cells, which he calls " proparenchyma cells," undergo a metamorphosis during the first year of post-natal life, which is usually completed by the end of the first year. The small proparenchymatous cells give rise to large cells with clear vesicular nuclei ; these are the " parenchymatous cells," and he believes that the fibrous elements are derived entirely from the connective tissue. Most authors agree with Krabbe in assigning the origin of the fibrous connective tissue to the ingrowth of mesoderm, which accompanies the penetration of vessels between the outgrowing buds of epithelium, and they believe that the parenchyma cells originate by transformation of the small darkly stained cells of which the epithelial outgrowths are primarily composed ; but it seems probable that the transformation of the indifferent epithelial cells into the large round cells with pale nuclei commences at a much earlier period than the post-natal, namely, about the middle of fœtal life, and that it only becomes a pronounced feature during the critical period of early infancy (1st to 2nd month). It is also generally believed that the small round cells give rise to a certain number of glial cells in addition to the parenchymal cells which in young subjects form the bulk of the tissues composing the pineal organ ; but they do not give origin to fibroblasts, these being wholly derived from the ingrowth of mesodermal tissue.

Later, a still further development takes place of the larger round cells, with clear vesicular nuclei, namely, the outgrowth of the characteristic processes of the parenchyma cells (see Fig. 218) ; and according to Dimitrowa and others the appearance of what they believe to be " secretory " granules in the nucleus and in the cytoplasm of these cells (Fig. 219).

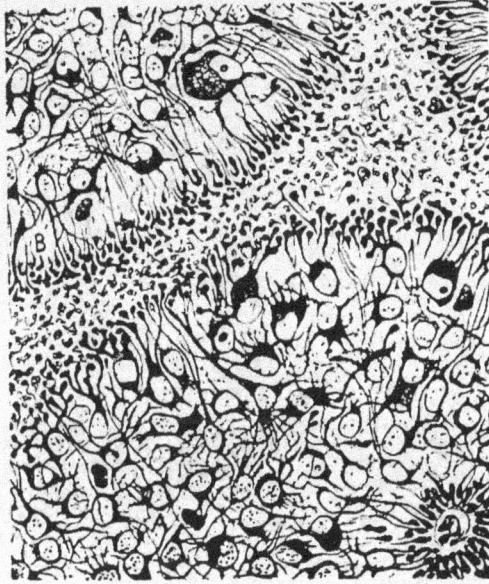

FIG. 218.—PINEAL BODY OF A YOUNG BOY, SHOWING BRANCHED PARENCHYMA
CELLS, PERIPHERAL PROCESSES OF WHICH END IN CLUB-SHAPED ENLARGEMENTS
IN THE INTERLOBULAR CONNECTIVE TISSUE OR IN THE SHEATHS OF VESSELS.
(AFTER DEL RIO-HORTEGA.)

A : parenchymatous cells.   *C :* interlobular tissue.
B : marginal claviform processes.   *D :* vessel with club-shaped processes in
                                              its adventitia.

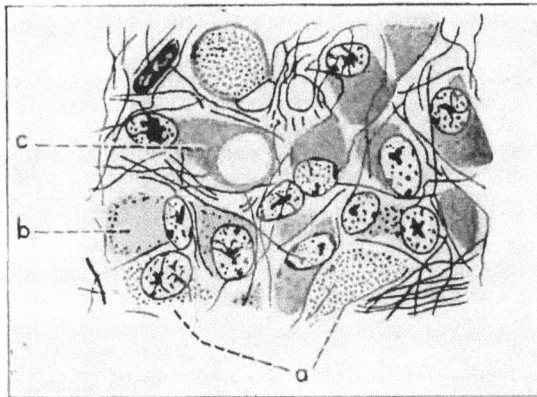

FIG. 219.—CELLS WITH GRANULAR PROTOPLASM FROM THE EPIPHYSIS OF BOS
TAURUS.

Some (*a*) have their whole body filled with granulations, others (*b*) have only a
thin peripheral layer showing granules ; (*c*) cell with a vacuole.
(Weigert's method. After Dimitrowa, 1901.)

The processes of the parenchyma cells are especially well seen in the marginal plexus, at the periphery of the pineal lobules (Fig. 220). According to the prevailing view held by the more recent authors, e.g. del Rio-

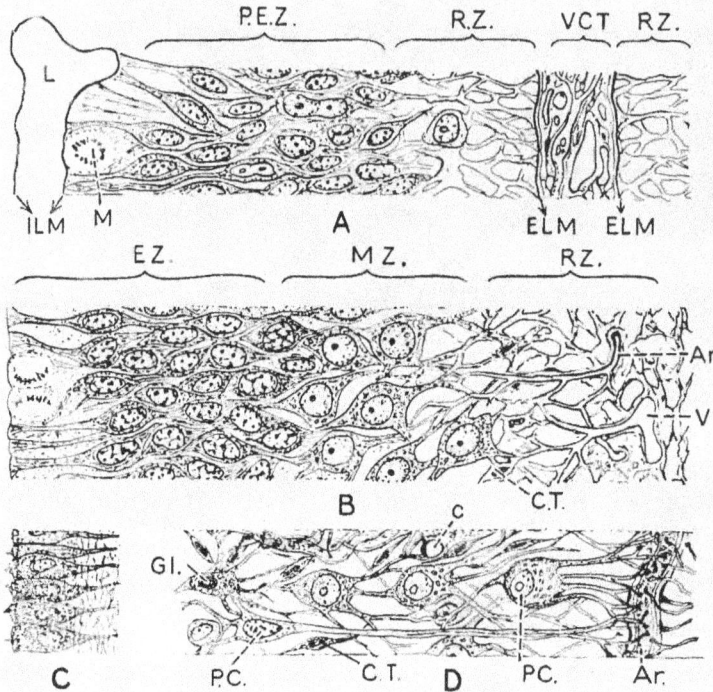

FIG. 220.—DIAGRAM REPRESENTING STAGES IN THE DEVELOPMENT AND DIFFERENTIATION OF THE PINEAL ORGAN.

A—Early stage, showing part of the epithelial wall of a lobule of the primary pineal diverticulum, with a vascular strand of connective tissue separating it from an adjacent lobule on the right.

B—Later stage, the external limiting membrane has disappeared, and the vessels with their connective tissue sheaths have penetrated the epithelial wall. A differentiation of the primary ependymal cells has now taken place, a middle zone of pale cells with vesicular nuclei now being present between the small darkly staining cells and the reticular zone.

C and D—The differentiated neuro-epithelial cells of the adult organ—ependymal, C ; glial and parenchymatous, D.

Ar. : arteriole.	I.L.M. : internal limiting membrane.
C. : capillary vessel.	M.Z. : mantle zone (large pale cells).
C.T. : connective tissue.	P.C. : parenchyma cells.
E.L.M. : external limiting membrane.	P.E.Z. : primary ependymal zone.
E.Z. : ependymal zone.	R.Z. : reticular zone.
G.l. : glial cell.	V.C.T. : vascular connective tissue.

Hortega, the majority of the processes end in club-shaped swellings which are attached to the walls of the blood-vessels running in the trabeculæ of connective tissue, while others join with each other in the formation of the central and marginal plexuses. It is not at all clear, however, what is the exact relation between the connective tissue elements and the processes of the parenchyma cells. According to the description by Studnička of the pineal organ in birds, and more especially in *Strix flammea* (see p. 297, Fig. 204), after the disappearance of the external limiting membrane at an early stage of development the connective tissue elements become inextricably blended with the branched processes of the ependymal cells which in birds line the follicles of the epithelial buds, and thus presumably correspond to the parenchyma cells of the mammalian pineal body, since the latter arise by transformation of the indifferent primary ependymal cells. In the adult both collagenous and glial fibres are found in addition to cellular elements having the distinctive characters of connective tissue cells and glial cells (astrocytes). Also, large areas, or " plaques," of degenerated glial tissue, containing few or no parenchyma cells are found in old subjects and sometimes even in children and infants only 4 months old. These areas are conspicuous owing to their being composed of a network of feebly stained, fine glial fibres, and by the sparseness and small size of the nuclei (Fig. 221, A, B, C, *Gli.*). The existence of these degenerate areas in the pineal bodies of young subjects, quite apart from any diseased condition of the central nervous system generally, appears to afford very strong evidence of the retrogressive nature of the pineal organ in the human subject. The regressive character of the pineal organ is also plainly indicated by the frequent formation of calcareous deposits, which occur in the parenchyma in the glial plaques, in the connective tissue capsule, and in the trabeculæ (Fig. 317, B, p. 465, *Ca.*, and Fig. 318, p. 466). The deposits are found in the pineal body and the surrounding vascular pia mater from early infancy to old age, and although they are not always present, their existence in or around the gland is sufficiently frequent to have led some authors to describe the condition as being normal in the adult (Fig. 222). The frequent onset of fibrosis and gliosis in early life and the great variability in the general appearance of the gland which is associated with these states are further evidences of involution. Although the maximum degree of differentiation is usually attained by about the seventh year, in many cases, judging from the microscopic appearances of the cells and of the supporting tissues, the development of the organ appears to have been arrested in early childhood or even in infancy.

The changes that take place in the normal development of the human pineal body in some respects are similar to those which take place in the development of the central nervous system generally, but in the pineal organ they do not reach the high degree of differentiation which occurs in the central nervous system, and in the pineal there is an outgrowth

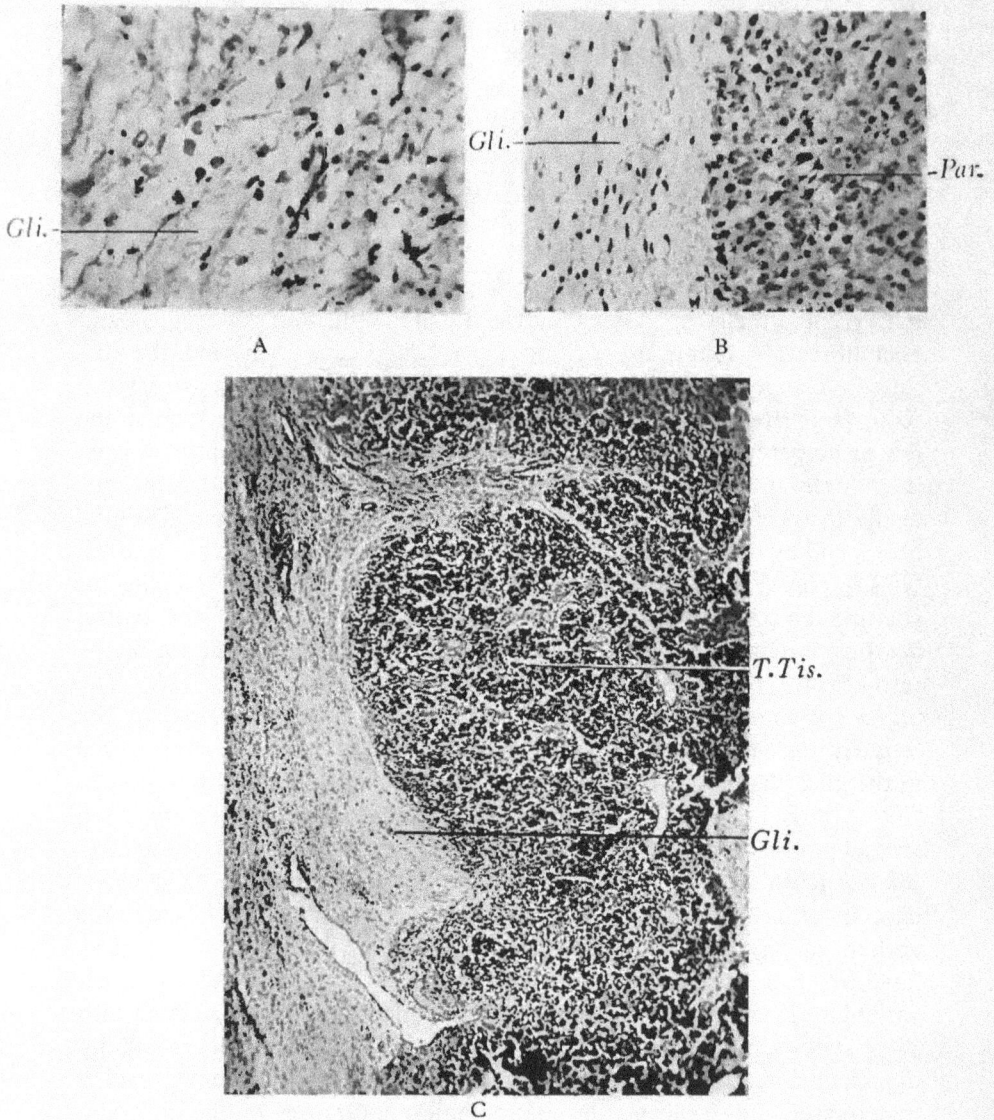

FIG. 221.

A—Section through a glial plaque of an adult human pineal gland showing
   sparsely scattered oval nuclei, imbedded in a reticulum of glial fibres.
   × 194 D.   *Gli. :* glial tissue.

B—Section through another part of the same gland as A, less highly magnified.
   The parenchymatous tissue, *Par.*, contains closely packed cells with large,
   deeply stained, round nuclei. The glial tissue, *Gli.*, on the left is devoid of
   parenchyma cells.

C—Section of pineal tumour showing lobules of tumour tissue, *T. Tis.*, on the
   right of the photograph and strands of degenerated glial tissue on the left, *Gli.*

of epithelial cords into the surrounding vascular connective tissue and an intimate blending of the epithelial and mesodermal elements. The resemblance lies chiefly in the mode of differentiation of the definitive cellular elements from the primary ependymal cells of the developing neural tube. It will be remembered that in the development of the central nervous system the medullary plate at first consists of a single layer of columnar cells, between which on the primarily superficial surface (Fig. 223, A), there are scattered here and there cells which are undergoing mitosis. The medullary or neural plate is soon converted into the neural

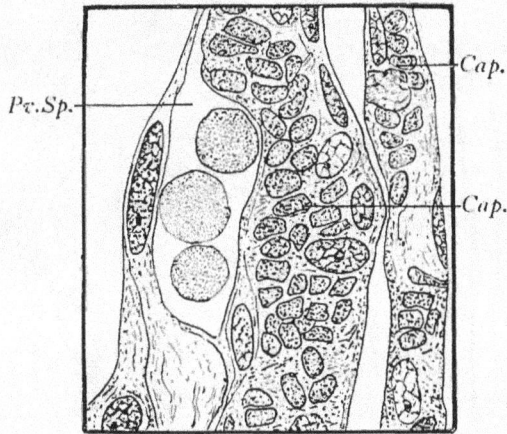

FIG. 222.—SECTION THROUGH A PERIVASCULAR SPACE IN AN ADULT HUMAN PINEAL ORGAN SHOWING MINUTE DROPLETS OF A FINELY GRANULAR MATERIAL PROBABLY OF A COLLOID NATURE AND INDICATING AN EARLY STAGE IN THE FORMATION OF A CORPUS ARENACEUM. (R. J. G.)

Cap. : capillary containing red blood corpuscles.
Pv. Sp. : perivascular space.

groove, which afterwards by fusion of its margins along the mid-dorsal line becomes the neural tube. The primarily superficial surface of the plate is now the internal or ventricular surface ; and the primarily deep or under surface is external and in relation with the vascular mesenchyme which will become the pia mater. The wall of the neural tube rapidly increases in thickness and the cell-elements lengthen out into protoplasmic strands containing small, oval, nuclei (Fig. 223, B and C) ; an external and an internal limiting membrane is developed and the mesenchyme lying outside the external limiting membrane condenses to form the pia mater. The radiating protoplasmic strands become joined by the union of lateral processes and thus give rise to a continuous network of fibres enclosing spaces. Imbedded in the radiating strands are deeply stained oval nuclei, which occupy the inner and middle zones ; whereas the large

21

cells showing mitotic figures are found next the internal limiting membrane. There is at first no definite limit demarcating the ependymal zone from the middle or mantle zone. The outer or marginal zone is, however, easily recognized (Fig. 223 B, *RZ*) by the absence of nuclei and the clear visibility of the glial fibres, which form the bed in which

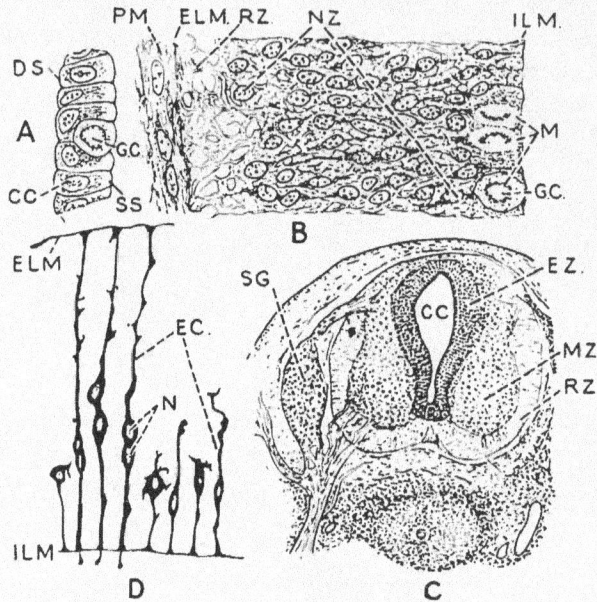

FIG. 223.—DIFFERENTIATION OF CELLS IN WALL OF NEURAL TUBE.

A—Section of medullary plate of rabbit embryo before closure of neural tube.
B—7-mm. pig embryo ×690, after Hardesty.
C—10-mm. human embryo showing ependymal, mantle and reticular zones.
D.—Ependymal cells from a part of the wall of the neural-groove of a first-day chick embryo ; Golgi preparation (Cajal).

C.C. : columnar cell or central canal.
D.S. : deep surface
E.C. : primary undifferentiated ependymal cells which will give rise to definitive ependymal cells, supporting glial cells (spongioblasts) and nerve cells (neuroblasts)
E.L.M. : external limiting membrane
E.Z. : ependymal zone.
G.C. : germinal cell

I.L.M. : internal limiting membrane.
M. : mitosis.
M.Z. : middle or mantle zone containing neuroblasts.
N. : nuclei of ependymal cells.
P.M. : pia mater.
R.Z. : reticular or marginal zone.
S.S. : superficial surface later becoming the internal or ventricular surface.

the white medullated fibres are afterwards developed. In a 10-mm. human embryo (Fig. 223, D) the three zones are distinct and consist of : (1) an inner primary ependymal layer, formed of undifferentiated cell-elements containing small, darkly stained nuclei, which are arranged in a radial manner round the central canal and are closely packed ; the nuclei are about five or six deep and are almost uniform in size ; (2) the middle or mantle zone—this is the forerunner of the grey matter and contains large, rounded cells with pale vesicular nuclei. These are the neuroblasts and are comparable with the large pale cells with vesicular nuclei of the pineal organ in late fœtal life and early infancy, both as regards their origin from the primary ependymal cells of the inner zone and with respect to their further differentiation, namely, the neuroblasts of the central nervous system into nerve cells ; the large pale cells with vesicular nuclei of the pineal organ into parenchyma cells with processes resembling the processes of nerve-cells, but lacking an axis cylinder or myelinated nerve-fibre. A differentiation also takes place of the primary ependymal cells into the definitive ependyma, consisting of cubical or columnar cells lining the ventricular cavities and central canal of the spinal cord, and the spongioblasts which develop into the supporting or neuroglial cells. The primary ependymal cells of the central nervous system thus give rise to three types of cells : (1) the definitive ependyma, (2) the neuroglial cells, and (3) neuroblasts which differentiate into nerve cells. In the pineal organ a similar differentiation takes place of three types of cell from the primary ependymal zone, namely : (1) the definitive ependyma, lining the pineal recess ; (2) spongioblasts giving rise to glial cells ; and (3) large pale cells with vesicular nuclei which give origin to the branched parenchymatous cells of the adult organ.

As a rule the lumen of the epiphysis in mammals and the cylindrical ependymal epithelium which lines it disappear entirely during the later periods of fœtal life ; remnants of the lumen may, however, persist in the adult animal, in the form of minute, often microscopic, cysts, of which an example is shown in the section of an epiphysis of an ox (Fig. 304 (Dimitrowa), Chap. 32, p. 452).

We do not propose to do more than allude here to some of the general relations of the pineal organ to neighbouring structures and to note some points of interest with regard to the relative size and form of the pineal organ in some types of the Mammalia, since the variations in microscropical structure can be most conveniently dealt with in the chapter on the structure of the human pineal organ.

Relations of the Pineal Organ in Mammals

The pineal body has been found to be present in nearly all species of mammalia, from the Prototheria or Monotremes, including the duck-bill or *Ornithorhynchus* (Fig. 224) and the spiny ant-eater or *Echidna*, up to man. Its attachment to the roof of the thalamencephalon between the anterior and the posterior commissures is always the same, but there are differences with regard to its general form. As a rule it is conical,

with the rounded base of the cone, corresponding to the root of attachment, lying just above the posterior commissure and the apex directed
backwards. In some cases, however, as in the rabbit, it may consist of a
terminal pyriform expansion which is attached by a long, narrow stalk
to the roof of the third ventricle in the usual situation (Fig. 225); while
in the rat the terminal vesicle becomes separated by rupture of the stalk,
and in the adult, as pointed out by Herring, all communication with the
habenular ganglia is cut off and the only connections of the organ with
the body generally are by means of the vascular and sympathetic systems.

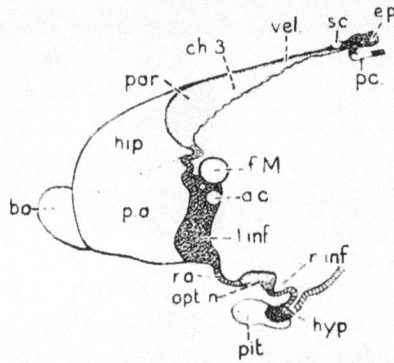

FIG. 224.—DIAGRAM OF A MEDIAN SECTION THROUGH THE FOREPART OF A BRAIN
OF A FŒTAL ORNITHORYNCHUS, SHOWING THE PINEAL BODY AND ITS RELATION
TO THE HABENULAR AND POSTERIOR COMMISSURES. (AFTER G. ELLIOT SMITH.)

a.c. : commissura anterior.	p.a. : precommissural area.
b.o. : bulbus olfactorius.	par. : paraphysis.
ch. 3 : choroid plexus of third ventricle.	p.c. : posterior commissure.
ep. : epiphysis cerebri.	pit. : pituitary gland.
f.M. : Foramen of Monro.	r. inf. : recessus infundibuli.
hip. : rudiment of the hippocampus.	r.o. : recessus opticus.
hyp. : hypophysis cerebri.	s.c. : superior commissure.
l. inf. : lamina infraneuroporica.	vel. : velum.
opt. n. : optic nerve.	

The pineal organ of the rabbit and of the rat thus differ markedly from
those of the sheep, ox, or horse, in which the organ has the usual conical
or oval form and is connected by well-defined superior and inferior
peduncles with the habenular and posterior commissures (Figs. 226 and
227).

Complete separation of the pineal organ from the central nervous
system in the adult animal, such as occurs in the rat, precludes any possibility of any secretory function being under the direct control of the
central nervous system; and if such a secretion exists, it can only be
regulated by the blood circulating through its vessels; thus it may be
supposed that the amount of blood passing through the vessels could be
influenced through the sympathetic system, and that the secretory

activity of the cell-elements might be stimulated by the action of hormones circulating in the blood, or by efferent inpulses reaching the organ by means of sympathetic nerve-fibres terminating in direct relation with the

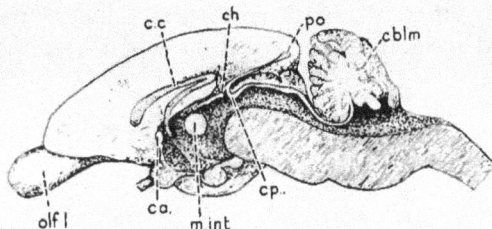

FIG. 225.—MEDIAN VERTICAL SECTION THROUGH BRAIN OF A RABBIT, LEPUS CUNICULUS, SHOWING PINEAL ORGAN WITH LONG NARROW STALK, SITUATED BEHIND THE SPLENIUM OF THE CORPUS CALLOSUM. (AFTER PARKER.)

ca. : anterior commissure.	*cp.* : posterior commissure.
cblm. : cerebellum.	*m. int.* : massa intermedia.
c.c. : Corpus callosum.	*olf. l.* : olfactory lobe.
ch. : habenular commissure.	*p.o.* : pineal organ.

parenchyma cells. The epiphysis in these rodents is, however, small and imperfectly developed with respect to its microscopical structure ; and it appears to be very doubtful whether true secretory nerve-fibres are actually present in direct association with the cell-elements. The

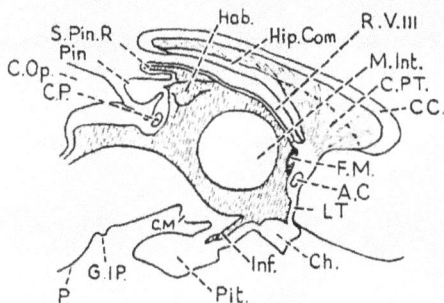

FIG. 226.—MEDIAN SAGITTAL SECTION THROUGH THE PINEAL REGION OF A SHEEP. (AFTER J. WILKIE.)

A.C. : anterior commissure.	*Hab.* : habenular ganglion.
C.C. : corpus callosum.	*Hip. Com.* : hippocampal commissure.
Ch. : optic chiasma.	*Inf.* : infundibulum.
C.M. : corpus mammillare.	*L.T.* : lamina terminalis.
C. Op. : colliculus opticus.	*M. Int.* : massa intermedia.
C.P. : posterior commissure.	*P.* : pons.
C.P.T. : corpus paraterminalis.	*Pin.* : pineal
F.M. : foramen of Monro.	*R.V. III.* : roof of third ventricle.
G. IP. : ganglion interpedunculare.	*S. Pin. R.* : suprapineal recess.

condition of the separated end-organ of the adult rat is very similar to that of Stieda's organ of the frog, namely, a degenerate vestige, which has lost the characteristic features of the parietal eye, and does not show the special characters of an actively functioning endocrine gland. The basal portion of the stalk or epiphysis in the frog, as was described in Chap. 19, p. 228, Figs. 161 and 166, undergoes a certain degree of development and differentiation; in the rat, however, this segment remains small and insignificant. It may be noted here that most of the

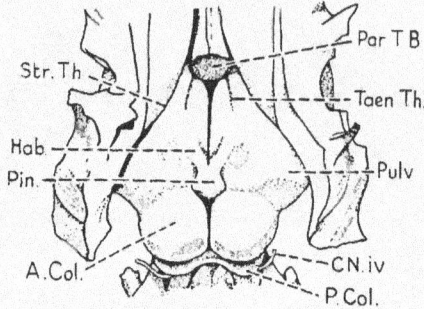

FIG. 227.—PINEAL ORGAN AND HABENULÆ OF A SHEEP'S BRAIN SEEN FROM ABOVE. (AFTER J. WILKIE.)

A. Col. : anterior colliculus.
CN. iv. : fourth cranial nerve.
Hab. : habenula.
Par. T.B. : paraterminal body.
P. Col. : posterior colliculus.

Pin. : pineal organ.
Pulv. : pulvinar.
Str. Th : stria thalami.
Taen.Th. : taenia thalami.

experimental work that has been carried out on rats has been by way of the injection of extracts of the epiphysis of the horse, or ox, or grafts of the epiphysis ; Kolmer and Löwy have, however, cauterized the pineal region in young rats, and Lehmann removed the gland in rats and mice without any positive results.

CHAPTER 23

THE GEOLOGICAL EVIDENCE OF THE EXISTENCE OF MEDIAN EYES IN EXTINCT VERTEBRATES

THE anatomical evidence of the existence of both median and lateral eyes in the extinct order of Palæozoic fishes known as the Ostracodermata, which lived in the Silurian and Devonian periods, is of great value not only with reference to the antiquity of the vertebrate eyes but also with respect to the constancy of the pattern formed by the relative positions of the cavities and impressions on the head-shields which lodged the sense-organs, namely : the small pineal impression in the centre ; the orbital cavities for the lateral eyes on each side ; the narial and hypophyseal apertures in front and the smooth " glabellar plate " forming the roof of the cranial cavity which contained the brain behind [1] (Fig. 228). Moreover, palæontology affords very strong evidence of the bilateral origin and nature of the pineal body, e.g. the existence of two impressions placed side by side on the *outer* surface of the pineal plate of *Pholidosteus* and *Rhinosteus*, recorded by Stensiö (Fig. 229) ; the two pits also placed side by side but on the *inner* surface of the pineal plate of *Titanichthys*, described by E. S. Woodward (Fig. 230), along with the heart-shaped foramen figured by E. S. Hill on the dorsal aspect of the skull of *Dipnorhynchus* (Fig. 140, Chap. 18, p. 200) and the similar heart-shaped pit on the intracranial aspect of the pineal plate of *Dinichthys intermedius* shown in the drawing reproduced from Adolf Heintz (Fig. 231). All these examples tend to confirm the similar conclusions with respect to the bilateral origin of the pineal which have been founded on the comparative anatomy and comparative embryology of living species and advocated by Cameron (pp. 292, 294), Dendy (p. 245), Gaskell (p. 187), Hill (p. 218), Kingsbury (p. 215), Locy (p. 202), and others. Further, the palæontological evidence of the position and relations of the orbital cavities and pineal impressions in fossil vertebrates, more especially in the head-shields of the Ostracodermata, taken along with other evidence of a more general character seems to indicate the existence at a very early period of a common ancestral stock from which arose the prevertebrate stem of these Palæozoic

---

[1] The glabellar plate corresponds to the " dorsal electric field, a slightly depressed spear-shaped area, which Stensiö considers may have lodged a dorsal median electric organ.

fishes and the main or parent stem from which certain extinct and living arthropods have descended. The resemblances are found chiefly in the head region and are most evident in the Eurypterida and Trilobites among the extinct classes, and in *Limulus*, *Apus*, and *Lepidurus* among living species. But the fundamental differences in the relative positions of the thoracic and abdominal viscera between vertebrates and invertebrates (Fig. 68, Chap. 11, p. 106) precludes the assumption of there being any

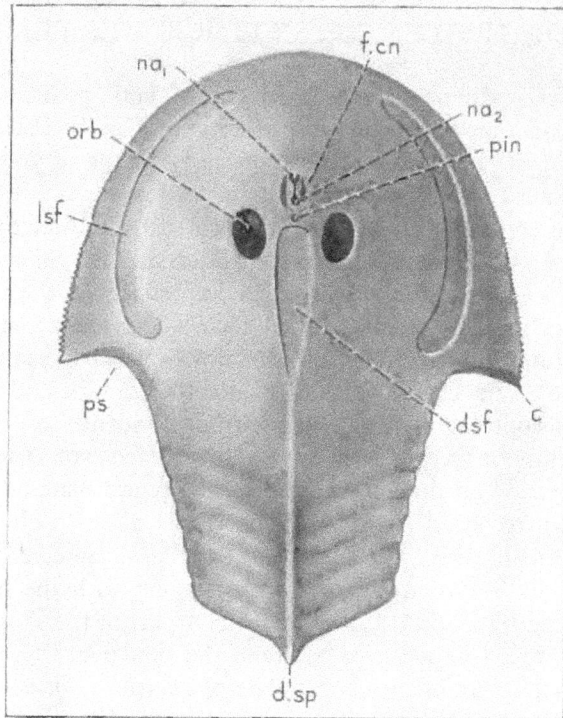

Fig. 228.—Restoration of Cephalic Shield of Kiæraspis auchenaspidoides. Dorsal View. (After Stensiö.)

c. : cornu.	na₁ : opening of hypophyseal sac.
dsf. : dorsal electric field.	na₂ : nasal opening.
d.sp. : dorsal spine.	orb. : orbital opening.
f. cn. : fossa circumnasalis.	ps. : pectoral sinus.
lsf. : lateral electrical field.	pin. : pineal foramen.

close relationship between these divergent types; and they indicate that the period during which the divergence of the vertebrate from the invertebrate stock and the primary changes in the evolution of their respective types of lateral eyes took place must have been infinitely remote and probably occurred in a very simple form of animal showing bilateral symmetry and paired ocelli of the simple upright type. Thus it may be conceived that the eyes of the prototype animal, from which by gradual differentiation the median and lateral eyes of both invertebrate and vertebrate animals have been evolved, resembled the simple paired

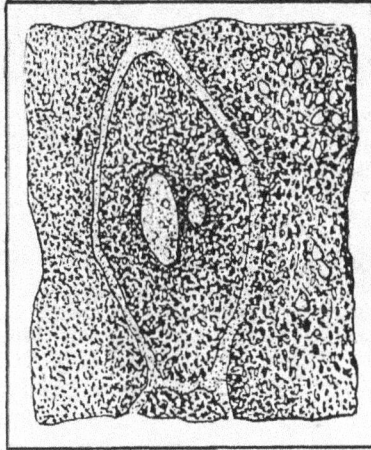

A

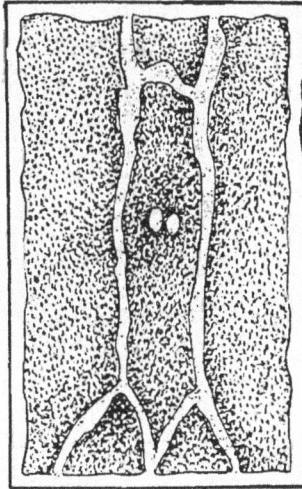

B

FIG. 229.—DORSAL ASPECT OF THE PARIETAL PLATES OF : A—PHOLIDOSTEUS ; B—RHINOSTEUS, SHOWING PAIRED PINEAL PITS. (AFTER ERIK-A-SON STENSIÖ.)

In *Rhinosteus* the left pit is completely preserved as an impression, whereas the impression of the right pit has been broken off.   (× 5 diameters.)

eyes of the type found in living Planaria and Turbellaria or in the Annelid *Hæmopis sanguisuga* (Fig. 16, Chap. 3, p. 21).   In these animals there is a bilaterally disposed nervous system ; the eyes lie on the dorsal aspect of the head, in or near the surface, and they are connected by nerve-fibres with a supra-œsophageal ganglion which represents the brain. Further, it is probable that the rudimentary eyes of this prototype animal, which were at first freely exposed on the dorsal surface of the head—no carapace or head-shield as yet having been evolved—as they gradually developed

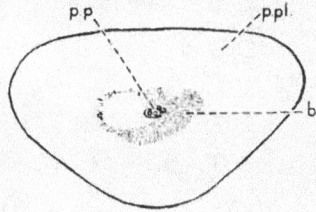

FIG. 230.—PINEAL PLATE OF TITANICHTHYS, FROM THE UPPER DEVONIAN OF OHIO, U.S.A. (INNER VIEW, ONE-HALF NATURAL SIZE). PAIRED PINEAL PITS OR OPENINGS ARE SEEN IN THE MIDDLE AREA OF THICKENED BONE. (AFTER A. S. WOODWARD.)

b. : radiating spicules of bone.   p.p. : paired pineal impressions.
p. pl. : pineal plate.

into more complex organs which, with the brain and other delicate parts of the head, required protection from injury, were afforded this protection by the deposition of a chitinous shield around the ocelli and over the surrounding soft parts, leaving a transparent epithelial or horny

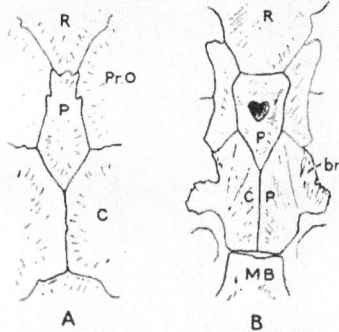

FIG. 231.—DINICHTHYS INTERMEDIUS.

A—Part of the roof of the skull, viewed from above.
B—The same area, seen from the inside, and showing the parietal pit on the inner aspect of the pineal plate. (After Heintz, A.)

C. : central plate.   P. : parietal or pineal plate.
C.P. : central part.   M.B. : median basal plate.
br. : branch of central part.   Pr. O. : preorbital.
R. : rostrum.

covering for the eyes, which became transformed into either a faceted or a continuous smooth cornea. Moreover, as the type of animal became more active and left the mud or sand at the bottom to swim in the water, the more lateral eyes, being more suitably placed than the median eyes, became more highly developed ; while the latter either retained their original simple character or degenerated, and in some cases when displaced towards the median plane, by the great development of the lateral eyes, the median pair of eyes fused with each other to form a cyclops eye, as in Tabanus (Fig. 20, Chap. 3, p. 26) and in many of the Crustacea. In the stem which branched off to form the vertebrates it may be supposed that in the evolution of the lateral eyes the simple optic pit which arose as a downgrowth from the medullary plate (Figs. 5 and 6) became transformed into a stalked vesicle which afterwards came in contact with the surface layer of epithelium, as occurs in the ontogenetic development of the typical lateral eyes of vertebrates, and that this stage was followed or accompanied by inversion of the retina and the development of an epithelial type of lens from the overlying ectoderm. Further, that at an early stage in the evolution of the lateral eyes a cartilaginous or bony capsule was formed around each, and served as a special protective covering corresponding to the similar nasal and otic capsules. When we examine the skulls of the earliest fossil fishes, such as the Anaspida of the Silurian

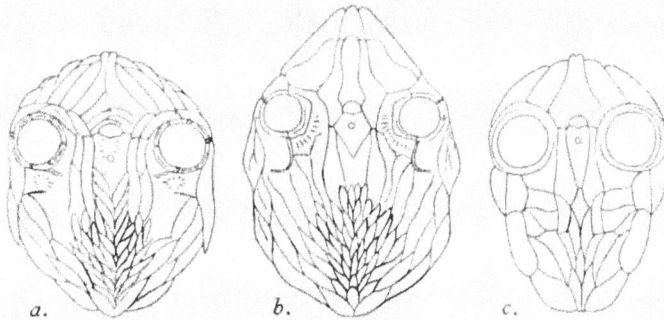

FIG. 232.—SCHEMATIC SKETCHES OF THE CRANIAL ROOF OF THE NORWEGIAN ANASPIDA, SHOWING THE PINEAL PLATE AND FORAMEN ; THE ORBITAL SCERAL PLATES AND GENERAL ARRANGEMENT OF THE SCALES. (AFTER KIAER.)
a. : Pterolepis.   b. : Pharyngolepis.   c. : Rhyncholepis.

period (Fig. 232) or that of Osteolepis (Fig. 132, Chap. 17, p. 182), a lobe or paddle-finned fish of the Devonian period, we find that the orbital cavities for the lateral eyes, are surrounded by a series of flat plates—in Pterolepis (Fig. 232) six in number on each side—and that there is a single pineal foramen in the centre between the two fused frontal bones. It seems probable, therefore, that the median eyes or their stalks were already fused, or possibly that one member of the pair had become suppressed owing to the more active growth of the other member of the pair. The median posterior part of the skull in these fishes (Fig. 132) was separated by an interval or articulation from the anterior part formed by the frontals, post-frontals, post-orbitals, and squamosals. This median part had grown backwards over the hinder part of the brain and formed the parietal, supratemporal, and occipital region of the skull, whereas the lateral horns which bounded the gap on each side gave rise to the squamosal plates and maxillæ. In the course of evolution of the brain it seems that the pineal region has—relatively to the cerebral hemispheres —been gradually displaced backwards ; thus the pineal foramen in the earlier types of skull such as *Osteolepis* lies in the same transverse plane as the orbital cavities for the lateral eyes and between the frontal bones. In later types the foramen lies between the parietal bones, where, owing to the formation of the median anteroposterior crest formed between the two temporal muscles and running backwards to the occipital region (Figs. 205, 206, Chap. 22, pp. 300, 301, and Fig. 233), it eventually becomes obliterated. The direction of the pineal foramen or plate seems also to have changed in the course of time. Thus in the restoration of the skull of

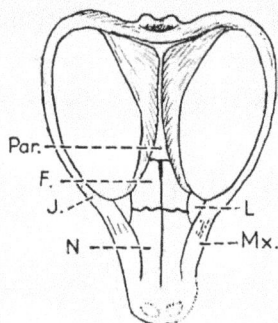

FIG. 233.—VIEW FROM ABOVE OF THE SKULL OF AN ICTIDOSAURIAN REPTILE, SHOWING THE MEDIAN PARIETAL CREST. ALL TRACE OF A PARIETAL FORAMEN HAS DISAPPEARED. THERE ARE TWO OCCIPITAL CONDYLES, AND OTHER MAMMALIAN CHARACTERISTICS. (AFTER BROOM.)

F. : frontal.	*L.* : lacrimal.	*N.* : nasal.
J. : jugular.	*Mx.* : maxilla.	*Par.* : parietal.

Dinichthys intermedius (Fig. 234) the plate seems to have been directed forward as well as upwards, in *Osteolepis* directly upwards ; while the apex of the pineal organ, inside the skull, in adult mammals is directed backwards over the quadrigeminal plate and towards the vermis of the cerebellum. The relative position of the pineal organ to the skull and the fore-brain is greatly affected in the human subject and in mammals generally by the growth of the hemispheres, which as they enlarge in a forward direction are also bent ventralward, thus forming the primary or cephalic flexure. The pineal organ remains for a time in close relation to the membranous capsule of the brain and skin at the summit of this flexure. In this primarily superficial position the pineal organ of amphibians and reptiles appears to have attained its highest degree of development, as is evidenced by the large size of the pineal foramen in certain of the extinct amphibia, e.g. *Protriton* (Fig. 170), and *Procolophon* (Fig. 170, a), Chap. 19, p. 237. Moreover in the more primitive types of living reptiles, such as *Sphenodon*, the organ is found to be more highly differentiated than in the less primitive ; but in all living reptiles, including *Sphenodon*, the pineal eye frequently shows signs of degeneration, such as the development of pigment in the lens or the frequent absence of its nerve in the adult animal, and judging from the large size of the pineal canal in some extinct amphibia and reptiles the organ in living species is relatively extremely small.

This difference in size of the pineal foramen suggests that in those extinct animals in which the foramen was large, the organ itself may have been not only larger but also more highly differentiated, and may even have served as a visual organ, as contrasted with a light-perceiving organ.

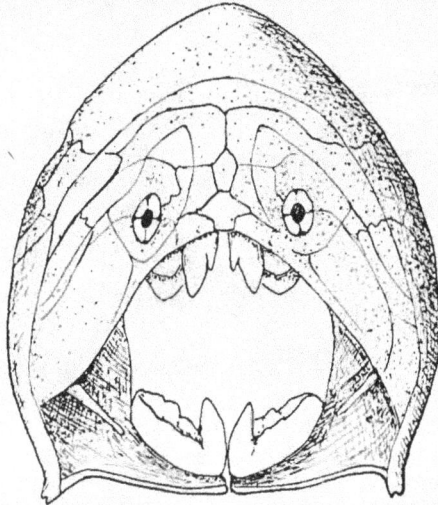

FIG. 234.—RESTORATION OF SKULL OF DINICHTHYS INTERMEDIUS, VIEWED FROM IN FRONT AND SHOWING THE POSITION OF THE PINEAL PLATE. (AFTER ANATOL HEINTZ.)

But in many of the fossil skulls of fishes, amphibians, and reptiles the foramen is closed or small and in some completely absent, indicating that the organ had become vestigial in these animals at a very early period of their evolution.

The pineal impression in certain of the ancient Ostracoderm fishes is, as we have already mentioned, seen only on the inner surface of the pineal plate, the outer or superficial surface in some cases being smooth (Fig. 234), while in others an external impression is also visible, but it is less deep than the pit found on the intracranial surface. These fossil markings correspond closely with the conditions which are found in many living examples of the more primitive types of cartilaginous and bony fishes, such as the spiny dogfish (*Spinax niger*) (Fig. 49) and the spoonbill (*Polyodon*) (Fig. 50, Chap. 3, p. 73, and Fig. 235). In these the pineal canal does not perforate the roof of the skull and open on the dorsal aspect, but ends blindly, and the pineal organ consists merely of the basal portion and the stalk. The distal end of the stalk is sometimes slightly expanded, but there is no differentiation of a definite eye, such as is seen in *Petromyzon*, and it is probable that the small pear-shaped vesicle at the distal end of the hollow stalk does not represent the parietal organ. The appearances in the fossil fishes may be accounted for by supposing that : (1) during the ontogenetic development of the cranial roof, the pineal diverticulum was not only surrounded circumferentially by the developing membrane-bone but also covered by it ; or, in other words, the pineal organ never pierced the skull (Fig. 235). Moreover, it may be

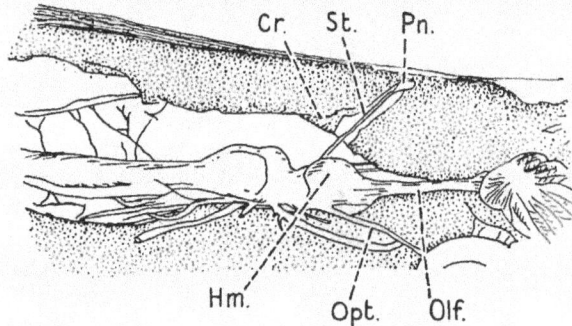

FIG. 235.—LATERAL VIEW OF THE BRAIN AND PINEAL ORGAN OF POLYODON FOLIUM. THE CRANIAL CAPSULE HAS BEEN OPENED FROM ONE SIDE. (AFTER GARMAN.)

Cr. : primordial cranium.	*Opt.* : optic nerve.
Hm. : hemisphere.	*Pn.* : end-vesicle of pineal organ.
Olf. : olfactory nerve.	*St.* : stalk of pineal organ.

inferred that the cases included in this category were : (*a*) those in which single or paired parietal sense-organs were developed but not fully differentiated as an eye or eyes (Fig. 177, p. 248) ; (*b*) those in which the regression or arrest of development was more pronounced and the pineal apparatus was represented merely by the unpaired base and stalk of the pineal organ (Fig. 49, Chap. 3, p. 73, and Fig. 153, Chap. 18, p. 219). (2) Those in which the growth of the pineal organ was more vigorous and in the development of the roof of the skull, the stalk of the organ was surrounded on all sides by the developing bone, but the pineal canal not being closed over superficially by a covering layer of bone, the terminal vesicle (or pair of vesicles) was left free to develop outside the skull in the subepidermal areolar tissue. Further, it may be inferred that the cases comprised in this second category may be subdivided into two groups : (*a*) those in which a more or less fully differentiated eye was developed with an optic nerve connecting it with the central nervous system (Fig. 134, Chap. 17, p. 188, and Figs. 183, 185, Chap. 20, pp. 259, 261), and (*b*) those in which the parietal sense-organ was constricted off from its stalk by the growth of the skull and was left as a vestigial cyst (or pair of such cysts) in the sub-epidermal extracranial areolar tissue (Figs. 162, 167). In the latter all connection with the central nervous system would have been severed and the parietal vesicle would have been quite functionless as a sensory organ. In some instances an impression or pair of impressions was left on the dorsal aspect of the pineal plate (Fig. 229); in others the development of the vesicles may have been less pronounced, and though they may have persisted in the adult animal—as is the case with Stieda's " frontal organ " in the frog—they left no impression on the outer surface of the skull.

On comparing the pineal pits and impressions which have been observed in the skulls of fossil Ostracoderm fishes with those in the skulls of living species, it may be concluded that certain of the more ancient extinct specimens fully confirm the evidence which has been independently obtained from both embryonic and adult specimens of the bilateral origin of the pineal body. The palæontological evidence also points to regressive changes having already commenced in some of the most primitive and earliest known fishes, and having continued in their descendants until the present time. Nevertheless vestiges of the pineal system have persisted in nearly all types of living vertebrates, and structural changes have taken place in the organ which have suggested the occurrence of an evolutionary transformation into an organ of internal secretion. These changes are, however, much more pronounced in the embryonic stages of development and the early post-natal period of life than they are in the adult animal, in which evidence of regression is nearly always present.

Now, it is interesting in connection with the general occurrence of regressive changes which have taken place in the pineal system since the period when it appears to have attained its highest degree of development, in the extinct amphibians and reptiles of the late Palæozoic and the Mesozoic periods, to recall that among the existing Dipnoan fishes—*Lepidosiren*, *Protopterus*, and *Ceratodus*—which in some respects appear to be intermediate between fishes and amphibians, their general features when compared with the early fossil fishes have remained essentially unchanged since the middle of the Devonian period, and such changes as have been observed are regressive rather than evolutionary. According to the description given of them by Smith-Woodward, " they have in the interval merely abandoned the fusiform shape which is adapted for a free-swimming life and become more or less eel-shaped in adaptation to a wriggling and grovelling existence at the bottom of the rivers into which the last survivors retreated at the end of the Mesozoic era." In the extinct Dipnoi (*Dipterus, Ctenodus, Sagenodus*) found in the Old Red Sandstone (Devonian) the general form of the animal resembles the primitive fish *Osteolepis* (Fig. 132, Chap. 17, p. 183), and the roof of the skull consists of numerous small, flat, dermal bones most of which are paired. No parietal foramen was, however, present in the extinct Dipnoi, nor is a pineal foramen present in *Ceratodus*, the most primitive of the living Dipnoi (Fig. 156, Chap. 18, p. 222), and in this animal it will be seen that extensive fusion of the bones of the skull has taken place, only two elongated bones being present in the median region of the roof of the

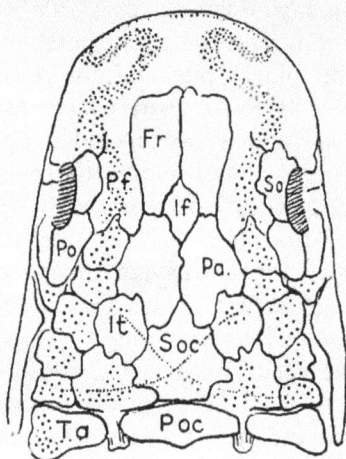

FIG. 236.—DORSAL VIEW OF HEAD OF DIPTERUS, SHOWING DERMAL BONES OF ROOF OF SKULL AND PORES OF THE LATERAL-LINE SYSTEM IN ONE OF THE EARLIEST KNOWN FISHES. (AFTER GOODRICH.)

Fr. : frontal.	*Po.* : postorbital.
If. : interfrontal.	*Poc.* : postoccipital.
It. : intertemporal.	*So.* : supraorbital.
Pa. : parietal.	*Soc.* : supraoccipital.
Pf. : prefrontal.	*Ta.* : tabular.

skull, namely the " ethmoid "—probably including the frontal, interfrontal, and prefrontal elements—and the " occipital," which is formed by the fusion of the parietals with the supraoccipital. The Dipnoi, therefore, although in other respects they constitute a very interesting primitive type of fish, are to be regarded as a degenerating side-branch and not likely to afford any clue as to the origin of the pineal organ, which even in the fossil types belonging to this order did not perforate the skull.

According to the description given by A. S. Woodward in 1922, the real links between the fishes and amphibians appear to be the paddle-finned fishes—Crossopterygii—including *Polypterus* and *Calamoichthys*, the ancestors of which, e.g. *Osteolepis* (Fig. 132, Chap. 17, p. 183) and

Diplopterus, showed a pineal foramen in the same position as in the skulls of the Stegocephala (Fig. 170, Chap. 19, p. 237). Some of these also resemble the Stegocephala in the possession of a ring of sclerotic plates around the lateral eyes. The skull of one of the living representatives of the order—*Polypterus*—shows no pineal foramen, but there is a well-marked pineal diverticulum in the embryo. Moreover, in the nearly related order Chondrostei—including *Acipenser* (sturgeon) (Figs. 147, 148, Chap. 18, p. 211) and *Polyodon* (spoonbill) (Fig. 235)—and in the order Holostei—which includes *Lepidosteus* (bony pike) and *Amia calva* (bow fin)—the pineal organ, although vestigial, is easily recognizable in the adult animal, and in *Amia* shows evidence of bilaterality (Fig. 149, Chap. 18, p. 213).

The position and relations of the pineal organ and foramen in living Crossopterygii and allied living orders, when compared with the extinct Osteolepis, appear to confirm the connection of the Crossopterygian fishes with the more ancient type of Osteichthyes, which on account of other general resemblances is considered to be close to the parent stock from which the Stegocephala and modern Amphibia have arisen. This is a point of very considerable interest, since it is in some of the Stegocephala and extinct reptiles of the Carboniferous, Permian, and Mesozoic periods that the pineal organ seems to have reached its greatest size and possibly highest degree of differentiation.

Among extinct Amphibia, the parietal foramen is found to be of very variable size. It is, relatively to the size of the skull, very large in *Protriton*, one of the smaller Stegocephala (Fig. 170, Chap. 19, p. 237). In this primitive animal the pineal foramen lies between the parietal bones in a transverse plane behind the orbital cavities. The lateral eyes were protected by a ring of bony plates in the sclerotic ; these are similar to those in *Ichthyosaurus*, and they probably indicate that either *Protriton* itself or its ancestors were able to dive to great depths in the water, and that they served to resist the pressure of the water on the eyeballs. In the skulls of *Branchiosaurus amblystoma* and *Metanerpeton* (Fig. 169, A, Chap. 19, p. 236), which represent primitive examples of the Stegocephala, the pineal foramen was also large.

The pineal foramen was, relatively to the size of the skull, of moderate size in *Eryops megacephalus* and in the curious snake-like *Dolichosoma longissimum* (Fig. 169, B, Chap. 19, p. 236), found in the Permian strata of Bohemia. In the skull of this animal the frontals and parietals are fused into a single elongated plate near the hinder end of which the circular pineal foramen is conspicuous owing to its margins being slightly raised above the general surface of the skull.

In *Diplocaulus magnicornis* (Fig. 168, Chap. 19, p. 235)—Permian of

22

Texas—the foramen is very small, and it is also small in *Palæogyrinus*—
Carboniferous—and in *Trematosaurus*. In the latter the foramen is
situated far back in the roof of the skull behind the central point of the
interparietal suture.

In the adult skulls of living Anura (*Rana*) and living Urodela (*Molge*)
the pineal foramen is usually absent, although a slight depression is
visible on the dorsal aspect of the skull, in the usual situation of the
foramen in the skull of *Cryptobranchus japonicus*.

Since some of the extinct Labyrinthodonts were of gigantic size—the
skull of *L. Jægeri* measuring more than 3 ft. in length and 2 ft. in breadth—
it may be presumed that the actual size of the pineal eye was proportion-
ately large and also more highly differentiated than in modern Amphibia,
in which the terminal vesicle is constricted off during the larval or tadpole
stage of development by the growth of the skull, and since it is completely
separated from its connection with the brain it can have no function as a
visual organ.

It is in some of the extinct carnivorous reptiles of the Mesozoic period
that the pineal foramen attained its maximum size, both relatively to the
size of the skull in some of the smaller animals and actually in some of
the larger types, such as the Ichthyosauri—Lias, Oolitic, Chalk (Fig. 190,
Chap. 20, p. 268). It was also large in the mammal-like or Theromorph
reptiles, including *Titanosuchus*, in which the diameter of the foramen
was approximately 1 centimetre (Watson) (Fig. 237).

The foramen is more circular in the primitive flat-headed types such
as *Conodectes* (Permian), *Captorhinus*, and *Procolophon* (Fig. 171, Chap. 19,
p. 237). It is more oval in form in those types in which the cranial cavity
is narrowed in association with elongation of the skull and a high degree
of development of the temporal fossæ with their contained masticatory
muscles, as in the Anomodont reptile *Dicynodon* (Broom) (Fig. 205, p. 300).
In *Dicynodon* the canines were very large, and in the dog-toothed Cynodont
reptiles in which incisor and molar teeth were also present both these
and the canines were well developed. Moreover, associated with this
development of the teeth there was a corresponding development of the
masticatory muscles, including the temporals, which grew upwards over
the roof of the skull, where they became attached to a median sagittal
crest, within which was the pineal canal. Finally, as the muscles increased
in size and the crest became deeper and narrower, the pineal canal within
it became obliterated, as in Ictidosaurus (Fig. 233, p. 332).

Having referred to the regressive changes which have occurred in the
pineal system, during the period which has elapsed since the Palæozoic
era, in the sub-classes Teleostomi and Dipnoi, with special references to
the supposed origin of the amphibians and reptiles from extinct repre-

sentatives of the Crossopterygian fishes, it will be necessary to consider the relations of the Cyclostomata to the fossil representatives of this order, and in particular to the Anaspida, Cephalaspida, and Palæospondylus. We have already seen that in amphibians and reptiles the pineal system attained a maximum development in the extinct Labyrinthodonts

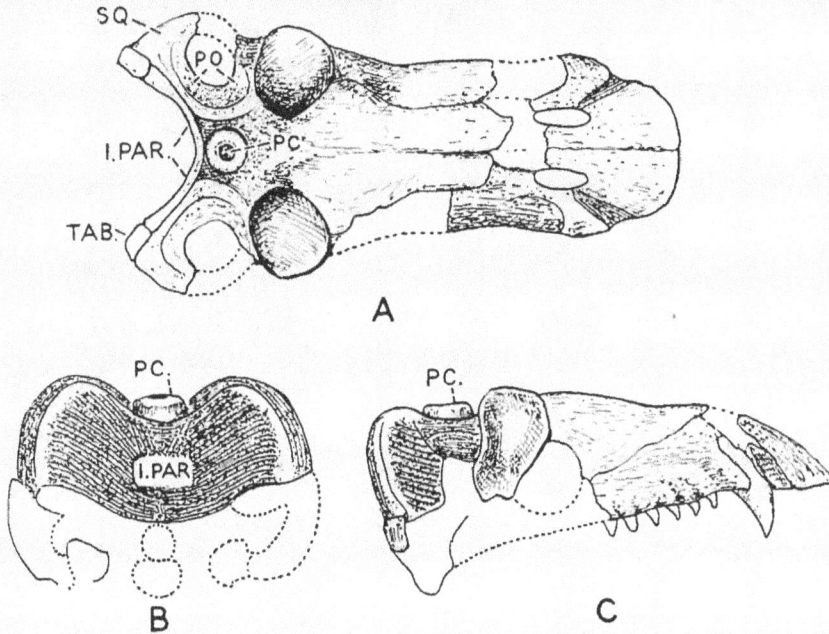

FIG. 237.—RECONSTRUCTION OF SKULL OF TITANOSUCHUS, A MAMMAL-LIKE REPTILE OF S. AFRICA. (AFTER D. M. WATSON.)

The specimen shows a large parietal canal for the pineal organ, "the walls of which form a special little projection raising the opening more than a centimetre above the general line of the surrounding bone."

A—Dorsal aspect of skull.   B—Posterior aspect.   C—Lateral aspect.

> I. PAR : interparietal.   SQ. : squamosal.
> PC. : parietal canal.   TAB. : tabulare.
> PO. : post-orbital.

In the account of another specimen (*Mormosaurus seeleyi*) belonging to the same order, Deinocephalia, Professor Watson describes the parietal canal as "a long cylindrical tunnel" which lies in the median suture between the two parietal bones.

and in the Ichthyosauri and Plesiosauri, during the late Palæozoic (Amphibia) and the Mesozoic periods (reptiles). Many of the extinct forms seem to have died out completely and left no representatives; while in the modern amphibians and reptiles the parietal sense-organ is less developed and shows signs of degeneration. Similar changes appear to have occurred also both generally and in the pineal system of Cyclostomes, and at one time it was thought that the Cyclostomes were a degenerate form of the true fishes. Now, although the older view that the Cyclostomes are degenerate fishes has been replaced by the modern conception that the living Cyclostomes, with their fossil representatives the Ostracodermi, constitute a separate and distinct branch of the phylum Vertebrata, there is no doubt that in many respects the living Cyclostomes are less highly developed than their fossil ancestors. Thus the living lampreys and hag-fishes have no exoskeleton, no pectoral fins, and in the hag-fishes not only are the lateral eyes vestigial and sunk beneath the skin, but the static organ has only one semicircular canal, as compared with two (anterior and posterior) in some of the Ostracodermi, and according to Studnička the pineal organ (at any rate in some specimens) is absent altogether.

In considering the markings found in the head-shields of the sub-class Ostracodermata it is necessary to inquire whether there is anything which corresponds to the head-shield of these most primitive extinct vertebrates among living species of vertebrates. Now Gaskell (1908) showed that the head-shield of the larval *Petromyzon* closely resembles that of the extinct Palæozoic fishes (Cephalaspidæ), not only in general form (Fig. 135, Chap. 17, p. 191) but in the structure of the mucocartilage, which forms the branchial skeleton and the dorsal and ventral head-plates of the *Ammocœtes* larva. This is a peculiar type of embryonic cartilage which consists of fibrils whose direction is mainly at right angles to the investing layers of perichondrium ; these fibres are intersected by others which run parallel to the surfaces of the plate. At the points of inter-section of the fibrils are star-shaped cells, and the spaces enclosed between the fibrils are filled with a semi-fluid mucoid material which stains a purple colour with thionin. A somewhat similar structure is seen in the head-shields of the extinct Cephalaspid fishes in which there is an appear-ance of spaces enclosed by osseous laminæ running at right-angles to each other. These appearances suggest the existence of a fibro-cartilaginous matrix which, having become calcified, formed a hard plate, different from bone in the absence of definite Haversian systems showing con-centric laminæ, surrounding the vascular canals.

Since Gaskell's time the structure of the head-shields of the Cephala-spids has been studied in detail by Stensiö (1927), who describes an exoskeleton consisting of superficial, middle, and basal layers (Fig. 238). The basal layer shows thin fibrous laminæ enclosing numerous cell-spaces, the fibres in each lamina being arranged in such a way that they are nearly at right-angles to the laminæ next above and below. He differs from Gaskell, however, in that he considers the basal layer is composed of true laminated bone. He further describes minutely the relation of the vascular canals contained in the three layers mentioned, with reference to certain polygonal areas and inter-areal grooves which are present in some of the specimens, and small pores which open on the smooth,

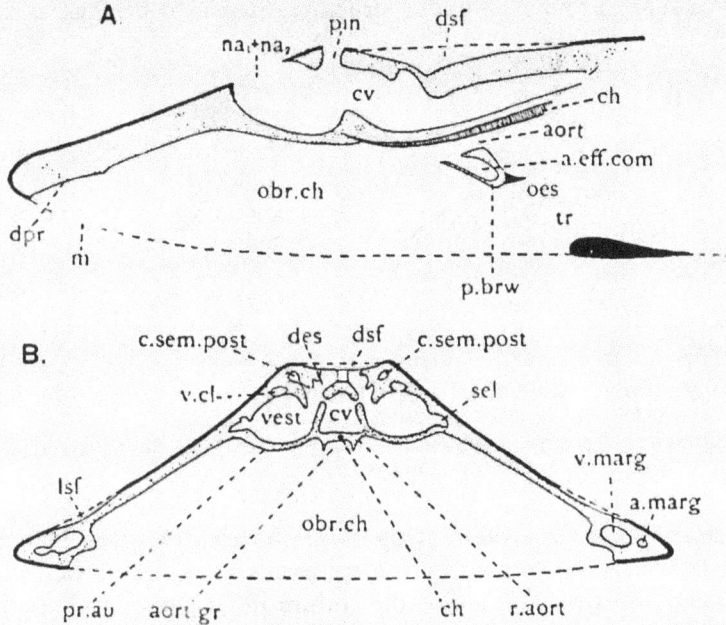

FIG. 238.—TWO SCHEMATIC SECTIONS THROUGH THE HEAD OF A CEPHALASPID FISH. (AFTER STENSIÖ.)

A—Median sagittal section.
B—Transverse section through the posterior part of the otic region. The exoskeleton shown with thick lines, and the perichondral-bone layers with fine lines, cartilage dotted.

a. eff. com. : space for the arteria efferens communis.
aort. : aortic canal.
aort. gr. : aortic groove.
a. marg. : canal for marginal artery.
ch. : notochord.
c. sem. post. : posterior semicircular canal.
c.v. : cranial cavity.
d.p.r. : area which bounded the mouth-cavity on the dorsal side.
d.e.s. : canal for the electric nerve to the dorsal electric field, *dsf*.
l.s.f. : lateral electrical field.

m. : mouth opening.
$na_1 + na_2$: nasal opening + the opening of the hypophyseal sac.
obr. ch. : oralobranchial chamber.
oes. + tr. : opening for the œsophagus and trachea + the truncus arteriosus in the posterior branchial wall.
pin. : pineal foramen.
pr. au. : otic prominence.
r. aort. : right aorta and aortic ridge.
sel. : nerve canal to lateral electrical field.
vest. : vestibular division of labyrinth cavity.

shining external surface, these appear to have transmitted the external branches from a series of radiating canals originating from a subepidermal vascular plexus. The superficial layer consists of dentine—orthodentine and osteodentine—which, as the dentine canals diminish in diameter as they course distally, acquires an enamel-like appearance. This agrees very closely with the enamel which occurs in the true fishes. Beneath the superficial layer are pulp-like cavities, from which radiating " dentinal canals " issue. From its minute structure Stensiö concludes that the

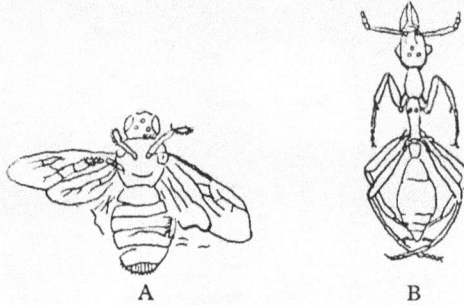

FIG. 239.

A—*Xylocopa senilis*. Miocene. Baden. (After Heer.) 1/1 Apis. A fossil bee, showing ocelli and lateral compound eyes.
B—*Prionomyrmex longiceps*. Oligocene, Baltic amber. 2/1 after Maye. Fossil ant, showing ocelli and compound eyes.
(From von Zittel.)

exoskeleton with the exception of the most superficial part of the superficial layer which was formed by the epidermis must have arisen in the corium, and also that it occupied the corium in its entire thickness. In

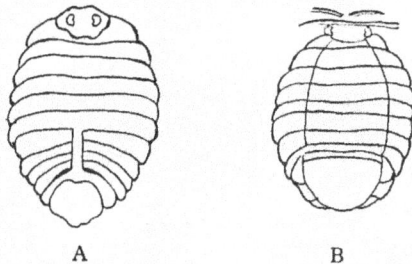

FIG. 240.

A—*Aracheoniscus Brodei*. Purbeck, Wiltshire. A small fossil crustacean similar in type to the wood lice of the living species. (After Woodward.)
B—*Eosphaeroma Brougniarti*. Middle Oligocene, Butte de Chaumont, near Paris. (After Quensted.) Order Edriophthalmia. Sub-order Isopoda. Both specimens show large sessile eyes on the sides of the head.
(From von Zittel.)

Thyestes verrucosus, the superficial layer is incomplete, and is limited to the tubercles, the middle layer being exposed in the inter-areal grooves.

Beside the exoskeleton there was beneath it a continuous bony endoskeleton, in which was lodged the brain, sense-organs, cranial nerves and vessels, and the branchial system ; and Stensiö considers that it is probable that the exoskeleton did not give rise to the endoskeleton, as has been generally maintained, but that the exoskeleton and the endoskeleton were formed simultaneously.

Moreover, since Gaskell's time the general architecture of the Ostracoderm fishes has been studied with great exactitude by Stensiö, Kaier, and other Norwegian palæontologists, who by the use of modern methods of research have been enabled to study the markings on the interior of the shields and obtain from serial sections reconstruction models representing complete casts of the cavity of the skull (Fig. 238, A and B, p. 341). Wax models of the interior of the skull have been made in much the same

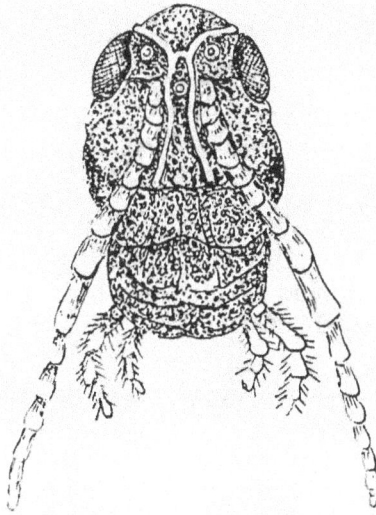

FIG. 241.—FRONT OF HEAD OF PORTHETIS SPINOSUS, TRANSVAAL, SHOWING THE THREE FRONTAL OCELLI, ARRANGED IN THE TYPICAL TRIANGULAR MANNER, ONE IN FRONT, TWO BEHIND. (REDRAWN FROM *Cambridge Natural History*.)

way as embryological material is reconstructed from serial sections by the wax-plate method of Born. The reconstructions made from serial sections of the fossil specimens are magnified sufficiently to allow of a detailed study being made of the main cavities which enclosed the brain and branchial system ; the minor cavities and canals which contained the cranial nerves, venous sinuses, and cerebral arteries ; the afferent and efferent vessels of the branchial apparatus ; also the orbital cavities ; labyrinth ; naso-hypophyseal canal ; pineal recess ; and the canals for the nerves and vessels leading to the impressions which Stensiö describes as the median " dorsal electrical field," and the marginal or " lateral electrical fields " on the dorsal aspect of the shield, Fig. 228.

From an extensive study of a very large amount of material obtained from the Downtonian and Devonian strata of Spitzbergen and other sources, Stensió has classed vertebrate Crania into two main branches, namely, those without jaws—Agnathi ; and those with jaws—Gnathostomi. The Agnathi comprise the Class Ostracodermi or Cyclostomata, which he subdivides into two subclasses with their respective Orders as shown in the following table :

VERTEBRATA CRANIATA

BRANCH I : AGNATHI
  Class : Ostracodermi (Cyclostomata)
  Subclass A : Pteraspidomorphi
   Order 1 : Heterostraci
    ,, 2 : Palæospondyloidea
    ,, 3 : Myxinoidea
  Subclass B : Cephalaspidomorphi
   Order 1 : Osteostraci
    ,, 2 : Anaspida
    ,, 3 : Petromyzontia

BRANCH II : GNATHOSTOMI

Stensiö concludes that the Ostracodermi constitute a group of primarily agnathous craniate vertebrates " which have nothing to do with either the Arthrodira or the Antiarchi, and are true fishes related to the Elasmobranchs."

Of the two living Orders of the Ostracodermi, the Myxinoidea (hagfish) is included in the pteraspid Subclass A and the Petromyzontia (lampreys) belong to the cephalaspid Subclass B.

In the subclass Pteraspidomorphi the rostral part of the head formed by the ethmoidal region and the common naso-hypophyseal opening lie on the ventral side of the head, close in front of the mouth, whereas in the subclass Cephalaspidomorphi the rostral part of the head is formed by the excessively developed upper lip, and is thus of visceral origin ; moreover, owing to the great development of the upper lip the nasohypophysial opening is carried upward on to the dorsal aspect of the head, where it lies immediately in front of the pineal foramen. Stensiö also concludes that the hag-fishes and lampreys being persistent representatives of the extinct Ostracoderms must be a primitively low type of agnathous craniate vertebrate and not degenerate descendants of the true fishes, but it is also quite clear with regard to the skeleton that they have undergone regressive changes, and that the absence of pectoral fins, which is characteristic of the living species, is one of these secondary regressive changes.

We may add, further, that the degenerate condition of the parietal sense-organs, more especially of the left pineal eye, is an additional fact in support of Stensiö's conclusion that the Myxinoidea and Petromyzontia have undergone regressive changes in their descent from the ostracoderm ancestral stock.

Now in the Downtonian strata of Ringerike, about 35 miles north-west of Oslo, there have been found, according to the description given

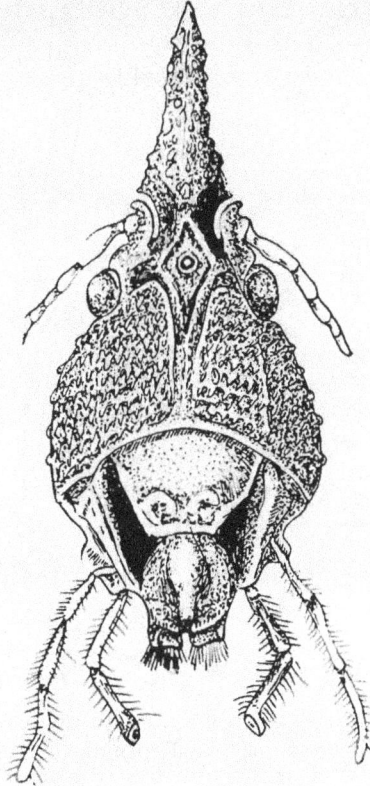

FIG. 242.—FRONT OF HEAD OF COPIOPHORA CORNUTA (FEMALE). DEMERARA—
LOCUSTIDÆ.

There is a high degree of development of the median frontal eye which forms a conspicuous feature of the Frons ; the other two ocelli are poorly developed and are placed one on each side of the curious frontal cone. (Redrawn from *Cambridge Natural History.*)

by Kaier, large quantities of the remains of fossil crustaceans belonging to the order Merostoma (e.g. small and giant Eurypterids). In close proximity to these, embedded in a stratum termed by him the "fish horizon," are found numerous examples of the Ostracodermi and more particularly of the groups Anaspidæ, Cephalaspidæ, Cœlolepidæ, the head shields of which are represented in a schematic manner in Fig. 232. Although the general exoskeleton of the Anaspidæ consists mainly of small lancet-shaped scales ; on the dorsal aspect of the head there is in the centre a well-defined median pineal plate perforated by a pineal foramen. The pineal plate lies between the orbital cavities, which are surrounded by a ring of orbital plates ; and in front is a single—naso-

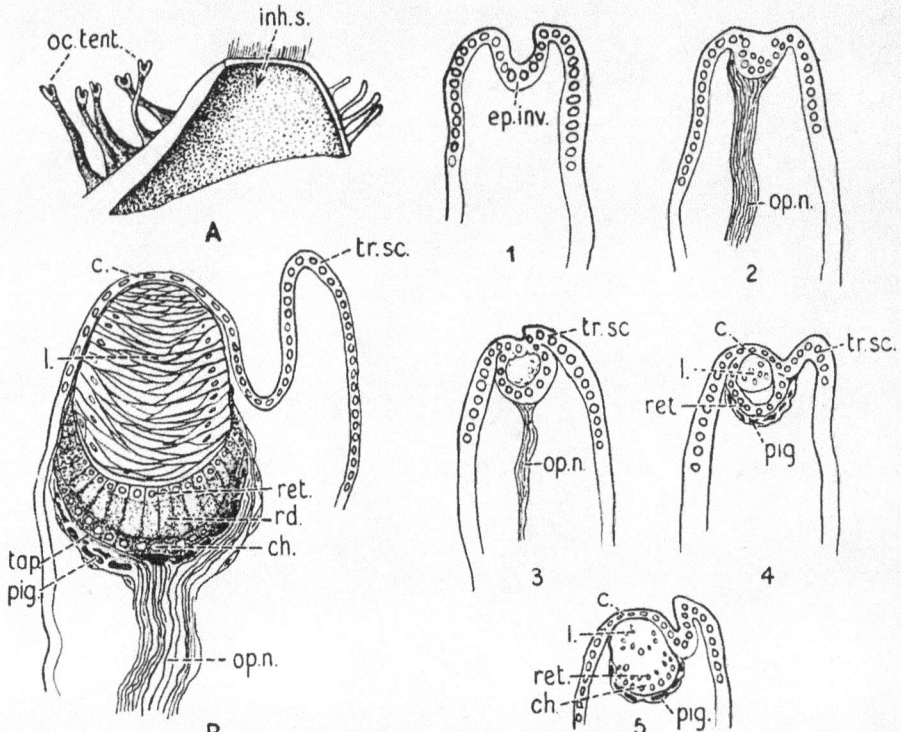

FIG. 243.—THE EYES OF CARDIUM NUTICUM.

A—tentacles bearing eyes around siphonal opening.

B—section through eye, showing the relations of the lens, retina, rods, " choroid," non-cellular tapetum, and pigment layers. 1, 2, 3, 4, 5 : stages in the development of the eyes.

c. : cornea.	pig. : pigment.
ch. : " choroid."	rd. : rods.
ep. inv. : epithelial invagination.	ret. : retina.
inh. s. : inhalant siphon.	tap. : tapetum.
l. : lens.	tr. sc. : triangular screen.
op. n. : optic nerve.	

(After Kishinouye.)

The structure and development of these eyes resemble in certain respects that of the lateral eyes of vertebrates.

hypophyseal—opening similar to that in *Kaieraspis auchenaspidoides* (Fig. 228). Moreover, behind the pineal plate there is an elongated oval area marked by small scales and corresponding to the glabellar plate or post-pineal area of *Auchenaspis verrucosus*. The Anaspida show no traces of a bony skeleton, although it is probable that a cartilaginous endo-skeleton did in reality exist, but it has left no evidence of its presence, the cartilage not having been fully calcified and thus not being preserved.

The strata, according to Kaier, appear to have been laid down rapidly at the estuaries of large rivers which in periods of floods deposited thick layers of mud, in which the fossils were imbedded and preserved *in situ*. The remains are thus in some cases remarkably complete and perfect, and although sometimes distorted, it is possible to reconstruct the parts and make comparisons of the different species, as shown in Fig. 244, in which it will be seen that a series or branchial apertures are present which resemble those in living species of Marsipobranchia or cyclostomes ; and also that pectoral spines were present which it is believed correspond to the pectoral fins of fishes. Moreover, since the olfactory organs of the cyclostomes, although opening on the surface by a single aperture, are,

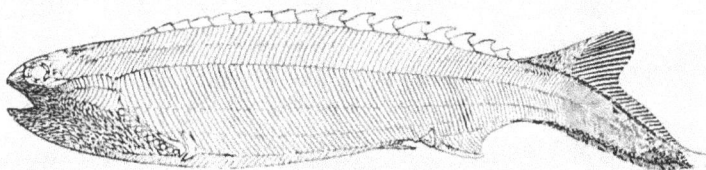

FIG. 244.—RECONSTRUCTION OF PTEROLEPIS NITIDUS. (AFTER KIAER.) DOWN-TONIAN STRATA. RINGERIKE, SHOWING ORBITAL SCLERAL PLATES, TEN BRANCHIAL APERTURES, RUDIMENTARY PECTORAL FIN, AND HYPOCERCAL TAIL.

as was strongly emphasized by Gaskell, truly bilateral in nature—there being paired olfactory nerves and paired olfactory lobes of the brain both in the living and extinct species of Cyclostomata—and since there is a close correspondence in the brain, sense-organs, cranial nerves, and many other structural points between the cyclostomes and fishes, it is obvious that they must have originated from a common stock ; and the circum-stance that the existence of a single nasal aperture in the class Cyclosto-mata has been employed as the basis of their classification as a separate branch—" Monorhina "—must not be thought to imply that they are totally different and have nothing to do with the class Pisces. Further, the presence of a pineal foramen located in the centre of a pineal plate which is situated between the orbital cavities and the proof of the bilateral nature of both the pineal and olfactory organs constitute along with other structural resemblances important evidence substantiating this conclusion.

Geological Evidence of the existence of Median Eyes in Invertebrates

In tracing the evolution of median eyes from the earliest known classes of fossil animals which show indications of such, we may consider first that great class of extinct animals the trilobites (Figs. 97, 100, 102, Chap. 11). These vary greatly in size and form, and they range from the Cambrian to the late Carboniferous and Permian eras. According to recent estimates of geologists the Cambrian age comprises a period from 500,000,000 to 750,000,000 years ago, and the Permian, which marks the

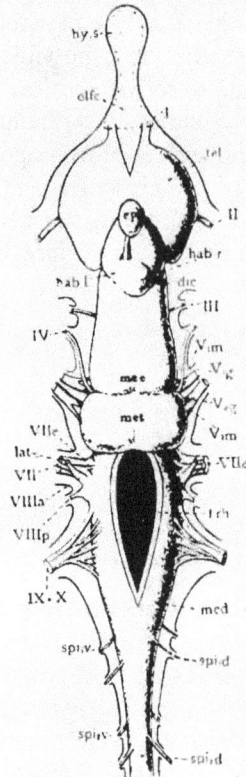

FIG. 245.—ATTEMPTED RESTORATION OF BRAIN OF KIAERASPIS IN DORSAL VIEW. (AFTER STENSIÖ.) COMPARE WITH FIG. 22, CHAPTER 3, p. 28.

dic. : diencephalon.
ep. : epiphysis.
f. rh. : fossa rhomboidalis.
hab. l. : left habenular ganglion.
hab. r. : right habenular ganglion.
hy. s. : hypophyseal sac.
lat. : roots of the prootic lateral nerves.

mec. : mesencephalon.
med. : medulla.
met. : metencephalon.
olf. c. : olfactory capsule.
sp. d. : dorsal roots of spinal nerves.
sp. v. : ventral roots of spinal nerves.
I. to X. : cranial nerves 1 to 10.

end of the Palæozoic period, from 215,000,000 to 280,000,000 years ago. When the first trilobites existed other invertebrate phyla were abundant, and it is considered that the trilobites and kindred types were preceded by a hypothetical class for which the name Protostraca has been suggested, the term signifying the earliest type of animals possessing a shell—the name " Palæostraca " being reserved for the whole group of known fossils which includes such primitive types of marine arthropods as the Gigantostraca, including *Eurypterus*, *Pterygotus* (Fig. 96, Chap. 11, p. 135), and *Stylonurus*, sometimes spoken of as the sea scorpions, and also the Xiphosura or Merostomata, of which *Limulus*, the king crab, is a living example (Fig. 69, Chap. 11, p. 108).

The trilobites have affinities with both the Crustacea and the arachnids, or spiders, and are usually allocated to a separate subclass or are classified as an appendix of the Crustacea or Arachnida, the trilobites being regarded as a precursor of both. The trilobites and all the marine fossil arthropods

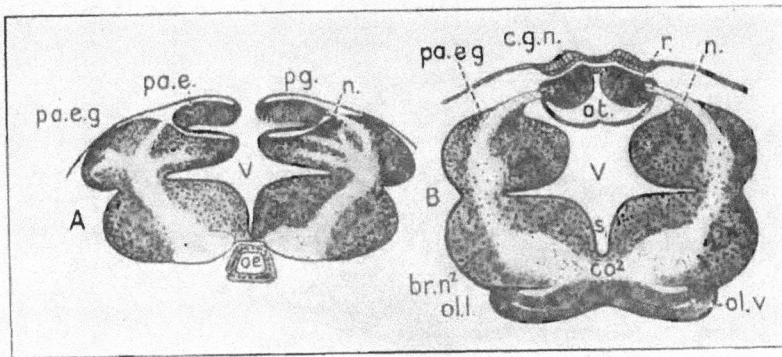

FIG. 246.

A—Section through the parietal eye vesicle of a scorpion (stage H), showing the approaching pallial folds previous to the union of the two retinas.

B—Section through the parietal eye of a newly born scorpion showing the parietal eye vesicles and the ventricle, *V*., bounded by the optic ganglia, the pallial folds and the neuromeres of the fore-brain. The ventricle extends downward and forward into the cavities of the olfactory lobes, *ol. v.*

at. : atrium, or cavity of parietal eye-vesicle.	*ol. v.* : olfactory ventricle.
	pa. e. : parietal eye.
br. n.² : dicephalon.	*pa. e.g.* : parietal eye ganglion.
c.g.n. : corneagen.	*pg.* : pallial groove.
co.² : commissure of dicephalon.	*r.* : retina.
oe. : œsophagus.	*s.* : median sulcus.
ol. l. : olfactory lobe.	*v.* : ventricle.

mentioned above, include types which either in the adult or larval form show indications of (1) both median and lateral eyes, (2) only median eyes, (3) only lateral eyes. In some, known as " blind trilobites," eyes are said to be absent. It is probable, however, that in many adult specimens which have been described as blind, median eyes may have been present in the larval form which disappeared and left no traces of their existence in the adult animal. The lateral eyes of trilobites are usually faceted or aggregate eyes. These are borne on the movable or lateral cheeks and, as have been described on p. 137, are of two types : (1) holochroal, in which the visual area is covered by a smooth, continuous film or cornea through which the lenses of the ommatidia are visible by trans-lucence—*Asaphus, Illænus, Calymene* (Fig. 97, A); and (2) schizochroal, in which the cornea is transected by protrusion of the sclera between the ommatidia and is limited to or present only on the surfaces of the omma-tidia (Fig. 97)—*Phacops, Dalmanites, ?Harpes*. Barrande recognized a third type which is exemplified in the genus *Harpes*, the eye of which is regarded as an aggregate of ocelli which are disposed in groups of two or three together, a circumstance which may be regarded as indicating a primitive stage in the evolution of compound faceted eyes in which the ommatidia are uniformly disposed, are close together and are covered

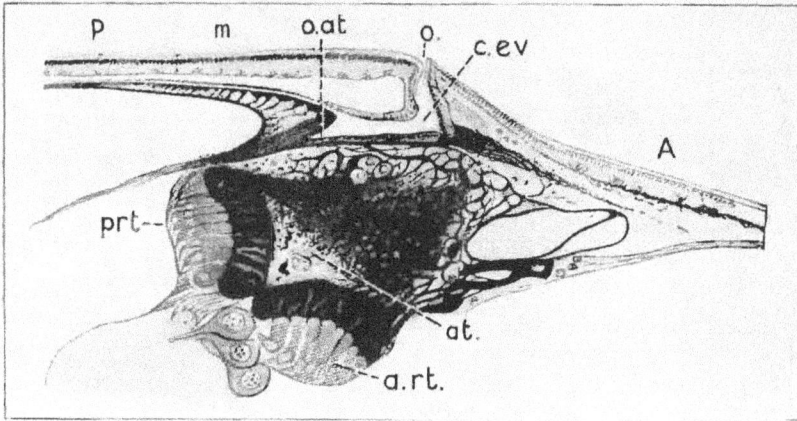

FIG. 247.—SAGITTAL SECTION THROUGH THE PARIETAL EYE VESICLE OF AN ADULT APUS. (AFTER PATTEN.)

A. : anterior.
a. rt. : anterior retina.
c. ev. : common cavity which encloses the lateral eye vesicles and into which the cavity, *at.*, of the parietal eye vesicle previously opened, at the recess marked *o. at.*
m. : fold covering the lateral eyes.

o. : opening of common cavity.
P. : posterior.
p. rt. : posterior retina. Each placode consists of a single row of large colourless columnar cells the distal ends of which are buried in a dense mass of pigment, their proximal ends being clear.

by a continuous cornea. *Harpes ungula* (Fig. 97, B), in which this primitive condition of the lateral eyes is met with, belongs to the Ordovician period, the age of which is estimated to be 480,000,000 to 590,000,000 years ago.

The three impressions on the glabella of *Æglina prisca* (Fig. 97, A), which are considered by some eminent palæontologists to represent ocelli, are arranged in the form of a triangle with the apex forward. In *Dalmanites socialis* (Fig. 104, A) a single impression is present. In a similar specimen of *Dalmanites* three impressions are found, disposed in the form of a triangle with the apex behind (Fig. 104, B), while in certain examples of Trinucleidæ there are five impressions on the surface of the median-eye tubercle arranged in a manner similar to the five of a playing-card. An almost identical disposition of ocelli in a group of three with the apex forward is found in certain recent fossil and amber-preserved insects, e.g. *Xylocopa senilis*, *Apis*, a fossil bee (Fig. 239, A), and *Priono-myrmex longiceps*, a fossil ant (Fig. 239, B), and this characteristic arrangement is maintained in the living representatives of the same species and other insects, e.g. *Porthetis spinosus* (Fig. 241) and *Copiophora cornuta* (Fig. 242). There is considerable difference of opinion among the older writers as to whether these markings really correspond to ocelli or not, but recent workers, e.g. Störmer, employing new methods of micro-scopical technique, have demonstrated not only the presence, but details of the structure of the median eyes in the glabella of several Norwegian species of Trinucleidæ both in the larval and adult specimens.[1] It is with his kind permission that we have been enabled to reproduce the following photographs, which serve to illustrate some of the more important points which he has described in this most interesting group of trilo-bites and of the frontal ocelli of insects in general, and of some arthropods.

Fig. 100 (Chap. 11, p. 139) shows the general position on the cephalon of the median-eye tubercle of *Tretaspis seticornis*, in the meraspid stage II, when viewed from the side as in B and as seen from above in A ($\times$ 80). C and D show the tubercle in adult specimens. Both in the meraspid stage and in the adult five impressions are visible on the dorsal aspect of the tubercle. The appearance of the tubercle when seen in section are well shown in Fig. 101, which is a transverse section through the median-eye tubercle of an adult *Tretaspis Kiaeri*, n. sp., and Fig. 102, which is from a photograph of a longitudinal section through the median-eye tubercle of *Trinucleus bucculentus*.

Störmer comes to the following conclusions :

(1) The median tubercle found on the top of the glabella in several Trilobites must be regarded as a true median-eye.

(2) The median-eye which has been found in four species of Trinu-cleidæ shows a different structure to the lateral eyes.

(3) The surface of the median-eye tubercle shows five distinct impressions, indicating four or five ocelli below.

(4) The structure resembles that of the median eyes in recent Phyllo-poda (*Apus*, Fig. 67, Chap. 11, p. 104, and Fig. 247, and Figs. 248, 250, Chap. 24, *Lepidurus*, Fig. 68, A, Chap. 11, p. 106).

(5) No lens such as that in the lateral eyes has been found.

(6) The ontogeny of the Trinucleidæ shows that the median eye is highly developed in the early larval stages, when the lateral eyes are small and little developed.

[1] Lief Störmer, *Scandinavian Trinucleidæ*, with Special References to Norwegian Species and Varieties, I to III, 1939, *Skrifter ut gitt av det Norske Videnskaps*, Akademi i Oslo.

CHAPTER 24

RELATION OF THE MEDIAN
TO THE LATERAL EYES

IN considering this question it will be necessary first to review briefly the development and structure of median and lateral eyes in the simplest forms of invertebrates, and to trace in living representatives of phyla in which bilateral symmetry has been evolved, the gradual differentiation and perfection of the paired lateral eyes of the higher types, in association with habits of life requiring accurate vision and quick perception, as for instance in the dragon-fly or cuttle-fish ; and to contrast the eyes of these with the type of eye which suffices for their free-swimming larvæ, or the adult animal of lower types which have not advanced much from the larval form, and in which the adult creature lives in an environment similar to that of the larva, e.g. as in some of the non-parasitic Turbellaria.

It will be necessary also to consider the conditions of life, which it may be assumed existed in the earliest stages of the ancestral history or phylogeny of these groups ; that is to say, before a terrestrial existence was possible or an active predatory and carnivorous life could have been maintained, either in the open sea, on land, or in the air. Such a life is possible only in animals with very highly evolved sensory organs, central nervous system, and organs of locomotion, such as fins, jointed-limbs, or wings. A comparison also may be made between the sense-organs of the more highly evolved types and those which live a burrowing life in the mud at the bottom of shallow waters, such as in ponds or tidal waters round the coast, or of those which lead a parasitic existence. If this is done, it will at once become evident that enormous periods of time must have elapsed in order to allow the evolutionary changes which have occurred in the higher types of animals to take place, and also that in tracing back the origin of any particular phylum, it is not the adult species of the more highly differentiated types of the orders that are likely to prove of value in assessing the relationship of different groups, but the larval forms and more particularly those species in which the larvæ have a free-swimming existence in the water or on moist herbage. These considerations limit the extent of the inquiry very considerably, and imply that there can be no very close relationship between such divergent and specialized types as those of the higher Crustacea and Mollusca ; or between the higher vertebrate classes and either of the two invertebrate phyla mentioned. At the same time a comparison of the very early stages of development does indicate a descent of these highly differentiated and specialized types from an extremely remote common stock, of which we have no geological record, but which it may be supposed existed as a simple form of animal adapted for life in water or in the mud or sand at the bottom of the sea, fresh water lakes, or estuaries of rivers. We may accordingly examine such types as are living to-day under similar conditions. As examples we may mention such animals as Planaria or simple forms of Annelids ; in these we find a type of sense-organ capable of reacting to light in an animal which shows bilateral symmetry of the body generally and more particularly of the central nervous system, e.g. as in Planaria or the Annelid *Hæmopis sanguisuga* (Fig. 16, Chap. 3, p. 21). The essential elements for the higher types of eye are present in these simple forms, namely : pigment, a refractive medium, and neuro-sensory cells connected by nerve-fibres with the central nervous system ; we see also in *Hæmopis* the commencement of the differentiation of a pair of aggregate lateral eyes, and between these two simple eyes formed by the modification of a single cell. It may be conceived that the lateral paired eyes, each consisting of a group of modified cells and being situated in a more favourable position than the median eyes, would in the process of time become still more differentiated, and that in place of single receptive or neuro-sensory cells containing pigment in one part, a clear refractive mucoid material in another, and terminating in a nerve-fibre, which originates from its deep aspect, special pigment cells and refractive cells would be set apart : the pigment cells for the absorption of superfluous rays of light, the clear refractive cells for the dioptric mechanism, e.g. " lentigen cells " and " cone cells," while others will serve as retinal or receptor cells and still others for the conducting of visual impulses through one or more optic ganglia to the brain.

As the requirements became greater, still further adaptive changes ensued ; thus a hard protective covering or scleral tunic was developed around the sensitive epithelial retina ; muscles were evolved to enable independent movements of the eyeball to take place ; also an outer chitinous or cartilaginous capsule which enclosed an orbital cavity, and which at the same time provided a framework for the attachment of the specialized orbital muscles (Figs. 91 and 92, Chap. 11, pp. 129, 130) in some instances, e.g. in *Sepia* (Fig. 36, Chap. 3, p. 50, and Fig. 121, Chap. 12, p. 164), a movable iris-like fold and intraocular muscles were developed for regulating the amount of light entering the eye, and possibly accommodation of the lens for near or distant vision ; also a " secondary cornea " growing as a fold over the front of the eyeball and enclosing a chamber,

23

resembling the anterior chamber of a vertebrate eye, but differing from it in its mode of formation and in communicating through an unclosed opening with the exterior and thus being filled with sea-water. We have thus, by means of what is termed " parallel development," an eye which resembles in many respects a vertebrate eye, yet differs from the vertebrate type in some very important structural details, which indicate that the differentiation and perfection of the cephalopod type of eye, must have taken many ages to complete and that the divergence of the parent stem of these higher molluscs must have taken place at a very early period in the phylogeny of the invertebrate stock. This conclusion is supported by reference to the ontogenetic development of *Sepia*, which was worked out by Koelliker and also by geological evidence. Embryology shows that there is a marked deviation in the course of development of the higher Mollusca from that of the simpler types, such as the Amphineura, which include *Chiton* (Fig. 115, Chap. 12, p. 157) and the Aplacophora, in which the bilateral symmetry of the central nervous system—which consists of paired lateral and ventral cords provided with serially arranged ganglia and united by transverse commissural bands, as in *Turbellaria*—remains undisturbed ; and, further, that the remarkable specialization in form which characterizes each of the higher classes of the Mollusca has not been evolved. While on the geological side, judging from the similarity of the phragmacone of living cephalopods to the ammonites, and belemnites of the Lias strata which belong to the lower series of the Jurassic period, it may be inferred that the Cephalopoda of that time were not only highly differentiated as regards their soft parts, including the eyes, but much larger than any living species. It seems obvious also that the period during which this remarkable differentiation took place in the higher types of the Cephalopoda must have extended much farther back than the Lias, in which it seems to have already attained a maximum.

If one were to judge from the higher types of Mollusca only, the differences which exist in the eyes and general anatomy of these types might lead one to think that the whole phylum of Mollusca was totally different from the phyla of other invertebrates. This is not so, however, as is most clearly seen in the ontogeny and in the adult structure of the Amphineura. The development of this class was specially studied by Kowalevsky in *Chiton*. In this animal the early stages of development show a typical blastocyst, gastrula, mouth (blastopore), proctodæum and anus, mesoderm formation, paired eyes and otocysts, cerebral ganglia, lateral (pleuro-visceral) and ventral (pedal) nerve cords—all of which point to a primary community of origin of the Mollusca, with other phyla of the invertebrates, and also indicate, when compared with similar stages of development in the embryos of vertebrates, that the pre-vertebrate stock from which the vertebrates arose passed through the same stages in development and had sensory organs and nervous system which was built up on essentially the same plan as that previously mentioned in connection with Planaria.

The study of the eyes of molluscs emphasizes another question bearing upon the history of the paired lateral eyes of the larva. In some instances in place of further development and differentiation taking place in the course of ontogeny, a reverse process is observed, namely degeneration. Thus in certain Lamellibranchia and in *Chiton*, cephalic eyes appear temporarily during the development of the larva and later disappear when, having become covered by the shell, they are rendered useless. This disappearance of the larval eyes is found chiefly in those animals which burrow in the mud, live in deep sea water, or are parasitic. In some cases they are replaced by eyes of a different type, which are secondarily acquired, e.g. the eyes on the edge of the mantle in some bivalve lamellibranchs, such as *Pecten* (Fig. 106, Chap. 12, p. 148) and on the back of *Chiton* (Fig. 115, Chap. 12, p. 157). In *Chiton* some of the megalæsthetes, or large sensory organs, become transformed into what appear to be eyes. Each of these eyes is covered by a pigmented layer of cells which envelops a modified æsthete ; superficially is an arched layer of the tegmentum which forms a cornea beneath which is a lens, and a cell layer which is regarded as a retina. The individual cells of the retina are connected by nerve fibres with the nerves of the ordinary æsthetes.

In connection with the degeneration of the larval lateral eyes of *Pecten* and *Chiton*, it may be noted that the simple form of eye found in *Nautilus* (Fig. 112, Chap. 12, p. 152), which consists of merely a spherical optic pit, opening to the exterior by a constricted orifice with neither lens, iris-fold nor cornea, is probably an instance of arrested development of a formerly more highly developed organ rather than the retention of a primitively simple form. It may be presumed that this arrest occurs at an early stage in its formation, and it may be regarded as an inherited condition which originated in association with a change in the habits of the adult animal from a creeping or possibly actively swimming creature to a passive state in which the animal floats about enclosed in the last compartment of its rigid spiral shell (Fig. 110, Chap. 12, p. 151).

The distinction between a simple structure, which is simple because it has retained its original simple form unchanged throughout its ancestral life-history, and one which is simple as the result of degeneration is in some cases very difficult and can only be decided by a very careful consideration of the animal as a whole, in all its bearings, structural and functional, embryological and phylogenetic. Unfortunately, as far as we are aware, the ontogenetic development of *Nautilus* has not yet been studied. The complicated structure of the adult tetrabranch *Nautilus* and a consideration of this structure in relation with the general principles and facts of comparative anatomy, combined with a study of the various types of extinct Nautilidæ, appear to warrant the general conclusion that the mobile shell-less forms with actively functioning eyes come first in the order of evolution, and that fixation or the development of a shell is usually followed by the degeneration of the locomotive organs and of the eyes. At the same time it is almost certain that the eyes of the Nautilidæ never attained the high degree of evolution which has been reached in the cuttle-fishes. The shell was developed at a very early period in the phylogenetic history of the Nautilidæ, which are pre-eminently Palæozoic in their distribution, and it seems likely that the truth lies between the two suppositions, and that the eye of *Nautilus* is simple partly because it has undergone degeneration and partly because it has retained its primarily simple form without having undergone a high degree of specialization.

Eyes of Mollusca

Among the various types of eye which are met with in the Mollusca it is worth while noting, with reference to the inverted eyes of *Pecten*, the singular compound eyes of the upright type which are found round the edge of the mantle of the " Noah's-ark " shell-fish (*Arca Noæ*). These appear on the summit of small rounded projections, and consist of a dome-shaped epithelial cap which covers and encloses a central meso-dermal core. In microscopical sections (Fig. 40, Chap. 3, p. 58) the epithelial cap is seen to be composed of a single layer of tall columnar cells, which are arranged in groups or units, each of which is composed of one central visual cell surrounded by six cylindrical pigment cells, thus forming an ommatidium resembling somewhat the ommatidia of certain arthropods. The ommatidia of *Arca* are, however, separated by slender unpigmented interstitial cells. The sensory or visual cells are conical in form, the base of the cone being slightly convex and directed outward, while the apex is directed inwards and rests on a subepithelial limiting membrane. A clear spherical nucleus is present in the super-ficial segment of the cell, whereas the tapering inner part of the cell has a rod-like structure. Although they resemble in certain points the simple forms of aggregate eyes of some arthropods, they are regarded as having been evolved independently and as having no genetic relation with these. Moreover, although there is a marked difference between the mantle eyes of *Arca* and those of *Pecten*, the single layer of columnar pigment cells which form the iris-like zone which surrounds the cornea and lens in *Pecten* resemble the columnar pigment cells of the ommatidia in the eyes of *Arca*, and they indicate a stage in the development of the eye previous to the differentiation of specialized visual cells from pigment cells. A comparison of the two types of eye also indicates the manner in which the eyes of *Pecten* can be developed from a simple type such as that of *Arca* by invagination of the superficial central area of modified epithelium into the subjacent mesodermal layer which forms the central core of the tentacle. This inference is confirmed by the work of Kishinouye on the development of the marginal or mantle-eyes of *Cardium nuticum* (cockle), which when fully developed closely resemble those of *Pecten*, but differ in the existence of a " choroid " layer between the retina and tapetum and by the mesoblastic origin of the pigment layer (Fig. 243). According to the description given by Kishinouye (1894), both right and left mantle edges are beset with dark-brown almost black pigment. They unite at the posterior end of the shell and form a triangular pigment area surrounding the siphonal openings. Over this area the right and left valves of the shell do not meet closely, but leave a rather wide gap. In this triangular interval the tentacles are arranged in irregular rows round the siphonal apertures. The larger and longer, which are about 100 in number, bear the eyes. They are bent away from the siphonal openings and each of them has a long band of black pigment on the siphonal side, i.e. the side exposed to the light. The eye appears as a black spot on the siphonal side of the tip of the tentacle, opposite the position of the eye in *Cardium edule*. A vertical section through the adult eye shows superficially a thin layer of pavement epithelium ; a central area of this epithelium, the " cornea," is unpigmented and clear ; this is surrounded by a zone of pigmented cells continuous externally with the general epithelium covering the tentacle. Beneath the cornea is a lens which is composed of flattened ectodermal cells. Its vertical diameter is considerably greater than the transverse diameter, and it is slightly constricted in the centre. In contact with the lower pole of the lens is a bilaminar, cup-shaped retina which consists of a superficial stratum of columnar cells, the outer deeper ends of which have a rod-like structure, whereas the inner segments of the cells, which are in contact superficially with the lens, are clear and contain a vesicular nucleus. The outer superficial stratum of the double-layered retinal cup is formed by a layer of cubical epithelial cells, which is continuous, at the margin of the cup, with the layer of visual cells. Kishinouye compared this layer with the outer layer of hexagonal pigment cells of the vertebrate retina, and speaks of it as the " choroid " layer. It is covered externally by a non-cellular layer or tapetum and a thin stratum of mesoblastic cells containing pigment. Both of these layers are pierced by the fibres of the optic nerve, which is connected with the viscero-parietal ganglion. Each eye is protected by a triangular fold of the epithelium, which forms an overlapping screen. The first stage in the development of these eyes is represented by a depression of the modified central area of epithelium at the apex of an ocular tentacle which forms a hollow cup. Later, by proliferation of the cells at the bottom of the cup, a solid mass of epithelium is formed which becomes differentiated into a superficial part, the lens, and a deeper layer, the retina, one side of the cup becomes raised to form the triangular protective screen, the inner limb of this fold is continuous with the opposite lip which covers the lens and forms the cornea. The retinal portion appears to be invaginated in much the same way as in the formation of the secondary optic vesicle in vertebrates.

This brief summary of the structure and development of the various types of molluscan eyes indicates that the higher orders of Mollusca have deviated very widely from the simple forms which represent the ancestral parent stock ; also that the eyes of different orders of the Mollusca differ very widely not only from each other but from those of other Phyla of the invertebrates and from the vertebrates. The eyes of the cuttle-fish show a high degree of differentiation and have a superficial resemblance to the eyes of vertebrates, but they lack the delicate mechanisms for accommodation of the lens and adaptation of the pupil, and they differ essentially in their mode of development and structure from the vertebrate eyes. Median eyes are only seen in the larval stages of the lower classes of Mollusca ; and the early stages of ontogeny having been abbreviated or suppressed, they have entirely disappeared in the cephalopods. In the phylogeny of the phylum Mollusca, different types of eye have been evolved in different regions of the body, such as the back and edge of the mantle, by methods which involve folding and invagination of the surface layers ; these are similar to those which occur in other phyla of the invertebrates and in the vertebrates, but have been evolved by processes of parallel development and are not genetically related, and it is only in the case of the paired eyes of the simpler types of molluscs and their trochophore and veliger larvæ that the genetic relation with other phyla can be traced with any degree of certainty.

The Median and Lateral Eyes of Arthropoda

It is with reference to certain classes of the Arthropoda that the most enthusiastic claims were made for the existence of a close relationship between vertebrates and invertebrates, and in view of the similarity in structure and position of the median eyes of invertebrates and the median or pineal eyes of vertebrates, it was thought that the common origin which was claimed for the Entomostracan and the pineal eyes constituted one of the most important pieces of evidence in favour of the vertebrate stock having arisen from an arthropod ancestor. The controversy was chiefly centred on the general resemblance in the form and structure of certain palæozoic Merostomata and their living representatives, e.g. *Apus*, *Limulus*, and *Scorpio*, to the Ostracodermata and their living representatives, namely, the cyclostomes. The Merostomata which were specially cited included *Bunodes*, *Eurypterus*, and Pterygotus, which along with the " trilobite larva " of *Limulus*, were compared with *Cephalaspis* and *Auchenaspis* (Thyestes). A closer study by recent workers (Stensiö, Kaier) involving the comparison of the central and peripheral nervous systems, the sense-organs, and other parts of living cyclostomes (see Fig. 22, Chap. 3, p. 28) with reconstructed casts of the cranial cavities of certain Palæozoic fishes (Anaspida, Cephalaspidomorpha, Fig. 245), has definitely shown that the claims made by earlier authors of a close relationship between these ancient fishes and the cyclostomes were well founded. Moreover, a more exact knowledge of the mode of development of the median and lateral eyes of invertebrates has led to a better understanding of the differences which exist between the fully developed eyes of different types of the adult animal ; also the mode of development of the more complicated types from the simpler, and the way in which an eye commencing as an epithelial pit and primarily purely dermal in origin may by a process of inrolling of the skin in the region of the neural crest be carried towards the median plane and ultimately included in the membranous roof of the fore-brain vesicle (Fig. 246), where later being cut off from the skin in the process of closure of the neural tube, it finally appears as a tubular evagination of the brain. The distal end of this tube, which corresponds to the bottom of the primary dermal pit, is usually dilated and forms a vesicle in the walls of which there are a variable number of retinal placodes (two, three, or four), which are commonly grouped or fused into a single median eye. These arise as one or two pairs, the tri-placodal type being formed by the complete fusion of one pair of placodes and the incomplete fusion of the other pair, which usually lie dorsal to the single placode (Figs. 248, 249). In the process of inrolling of the ocellar pit either the superficial or the deep limb of the fold may be developed as the sensitive or retinal layer (Fig. 246, A and B). If the deeper limb of the fold is modified to form the retina the superficial or pre-retinal layer may atrophy or it may be utilized in the formation of a lens. Whereas if the more superficial limb of the fold is transformed into the sensitive layer, the deeper or post-retinal stratum may give rise to a pigment layer or a reflecting membrane (tapetum). A more common arrangement is for only the deeper part of a symmetrically formed optic pit to be modified as a sensitive or retinal area, the cells at the sides of the pit becoming elongated and transformed into lentigen, or vitreogen cells, which secrete a clear, viscous fluid. This condenses and forms a non-cellular or vitreous lens in the cavity of an ocellar pit which is usually closed by the union of the margins of the fold over the mouth of the pit and the formation of a cuticular and cellular lens superficial to the vitreous lens (Fig. 248).

Now in *Apus* and *Branchipus* Patten has demonstrated a very interesting phase of the development of the triplacodal type of median or " Ento-

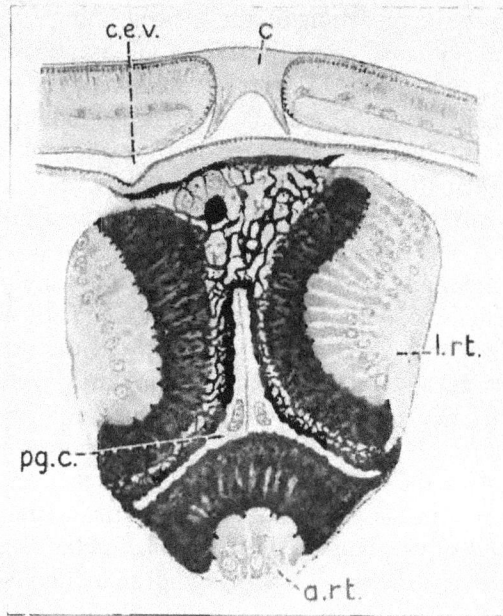

FIG. 248.—CROSS-SECTION OF PARIETAL EYE VESICLE OF APUS. (AFTER PATTEN.)

a. rt. : anterior retina.

c. : chitinous plug closing the opening of the common cavity to the exterior.

c.e.v. : common cavity of lateral and parietal eye vesicles.

l. rt. : left retina.

pg. c. : large pigment cells bounding cavity of parietal eye vesicle.

mostracan eye." The retinal placodes, which are four in number and purely dermal in origin, are depressed so that they come to lie at the bottom of separate pits, below the general surface of the surrounding ectoderm. They approach the median plane and become infolded so as to lie in the walls of a small common pit which opens into a larger common chamber which is enclosed by the forward growth of a transverse fold of the skin. This covers over both the median and the lateral eyes. The narrow mouth of this common chamber, which appears as a small pore in the skin, becomes closed by a chitinous plug (Fig. 248), and the

opening of the smaller pit in the walls of which the retinal placodes of the
median eye are imbedded also becomes closed, only a small recess in the
floor of the larger common chamber being left as an indication of the
site of the original communication (Fig. 247). The median or parietal eye
of *Apus*, according to Patten's description, forms a closed chamber with
a retinal placode on each side wall, and two unpaired placodes one on its
posterior and the other on its inner wall. Each placode consists of a
single row of large colourless, columnar cells. Their distal ends are
buried in a dense mass of dark brown or black pigment, their proximal
ends are colourless. As in *Branchipus*, there are two large cells which

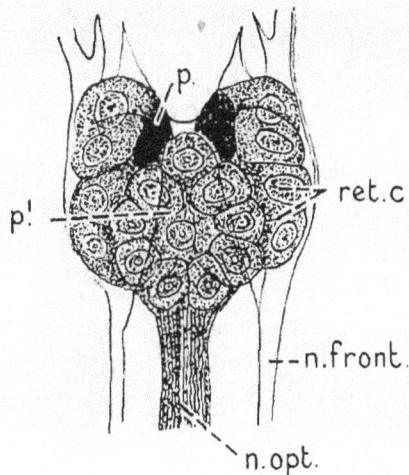

FIG. 249.—TRIPLE EYE OF CALANELLA MEDITERRANEA, A FREE-SWIMMING COPEPOD
CRUSTACEAN. ♀ *jun.* : FROM BELOW. (AFTER GRENACHER.)

n. front : frontal nerve.
n. opt. : optic nerve.
*p.*¹ : pigment plate of unpaired portion.
p. : pigment plates of the paired eyes.
ret. c. : retinal cells.

appear to give rise to the greater part of the pigment that fills the cavity
of the vesicle. When the pigment is partially dissolved it is seen that
each retinal cell is capped with a large brush-like mass of fine fibres
(retinidium).

Before commencing the detailed comparison of the median with the
lateral eyes of arthropods it will be necessary to define the different types
of eye which are met with in this phylum, which includes the Crustacea,
Insecta, and Arachnoidea. Patten subdivided the eyes of Arthropoda
into four types, namely :

1. Paired larval ocelli.
2. Parietal eyes.
3. Frontal ocelli or stemmata.
4. Lateral or compound eyes.

Other authors combine Patten's second and third types into a single group, namely *median eyes*, or speak of Patten's second group as the Entomostracan eye, and the third group as the hexapod type or frontal eyes of insects.

Patten contrasted the principal characters of his four types in the following manner :

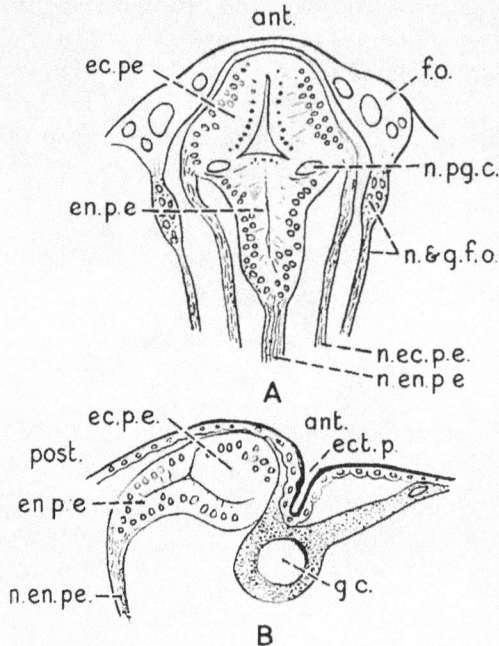

FIG. 250.—TRIPLACODAL PARIETAL EYE OF BRANCHIPUS. (REDRAWN FROM PATTEN.)

A—Axial section from front to back.
B—Median sagittal section. The three-lobed vesicle consists of right and left ectoparietal eyes and a single (probably bilateral) entoparietal eye. The cavity is completely cut off from the exterior in the adult animal. The distal ends of the retinal cells, which contain imperfectly formed rods, are turned towards the lumen of the cavity.

ant. : anterior end.
ec. p.e. : ectoparietal eye.
ect. p. : ectodermal pit.
en. p.e. : entoparietal eye.
f.o. : frontal organ.
g.c. : ganglion cell.

n. ec. p.e. : nerve of ectoparietal eye.
n. en. p.e. : nerve of entoparietal eye.
n. & g.f.o. : nerve and ganglion of frontal organ.
n. pg. c. : nucleus of pigment cell.
post. : posterior end.

1. " The *larval ocelli* (Fig. 78, Chap. 11, p. 117), of which there may be six pairs. These are present in the active larvæ of most insects, but disappear during the metamorphosis (Coleoptera, Lepidoptera, Neuroptera, Hymenoptera). They are cup-like infoldings of the ecto-derm, with upright or horizontal retinal cells or rods."

" In the insects the retinal cells are never completely inverted, and

RELATION OF MEDIAN TO LATERAL EYES

the ocelli never form unpaired eyes enclosed in a common chamber or vesicle."

2. " The *parietal eye* (Entomostracan eye) (Fig. 250). In the Crustacea and Arachnida two pairs of ocelli unite to form an unpaired ocellar vesicle or parietal eye. The ocellar placodes remain more or less distinct and form the side walls of the dilated anterior or distal end of the vesicle. The proximal or posterior end is generally tubular, and may open on the outer surface of the head or it may merge with the pallial folds and open into the forebrain vesicle. The parietal eye usually persists through life, and it may be the largest and most important one functionally."

3. " The *frontal eyes* or *stemmata* (Figs. 241 and 242, Chap. 23, pp. 343, 345) of insects consist of two pairs of placodes that form a median triocular group. They arise during the metamorphosis, or at any rate after the embryonic period, and are quite independent of the primary ocelli. They are never involved in a pallial fold or a common vesicle, and the retinal cells are apparently always upright. They are functional eyes only in adult insects, or in the late larval stages."

" In the arachnids and crustacea (phyllopods, Entomostraca) the frontal eyes are present in a highly modified form as two sets of frontal organs, two paired and one unpaired. In *Limulus* they become the olfactory organs. In spiders and scorpions they are apparently absent. Their nerve-roots arise from the median anterior surface of the forebrain or from the anterior surface of the optic ganglia and hemisphere."

4. " The *lateral* or *compound eyes* are found in adult Insecta, Crustacea and Arachnida, including the trilobites and merostomes. Like the stemmata, their relation to the primary head segments cannot be easily determined, because at the time that the cephalic lobes are most clearly segmented, as in the embryonic stages of *Acilius* and the scorpion, the lateral eyes are absent and they do not appear, if at all, until near the close of larval life. In *Limulus* they belong to the cheliceral segment; in insects they appear to belong to the antennal segment. The development of the lateral eyes is essentially the same in all arthropods. They are developed from large, crescentic placodes lying near the postero-lateral margin of the cephalic lobes, close to the infolding for the optic ganglion, but they never lie inside the fold, and the visual cells are never inverted. The entire visual layer is formed from a single layer of primary ectoderm. The placodes are frequently divided, or may be entirely separated into two distinct parts, which differ in their histological characters and in function (Hymenoptera, Neuroptera, Coleoptera). One part may be especially well developed in males (Ephemeridæ), or one may serve for vision under water and the other for vision in air."

Now Patten in using the term " parietal eye " to denote the entomo-

stracan type of median eye, definitely assumed not only that this type
of invertebrate eye resembled in its structure and mode of development
the parietal eye of vertebrates but that this correspondence of the parietal
eyes was merely one of many structural and developmental resemblances
between the entomostracan and vertebrate phyla. He, further, presumed that there was a long period of functional activity of the median
eye or eyes of vertebrates, during which the lateral eyes passed through a
corresponding period of inactivity while they were evolving and before,
as he states, "they again became functional." During this period he
believed that the parietal eyes were the only functional visual organs.
This latter concept is, we believe, for many reasons untenable, of which
we may mention : (1) that the general tendency is for inactive or non-
functioning organs to regress rather than evolve ; and (2) that the oldest
fossil fishes which are known, such as the Anaspidæ and Cephalaspidæ,
lived during the same period side by side with the giant forms of marine
Merostomata, e.g. *Eurypterus* and *Pterygotus*. In both the ostracoderm
fishes and the Merostomata many of the principal distinguishing characters
of the two phyla were already developed, including those relating to the
cranial skeleton, the brain and cranial nerves, the sense-organs, branchial
and vascular systems (Figs. 238, 245), and we may therefore conclude
that although the parietal eyes of living Cyclostomes and Entomostraca
resemble each other in certain respects and their special characters appear
to have persisted for an immensely long period without undergoing any
essential changes in structure, there has during this period been a
simultaneous and gradual evolution with differentiation of the lateral
eyes of both invertebrates and vertebrates. As the differentiation of each
type became more pronounced, namely, the invertebrate and vertebrate
types, so they diverged more and more from the simple form of eye,
from which they both originated, and from each other ; whereas the
median or parietal eyes tended to regress rather than evolve, except in
certain genera among Arthropoda, Monorhina, Amphibia, and Reptilea.
These evolutionary changes have resulted in two widely different types
of eye, one of which is upright and faceted, while the other has an inverted
retina and single lens protected by a smooth transparent cornea. Thus
at the present day it is difficult to believe that these two types of eye could
have arisen from a common ancestral form. Intermediate stages are
found between simple ocelli and the compound faceted eyes of invertebrates, but the special characters of the vertebrate eye seem to have been
already evolved in the earliest fishes of which we have any geological
record. It is true that the geological evidence is circumstantial rather
than direct, but the close agreement in the structural details of the cranial
skeletons of many of the extinct Palæozoic fishes with their living repre-

sentatives—showing that the brain, cranial nerves, vestibule, and semi-circular canals along with the branchial and vascular systems were in essential points alike—fully warrants the assumption that the lateral eyes of the extinct ostracoderm fishes and living Cyclostomata were essentially alike. In other words, that the lateral eyes of the cephalaspid and other fossil fishes were of the inverted type found in living species, and that they were functional. Moreover, judging from the small size of the parietal foramina or impressions in many of the extinct Palæozoic fishes as compared with the size of the orbital cavities ; and that in many cases the parietal canal did not even pierce the roof of the skull, it must be concluded that the lateral eyes were the chief organs of vision, and that in those cases in which the parietal canal did not pierce the vault of the skull, the parietal eye was completely functionless as a visual organ.

The replacement of the simple ocellar eyes of the larva by the compound eyes of the imago has been clearly demonstrated in the water beetle, *Dytiscus marginalis*, by Günther, and has already been alluded to, p. 117. It will be necessary, however, to describe in detail the differentiation of the crescentic or kidney-shaped area of epithelium called the " optic plate " or " rudiment of the lateral eye " in order to compare the ommatidia of the lateral eye with the ocelli which precede it (Figs. 78, 79, 80, 81, Chap. 11, pp. 117–119). The cells of the optic plate elongate and also proliferate and those in the centre of the plate become grouped into cylindrical unit-systems or *retinulæ*. Their protoplasm becomes clear, and some of the nuclei assume a deeper position. Each group consists of eight cells, one central and seven peripheral. The central cell and six of the peripheral cells take part in the formation of a retinula, while the seventh cell of the peripheral series is pushed out of the system. The central cell, which is flask-shaped in its basal portion where the nucleus is situated, tapers into a fine rod as it approaches the surface. The remaining six cells with the central basal cell form the visual portion of the retinula or *rhabdome*. Superficial to each retinula and between it and the ectoderm are especially modified clear ectoderm cells containing vacuoles, which give rise to the *crystalline cones* and together with these form the *ommatidia*. Each crystalline cone is formed by the amalgamation of four clear rods and each of these rods is derived from a refractile vesicle which is contained in one of the clear ectoderm cells. Later the four rods cohere and give rise to a crystalline cone, as in the crustacean, *Palæmon* (Fig. 37, Chap. 3, p. 52). The cells between adjacent ommatidia extend through the entire thickness of the ectoderm and secrete pigment, while superficially the cuticle, which covers the whole area, is secreted by small corneagen or lentigen cells. The cuticular layer is thickened over the distal ends of each ommatidium to form a plano-convex cuticular lens.

Now in comparing the compound lateral eyes with the simple eyes of the larva, it may be presumed that each ommatidium of the compound eye represents an ocellus and that the whole compound eye is formed by an aggregate of modified ocelli. The process of pit formation by a downgrowth of epithelial cells, however, appears to have been abbreviated in the ontogenetic development of the ommatidia, and although a potential lumen may be considered to exist in the central axis of each ommatidium, there is no actual cavity containing a vitreous mass, as in the simple ocellus (Fig. 38, Chap. 3, p. 53). There is nevertheless a distinct resemblance between the single basal cell of the rhabdome surrounded by the six peripheral cells of each retinula of the compound eye and the two large visual cells, with the adjacent long, slender cells surrounding it, which lie at the bottom of the pit of the simple ocellus. The probability of compound eyes being formed by an aggregation of simple ocelli is, moreover, supported by intermediate conditions between compound and simple eyes, such as are seen in the lateral and central eyes of *Euscorpius* (Figs. 94, 95, Chap. 11, pp. 132, 133) and *Limulus* (Figs. 86, 87, Chap. 11, pp. 124, 125), in both of which there is a combination of retinular or rhabdome formation with a continuous corneal surface, suggesting fusion of phylogenetically separate ocelli. The schizochroal eyes of *Phacops*, a Trilobite of the Devonian period, also support the view that the compound lateral eyes arise phylogenetically by fusion of adjacent ocelli into a single optic plate, for in *Phacops* the ommatidia are definitely isolated and separated by interstitial areas of the test (Fig. 98, Chap. 11, p. 137), the corneal facets thus being discontinuous, as contrasted with the more common continuous corneal surface of the holochroal type.

The various stages by which the simple upright eyes of the lower types of arthropods appear to have been transformed in the course of phylogeny into the paired compound eyes of the higher types has been studied by Lankester, Parker, Patten, Watase, and others, who have also endeavoured to fill in and explain certain intermediate stages between the larval and adult forms, which are often absent in those arthropods in which there is a definite metamorphosis in the life history of the animal, as for instance in many of the Insecta. In tracing these changes, it will be necessary first to review briefly some of the causes of these alterations in form and structure.

Starting with the assumption that the effect of light on protoplasm is to produce a chemical change that results in the formation of pigment, and further that this process renders the cell at once capable of absorbing light and reacting to it, we may note next that this reaction is a chemical change which is accompanied by decomposition of a part of the protoplasm of the cell during the manufacture of the pigment, and further that the work done by the action of the rays of light involves an expenditure of energy which affects the nerve-endings in the base of the cell. Thus one part of the cell becomes differentiated as a receptor and transmitter of nerve-impulses, and another the pigmented part for the absorption of light. Later special cells or parts of cells are differentiated to form the refractile elements, namely, the vitreous, the cuticular lenses or facets, and the rods and cones ; these lie for the most part superficially and at the clear distal ends of the cells or of the ommatidia. The intracellular pigment or the specialized pigment cells are displaced towards or are formed in the peripheral parts of the cells, or ommatidia ; whereas the neuro-sensory cells tend to sink beneath the level of the surrounding epithelium, and in this way a pit or downgrowth of epithelium is produced from which nerve-fibres pass to a sub-epithelial plexus or join to form an optic nerve. This process of pit-formation or downgrowth of the neuro-sensory cells may occur singly as in the formation of a simple ocellus, or as an aggregate of unit systems within a definite optic area. The unit systems or retinulæ may lie close together, being covered by a continuous layer of the cuticle, which in some cases is thickened over each retinula so as to form a corneal lens, as in the lateral eyes of *Limulus* (Fig. 86, Chap. 11, p. 124), or to a less extent as in the minute plano-convex lenses which are present in the adult lateral eyes of *Agelena* and *Dytiscus marginalis* (Fig. 81, Chap. 11, p. 119), or again in the faceted eyes of many insects. In some cases the units may be widely separated from each other, as in the schizochroal type of trilobite eye (Fig. 98), this form being generally regarded as the more primitive as compared with the holochroal forms in which the corneal lenses form a continuous surface. In many cases there lies in front of or superficial to the retinular layer, and between it and the cuticle, a stratum of modified epithelial or " hypodermal " cells. This layer is usually produced by the infolding of the epithelial cells surrounding the mouth of a single visual pit, as in the larval eye of *Dytiscus* (Fig. 4, Chap. 3, p. 10), or as in the median eyes of *Limulus* (Fig. 87, Chap. 11, p. 125), and *Scorpio* (Fig. 251), by a single layer which covers the whole sensory placode. In these cases the retinal layer of the larva is, when first formed, frequently inverted, and the eye consists of three layers, pre-retinal, retinal, and post-retinal, a condition which is somewhat similar to that found in the lateral eyes of vertebrates, but which must not be regarded as foreshadowing the evolution of the lateral vertebrate type, as the two types of eye occur at the ends of two widely divergent stems or phyla of the animal kingdom, and have most probably arisen independently.

The folding of the epithelial layers which has produced the reversal of the retinal layer must be considered as a mechanical process which in the invertebrate phylum Arthropoda has involved the median paired eyes of certain groups—for instance *Apus, Branchipus, Scorpio, Limulus*— whereas in other examples the median paired eyes have retained the primary upright character, as in *Acilius* (Fig. 82, Chap. 11, p. 120), the blowfly (Fig. 9, Chap. 3, p. 14), and the median or parietal eyes of verte- brates (Fig. 134, Chap. 17, p. 188, Fig. 183, Chap. 20, p. 259, and Fig. 252.

Besides this differentiation in the extent of the superficial area of the

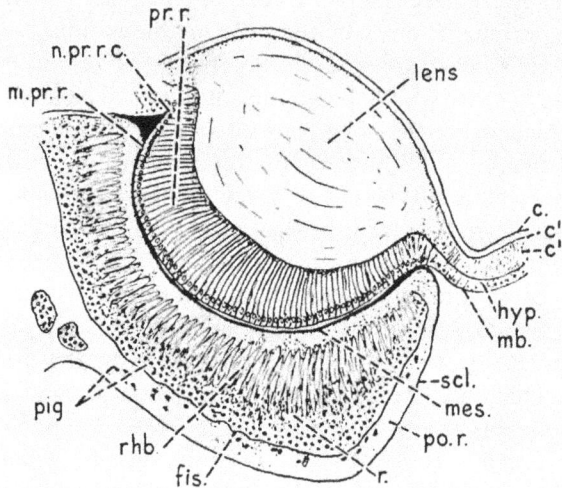

FIG. 251.—A TRANSVERSE SECTION OF THE RIGHT MEDIAN EYE OF AN ADULT SCORPION. (AFTER G. H. PARKER.)

Compare with Fig. 253, D. The primary cavity has been obliterated by adhesion of the retinal and post-retinal layers, along the line marked *fis*.

c., c'., c." : outer, middle, and inner layers of cuticle.
hyp. : hypodermis.
lens : cuticular lens.
mb. : basement membrane.
m. pr. r. : pre-retinal membrane.
mes. : thin mesodermal layer between retina and pre-retina.

n. pr. r.c. : nucleus of pre-retinal cell.
pig. : pigment.
po. r. : post-retina.
pr. r. : preretina (lentigen or vitreous layer).
r. : retina.
rhb. : rhabdites.
scl. : sclera.

derma which is involved in the formation of an optic placode, there is a tendency in the more highly differentiated eyes to increase in depth. The central neuro-sensory cells become more and more depressed and at the same time elongated ; moreover, their distal ends become modified to form vertical rods, whereas the distal ends of the cells lining the sides of the pit form short rods which tend to become horizontal, and near the mouth of the pit secrete a vitreous mass which serves as a lens. In the adult eyes of the higher types of insects and many of the Crustacea the unit systems or ommatidia tend to elongate still further and undergo further specialization. In some cases this elongation of the ommatidia is attended by cell division, so that the retinal layer becomes changed from the primary single layer of epithelial cells to one consisting of two or more layers of cells, while in others the increase in depth is considered to be brought about by simple elongation of the cells, which extend the whole distance from basement membrane to cuticle (Patten). In the eyes of many of the Crustacea there is an extension outward so that the retinal layer becomes raised on the summit of a movable stalk which contains a

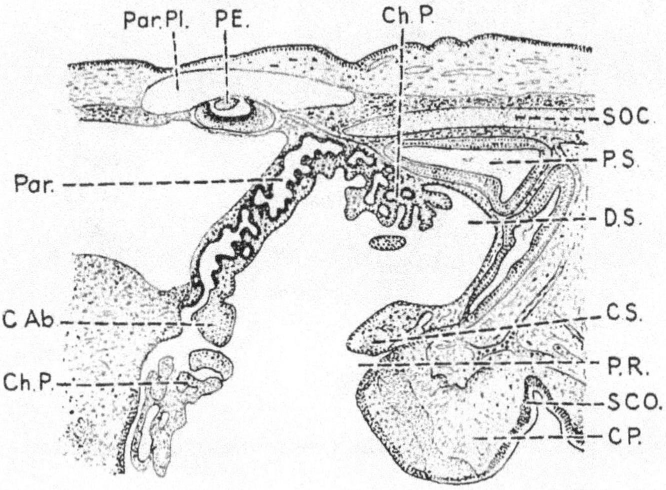

FIG. 252.—LONGITUDINAL SECTION OF SPHENODON EMBRYO (II, STAGE S[1]). (AFTER DENDY, SHOWING PINEAL REGION.)

C. Ab. : commissura abberans.
C.P. : commissura posterior.
C.S. : commissura superior.
Ch. P. : choroid plexus.
D.S. : dorsal sac.
Par. : paraphysis.

Par. Pl. : parietal plug.
P.E. : pineal eye.
P.R. : pineal recess.
P.S. : pineal sac.
S.C.O. : subcommissural organ.
S.O.C. : supraoccipital cartilage.

series of secondary neurones ; these form one, two, or three optic ganglia which connect the retinal ganglion with the supra-œsophageal ganglion or fore-brain. Intermediate conditions are found between the more primitive and less specialized types in which only one optic ganglion is present, as in Branchipus, and the more highly evolved genera such as *Astacus*, in which three are present.

In the median eyes (parietal or entomostracan) the development of the placodes does not extend beyond the one-layered simple type of retina, and in some the visual layer becomes inverted and the placodes of opposite sides become fused in the median plane.

[1] See reference, p. 262.

24

G. H. Parker, in his description of the eyes of scorpions (1886), made some important observations on their mode of development and of the changes which take place in the relation of the fibres of the optic nerve

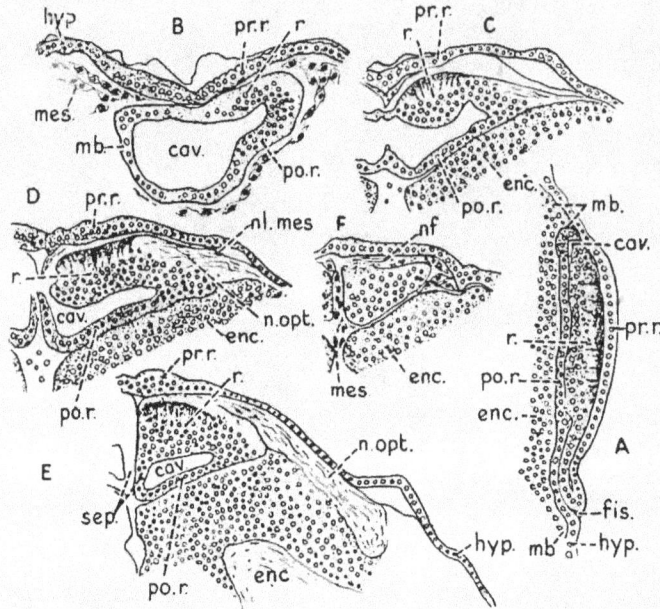

FIG. 253.—SECTIONS ILLUSTRATING THE DEVELOPMENT OF THE MEDIAN EYES OF A SCORPION. (AFTER G. H. PARKER.)

A—Right face of an approximately vertical section of a young embryo. The lower part of the section is in the median plane ; the upper part is slightly to the right of the median plane. The opening of the cavity has commenced and is seen at the upper part of the fissure. The retina is inverted, its morphologically superficial surface being situated on its deep aspect and directed towards the brain, from which it is separated by the post-retinal layer.

B, C, D, E, F—Transverse sections at successively higher levels, through the same region of a slightly older embryo, when the cavity has been fully opened out. It shows the division of the stem of the Y-shaped cavity into two limbs, which constitute the cavities of the right and left median eyes. It also shows the emergence of the fibres of the optic nerve from the superficial aspect of the retina. In the adult scorpion this relation is reversed.

cav. : cavity.	*n.f.* : nerve-fibres.
enc. : brain.	*nl. mes.* : nucleus of mesoderm cell.
fis. : lower end of cleft-like fissure beneath the fold forming the retina and pre-retina.	*n. opt.* : optic nerve.
	po. r. : post-retina.
	pr. r. : pre-retina.
hyp. : hypodermis.	*r.* : retina.
mb. : basement membrane.	*sep.* : septum.
mes. : mesoderm.	

in the transitional period between the larva and the fully developed animal. He also made some interesting comparisons between the median and the lateral eyes. He noted that the median eyes are situated close to the sagittal plane a little in front of the centre of the shield ; they are two in number and always symmetrically placed. The lateral eyes form two isolated groups one on either side at the edge of the shield, where its anterior border meets its lateral margin. In different genera the number of eyes in each group varies from two to seven. Two kinds of lateral eyes can be distinguished, the larger or "principal" and the smaller or "accessory." No essential difference exists between these two groups. As in the spiders, the vitreous and retinal layers are separate (Fig. 251). These apparently two-layered eyes were described by Lankester and Bourne as diplostichous. Locy and Patten, however, recognized that these eyes are in reality three layered or triplostichous. Patten (1886) also claimed that the median eyes of scorpions were formed from a cup-like involution of the ectoderm. Parker fully confirmed

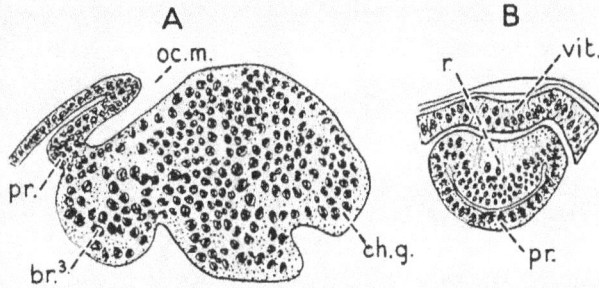

FIG. 254.—A—SECTION THROUGH EARLY STAGE OF ONE OF THE DEVELOPING MEDIAN EYES OF AGELENA. B—SECTION THROUGH A LATER STAGE OF A DEVELOPING MEDIAN EYE. (AFTER KISHINOUYE.)

br.[3] : third lobe of brain.
ch. g. : cheliceral ganglion.
oc. m. : mouth of ocellar pit of median eye.

pr. : post-retinal layer.
r. : retina.
vit. : vitreous.

these earlier observations, and showed that inversion of the retina takes place during the development of the median eyes of the scorpion, *Centrurus*, as has been demonstrated in the median eyes of the spider *Agelena* by Locy and Kishinouye (Fig. 254, A), but in the scorpion the two optic pits or sacs are united by a common stalk (Fig. 253, B, C, D, E, p. 370), whereas in the spider they appear as independent involutions. In the scorpion the fibres of the optic nerve arise at first from the superficial surface of the retinal layer (Fig. 253, D, E, F), and pass out beneath the superficial layer of the fold of ectoderm which covers the retina (Fig. 253, A, *pr.r.* and F, *n.f.*). This superficial layer of the fold is known as the pre-retinal layer, and gives rise to the vitreous or lentigen stratum. During the later stages of development there is little change in the point of exit of the fibres of the optic nerve ; it simply shifts from the embryonic postero-lateral position to the postero-ventral position of the adult. There is, however, a very important and significant change in the course of the intracapsular fibres, which apparently shift from an attachment at the outer ends of the retinal cells to the inner or deep ends of these cells, which is the position they occupy in the adult. The migration of the fibres takes place at the same time that the nuclei recede into the deeper parts of the eye, and seems to be controlled by the growth of the rhabdomeres. The exact process by which the change from the inverted embryonic position of the retina to the final adult position takes place are still obscure ; but it is quite clear that as a result of the involution of the retinal area its morphologically deep surface, from which the nerve-fibres primarily arise, becomes turned towards the light, and that its originally superficial surface, in which the clear refractile rods become developed in upright eyes, is in the early larval stages turned away from the light. This apparently anomalous condition is changed during the later stages of development, so that eventually the nerve-fibres are found leaving the deep ends of the retinal cells, and in the adult animal the rods or rhabdomeres are pre-nuclear and directed towards the light. It is also certain that the retinas of both median and lateral eyes are strictly hypodermal in origin and not neural. Owing to the manner in which the involution takes place the median eye is of the three-layered, tri-plostichous type, the superficial layer of the hypodermis or pre-retina giving rise to the vitreous body and cuticular lens ; the middle layer forming the inverted retina and the third or deep layer forming the sclera, which becomes intimately fused with the retina. The retina contains two kinds of cells, the visual or neuro-sensory cells and pigment cells. Pigment is also contained in the neuro-sensory cells. The walls of these cells develop pre-nuclear rhabdomeres, and a nerve-fibre emerges from their deep ends.

Parker draws the following conclusions with regard to the adaptive structural changes which follow the inversion of the retina in the median eyes of scorpions and spiders : " The striking similarity in the structure and development of the median eyes of scorpions and the median eyes of spiders has already been indicated. In both cases the retina by a process of involution has become inverted. The question whether the retina was functional during the involution of the eye was answered in the affirmative by the phases noted in the development of the optic nerve. At least the fact that the fibres of the optic nerve are at first attached to the morpho-logical deep ends of the retinal cells, and only at a later date come to emerge from the opposite end, is most easily explainable on the sup-position that the retina was functional before involution. The primitive eye would then consist of a single layer of retinal cells, from the deep ends of which the nerve-fibres emerge. Admitting that in the ancestral eye the rhabdomes were in their usual position, namely, at the outer end of each retinal cell, an inversion of the retina would not only place the optic fibres on the front face of the retina, but the rhabdomeres would come to occupy the deep ends of the cells. The prenuclear rhabdomeres of the median eyes in scorpions must then be secondary structures, developed in such a way as to replace functionally the older post-nuclear structures. The sphæospheres, as Mark has suggested, may represent the remains of post-nuclear rhabdomeres. These are then to be regarded as disappearing, and the fact that in some species of scorpions they are present while in others they are absent, would favour this view."

" The possible relation of the median eyes to the lateral eyes in scorpions has already suggested itself, for in pointing out the probable

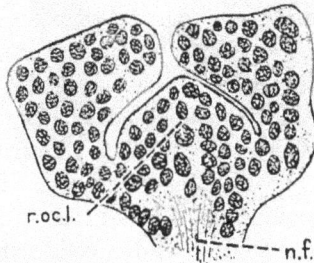

FIG. 255.—SECTION THROUGH ONE OF THE DEVELOPING LATERAL EYES OF A SPIDER, AGELENA. (AFTER KISHINOUYE.)

The retina is upright, and the nerve-fibres issue from the base of the retinal papilla.

    n.f : nerve-fibres.   *r. oc. l.* : retina of lateral eye.

nature of the phylogenetic antecedent of the median eyes a condition has been implied which agrees with the essential features of the lateral eyes. Of all the eyes in spiders and scorpions, the lateral eyes in scorpions are undoubtedly the least complicated, and they may be looked upon as deviating least from the ancestral type."

These considerations, taken in connection with papers published by Mark (1887) and Patten (1889) on the mode of development of the eyes of *Apus, Branchipus*, spiders, and scorpions, provide a clear explanation of the means by which a pre-retinal cellular and cuticular lens are formed in continuity with a retinal and post-retinal layer, by a simple folding of the hypodermis in such a way that the developing eye appears in transverse section as an S-shaped bend (Fig. 254, A : compare Fig. 255, which shows the position of the nerve-fibres in the upright lateral eyes of the spider *Agelena*). The middle segment of the bend is inverted and becomes the retina, and when the visual cells become differentiated their outer ends, which give rise to the rods and which were primarily directed towards the surface, become deep; whereas their inner ends, which terminate in nerve-fibres, become superficial and lie in contact with the cellular or vitreous lens which is developed as a modification of the ordinary hypodermal cells where they cover the retinal layer. The lower limb of the S-shaped bend or post-retinal layer, may become condensed so as to form a protective capsule (Fig. 251) or it may become pigmented. Further, as described by Parker in the later stages of development of the median eyes of scorpions (and spiders), the reversal of the cell-elements caused by the infolding of the retina is corrected by migration of the nerve-fibres to the deep surface of the retina and the development of secondary rods at the primarily inner ends of the cells, which as a result of the inversion are now superficial.

We shall see later that the same processes which occur in the development of certain invertebrate eyes also take place in the evolution and development of vertebrate eyes. With certain modifications as regards details, there are to be noted a similar infolding of the ectoderm and inclusion of the optic plates within the neural tube; there is also a similar differentiation of the retinal ectoderm into dioptric, receptive, and pigment cells (Fig. 256; and Fig. 10, Chap. 3, p. 15). There is, moreover, the same migration of cell-elements or their nuclei within the retina, and a similar connection of the visual receptive cells with the cortex of the brain by means of nerve ganglia and intervening plexiform bands or tracts of nerve-fibres.

In a work limited to the study of the morphology of the pineal organ it would be inexpedient to do more than allude to the controversial points which have been raised in the past by such authors as Patten and Gaskell in relation to the important bearing which it has on the whole problem of the evolution of vertebrates. But in this discussion on the relation of the median and lateral eyes of vertebrates and invertebrates, it is necessary that the reader should have a concise statement of these views in order that he may judge for himself the principles that are concerned in coming to a decision on this complex biological problem, and which we shall endeavour to summarize in our concluding chapter.

We propose in the first place to give a summary in his own words of some of the more important views of Patten on the parietal eye of vertebrates, which, as we have already stated, he regards as homologous with the median eyes of the Entomostraca.

1. " In vertebrates we recognize as belonging to the forebrain the median or parietal eyes, the lateral eyes, and the olfactory organs. At an early embryonic period they lie on the outer margins of the open neural plate in similar positions to the ones they occupy in arthropods.

2. " *The parietal eye :* there are probably two pairs of ocellar placodes that for a short time occupy this marginal position (Fig. 257). Later they are caught in the pallial overgrowth and carried on the inner limb of the closing neural crests to the median line. There they form a group of one, two, or three placodes lying in the membranous roof of the brain. During or after the closing of the cerebral vesicle the brain roof is evaginated at the place where the ocelli are located, thus forming a sac or

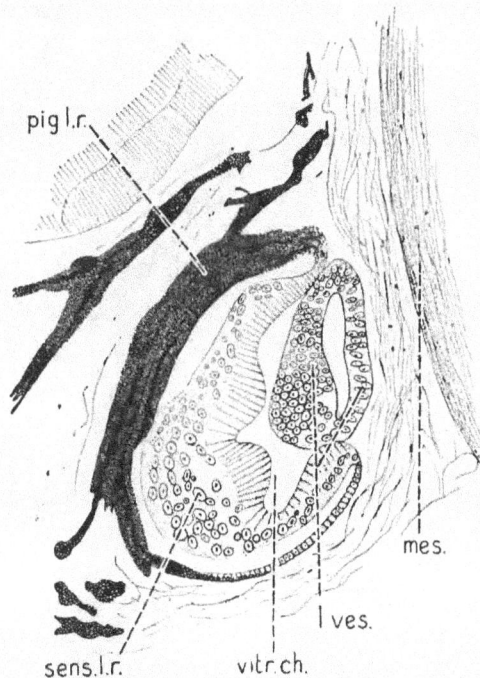

FIG. 256.—SECTION THROUGH A DEVELOPING LATERAL EYE OF AMMOCŒTES, SHOWING THE INVERSION OF THE OPTIC CUP ; AND THE LENS VESICLE, SUPERFICIAL TO WHICH IS A THICK LAYER OF MESENCHYME. (AFTER BEARD.)

l. ves. : lens vesicle.	*sens. l.r. :* sensory layer of retina.
mes. : mesodermal layer of cornea.	*vitr. ch. :* vitreous chamber.
pig. l.r. : pigment layer of retina.	

tube in the blind end of which the ocellar placodes lie. The development is essentially like that of the parietal eye of *Limulus* and the scorpion. This fact demonstrates that the parietal eye of crustaceans and arachnids is a true cerebral eye in the vertebrate sense, and is identical with the eye of vertebrates.

3. " *The lateral eyes of vertebrates :* these represent the compound or convex eyes of arthropods that have been transferred to the interior of the cerebral vesicle. In the arthropods the lateral eyes lie near the margin of the cephalic lobes on the outer edge of a deep ganglionic infolding.

In invertebrates they are seen in a very similar position on the lateral margin of the open medullary plate. Later they are swept into the infolding brain, turning the retinas inside out. They then grow out laterally on the end of membranous tubes in much the same manner as the median eyes. In arthropods the lateral eyes usually have a crescentic or kidney-shaped outline ; in vertebrates this shape is retained, giving the retinas their characteristic crescentic outline during the early stages. When the two limbs of the crescent unite a circular retina is produced, giving rise to the choroid fissure and the centrally located optic nerve, that, together with the inverted rods and cones, have long been such inexplicable features of the lateral eyes of vertebrates.

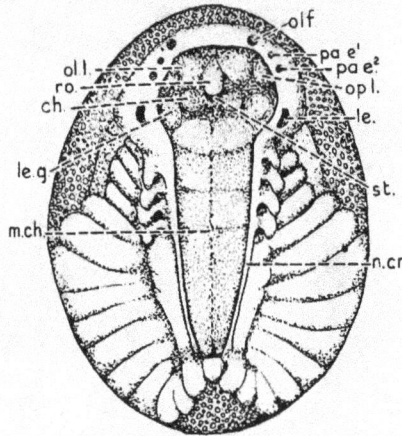

FIG. 257.—EMBRYO SPIDER. (AFTER PATTEN.)

Showing the primary position of the olfactory placodes, *olf.*, the parietal eye placodes, *pa.e¹*, and *pa.e²*, and the lateral eye placodes, *le.* These are situated on the edge of the neural crest, *n. cr.*

ch. : cheliceral ganglion.	*op. l.* : optic lobe.
le. g. : lateral eye ganglion.	*ro.* : rostrum.
m. ch. : median chord.	*st.* : stomodæum.
ol. l. : olfactory lobe.	

4. " *The parietal eye :* all vertebrates possess remnants more or less distinct of a median or parietal eye, which in some forms contains true retinal cells and visual rods, and is connected by several (? four) distinct nerves with as many ganglia.

5. " There is but one median or parietal eye, consisting, however, of several parts.

6. " The eye proper consists of three or four sensory placodes, each one representing the retina of a simple ocellus of the arthropod type. The placodes form the walls of a sac on the end of a membranous tube projecting from the roof of the ' tween-brain.'

7. " The placodes have a paired arrangement and probably represent two pairs of ocelli, located originally in the ectoderm just outside the lateral margins of the open medullary plate.

8. " They were ultimately forced into or carried into the brain chamber by the same forces which produced the brain infolding. The placodes are carried on the crest of the brain, infolding towards the median line, meanwhile shifting from the outer to the inner limb of the fold (Fig. 246, p. 349). When the crests unite, the four placodes form a compact group on the membranous roof of the brain. At that point a tubular outgrowth of varying length is formed, which has a vesicle or dilatation at its distal end, in the walls of which the placodes lie (Figs. 247,

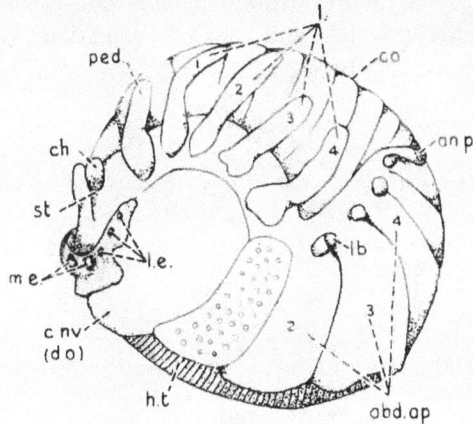

FIG. 258.—EMBRYO SPIDER SEEN FROM THE SIDE, SHOWING THE POSITION OF THE PLACODES WHICH WILL GIVE RISE TO THE MEDIAN AND THE LATERAL EYES. (AFTER PATTEN.)

abd. ap. : 2, 3, 4 : abdominal appendages.	*l.* 1, 2, 3, 4 : legs.
an. pl. : anal plate.	*l. b.* : lung book.
ch. : chelicera.	*l. e.* : lateral eyes.
c. nv. : cephalic navel (do. dorsal organ).	*m. e.* : median eyes.
co. : commissure.	*ped.* : pedipalp.
ht. : heart.	*st.* : stomodæum.

p. 350, and 248, p. 360). This vesicle with its four placodes is the parietal eye. The primary vesicle may now be constricted, forming two unpaired lobes, or the lobes may separate, forming two separate sacs, a larger anterior and outer one, the ' ectoparietal eye,' containing the two most highly developed placodes, and an inner posterior one or ' entoparietal ' eye containing the remaining two placodes completely united into one organ and with greatly reduced structural details.

9. " The membranous tube or epiphysis may disappear in whole or in part, leaving the terminal eye-sacs either isolated or united by distinct nerves with the parietal eye-ganglia or habenular ganglia (Fig. 250, p. 362).

10. " The parietal eye of vertebrates is homologous with the parietal

eye of such arthropods as *Limulus,* scorpions, spiders, phyllopods, copepods, trilobites, and merostomes, but not with the frontal stemmata or
other ocelli of insects.

11. " In the arthropods various stages in the evolution of a cerebral
eye are shown in detail, from functionless eyes on the outer margin of
the cephalic lobes to a median group of ocelli enclosed within a tubular
outgrowth of the brain roof.

12. " The most primitive type of a parietal eye is shown in the nauplii
of phyllopods and Entomostraca, where the eye is a pear-shaped sac
opening by a median pore or tube on the outer surface of the head (Fig.
247, p. 350). In the higher arachnids the process of forming an eye vesicle
is merged with the process of forming a cerebral vesicle, the external
opening of the forebrain vesicle and that of the parietal tube forming a
common opening or neuropore.

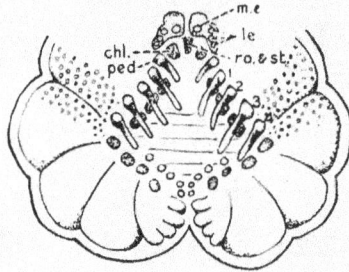

FIG. 259.—ANTERIOR AND VENTRAL ASPECT OF AN EMBRYO SPIDER, SHOWING
THE POSITION OF THE MEDIAN (PARIETAL) EYES AND THE LATERAL EYES.
(AFTER PATTEN.)

chl. : chelicera.	*ped. :* pedipalp.
l.e. : lateral eyes.	*ro. & st. :* rostrum and stomodæum.
m.e. : median eye.	1, 2, 3, 4 : first to fourth legs.

13. " The parietal eye of arthropods is an important visual organ
until the lateral eyes which represent a later product are fully developed.
It may then diminish in size and in activity, but it rarely if ever wholly
disappears.

14. " During the evolution of vertebrates from arachnids there was
a considerable period during which the lateral eyes were adjusting themselves to their new position inside the brain chamber, when they were in
functional abeyance. At this period ancestral vertebrates were monoculate,
that is, they were dependent solely on the parietal eye, which had come to
them from their arachnid ancestors as an efficient and completely formed
organ. When the lateral eyes again became functional the parietal eye
began to decrease in size and effectiveness.

15. " The parietal eye is the only one now present in tunicates (Fig.
260). In the oldest ostracoderms, like *Pteraspis, Cyathaspis, Palæaspis,*

the lateral eyes are absent or at least do not reach the surface of the head ; the functional one being the parietal eye, which is of unusual size.

16. " In the lampreys we see the same conditions, the parietal eye being well developed in the larvæ, while the lateral eyes are deeply buried in the tissues of the head and are useless. During the transformation the lateral eyes again become functional and the parietal eye begins to atrophy, finally losing many of its structural details and its function, although still retaining very nearly its original form."

From this brief summary of some of the more important observations and conclusions relating to the morphology of the parietal eye of vertebrates and of the parietal eyes of the Entomostraca, it will be obvious that

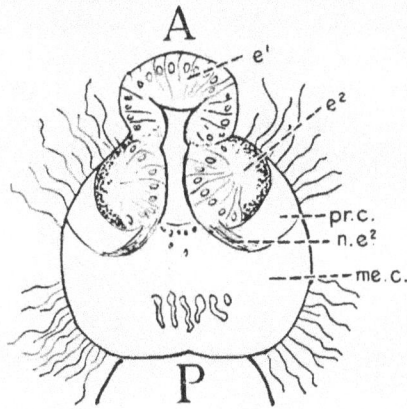

FIG. 260.—VENTRAL CORD AND OCELLI OF ADULT CYCLOSALPA. SEEN FROM NEURAL SURFACE. (AFTER PATTEN.)

A. : anterior end.
e^1, e^2 : anterior and posterior ocelli.
me. c. : mesocephalon.

$n.e.^2$: nerve of posterior ocellus.
P. : posterior end.
pr. c. : procephalon.

Patten believed not only that there was a close connection between the arthropod stock and the Ostracodermi but that the vertebrate phylum actually originated from arachnids (p. 378, para 14). Further, it is clear that he believed the evidence afforded by his observations on the parietal eyes in the two groups strongly supported this conclusion which he had come to from his extensive study of eyes in general and of other systems and organs in various classes of invertebrate animals, of which we may specially mention that of the eyes of *Acilius, Vespa, Pecten,* and *Arca.* This material, taken along with that afforded by other pioneer workers such as Reichenbach, Huxley, Grenacher, Bertkau, and Lowne, and more recent writers on the Palæozoic fishes and merostomata, provides a basis for more accurate generalizations on the main principles which are concerned in the evolution of the different types of eye, and of evolution in general, than it was at the close of the nineteenth century. It is, we believe, now more generally appreciated that many of the striking similarities which undoubtedly exist in certain of the more highly differentiated animals which belong to otherwise dissimilar or divergent classes are not necessarily to be regarded as evidence of a close relationship between these classes; and that if the environmental conditions remain similar, functioning organs which are well adapted to their environment and requirements may continue with little change for immensely long periods of time. While, on the other hand, differences such as exist between the more highly differentiated types of the principal phyla and classes also require an immensely long period of time to evolve. Moreover, the differences which constitute class distinctions were in many cases already established in the earliest known fossil representatives of the classes concerned, e.g. to take a concrete instance, between the Merostomes and Ostracodermi. This indicates that the period in which the hypothetical common ancestral stock existed must have extended many ages further back than that of which we have definite geological evidence.

CHAPTER 25

THE HUMAN PINEAL ORGAN

Development and Histogenesis

THE stages in development of the derivatives of the primary ependymal elements of the brain and spinal cord, which we have described in Chapter 22, are of great importance in connection with the study of the structure of the fully developed pineal body. In the early phases of development it was shown by Cajal that the ependymal cells extend through the whole thickness of the wall of the neural tube, as is seen in Golgi preparations of the chick embryo at the third day of incubation. At a later stage, when the width of the neural tube has increased, there is a tendency for the central part or body of the cell, which contains the nucleus, to separate from its attachment to either the internal or the external limiting membrane, or it may lose its connection with both of these membranes. In the latter case the cell is said to be liberated, and it may form a branched neuroglial cell of the astrocyte or oligodendric type. In those cases in which the attachment of the inner end of the cell element to the internal limiting membrane is retained, the cell may develop into a definitive ependymal cell, lining either the central canal of the spinal cord or a ventricle of the brain (Fig. 261, *a*), whereas if the internal connection is lost (Fig. 261, *c*) and the cell body remains anchored to the external limiting membrane or to the glial membrane covering the pial sheath of vessels penetrating the substance of the brain or spinal cord, the cell may differentiate into a subpial astrocyte, e.g. the cells or fibres of Bergmann, in the molecular layer of the cerebellum, or into a fixed " vascular " astrocyte, as contrasted with the free unattached type, which appears to be connected by its processes with those of neighbouring astrocytes. Besides these three principal types, intermediate forms are frequent : thus, one large process of an astrocyte provided with an expanded foot-plate may preserve its attachment to the sheath of a vessel, while the other small branched processes appear in Golgi preparations to end in free extremities.

There is, however, a considerable amount of doubt as to whether the apparent continuity of the neuroglial cell-elements is a true uninterrupted connection of one glial cell with another, since many of the modern neurologists hold the view that both the glial cells and the nerve cells are independent units. The discussion of this interesting and fundamentally important problem presents many difficulties, and we do not propose to enter into the question here, since, apart from its general bearing on the structure of nervous tissue, it does not specially affect the study of the pineal organ ; for, whether the processes of the glial cells are merely in contact or are continuous with each other, there seems to be a functional continuity in the framework as far as support is concerned.

At this point it will be necessary to refer to the view which was originally taken by His with respect to the origin of neuroglia cells and neuroblasts. He believed that the medullary plate is primarily formed

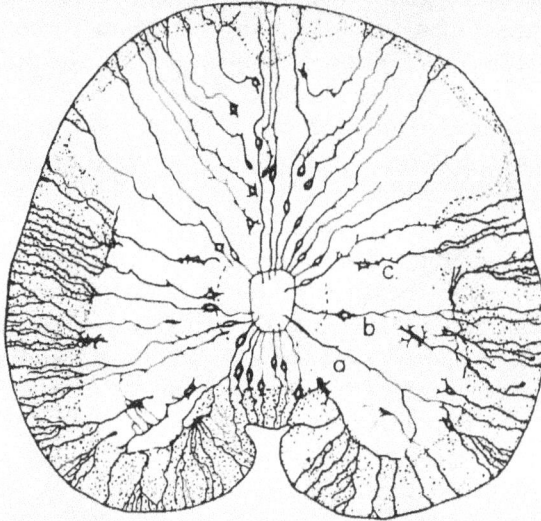

FIG. 261.—TRANSVERSE SECTION THROUGH THE SPINAL CORD OF A TEN-DAY CHICK EMBRYO, SHOWING THE SUPPORTING CELLS. (AFTER LENHOSSÉK, 1895.)

a. : ependymal cell.
b. : supportive spongioblast.
c. : astroblast, or displaced epithelial cells.

of undifferentiated cells which give rise to " germinal cells " and " spongioblasts." The former in his opinion gave rise to neuroblasts and ultimately to nerve cells, whereas the spongioblasts developed into the supporting neuroglial tissue and ependyma. The germinal cells or the cells next the internal limiting membrane which are undergoing mitosis give rise to two daughter cells, both of which, he thought, migrated outward through the spongioblasts into the mantle zone, where they could be distinguished by their large size and pale vesicular nucleus, and were spoken of as " neuroblasts." Schaper, in 1897, contended that the germinal cells gave origin to both neuroblasts and spongioblasts, and that the indifferent cells which resulted from their division were capable of producing either neuroglia cells or nerve cells even after the outward migration of the indifferent cells from the internal limiting membrane had already occurred. Whether an actual migration of whole cells takes place or simply an outward movement of the nucleus along a protoplasmic strand which has grown out as a process from the body of the cell is a much debated question, but we are inclined to believe that the latter alternative is the correct interpretation of the changed position of the nuclei. The migration by amœboid movements of microglial cells has, however, been definitely proved and recorded on cinematograph films.

It has been demonstrated by Cajal that at an early period of embryonic life the spongioblasts send out a process which on reaching the external limiting membrane expands into a conical swelling or foot-plate, while the inner end, retaining its attachment to the internal limiting membrane, develops one or more processes resembling cilia which project into the central canal or a ventricle of the brain (Fig. 223, Chap. 22, p. 322, and Fig. 261). The foot-plate at the outer end is in relation with the vessels of the pia mater outside the external limiting membrane, and it is believed that it serves to absorb material from the blood for the nourishment of the nerve tissue, for in the earlier stages of development the latter does not possess the rich blood supply which it has in late embryonic stages and in fœtal life. In these later stages, when the central area of the nerve tissue has become vascularized, foot-plates are developed on those processes of the neuroglia cells which come into relation with the sheaths of ingrowing vessels (Fig. 220, p. 318), and it is said that with further evolution there is a tendency for the sub-pial expansions to disappear and eventually for the attachment of the inner end of the cell to the internal limiting membrane to be lost. Branched lateral processes from the body of the cell have in the meantime been developed, and eventually one or more thick processes of the cell which have become attached by a foot-plate to the sheath of a vessel constitute what are known as its vascular processes, while the others, namely, the dendritic processes, either end freely or communicate with similar processes of adjoining neuroglia cells. The foot-plates on the vascular processes of the neuroglia cells are somewhat like the club-shaped expansions of the parenchyma cells of the pineal body (Fig. 218, Chap. 22, p. 317), and it is possible that serving as points of attachment, the latter have the same function as the foot-plates, namely, that of absorbing nourishment from the blood circulating in the vessel to which the expansion is attached.

In both neuroglial and pineal parenchyma cells the terminal expansions are frequently conical or trumpet-shaped, but the expansions of the neuroglial processes more often have the form of flat oval plates applied to the surface of the vascular sheath (Fig. 262), whereas the ends of the processes of the pineal cells are more typically club-shaped and the cells usually give off several processes each of which terminates in an expansion.

At a later period of fœtal development, and especially at about the

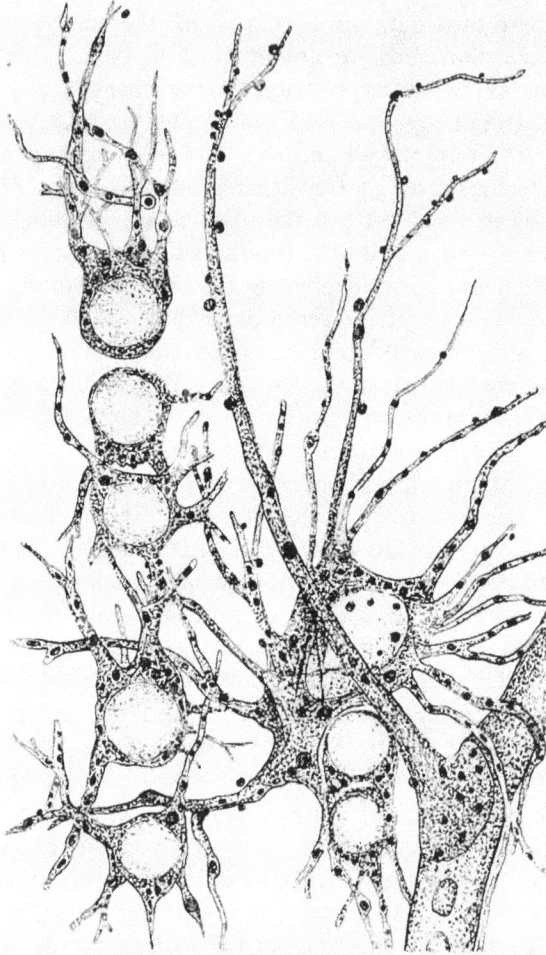

FIG. 262.—FOOTPLATE OF NEUROGLIAL CELL ATTACHED TO SHEATH OF BLOOD VESSEL : RABBIT. (AFTER PENFIELD.)

The drawing shows two rows of cells of the oligodendroglia type ; these are situated between myelinated fibres of the cerebral white matter. One large fibrous astrocyte is seen above two oligodendroglial cells. Gliosomes stained by the method of Del Rio-Hortega are seen in relation with the cell-bodies and processes of both types of cell.

time of birth, small cells with few and slender processes are developed between the medullated fibres of the white matter in the brain and spinal cord. These are termed oligodendrocytes, and their small round nuclei, lying in rows between parallel nerve-fibres, have long been recognized in specimens stained with the ordinary nuclear dyes such as iron hæmatoxylin. The appearance of these small cells in rows between the nerve-fibres is strongly suggestive of multiplication by amitotic division, more especially as mitotic figures are not often seen at this stage of development and the nuclei frequently lie in pairs. It also seems possible that they represent a modified or immature form of astrocyte rather than a distinct type, the modification from the usual astrocyte form into the interfascicular type of cell found in the white matter being due to the presence of the medullated white fibres, which limit the expansion and formation of processes in certain directions. The existence of transitional forms between the oligodendrocytes and the astrocytes among the cells in the aforementioned rows is an additional point in favour of this interpretation. Oligodendrocytes are also found in relation with large nerve-cells, such as those in the anterior cornua of the spinal cord and the pyramidal cells of the cortex cerebri (Fig. 263). These are often spoken of as satellite cells or perineuronal cells, whereas the oligodendrocytes found between the medullated nerve-fibres of the white matter in the brain and spinal cord are known as interfascicular cells. The small round granules lying in or on the processes of both types of oligodendrocyte which are termed gliosomes are believed to be concerned in the formation of the myelin sheath of nerve-fibres, and the relation of the perineuronal and interfascicular oligodendrocytes to the nerve cells and nerve-fibres suggests an homology of the oligodendrocytes of the central nervous system with the ganglionic capsular cells and the cells of the sheath of Schwann in the peripheral nervous system. The small branched cells with acidophil granules which are found in relation with the parenchyma cells of the pineal body possibly represent oligodendrocytes in this organ.

The mode of development of neuroglial fibres and the question of the existence of an intercellular substance we shall discuss later in the description of the structure of the normal pineal organ and the changes which it undergoes in disease or as a result of involution, but, as we have thought it advantageous to allude to some of the characteristic features of neuroglial tissue in the central nervous system before entering on the description of the pineal organ itself, so also we think that it will be profitable to discuss now the structure and some of the principal modifications of the normal ependyma of the brain and spinal cord, and the changes which it undergoes in disease or as a result of degeneration.

In the fully developed pineal organ the definitive ependyma is limited to the cells lining the pineal recess, but under certain conditions remnants of the original ependymal lining of the primary cavity of the pineal diverticulum or of its secondary outgrowths may persist as the lining

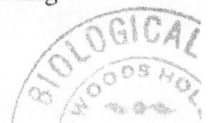

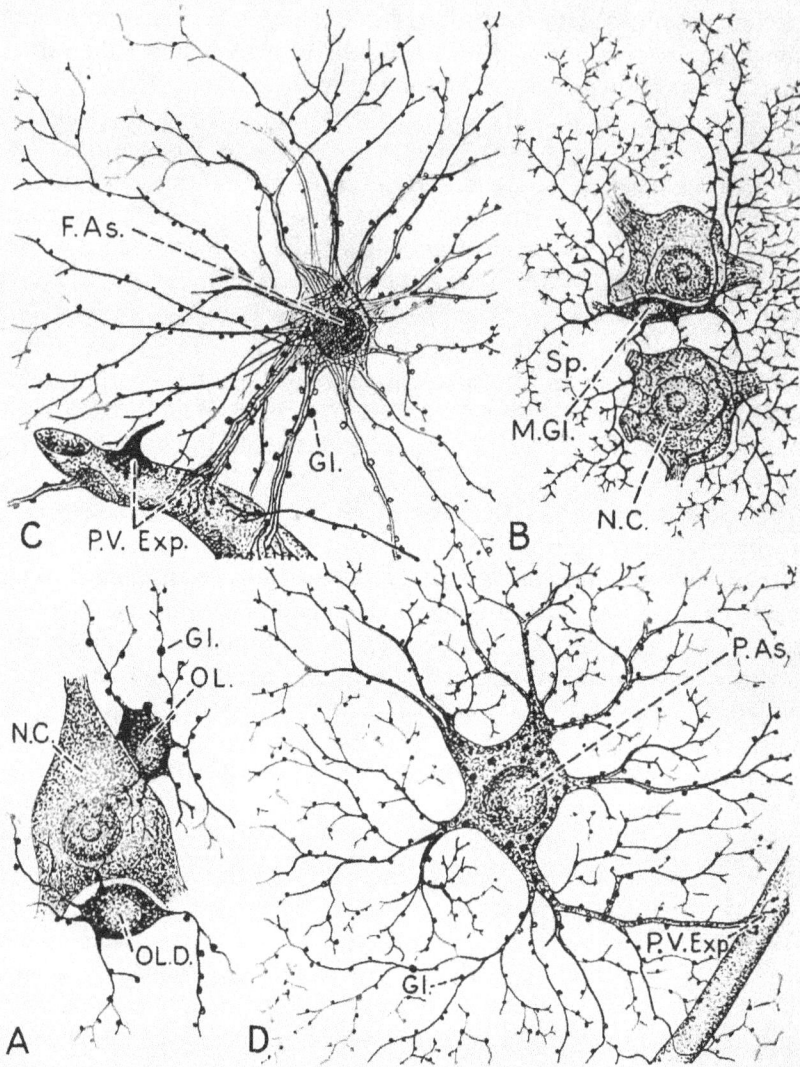

FIG. 263.

A—Oligodendrocytes in relation with pyramidal cell of cerebral cortex : human.
B—Microglial cell, in relation with nerve-cell of grey matter. C—Fibrous
astrocyte, showing perivascular feet and gliosomes. D—Protoplasmic
astrocyte, also showing perivascular expansions and gliosomes.

F. As. : fibrous astrocyte.	*OL., OL.D.* : oligodendrocytes.
Gl. : gliosome.	*P. As.* : protoplasmic astrocyte.
M. Gl. : microglial cell (mesoglia).	*P.V. Exp.* : perivascular expansion.
N.C. : nerve cell.	*Sp.* : spines.

(After Penfield and Cone, redrawn from Cowdry's *Special Cytology*.)

membrane of one type of pineal cyst, and it seems possible that even after the full development of the organ has been attained and all traces of the original cavity have disappeared, certain cells which resemble the embryonic spongioblasts or primary ependymal cells retain the power of differentiating into either ependyma or neuroglia. This supposition may also apply to the development of ependymal cells lining the cavities in certain cases of syringomyelia, but when epithelium is found lining cysts in the pineal body or the cavities in the grey matter of the spinal cord it is usually of an irregular type—pseudo-ependymal—and the typical ependyma of the tall columnar form is seldom seen. The variations which occur in the normal ependyma and choroidal epithelium of the ventricles and central canal of the spinal cord are very considerable. These changes in the structure and form of the epithelium are related to varying mechanical and other conditions which are present in different parts of the brain and spinal cord. Thus the lining epithelium may be modified in one situation to form a sensory epithelium, e.g. the retina of the lateral eyes, and in another to form a secretory organ, as in the choroidal epithelium of the ventricles ; and since ependyma enters largely into the composition of the pineal organ as a whole, we propose to give a short summary of the morphology and functions of the ependyma in general, with the view of gaining a better insight into the structure and possible functions of this tissue as it occurs in the epiphysis of mammals. The morphology of the ependyma has been specially studied by Agduhr and Studnička, and the following brief note is largely based on Agduhr's account of the ependyma in Penfield's *Cytology of the Nervous System.*

The ependyma is seen in its simplest form in the central nervous system of *Amphioxus* and of cyclostomes, in which the supporting tissue of the central nervous system is said to be wholly epithelial throughout life. The term " ependyma," as usually understood, is applied to the epithelial lining of the ventricular cavities of the brain and central canal of the spinal cord, but in the embryonic condition in all vertebrates, before the development of nerve cells and nerve-fibres, it extends through the whole thickness of the wall of the neural tube and takes part in the formation of the internal and external limiting membranes. Later, when the differentiation of this wall into zones has taken place, the term " ependyma " is often applied to the inner zone, which consists of several layers of spongioblasts, or " primary ependymal cells." This inner zone at a later stage is seen to be further differentiated into the definitive ependyma, glioblasts or astroblasts, and neuroblasts. Still later, the supporting function of the neuroglial tissue is supplemented by the ingrowth of vessels with their connective tissue sheaths.

From the morphological standpoint it must be remembered also that the lining membrane of outgrowths from the cerebral vesicles is homologous with the ependyma, and thus the epithelial lining of the following parts is ependymal in origin : the olfactory lobes ; the optic vesicles, including the pigment and sensory layers of the retina ; the infundibulum of the hypophysis ; the choroidal epithelium ; the para-physis ; the epiphysis and the subcommissural organ ; also the lamina terminalis and the roof and floor-plates of the brain and spinal cord. The shape, the structure, and the function of the ependymal cells in these different situations varies. Thus the cells may be flattened, cubical, or columnar in form. They may be club-shaped, flask-shaped, or bottle-shaped. They may be specialized in form, as in the hexagonal pigment cells, or rod and cone cells of the retina ; they may be glandular in type, as in the choroidal epithelium or in the paraphysis. They are, in some situations, devoid of cilia, in others they possess well-defined cilia, having minute rod-like particles or blepharoplasts at their bases, and their free ends converging to a point from the wide basal or ventricular end of the cell. The cells may be close together or separated by an interval. The basal ends of the cells may be joined by intercellular bridges so as to form an internal limiting membrane or separated so that the spaces between the cells open into the ventricular cavities or central canal of the spinal cord.

Large intra- and inter-ependymal nerve cells have been demonstrated by Agduhr (1922) in the ependyma lining the central canal of the spinal cord in the human subject and in various mammalian animals. These cells frequently end in a club-shaped process which projects into the central canal and resembles the club-shaped projections of the sensory cells described by Dendy and Studnička in the parietal organ of cyclo-stomes and fishes. These cells have been beautifully demonstrated by the Nissl method of staining, and Agduhr has shown connections (synapses) between peripheral processes of intra-ependymal cells and the processes of cells lying in the nerve substance external to the ependyma.

The Functions of the Ependyma

These may be enumerated in the following order :
Generative.
Supporting.
Lining membrane for protection and limitation of the nerve-tissues.
Causation of currents in the cerebrospinal fluid by means of its cilia.
A membrane concerned in dialysis and filtration, or serving as a limiting barrier.

Secretory.

Pigment formation.

Special sense.

Receptive cells concerned in reflex mechanisms.

The generative capacity has already been referred to in connection with the differentiation from it of spongioblasts, neuroblasts, and the definitive ependyma, as has also the supportive character of the early ependymal elements. The limiting function of the definitive ependymal layer is, moreover, obvious, and the supposed action of the cilia in producing movement of the cerebrospinal fluid is well known. The special problems concerning dialysis, filtration, and the formation of a barrier to the passage of certain fluids or substances, whether normal or extraneous, into the cerebrospinal fluid are familiar to neurologists.

The secretory function of the modified ependymal epithelium which covers the choroidal plexuses is well established, and is definitely proved by inferences made in cases of obstruction to the outflow of cerebrospinal fluid from the ventricles and by direct observation of secretion of the fluid on the surface of the choroid plexus—in the human subject by Mott and Cushing, and in animals by Dandy and Blackfan. It is generally thought that the ependyma in other situations has a limited power of secretion of cerebrospinal fluid, but normally only to a very small extent. The question of the power of the ependymal cells to absorb cerebrospinal fluid has been studied by Nañagas and others. According to Nañagas a very small amount of cerebrospinal fluid may be absorbed through the ependyma lining the ventricles of the brain in normal animals (kittens), and evidence obtained from post-mortem examinations shows that obliteration of the lumen of the central canal of the spinal cord, which sometimes occurs in old age, is not followed by distension of the cana below the obstruction.

We have already considered the formation of pigment in the outer layer of the retina, in nerve tissues, and in the epidermis, and it will thus be only necessary to recall its frequent presence in the parenchyma cells and fibro-glial tissue of the pineal body : a condition which may be partly due to degenerative changes setting in at an early age, before degeneration has commenced in the nerve tissues as a whole, either as a result of disease or old age ; or it may in part be due to an hereditary trait, which has been preserved from the remote period when it may be inferred pigment was normally present in large quantity in the parietal sense-organ of our reptilian ancestors.

The possible function of the ependyma as a sensory layer containing receptive nerve-cells which are concerned in reflex action is strikingly suggested by Agduhr's demonstration of nerve cells in the ependyma lining the central canal of the spinal cord and brain stem in animals and the human subject. The existence of nerve cells in the ependyma which are connected by their peripheral processes with nerve cells in the adjacent grey matter suggests that impulses originating in the ependyma may be transmitted to ganglion cells in the grey matter of the spinal cord or brain stem. Whether the impulses are transferred to the cortex of the brain and give rise to a conscious sensation or not, it seems quite possible and even probable that they may originate reflex actions.

The function of the subcommissural organ, which is developed as a thickening of the ependyma below the posterior commissure and inferior peduncle of the pineal body (Fig. 185, B, p. 261), is not known, nor is that of Reissner's fibre, which is developed in relation with the subcommissural organ (Fig. 134, p. 188).

Microglia

Any investigation into the structure and pathology of an organ such as the pineal body, which is derived as an outgrowth from the central nervous system would be incomplete without a reference to the nature and origin of microglia as it occurs in the cerebrospinal system generally. The microglia or mesoglia is sometimes alluded to as the " third element " in the composition of nervous tissue. This name was originally given by Cajal (1913) to a group of small non-nervous elements which were afterwards differentiated by the special staining methods of Del Rio-Hortega into oligodendrocytes and microglia, the former neuroglial in nature, the latter mesodermal. Hortega accordingly proposed to restrict the application of the term " third element " to the microglia, and allocate the oligodendrocytes to the neuroglial constituents or " second element." Thus, of the three constituents of nerve tissue excluding the connective tissue and vessels, the " first element " comprises the nerve cells ; the " second element " the neuroglia, including both astrocytes and oligodendrocytes ; and the " third element " is represented by the microglia. The microglia cells are small branched elements with minute nuclei of irregular form which stain deeply by Nissl's method ; the ordinary nuclear dyes such as hæmatoxylin ; and the silver carbonate method of Del Rio-Hortega which also brings out clearly the cell-body and processes. The latter are irregular in form and size and are characterized by small thorn-like spines. The cells have phagocytic properties and are under certain conditions capable of amœboid movements. Thus, according to the descriptions of Hortega, during the migratory phase in the development of the microglia, throughout the nervous tissue, it consists of roundish cells with pseudopodia, the various shapes of which indicate the motility of the cells. " After this initial phase the cells become branched, and when they take up their positions in the tissue they have small dark nuclei, surrounded by scanty cytoplasm prolonged into two or more thin, wavy, branched processes beset with spines which end freely, that is, they are not anastomosed among themselves nor are they connected with the neuroglia elements." He also holds the view that in a broad sense the microglia of the central nervous system represents from the functional standpoint the reticulo-endothelium of mesodermal tissues. It has been known to fix certain colloids to phagocytose erythrocytes and cellular debris, and it is believed to be concerned in the elimination of substances resulting from metabolism and degeneration of nerve cells. Thus, it is found to participate actively in inflammatory and destructive processes involving the central nervous system, and as a result of the motility of the cells and their increase in size under pathological conditions they assume various forms, becoming rod-like, lamellar, or rounded in shape, and frequently contain fat granules.

Development of Microglia

The microglia, according to the description of Del Rio-Hortega, does not appear until the last period of embryonic life. In fœtuses at term and in new-born animals it is abundant both beneath the pia mater and spreading inward along the course of the vessels of the brain and cerebellum. It is developed later than the neuroglia, at the time when the vessels of the pia mater have reached their full development. The cells which give rise to the microglia are believed to be mesodermal in origin and are first visible immediately beneath the pia mater on the surface of the brain and spinal cord; they are found also in relation with the tela choroidea of the third ventricle below the corpus callosum and fornix, and also beneath the pia mater covering the white matter of the cerebral peduncles. It is also abundantly formed in connection with the vascular folds of the tela choroidea inferior and on the surface of the cerebellum.

Originating as a layer of rounded or flattened cells beneath the pia on the surface of the brain, the microglial cells afterwards develop pseudo-podia and migrate deeply into the substance of the white and grey matter, and eventually they reach the ependyma lining the ventricles or central canal of the spinal cord.

The cells beneath the pia are at first rounded, cuboidal, or flattened; they increase in size and develop irregular bulbous processes; later, when they reach their ultimate destination, they become fixed and dendrites are formed, on which later the characteristic spines are developed. The cells are said by Hortega to lie in the neuroglia, and their processes do not communicate with each other.

The nuclei in the early stages of development are easily visible in specimens stained with the ordinary nuclear dyes. They form two or three layers beneath the pia and resemble the nuclei of lymphocytes and proliferating endothelium, and in cases of injury or disease may be readily mistaken for these.

The microglia cells having attained their full development become " fixed " and are described as being in the resting condition. They are found throughout the nervous system in the grey and white matter, being, however, more abundant in the grey matter than in the white. It is probable that the normal number of cells is maintained during adult life by amitotic division of the nuclei, although mitotic figures have occasionally been seen (Del Rio-Hortega). Having reached their full development and entered the resting phase, in a fixed position, they may retrace their stages of development in reverse order ; the processes gradually thickening and becoming shorter, until they assume the form of pseudopodia, and the body becomes rounded. This process of devolution is seen in cases of injury to the brain, when the cells having assumed amœboid characters, migrate towards the focus of inflammation, hæmorrhage, or degeneration and there act as phagocytes, engulfing leucocytes, erythrocytes, and broken-down nerve tissue. Their function is, therefore, similar to that of leucocytes and the cell-elements of the reticulo-endothelium, and before the ordinary methods of staining were supplanted by the special methods of staining with silver carbonate, the appearances were interpreted as those of inflammation as it occurs elsewhere in the body generally and attended by the accumulation of leucocytes and proliferation of endothelium.

Relations of Microglia to Nerve-cells and Vessels

Microglial cells, like oligodendrocytes, are found as satellite cells of large neurones, such as the Purkinje cells of the cerebellar cortex. They may be associated either with the body of the cells or with its processes. They may be distinguished from oligodendrocytes by their small, deeply stained, and irregularly shaped nuclei and by the spines on their processes. Microglia cells are also found in relation with the adventitia of the vessels lying in the white or grey matter.

As might be expected, microglial cells are present in the retina and in the optic nerve, and they have been found in the fibrous plaques of the human pineal organ.

CHAPTER 26

STRUCTURE OF THE FULLY DEVELOPED HUMAN PINEAL ORGAN

As previously mentioned, the structure of the pineal body varies considerably at different ages and in different individuals, and like some other embryonic and infantile organs which develop up to a certain degree of perfection and then degenerate, e.g. the pronephros, the greater part of the mesonephros, and the thymus gland, the pineal body normally attains its maximum of development before the individual has reached maturity. This maximum, according to the general estimate, occurs somewhere between the ages of 5 and 7 years. Signs of degeneration are, however, frequently evident before this period, and the uniform alveolar appearance which is present in early infancy usually becomes less pronounced at the end of the second year, and signs of degeneration and replacement of parenchymal cells by fibroglial tissue are often seen in quite young children. The parenchymal tissue becomes surrounded by ingrowths of fibrovascular septa which are continuous externally with the capsule. These break up the parenchymal tissue into rounded lobes, as seen in Fig. 264, the pineal body of a child aged 5. This specimen may, however, be regarded as exceptional with regard to the age at which degenerative changes, accompanied by ingrowth of thick fibrovascular septa from the capsule, have taken place, and there are instances in which the uniform structure of the pineal organ present in the infant is retained even in advanced age. Speaking generally, however, it is commonly admitted that, although exceptions occur, there is an increase in the proportion that the fibroglial constituents have to the parenchyma from childhood onwards to old age. We shall, therefore, describe first the structure of the pineal organ as it appears in children between 3 and 6 years of age, in preference to commencing the description of the organ of adult individuals, in which both the parenchyma cells and the supporting tissue usually show signs of degeneration.

Besides variations in structure due to age changes there are differences in appearance which are brought out by different methods of preparation, and we propose, before dealing with the selective actions produced by the use of special methods of modern technique, to give a short description of the microscopic appearance of a section of the pineal gland of a child

5 years of age stained by the ordinary hæmatoxylin and eosin method. We shall then endeavour to interpret the appearances seen at this stage of development and in the organ of adult individuals by a reference to the earlier stages of embryonic and fœtal development and by the microscopic pictures brought out by the use of differential stains. The pineal organ at this stage is invested by a fibrovascular capsule, derived from the pia mater and lined internally by a glial stratum. This capsule sends trabeculæ containing blood-vessels into the substance of the gland. The trabeculæ pass inwards and partially surround the peripheral part of a branched system of lobules which primarily originate from the ependymal epithelium of the embryonic pineal diverticulum. The epithelial tissue of the lobules is, however, penetrated throughout by fine trabeculæ of intra-lobular connective tissue containing capillary blood-vessels. The lobular areas between the larger trabeculæ which grow inward from the capsule communicate with each other in the central part of the gland so that the lobules as a rule are not completely enclosed in separate compartments, but are continuous with a central mass of parenchymatous tissue which is more uniform in appearance than the lobulated peripheral zone. The lobules consist of a supporting glial tissue which has the character of a fibrillated sponge-work or reticulum enclosing clear intercommunicating spaces. Some of the spaces contain parenchyma cells with vesicular nuclei, while others appear empty. The reticulum is especially noticeable beneath the capsule and in relation with the larger trabeculæ. The cell-elements of the reticulum have the appearance of being continuous with each other, no intercellular septa or intervals ever being visible with the ordinary methods of preparation. The network thus seems to be formed

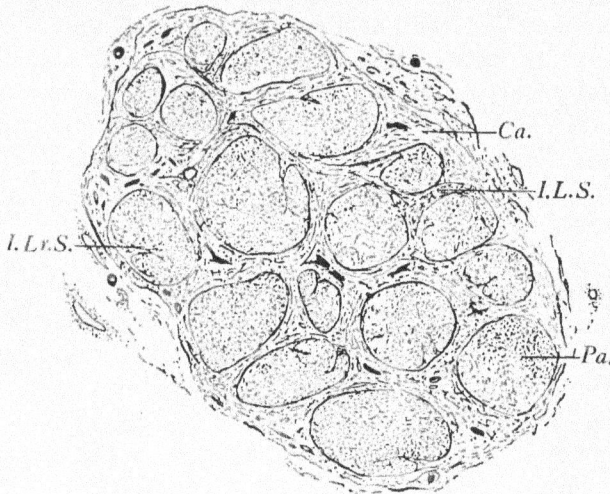

FIG. 264.—TANGENTIAL SECTION OF THE PINEAL GLAND OF A CHILD, SHOWING THE FIBROUS CAPSULE, LOBES, AND INTERLOBAR SEPTA. (R. J. G.)

Ca. : capsule.
I.L.S. : interlobular septum.
I.Lr. S. : intralobular septum.
P. : parenchyma.

of a plasmodium or spongioplasm within which the nuclei of the cell-elements are imbedded. In many of the spaces of the network branched parenchyma cells containing pale vesicular nuclei are present. The processes of these cells appear to be :

(1) Continuous with processes of similar adjacent cells.

(2) Continuous with the matrix of the general neurospongium.

(3) Spread out on the perivascular sheaths of the vessels contained in the trabeculæ or fibrous capsule.

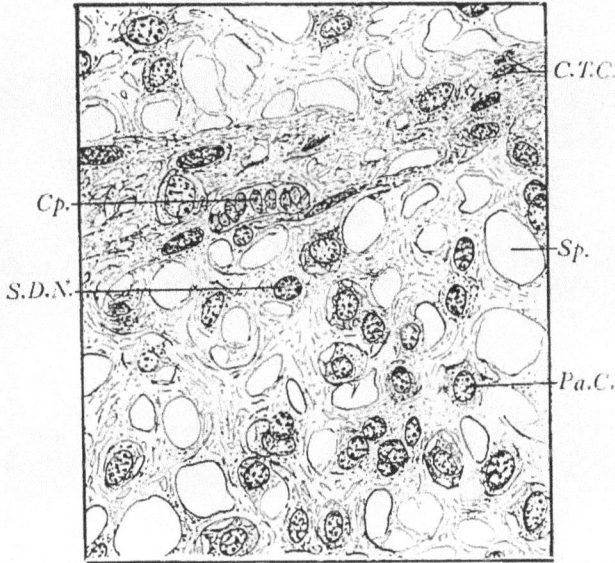

FIG. 265.—SECTION OF AN ADULT PINEAL GLAND STAINED BY VAN GIESON'S METHOD AND EOSIN, SHOWING THE APPARENT CONTINUITY OF THE RETICULUM IN WHICH THE PARENCHYMA CELLS ARE EMBEDDED ; AND ALSO THE RELATION OF THE PARENCHYMA CELLS TO THE SPACES OF THE RETICULUM AND THE SUPPORTING TISSUE OR NEUROSPONGIUM. AN INTERLOBULAR SEPTUM SHOWING CAPILLARY BLOOD VESSELS AND NUCLEI OF FIBROUS CONNECTIVE TISSUE CROSSES THE UPPER PART OF THE DRAWING OBLIQUELY. (R. J. G.)

Cp. : capillary vessel.
C.T.C. : connective tissue cells.
Pa. C. : parenchyma cell.

S.D.N. : small darkly stained nucleus.
Sp. : space.

The cells with the pale vesicular nuclei belong to the fully developed type of pineal or parenchymal cell ; many of the parenchyma cells, however, are embedded in the spongioplasm, and in this situation the nucleus is usually smaller and more deeply and uniformly stained than those of the cells just described. Between these two extreme types, in young as well as in adult specimens, there are numerous intermediate forms (Fig. 265), both with respect to the type of the nucleus and the

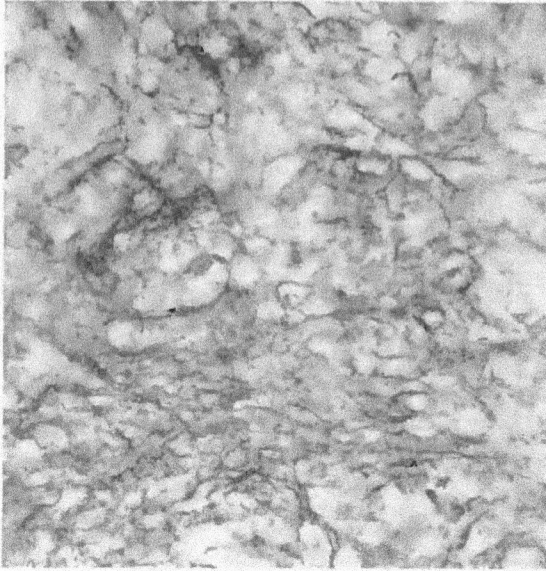

FIG. 266.—PINEAL BODY. × 350.

Median vertical section, through the peduncle, of a human pineal body prepared by the Blair-Davis modification of Ranson's pyridin method. The larger,
deeply stained fibres forming a network between the pineal cells are probably
glial, the finer fibrillæ in the centre of the photograph are indistinguishable from
nerve-fibres, and possibly represent the axis-cylinders or nerve-fibres reaching
the pineal body from the superior and posterior commissures.

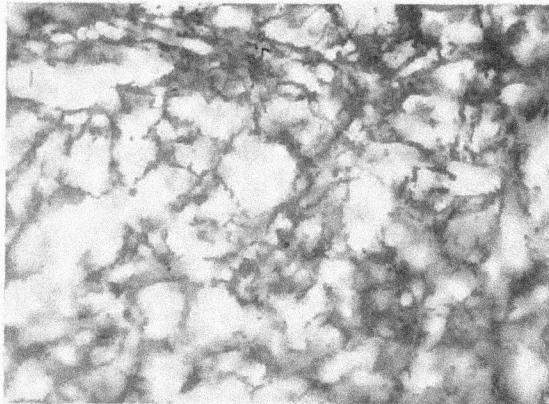

FIG. 267.—PINEAL BODY. × 350.

Section through the cortical zone of the same specimen as Fig. 266. The
larger fibres forming a network surrounding the pineal cells are probably glial.
The finer fibres between the cells and surrounding the capillary vessels are probably nerves of the sympathetic system.

position of the cell-element, namely, wholly contained within the spongio-plasm, protruding from this into a space, or completely extruded into the space and connected to the surrounding structures merely by fine, taper-ing processes.

In adult specimens, however, when specifically stained for neuroglia, the distinction between glial cells and the general plasmodium or syncytial reticulum in which they are imbedded is quite definite, and it is at once evident that the slender astrocytes and glial fibres in no sense form the principal constituent of the supporting tissue of the lobules.

The former appear as very sparsely scattered branched cells, chiefly of the astrocyte type (Fig. 272, p. 403), with fine delicate processes lying in a tissue which when specially stained by Hortega's silver impregnation method is seen to be principally composed of branched parenchyma cells which he believes to be separate and in-dependent units.

By combining the knowledge gained by the different specific methods of silver im-pregnation with that obtained by the best nuclear and cytoplasmic stains we are able to distinguish in the par-enchymatous tissue of

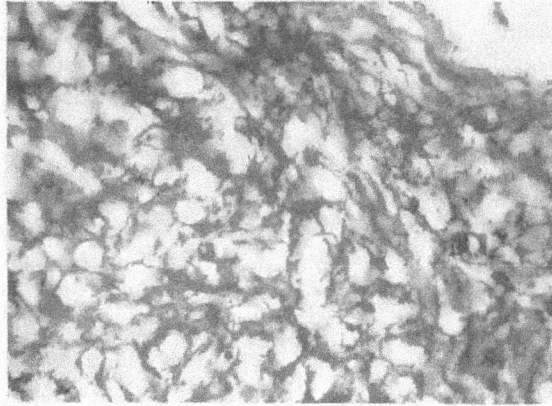

FIG. 268.—PINEAL BODY. × 350.

Section through the central region of the same specimen as Figs. 266, 267. Two types of fibres are visible, as in Fig. 267. The finer fibres appear to form a network on the walls of the capillary vessels.

the adult human pineal organ three principal elements, namely :

(1) A glial component, formed by the cell-bodies and slender branched processes of a relatively small number of astrocytes.

(2) The parenchyma or pineal cells, distinguished by their large, pale vesicular nuclei. These are much more numerous than the astrocytes and form the main bulk of the tissue.

(3) The mesodermal elements which consist of (a) the fibrous capsule and trabeculæ, derived from the pia mater, and (b) minute profusely branched cells which are present beneath the pia mater, in relation with the perivascular sheaths, and distributed in the lobules. These are the microglia or mesoglia cells of Del Rio-Hortega, and are only clearly demonstrable by means

of his silver carbonate process, though their nuclei are recognizable with other methods of staining, especially in glial
plaques.

(4) Cells and fibres, which resemble nerve-cells and nerve-fibres
but are in many cases only with difficulty distinguished from
the parenchyma and glia cells and the processes of these cells
(Figs. 266, 267, 268).

(5) Arterioles, capillaries, and venules.

The Parenchyma Cells

The form and full extent of the branches of the parenchyma or pineal
cells is only fully revealed by the silver methods of Del Rio-Hortega,
upon whose description the following account is largely based.   The
pineal cells of an adult human subject thus shown (Fig. 218, Chap. 22,
p. 317) are characterized by an irregularly shaped body containing a
clear vesicular nucleus.   The amount of cytoplasm varies, in some cells
being abundant, in others scanty.   The cells thus differ greatly in size.
The cell-body is usually branched, and the branches vary in number,
size, and complexity.   Thus the cell may be unipolar, bipolar, or multipolar.
The main branches may give off a group of slender processes which may
subdivide and end freely, or more commonly terminate in club-shaped
swellings implanted on or in the sheath of a vessel wall.   The free ends
of the smaller branches are said by Del Rio-Hortega not to communicate
with similar branches of neighbouring pineal cells.   The processes of the
cell may be polarized in one direction or they may be distributed irregularly
in any direction.   In the former case they are usually directed towards
a vessel lying in the periphery of a lobule, and lie in what is termed the
marginal zone, where they are radially disposed ;   in other cases, more
particularly in the centre of a lobule, the cells tend to be multipolar and
stellate in form, the branches appearing to form a plexus ;   the terminal
branches of these cells may end in club-shaped swellings on the sheaths
of endolobular vessels, or they may extend to the periphery of the lobule
and become attached to the sheath of an interlobular vessel.

Typical branched cells with club-shaped endings are seldom seen in
children below the age of eight years, and the complexity of the branching
and the size of the club-shaped swellings appear to increase with the
advance of age.

Although the general form and terminal processes of the pineal cells
can only be clearly demonstrated by means of the silver methods of
impregnation, very little of the structure of the cells and their content is
seen in these preparations ;   and in order to form a true estimate of the
nature of these cells it is necessary to adopt special methods which will

bring out particular characters, such as cytoplasmic granules, vacuoles, lipoid material, and other contents ; also mitochondria, blepharoplasts, the centrosome, and Golgi apparatus. Thus by staining frozen sections with Janus green, small rod-like mitochondria may be demonstrated in the pineal organ of such animals as the horse, ox, and sheep. The rods are most abundant around the centrosome and the part of the cell body which relative to the nucleus is the widest. Occasionally long rods or chondriocontes have been observed, and one or more thick rods close to the nucleus arranged in the form of crosses or bundles. Hortega states that in children the rods are short, while in adults and old subjects they have become elongated, their elongation coinciding with involutive changes.

The cytoplasm normally has a reticular structure, and frequently shows vacuoles which may be demonstrated by the use of neutral red. Lipoid material is also sometimes present. Granules of varying type are normally present. Some of these have been described as secretory (Dimitrowa, Rio-Hortega, Pastori, and others). There are also spherules which have been thought to correspond to the " gliosomes " found in the central nervous system. Some granules are apparently the result of degenerative changes and are seen abundantly in the pineal cells of aged subjects. Pigment granules, usually of small size, but sometimes large, are found in old subjects, and like the non-pigmented granules mentioned above are in some specimens due to involutive changes. These granules are of a yellow-brown colour, and differ considerably from the dark melanin granules which are also sometimes found in the pineal organ and may be of morphological interest (see pp. 61–63). These are chiefly found in the connective tissue elements, trabeculæ, capsule, and the surrounding pial tissue.

The nucleus of the parenchyma cells of adult subjects is typically spherical, of large size, and owing to its small chromatin content appears clear. A well-defined nucleolus is usually present and the nuclear membrane is conspicuous. The nucleus of the parenchyma cells is large, even in those in which the cytoplasm is scanty and the cell as a whole is small as compared with the average size of these cells ; and it is also large when compared with the small deeply stained nuclei of the fibroglial tissue. Under certain conditions spherular formations described by Dimitrowa as secretory in nature are present within the nucleus (Fig. 219, Chap. 22, p. 317). These spherules have been found in the human subject, the ox, lamb, and other animals. They appear as clear droplets which are stained red by Van Gieson's methods, a grey colour in Weigert preparations, and pink with saffranin. Dimitrowa regarded the existence and appearance of these spherules as undoubted evidence of secretory activity, and she believed that the nucleus produces a substance the chemical composition of which is unknown and which is periodically discharged into the cytoplasm. The spherules were stated to approach the nuclear membrane, pass through this into the cytoplasm, and afterwards disappear. The nuclear membrane was then said to be regenerated. Similar appearances have been described by other authors, e.g. Krabbe, who reported the presence of the nuclear spherules in the human subject commencing about the eighth year, reaching a maximum during the fourteenth year, and persisting in old age. Uemura and Weinberg have seen the spherules in the pineal body of a child of 4 years and under 3 years of age. The secretory nature of the nuclear spherules has, however, been doubted by many authors, more particularly by Achúcarro and Sacristan, Biondi, Josephy, and Walter. Intranuclear granules and spherules, wrinkling, outpocketing, and inpocketing of the nuclear membrane are quite common occurrences in cells with large nuclei in many structures besides the pineal body. Moreover, the small recesses between the folds of a wrinkled nuclear membrane may enclose granules of protoplasm which stain with hæmatoxylin and the various stains mentioned above in a similar way to the spherules of the parenchyma cells. Nevertheless the abundant granules which were demonstrated by Hortega within the nucleus in the cell-body and around the parenchyma cells by means of his silver carbonate method, in the pineal body of the ox, sheep, and human subject, must be regarded as histological evidence of a granular deposit of some stainable substance differing in its chemical composition from that of the unmodified nucleus and cell-body. Whether the chemical changes indicated by the presence of these granules is evidence of an internal secretion seems as yet to be indecisive, and more particularly is this the case since, as far as we are aware, the presence of the granules has not been noted in the capillary vessels.

The Supporting Tissues of the Pineal Organ

In our general description we have already alluded to the fibrous connective tissue elements comprising the capsule, the trabeculæ, and the delicate intercellular connective tissue derived from the sheaths of the intralobular vessels. Besides the ordinary connective tissue, there are occasionally seen the branched microglial elements which have been described in connection with the central nervous system ; these are sometimes present in plaques of glial tissue, and more especially in certain pathological states. The microglial elements probably enter the tissue of the pineal body in the same way as they pass into the central nervous system, namely, as independent units which are first seen beneath the pia mater in the form of small rounded cells, with deeply stained nuclei, which afterwards assume amœboid characters and migrate into the deeper

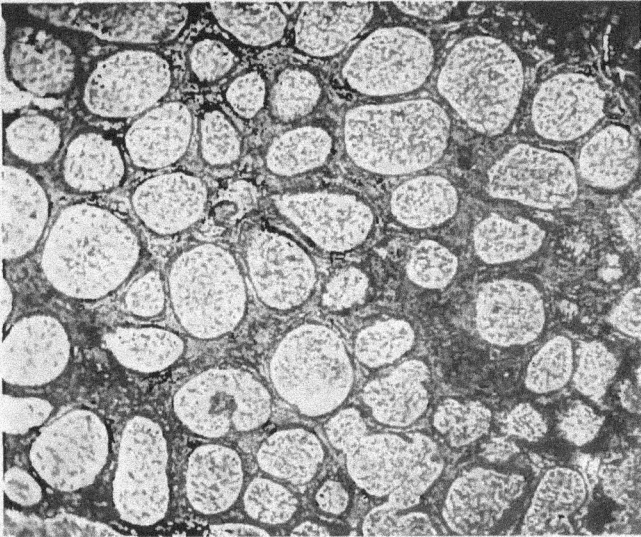

FIG. 269.—PINEAL GLAND OF A WOMAN AGED 40.   (AFTER R. AMPRINO.)

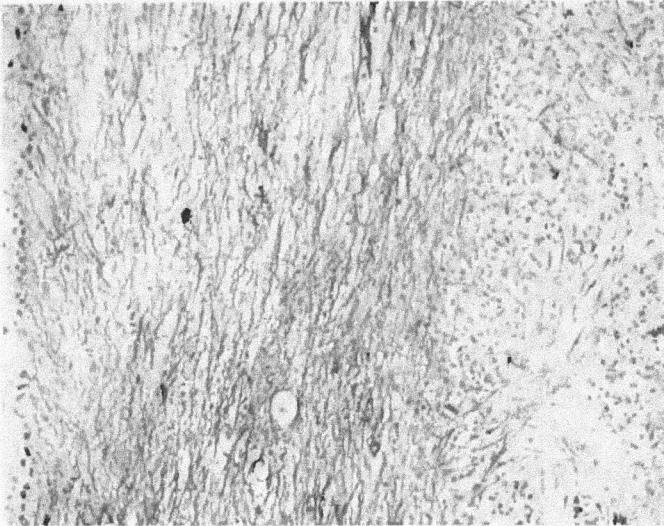

FIG. 270.—PINEAL GLAND OF A MAN AGED 76.   (AFTER R. AMPRINO.)

central parts of the organ, and there may develop a phagocytic function. There remain to be considered certain non-cellular elements, namely, a supposed intercellular substance; forming what has been termed a

26

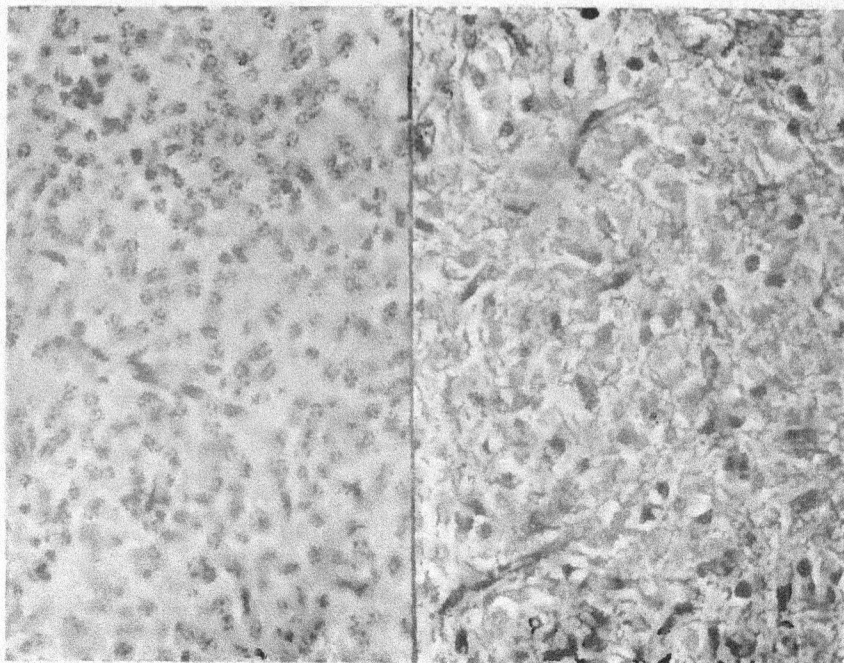

A   B

FIG. 271.—A—PINEAL GLAND OF A NEWLY BORN LAMB. B—PINEAL GLAND OF
A SHEEP AGED 4 YEARS. (AFTER R. AMPRINO.)

glial syncytium ; glial fibres ; and the tortuous thick fibrils which have
been specially described and figured by Amprino (1935) (Figs. 269, 270,
271, 272).

An intercellular substance is difficult to demonstrate with certainty,
and possibly in the living subject simply exists as an albuminous semi-fluid
material which everywhere fills the intercellular spaces. It is also probable
that in the preparation of specimens for microscopic examination the
coagulable material present in the interstitial tissue-fluid is concentrated
on the cellular elements and fibres, so as to form on these a continuous
membrane-like covering, such as was described by Held as the " grenz
membran." On the other hand, it is quite possible that a similar process
may occur normally during life and a more solid constituent be separated
out from the more liquid intercellular tissue-fluid, the more solid material
being deposited on the surface of the cellular elements and fibres and
thus forming a continuous membrane-like covering or, when it completely
fills the spaces, an intercellular ground substance. Such a conception is
important in connection with the passage of nutritive material, or possibly
secretory products, into or out of the cell-bodies and their processes—

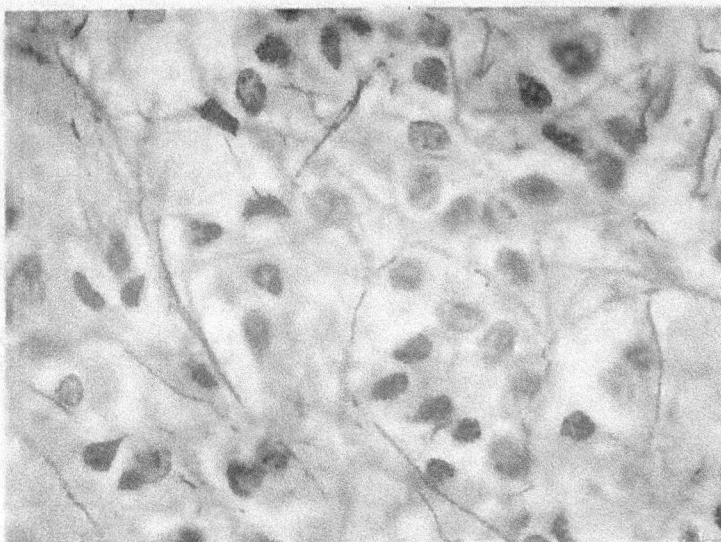

FIG. 272.—PINEAL GLAND OF A MAN AGED 40, SHOWING ASTROCYTE CELLS AND NEUROGLIAL FIBRES. (AFTER R. AMPRINO.)

or in other words, furnishing the means by which osmotic processes can take place between the cells and the tissue-fluid.

The Nerves of the Parietal Organ and Pineal Body

The study of the nerve supply of the human pineal organ necessarily involves a preliminary consideration of the pineal nerves, commissural fibres, and the associated ganglia of lower types of animals in which the parietal sense-organs, pineal sac, and pineal stalk are more highly evolved than they are in mammals, and in which the nerve tracts have been definitely traced from their origin in the sensory-cells of the retina of the pineal eye or the wall of the pineal sac to their termination in the nerve tracts and ganglia of the brain.

A feature of special interest in connection with the nerve supply of the pineal eye is the bearing that this has upon the question of the bilateral original of the pineal system, and the closely related problem of the homology of the pineal organ of birds and mammals with reference to the " parapineal organ " of cyclostomes and the pineal sac and pineal stalk of amphibia and reptiles. The nerve supply of the pineal eye and pineal sac in *Sphenodon* was specially studied with reference to this question by the late Professor A. Dendy (1911, *Phil. Trans. Roy. Soc.*, Ser. B., Vol. 201, pp. 228–339) (Figs. 183, 184, 185, A, Chap. 20, pp. 259, 260, 261). Unfortunately this important work appears to have escaped the attention of many modern writers on this subject, owing to the cir-

cumstance that only his earlier works have been quoted in many of the
published references to the literature of the pineal system, and these
authors have most probably been unaware of the existence of his later
publications. Dendy, as is well known from his earlier communications,
regarded the pineal eye of *Sphenodon* as the left pineal organ and the
pineal sac (epiphysis) as the right pineal organ of a paired system which
included the pineal eye and pineal sac, the pineal stalk, and the associated
vessels and nerves. He also considered that the primarily right and left
components of this system have, in the course of evolution, become displaced towards or into the median plane, so that the left organ has become
anterior and the right posterior. The latter or pineal sac of *Sphenodon*
has also become more degenerate than the left, which is separated off as
the parietal organ and presumably has retained, to a much greater extent,
the original structure of the ancestral pineal eye. In his later memoir,
published in 1911, Dendy clearly demonstrated that the wall of the pineal
sac of *Sphenodon* has a nervous structure which is essentially similar to
that of the pineal eye, and that although less highly differentiated it shows,
as in the pineal eye, internal and external limiting membranes, radial
supporting or glial fibres, which are comparable to Müller's fibres in the
retina of the lateral eyes of vertebrates, also neuro-epithelial cells which
he regarded as sensory in nature, ganglion cells, nerve fibres, and at its
distal extremity pigment cells. In one of his specimens this apical part
was partially constricted off from the main diverticulum so as to form a
thin-walled sac, containing pigment cells in the wall of the main sac.
He regarded this sac as being comparable to the accessory parietal organs
described by Leydig and Studnička, and as supporting his view that " the
structure of the pineal sac is fundamentally identical with that of the
pineal eye."

In cyclostomes (Studnička, Gaskell, Dendy) there is the same fundamental similarity in structure of the pineal eye and the parapineal organ
as is met with in the pineal eye and the pineal sac or epiphysis of reptiles.
Both in fishes and reptiles there are sometimes two outgrowths, one of
which, Epiphysis I, is anterior, while the other, Epiphysis II, is posterior.
In both fishes and reptiles the anterior epiphysis is usually to the left of the
median plane. In fishes, however, the posterior organ is the more highly
evolved and in cyclostomes it forms the pineal eye, whereas in reptiles the
anterior organ is the more highly evolved and forms the pineal eye or
parietal organ.

In *Geotria* Professor Dendy demonstrated non-medullated nerve-
fibres which apparently arose from the ganglion cells of the retina of the right
or posterior pineal eye ; these converged towards the optic stalk and then,
forming a nerve bundle in the stalk, coursed backwards to end in the right

habenular ganglion, the right bundle of Meynert, the ependymal groove or "subcommissural organ," and, he believed, also in the posterior commissure (Fig. 134, Chap. 17, p. 188). He likewise traced the connections of the nerve-fibres issuing from the parapineal organ (anterior or left pineal eye) to the left habenular ganglion, habenular tract, or superior commissure, and the left bundle of Meynert, which is much smaller than the corresponding bundle of the opposite side, which receives the larger pineal nerve coming from the more highly evolved right pineal eye. In his concluding remarks he states that " the connection of each of the two sense-organs with the corresponding member of the habenular ganglion-pair need no longer be questioned "; and, further, " the

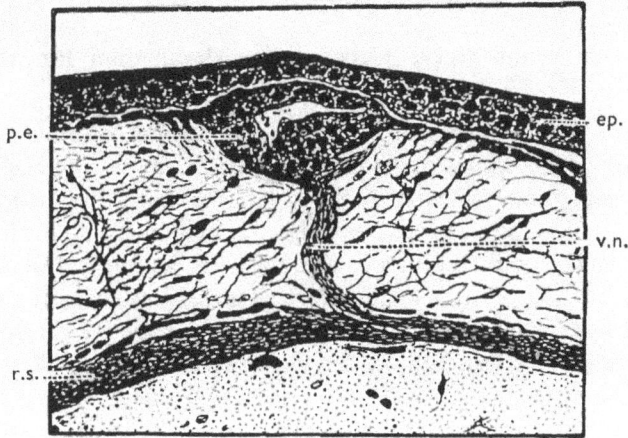

FIG. 273.—SECTION THROUGH THE VESTIGIAL EYE OF A FROG TADPOLE.   × 168.
(AFTER DENDY.) (From a photograph).

ep. : epidermis.	*r.s.* : roof of skull.
p.e. : pineal eye.	*v.n.* : vestigial stalk and nerve.

marked asymmetry in point of size of the two habenular ganglia and of the two bundles of Meynert corresponds exactly to the unequal development of the two parietal sense-organs with which they are connected, and leaves no doubt as to the paired character of the whole system."

Without entering further into this highly controversial question, we may conclude that these observations are highly suggestive of a system of nerve tracts with commissures passing from the parietal sense-organs to receptive centres in the brain, which in some respects is comparable to that of the paired lateral eyes—in other words, a system of afferent fibres of a sensory nature ; but, as might be expected from the vestigial condition of the receptive organs in these animals, the fibres are usually unmyelinated.

The nerve-fibres of the functional lateral eyes in the human subject are unmyelinated until a late period of fœtal life, and do not become myelinated until shortly before birth (Lucas Keene and Hewer, Langworthy, O.R.). In the pineal eye of *Geotria* and *Sphenodon* the nerves remain unmyelinated even in the adult animals, a condition which is to be expected in organs which even in these species are degenerate and apparently have little or no function. In other types, for instance in many reptiles and amphibia, the pineal nerve or tract, though present in early embryos (Fig. 187, Chap. 20, p. 264, and Fig. 273), usually disappears later, when the terminal vesicle (parietal organ) becomes separated from the pineal sac and its peduncle (Béraneck, E., p. 246 ; Dendy, A., p. 261 ; Klinckowström, A. de, pp. 241, 243).

The Nerve-fibres and Nerve Cells of the Mammalian Pineal Organ

Both in the past and recently, and in addition to the work done on the nerve supply of the pineal system in fishes, amphibia, and reptiles, a large amount of work has been devoted to the study of the sensory cells, nerve cells, and tracts of nerve-fibres belonging to the pineal system in the human subject and in various types of mammals. This has been carried out largely with the object of demonstrating an anatomical basis by which it may be presumed the pineal organ or epiphysis is capable of being influenced by afferent impulses and can function : either by means of specific hormones secreted by the pineal cells and carried to distant organs in the circulating blood or by means of efferent nerves issuing from the gland and joining the habenular ganglia and other nerve centres of the brain or the intracranial sympathetic system—exerting through these systems a direct influence on other organs, e.g. the secretory cells of the choroid plexuses, or an indirect influence on these cells, by means of vasomotor nerves regulating the circulation of blood in the vessels of the organs supplied by them.

The anatomical demonstration of the distribution of the nerve-fibres has been greatly facilitated by the various methods of silver impregnation, and the definite results obtained by Retzius, Studnička, Cajal, Pastori, and other workers have done much to establish the existence and connections of nerve-fibres, which are presumably afferent and efferent and may form the basis of a reflex mechanism by which it is possible for the pineal body to be influenced apart from the action of hormones reaching it through the circulating blood.

Theoretically one may postulate the existence of a pineal nerve supply consisting of a double central and a double sympathetic system, thus :

Central nervous system $\begin{cases} \text{Afferent nerve-fibres to the pineal body.} \\ \text{Efferent nerve-fibres from the pineal body.} \end{cases}$

Sympathetic system $\begin{cases} \text{Afferent nerve-fibres to the pineal body.} \\ \text{Efferent nerve-fibres from the pineal body.} \end{cases}$

Also one might expect to find in connection with these fibres sensory or receptive cells and ganglion cells, the latter giving rise to efferent fibres which leave the pineal organ and pass to such ganglia as the habenular or optic thalami, or to the plexuses of sympathetic nerve-fibres on the surrounding blood-vessels. Moreover, one might look for two types of nerve-cells, a large ganglion-cell belonging to the central nervous system and a small type of nerve-cell having the characteristics of the sympathetic system.

Actually, it appears that if observations on the pineal system through-out the whole series of vertebrate animals are included, all these different types of sensory epithelial cells, nerve cells, and nerve-fibres have been seen and described by competent observers. The pineal system, especially that of the mammalia, is, however, vestigial in structure and has undergone marked modifications, and as a consequence the full complement of nerve cells and nerve-fibres is not found in any one species. Nerve cells, in particular, are rare, and when present are usually not fully developed. Such cells have been described as " neuronoid cells " or " amacrine nerve-cells." Moreover, the existence of typical nerve cells showing both Nissl granules and axis cylinder process as a normal constituent of the human pineal organ has been not only doubted but denied by some recent workers, who regard the occasional occurrence of such cells as anomalous.

There seem, however, to be transitional stages between nerve cells and typical parenchyma cells, and it is probable that in some cases branched pineal cells with bulbous extremities have been mistaken for fully developed nerve cells. True nerve cells, apparently belonging to the sympathetic system, are occasionally seen on or near the surface of the organ or in close relation with the vessels contained in the trabeculæ, and in our opinion a distinction should be made between these cells and the transitional or " neuronoid cells " seen in the parenchyma. It is possible that the latter indicate a stage in the differentiation of true nerve cells from the indifferent neuro-epithelial cells which form the primary elements of the developing organ, and which may give rise to neuroglial cells, parenchyma cells, or very occasionally to either imperfectly or fully developed nerve cells.

The question of whether the parenchyma cells themselves are sensory in nature and capable of transmitting a sensory impulse from an afferent pineal nerve to an efferent pineal nerve is one of practical interest. Should they possess this function, their anatomical connections fully warrant the assumption that a reflex mechanism may exist within the pineal organ, which is capable of being influenced by impulses reaching it through its afferent nerve-fibres and transmitting such impulses by efferent fibres (e.g. sympathetic) to the organs or regions to which these nerves are distributed.

A general survey of the comparative anatomy of the pineal region, with detailed descriptions of the nerve cells and nerve-fibres of the pineal system in special types of animals, was published in 1905 by Studnička Die Parietalorgane. Oppel. Teil V.), and recent accounts with references to the literature in such works as L'Épiphyse, by J. Calvet, a special article on the pineal gland by del Rio Hortega in Cowdry's Special Cytology, Penfield (1928), and various articles such as those by Béraneck, Clarke, Darkschewitsch, Dendy, Dimitrowa, Herring, Pastori, and others. It will be realized on studying these contributions to the innervation of the pineal system that substantial agreement has been reached on the following points :

1. Tracts of nerve-fibres described as the nervus pinealis, nervus parietalis, tractus pinealis, and tractus habenularis have been traced from receptive sensory cells or ganglion cells in the retina of the parietal organs (namely, the pineal eye and end-vesicle of the parapineal organ) and found to terminate in or traverse the habenular ganglia, the superior and posterior commissures, and Meynert's bundles. These fibres have been observed in cyclostomes and other fishes, amphibia, and reptiles. They may be situated in the stalk of the vesicle, and thus resemble the optic nerve-fibres of the lateral eyes of vertebrates ; or they may course as an independent tract through the areolar connective tissue in the neighbourhood of the stalk ; or, after the disappearance of the stalk, they may lie in the region formerly occupied by the stalk. The nerve-fibres may be present only in the larval stages or they may persist in the adult animal.

2. Similar tracts of nerve-fibres may arise from sensory cells in the wall of the pineal sac or the epiphysis in elasmobranch and teleostean fishes, amphibia, reptiles (saurians and snakes), and in mammals. These fibres terminate for the most part in the posterior commissure, but connections are established in some species also with the internal capsule, striæ medullares thalami, Meynert's bundles, habenular commissure and ganglia, and the optic tracts (Darkschewitsch).

There is, however, a considerable amount of variation in different species of mammals, e.g. Herring states that occasional nerve-fibres may enter the pineal body from the habenular commissure in the cat, monkeys, and man, but have probable no functional significance ; whereas in the rat the pineal body is anatomically widely separated from the habenular commissure, and no nervous connection persists between them. In the adult rat the pineal body is an isolated organ which lies on the surface of the brain between the cerebral hemispheres and cerebellum. Its only apparent functional connection with the organ is vascular, and its nerve supply reaches it only in the form of non-medullated fibres accompanying the blood-vessels (Cajal).

The direction in which nerve impulses travel in the fibres connecting the epiphysis with the habenular ganglia, optic thalami, and the superior and posterior commissures is difficult to determine in mammalia, owing to the absence of experimental evidence. It seems, however, to be generally assumed that impulses travelling from the central fibres coming from the posterior commissure through the " tractus intercalaris " not only enter the stalk of the epiphysis, but are also distributed in the parenchyma of the epiphysis.

Pastori states that in some species of mammals (e.g. man and dog) the nerve-fibres coming from the optic thalami and habenular ganglia partly decussate in the inter-habenular commissure ; while in other species of mammals (e.g. the cat) the corresponding nerve-fibres remain homolateral and travel directly from the optic thalamus and habenular ganglion into the parenchyma of the epiphysis, that is to say, without decussating.

On the other hand, the primary direction in which the nerve impulses travel in the lower classes of vertebrates is apparently from the sensory cells of the pineal eye, pineal sac, or epiphysis to the central ganglia—vide Béraneck, Dendy, Gaskell, Klinckowström, Studnička, and others. Moreover, some writers have supposed that the parenchyma cells of the human epiphysis may be sensory, or receptor, cells ; and it has also been suggested that they may be specially sensitive to pressure, and, further, that they may function in regulating the pressure of the cerebrospinal fluid, either through the direct action of the sympathetic system on the choroidal epithelium or by an indirect action on the epithelium through the choroidal blood-vessels.

These considerations suggest that relays of nerve-fibres which originally carried impulses from the receptive organs of the pineal system to ganglia of the central nervous system have been either wholly or partially supplanted by nerves which are afferent to the epiphysis, and also that impulses arising by stimulation of the parenchyma cells of the epiphysis may be transferred to fibres of the sympathetic system.

An anatomical basis which affords support for the latter hypothesis is furnished by Pastori's recent work on the nervous connections of the epiphysis. He has demonstrated in the human subject and in the dog the constant presence of a sympathetic ganglion situated in the membranes just behind the posterior pole of the epiphysis. This ganglion is connected by a large number of very fine nerve-fibres with the epiphysis, and also by less numerous but coarser nerve-fibres, which form a definite bundle which joins the plexus of nerve-fibres on the great cerebral vein and its tributaries. The bundle is the *nervus conari* of Kolmer. Pastori describes both the fine and the coarse nerve-fibres as arising from small sympathetic nerve-cells situated in the ganglion. The fine fibres enter the epiphysis with the vessels contained in the trabeculæ.

It is thus possible that some of the fibres may be efferent nerves from the ganglion to the gland, and others afferent from the gland to the plexus of nerve-fibres on the neighbouring vessels, and that these furnish a means by which the epiphysis may be influenced by or act upon the sympathetic system.

The Vascular Supply of the Pineal Organ

The arteries of the pineal body are derived from the posterior choroidal branches of the two posterior cerebral arteries. The posterior choroidal artery on each side enters the transverse fissure of the brain between the two layers of the tela choroidea, and gives off small branches near its origin to the pia mater investing the pineal body ; from these branches numerous arterioles enter the capsule and trabeculæ of the organ, and ultimately give off capillary vessels for the supply of the parenchyma. The capillary net is drained by venules which passing through the trabeculæ and capsule unite to form a vessel which joins the great cerebral vein of Galen. This terminates in the anterior part of the straight sinus.

Since a tumour of the pineal organ may by pressure obstruct the great cerebral vein, it is important to know the exact course of this vessel. It will be remembered that the internal cerebral vein on each side is formed in the region just behind the interventricular foramen of Monro by the union of the anterior choroidal vein with the terminal or striate vein, and that the two internal cerebral veins course backwards below the fornix and between the two layers of the tela choroidea or velum interpositum. Here they receive tributaries from the choroid plexus of the third ventricle and optic thalami. They unite near the base of the pineal body to form the great cerebral vein of Galen, which curves upwards in the cisterna venæ magnæ cerebri around the splenium of the corpus callosum (Fig. 274). Here after receiving the right and left basal veins and the internal occipital veins, it opens into the anterior end of the straight sinus, the latter vessel commencing as a continuation of the inferior sagittal sinus. It is important to remember also that some of the superior cerebellar veins run inwards to terminate in the straight sinus or in the internal cerebral veins.

The opening of the right and left basal veins into the great cerebral vein of Galen has a practical bearing in connection with occlusion of the great vein, for unless the pressure on the great cerebral vein involves its terminal part and the openings into it of these two vessels, any resulting congestion of the choroidal veins which might result from an obstruction at the commencement of the vein would be relieved by the anastomoses between the tributaries of the basal veins and the choroidal veins in the inferior horns of the lateral ventricles. For detailed description of the

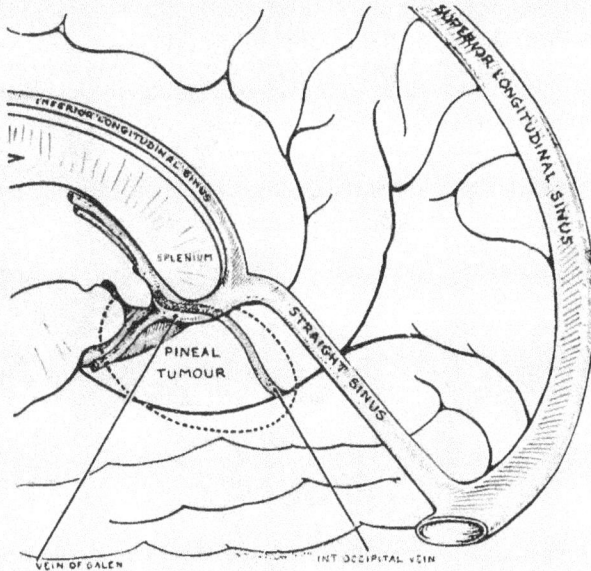

FIG. 274.—DIAGRAM SHOWING THE PRINCIPAL TRIBUTARIES AND RELATIONS OF THE GREAT VEIN OF GALEN, AND THE POSITION OCCUPIED BY A PINEAL TUMOUR.

anatomy of these veins in connection with the production of hydrocephalus the reader should consult articles by Dandy and Blackfan (1914), Stopford (1926, 1928), and Bedford (1934).

Since no lymphatic vessels are present in the central nervous system of which the pineal organ is a part, it is probable that secretory or waste products contained in the tissue-fluids of the pineal body would, like the cerebrospinal fluid, be absorbed directly into the venous system through perivascular channels which are in communication with the tissue spaces.

CHAPTER 27

RELATIONS OF THE ADULT PINEAL ORGAN

SOME of the more important relations are seen in Fig. 276, which is an X-ray photograph of a patient aged 50, showing a calcified pineal, and Fig. 1, p. 2, also of a calcified pineal organ. Fig. 277 is from a section of the pineal region made in the median sagittal plane, and Fig. 278 a transverse section of a brain containing a tumour in the pineal region. Fig. 274

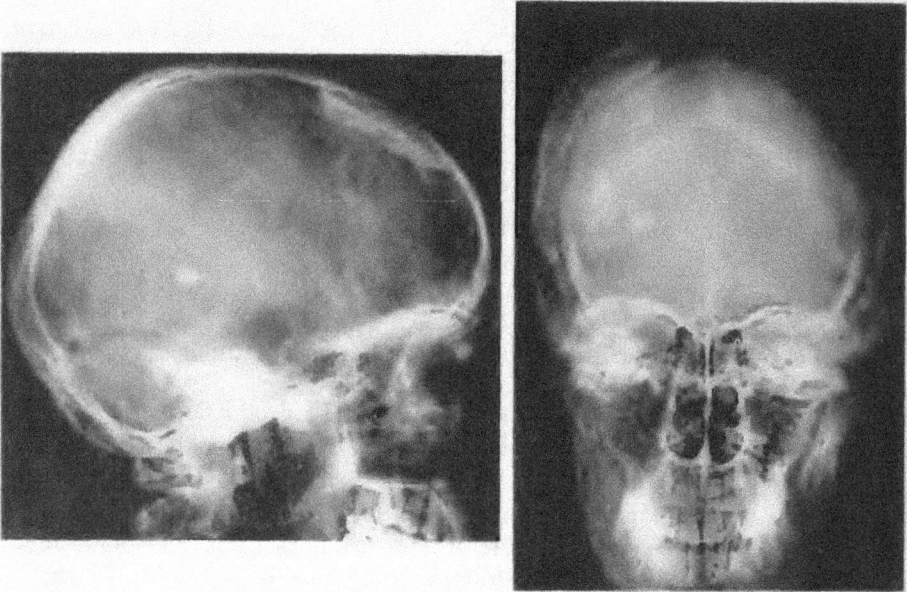

FIG. 275.—RADIOGRAPHS OF SKULL, SHOWING CALCIFICATION IN THE CHOROID PLEXUS.

also shows diagrammatically the position of the great cerebral vein, basal vein, and internal occipital vein to the pineal body ; the relations that a pineal tumour growing backwards beneath the tentorium cerebelli would have to the splenium of the corpus callosum ; the junction of the great cerebral vein with the inferior sagittal sinus to form the straight sinus, and the convolutions and sulci on the adjacent tentorial surface of the brain. The falx cerebri, tentorium, and falx cerebelli, the cerebellum

412

and pons Varolii are not represented in the diagram. The drawing can thus show the internal occipital vein which lies above and external to the tentorium. Here it issues from the parieto-occipital fissure ; near its termination it crosses the free border of the incisura tentorii and joins the great cerebral vein between the splenium of the corpus callosum above and the pineal body which lies below and internal to it. In this position it would be in direct relation with a pineal tumour. Fig. 279, a transverse and approximately vertical section, gives a notion of the parts in close relationship to the pineal body very different from that obtained from Fig. 278, since it passes through the posterior part of the fornix and great cerebral vein, which lie above, the pulvinares of the optic thalami, which are lateral, and the superior colliculi and aqueduct, which lie below. The close relation of the cavity of the lateral ventricle, choroid plexus, fimbria, and tela choroidea

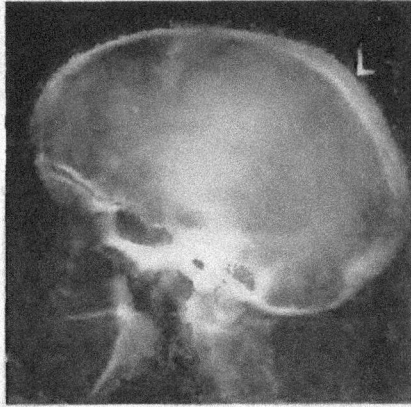

FIG. 276.—LATERAL RADIOGRAPH OF THE SKULL OF A PATIENT, AGED 50, SHOW-ING THE TYPICAL APPEARANCE OF CALCIFICATION OF THE PINEAL GLAND.

are also readily appreciated in this section.

The exact position and relations of the pineal body are specially well seen in Fig. 280. It is approximately conical in form, slightly flattened from above downwards, and averages about 8 mm. in length. The base of the gland is directed forwards

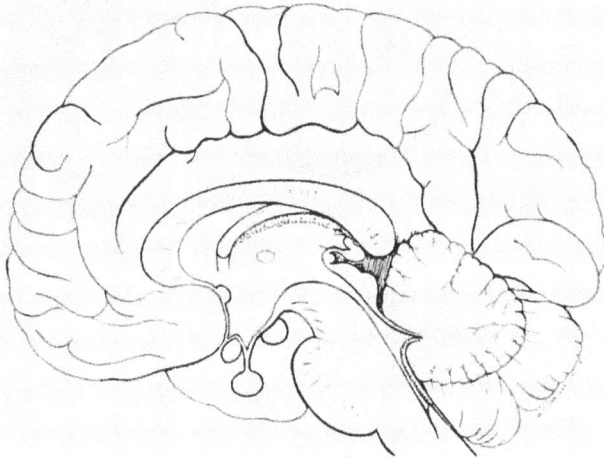

FIG. 277.—MEDIAN SAGITTAL SECTION OF BRAIN.

and slightly upwards. Its position, which is very constant, is primarily determined by that of the superior or habenular commissure and the posterior commissure, which lie respectively in its superior and inferior peduncles. The body lies in the groove between the superior colliculi of the quadrigeminal plate, and the apex is directed backwards and slightly downwards. The organ receives a partial covering of pia mater, which is derived from the lower layer of the tela choroidea or velum interpositum. The anterior third or half of its upper surface is covered by the layer of ependyma which forms the floor of the dorsal diverticulum or suprapineal recess. This is continuous with the ependyma lining the

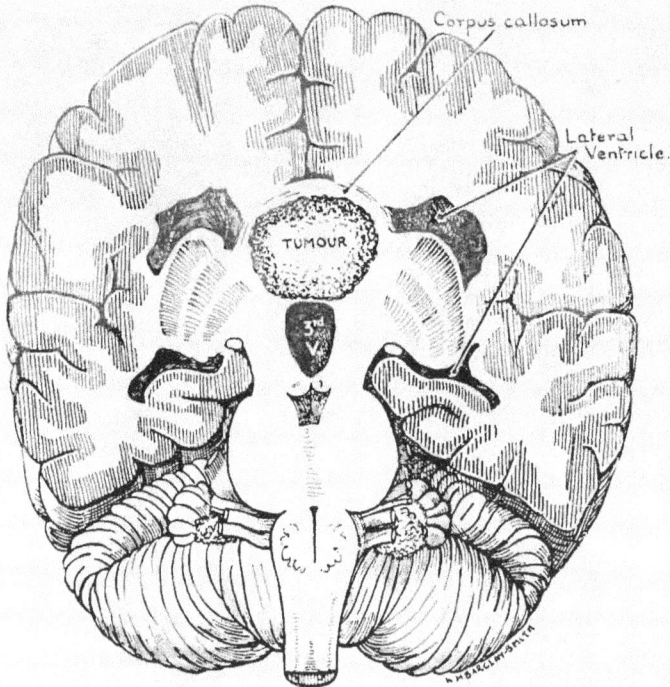

FIG. 278.—TRANSVERSE SECTION OF A BRAIN CONTAINING A TUMOUR OF THE PINEAL ORGAN.

cavity of the third ventricle, and is reflected anteriorly over the superior commissure and into the pineal recess. The roof of the superior pineal recess is continuous with that of the third ventricle, and has numerous choroidal villi hanging downwards from it and resting on the upper surface of the pineal body. The posterior two-thirds or half of the upper surface is covered by the lower layer of the tela choroidea which is firmly adherent to its capsule. It is in close relation with the great cerebral vein which separates it from the corpus callosum and commissural fibres of the fornix. The splenium projects backwards beyond the apex of the pineal body. The nerve-fibres of the splenium course outward and backward over the roof and lateral wall of the posterior horn and hinder part of the inferior horn of the lateral ventricle ; in this situation they form a thin lamina, the " tapetum," inside the fibres of the optic radiation. The latter consist of afferent and efferent fibres which connect the lower visual centres of the lateral geniculate body and superior colliculus with the occipital cortex.   It is said that no commissural fibres belonging to

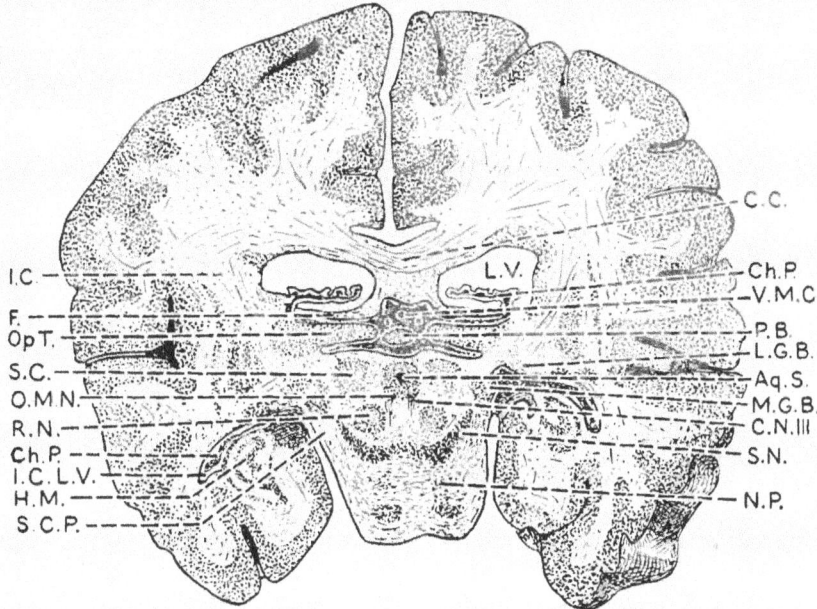

FIG. 279.—TRANSVERSE SECTION OF BRAIN SHOWING RELATIONS OF PINEAL BODY.

Aq. S. : aqueduct of Sylvius.
C.C. : corpus callosum.
Ch. P. : choroid plexus.
C.N. III. : third cranial nerve.
F. : fornix, beneath which is the great transverse fissure.
H.M. : hippocampus major.
I.C. : internal capsule.
I.C.L.V. : inferior horn of lateral ventricles.
L.G.B. : lateral geniculate body.
L.V. : lateral ventricle.

M.G.B. : medial geniculate body.
N.P. : nuclei pontis.
O.M.N. : oculo-motor nucleus and medial longitudinal fascicle.
Op. T. : optic thalamus.
R.N. : red nucleus.
S.C. : superior colliculus.
S.C.P. : superior cerebellar peduncle (brachium conjunctivum).
S.N. : substantia nigra.
V.M.C. : vena magna cerebralis.

the visual area of the cortex cross in the corpus callosum.   So far as we are aware, little is known about the function of the fibres of the tapetum and the fibres of the forceps major which cross in the splenium of the corpus callosum, and injury to these fibres does not appear to give rise to any definite symptoms or disability.

The under surface of the pineal body is typically separated from the groove between the superior colliculi by a fold of pia mater, which forms a recess called the subpineal *cul de sac* of Reichert. This may reach forward as far as the posterior commissure or it may become obliterated by adhesions. The lateral surfaces are also covered with pia mater which

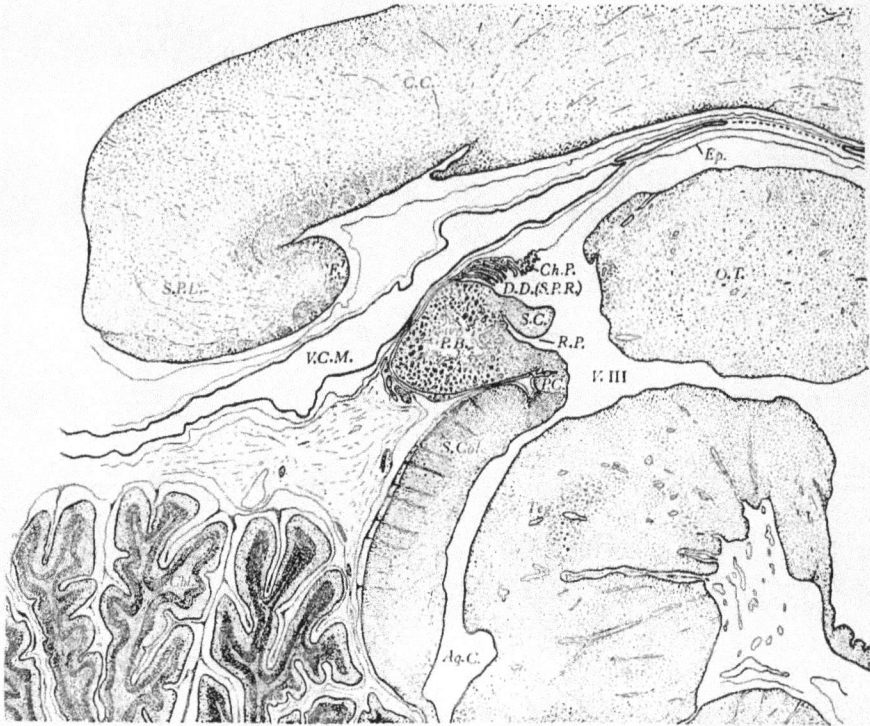

FIG. 280.—DRAWING OF A MEDIAL LONGITUDINAL SECTION THROUGH THE PINEAL REGION OF A HUMAN SUBJECT SHOWING THE RELATIONS OF THE PINEAL ORGAN TO THE CORPUS CALLOSUM, FORNIX, GREAT CEREBRAL VEIN, DORSAL DIVERTICULUM, AND CHOROID PLEXUS, SUPERIOR AND POSTERIOR COMMISSURES, QUADRIGEMINAL PLATE, AND THE MEMBRANES AND BLOOD-VESSELS AT ITS POSTERIOR POLE. (R. J. G.)

Aq. C. : aqueductus cerebri.
Cbl. : cerebellum.
C.C. : corpus callosum.
Ch. P. : choroid plexus.
D.D. (S.P.R.) : dorsal diverticulum (superior pineal recess).
Ep. : ependyma.
F. : fornix *P.B.* : pineal body.
P.C. : posterior commissure.
O.T. : optic thalamus.
R.P. : recessus pinealis.
S.C. : superior commissure.
Spl. : splenium.
S. Col. : superior colliculus.
Teg. : tegmentum.
V.C.M. : gr. vein of Galen.
V. III. : third ventricle.

may be continued backward from the sides and apex of the organ as a fold which contains between its layers vessels, nerves, and the ganglion conari (Kolmer, Löwy, and Pastori). The nerve-fibres are described as being of two kinds—" fine," which are the more numerous, and " coarse," both sets of fibres belong to the sympathetic system. This fold has been described as the posterior ligament (Calvet), whereas the reflections at the side are styled the lateral ligaments. In some cases the body and apex of the pineal organ are completely surrounded by a plexus of vessels lying in the subpial tissue and containing calcareous concretions. In old subjects this tissue is often very dense and thick, so that considerable difficulty may be experienced in freeing the body from its surroundings.

At the base of the organ are the superior and inferior peduncles and an intermediate or lateral peduncle (Calvet) which connects the pineal body with the medial surface of the thalamus. The superior peduncle contains medullated nerve-fibres belonging to the superior or habenular commissure, and the inferior peduncle conveys similar fibres of the posterior commissure ; between the two commissures is the pineal recess.

The superior peduncle is continued forward on each side as the habenula (Fig. 281). This forms the inner boundary of the trigonum habenulæ, and anteriorly is continuous with the tænia thalami, which marks the lateral limit of the roof of the third ventricle and the line along which the ependyma on the lateral wall of the ventricle leaves the medial surface of the thalamus. The habenular ganglion is situated in relation with the posterior and median part of the optic thalamus, beneath the trigonum habenulæ. It receives afferent fibres from the stria medullaris thalami, which if traced backwards divide into two bundles, of which one joins the ganglion of the same side while the other crosses in the habenular commissure to the ganglion of the opposite side. The stria medullaris is connected in front with the anterior pillar of the fornix, these fibres being derived from the cells in the hippocampal cortex, whereas a ventral bundle of fibres comes from a collection of cells in the anterior perforated substance. It is believed, therefore, that in the human subject the habenular commissure is chiefly composed of decussating fibres belonging to the olfactory system and that each habenular ganglion receives relays of fibres from the olfactory organ of both the right and left side. In lower vertebrates, however, such as the cyclostomes, in which definite pineal sense-organs are present, the habenular ganglia receive afferent fibres which arise in the ganglion cells of the retinæ of the pineal eyes, and in the human subject some of the fibres of the habenular commissure appear to terminate in the basal part of the pineal body (see p. 408).

The posterior commissure : in spite of the position of the posterior commissure, as seen in median longitudinal sections of the brain, being so familiar and such a valuable landmark, it has been found difficult to trace its connections with certainty, and there is considerable difference of opinion with regard to the origin of its fibres. Most authors are,

27

however, agreed that in the human subject some of its fibres arise in the nucleus interstitialis or nucleus of origin of the median longitudinal

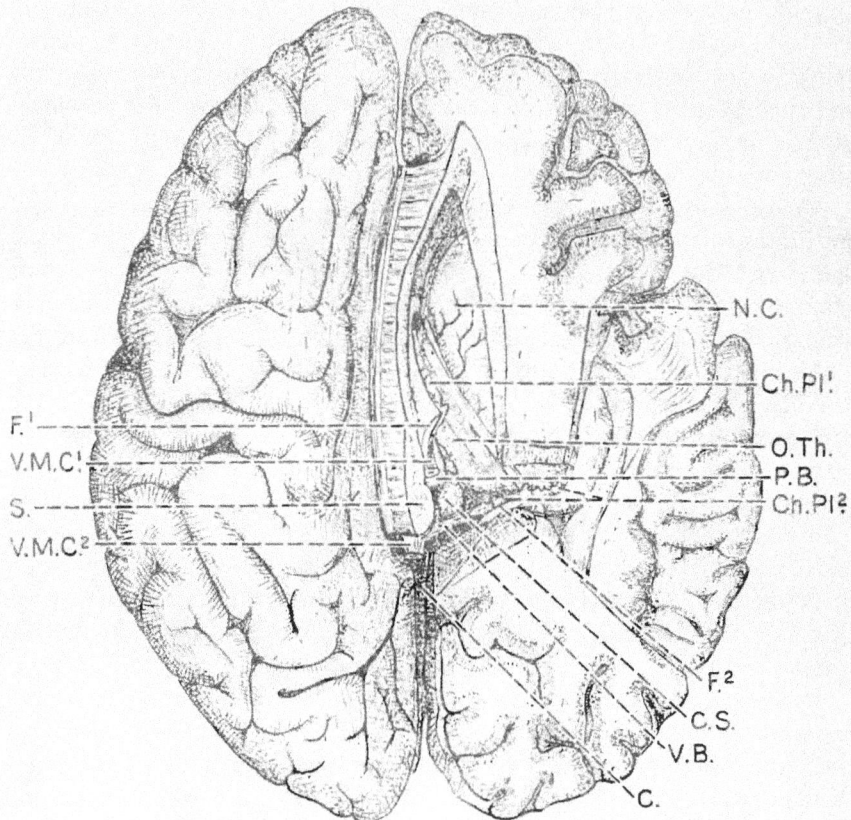

FIG. 281.—PINEAL REGION VIEWED FROM ABOVE.

The upper part of the right hemisphere of the brain has been removed and the right lateral ventricle opened by removal of portions of the corpus callosum and the roof of the posterior and inferior cornua. A part of the fornix and tela choroidea were then cut away so as to expose the pineal body, habenular region, and superior colliculus. The pineal body of the adult lies between 5 and 6 cm. directly below the supero-medial border of the hemisphere, and its apex is 1 cm. in front of the posterior end of the splenium of the corpus callosum. The great cerebral vein lies in the velum interpositum (T. Ch.) between the pineal body below and the fornix and corpus callosum above.

C. : cerebellum.	O. Th. : optic thalamus.
Ch. Pl¹ and ² : choroid plexus.	P.B. : pineal body.
C.S. : colliculus superior.	S. : splenium of corpus callosum.
F.¹ and ² : fornix.	V.B. : vena basilaris.
N.C. : nucleus caudatus.	V.M.C.¹ and ² : vena magna cerebralis.

(Original : R. J. G.)

fasciculus, and that the decussating fibres have connections through this tract with the nuclei and nerve-fibres of the eye muscles. The commissure also appears to contain fibres which originate or end in nuclei situated in the tectum opticum.

In cyclostomes, e.g. *Petromyzon*, in addition to fibres which are associated with the pineal system, fibres of the posterior commissure arise from cells which are widely scattered through the dorso-caudal part of the thalamus and tectum opticum. In *Geotria*, the Australian lamprey, according to Dendy the larger of the two organs, the right parietal organ (Epiphysis II or posterior pineal organ) is connected by a well-defined tract, the pineal nerve with the right habenular ganglion, and also sends fibres to the posterior commissure and right bundle of Meynert; whereas the smaller deeply placed left parietal organ (Epiphysis I or parapineal organ of Studnička) is joined by a few short fibres with the left habenular ganglion which lies immediately beneath it, and also sends fibres to the posterior commissure and the left bundle of Meynert. The morphology of the pineal tract and of the habenular commissure in cyclostomes is discussed on p. 193. Briefly summarized it may be stated that two organs or pairs of organs have been considered by some authors to be comprised in the pineal system, of which the anterior organ or Epiphysis I is related to the habenular ganglia and the habenular commissure, and the posterior organ or Epiphysis II is connected with the posterior commissure. It is this Epyphysis II in a modified form which is said to be represented by the epiphysis of amphibia; the pineal sac or epiphysis of reptiles; and the epiphysis of birds and mammals.

Having considered the immediate relations of the pineal body and the principal connections of the habenular and posterior commissures, it will be advantageous to examine the structures which lie around the pineal zone, and which are liable to be compressed by a tumour originating in these regions, or would have to be borne in mind when approaching the organ with the object of removing a tumour. A glance at the transverse section (Fig. 279) will show the relations of the tela choroidea with its contained vessels to the transverse fibres and fimbriæ of the fornix and also the connection of the latter with the body of the corpus callosum. Overlapping the fimbria of the fornix on each side is the choroid plexus, which projects into the lateral ventricle. The size, vascularity, and density of the plexus varies considerably in different individuals. In the specimen drawn the lateral ventricle is of moderate size, but in cases of obstruction to the aqueduct of Sylvius the ventricle may be greatly distended or, if emptied, the walls may be collapsed. On either side of the pineal body is the pulvinar of the optic thalamus. This is separated from the pineal body, superior colliculus, and superior brachium by pia mater containing blood-vessels. Lateral to the pulvinar is the internal capsule, passing between the caudate and lenticular nuclei and coursing downward into the crura cerebri. Immediately beneath the pineal body is the roof of the aqueduct, containing the tecto-spinal and tecto-bulbar nuclei. Around the aqueduct is the central grey matter and below it the various nuclei of the third nerve, the nuclei of the fourth nerve, and the medial longitudinal fasciculi (Fig. 279, p. 415), which if traced downwards are found to be connected on each side with the superior olive, the nucleus of the sixth cranial nerve, and that of the vestibular nerve. Ventral to the nuclei of the third nerve are the red nuclei, the decussation of the rubro-spinal tract, and the substantia nigra ; while dorso-lateral to the red nucleus is the medial lemniscus. Ventral to the red nuclei is the substantia nigra and near the outer borders of this are seen the medial geniculate bodies. Passing upwards round the outer side of the crus cerebri are the posterior cerebral and superior cerebellar arteries, with the fourth nerve running ventrally and forwards between them. The basal vein also, as mentioned previously, occupies the recess between the crus cerebri and medial geniculate body on the inner side, and the tail of the caudate nucleus, inferior horn of the lateral ventricle, choroidal fissure, fimbria, and hippocampus are on the outer side. Finally the apex of the pineal body is seen in a medial section (Fig. 280) to be in close relation to the superior vermis of the cerebellum, and if the organ is enlarged it may exert direct pressure on this and the superior peduncles or brachia conjunctivæ. Should a tumour of the pineal body enlarge forward into the third ventricle it may exert pressure on the interpeduncular and subthalamic regions and upon the optic thalami laterally.

CHAPTER 28

THE FUNCTIONS OF THE PINEAL BODY

WE do not propose to deal at length with the controversial question of the function of the mammalian pineal organ, which has been very fully discussed in publications specially concerned with the endocrine glands ; nor do we propose in this section to discuss the various functions attributed to the pineal organs of fishes, amphibia, and reptiles, which we have already alluded to (pp. 6, 46, 230) ; but from the practical standpoint of whether the use of pineal extracts as a therapeutic measure should be continued or should be discontinued, we believe that the present time is ripe for a short review of the principal results which have been obtained from recent experimental work on the function of the pineal gland in birds and mammals.

The evidence which is often contradictory may be classified under two principal headings, namely :

A—The results of experimental work on animals.

B—Observations on the human subject.

A. *Experimental Work on Animals.*—The biochemical aspect of this subject has been fully dealt with in numerous articles in the physiological and pharmaceutical journals and is beyond the scope of the present treatise ; we shall therefore limit our description to the consideration of the general results of experimental work under the following categories :

1. The results of pinealectomy.
2. The effects of feeding with pineal substance and injection of pineal extracts.
3. The influence of pineal grafts.

In the consideration of each of these subdivisions we shall allude first to results which are deemed to be of a positive character and afterwards to those which are negative. We shall also limit ourselves to a brief discussion on the more important and typical results which have been obtained by authoritative workers, and we shall not attempt to make a complete record of the numerous papers of an indecisive nature which have been published on this subject, references to which will be found in the larger monographs dealing with the organs of internal secretion and the principal journals on endocrinology.

Pinealectomy

Assuming that the pineal organ exerts an inhibitory influence on body growth and the development of the sexual organs, perhaps the most striking positive results which have been obtained in support of this view were those described by Foa in 1912 and Izawa in 1922. Foa performed the difficult operation of removing the pineal gland in young chicks between the ages of 5 and 7 weeks. The mortality was large and only a small number of chicks survived. After a period of 3 months the latter showed that the general development of the body had been much more rapid in the experimental birds than in the controls, and also

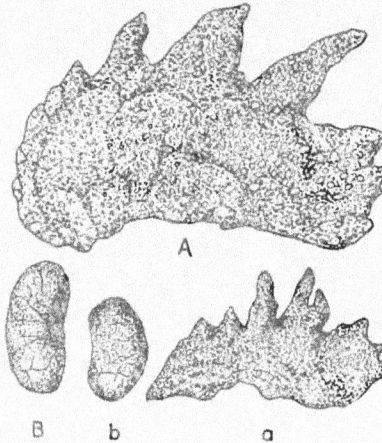

FIG. 282.—A—CREST, AND B—TESTICLE OF A COCK FROM WHICH THE EPIPHYSIS HAD BEEN REMOVED THREE MONTHS PREVIOUSLY ; a—CREST, AND b—TESTICLE OF A NORMAL CONTROL SPECIMEN OF THE SAME AGE.

The development of the experimental animals was much more rapid than the controls, and the development of the secondary sexual characters (crow, crest, spurs) was equally precocious.

(After Foa ; redrawn from L'Epiphyse, J. Calvet.)

that the development of the secondary sexual characters had been more precocious and active in the experimental animals, namely, the growth of the comb and spurs and the early occurrence of crowing (Fig. 282). Moreover, at the age of 10 to 12 months Foa examined the testicles of the pinealectomized birds and found that they were not only increased in size, but also showed that the general increase was due to the hypertrophy of both the interstitial tissue and the seminiferous tubules. He obtained similar results by repeating these experiments on rats and mice and another series of young chicks. In the latter series he noted that the size was not so markedly influenced as in the first series, and also that pinealectomy had no effect on hens.

Izawa performed pinealectomy on 36 chickens ranging from 4 to 5 weeks of age, and besides these 11 others of the same age and weight as those operated on were used for comparison. Aseptic precautions were taken, and no cases of infection occurred. Most of the experimental animals died shortly after the operation. Only four—three males and one female—survived the operation for any length of time. These were fed under the same conditions as the control animals and the effects observed. Compared with the controls, the pinealectomized animals showed a retarded growth for a few weeks following the operation, but about a month later they grew more rapidly than the controls, their body-weight becoming greater and their legs longer than those of the controls. In the two males whose pineal bodies were completely removed, the rapid development of the comb and the premature crow deserve special notice, and Izawa stated that they gave evidence of sexual instinct 31 and 50 days earlier than the controls. There was also a marked increase in the size of the testes.

In the female pinealectomized bird there was a remarkable increase in the size of the ovary and of the Fallopian tube, the latter showing a great increase in the length of the tube with increase in the width of its ampullary portion, which was described as voluminous, while the Fallopian tubes in the control were not only short but uniformly slender throughout their whole length.

Zoia and Horrax also report positive results following pinealectomy. The latter states that pinealectomized hens tend to breed earlier than controls of the same age and weight ; on the other hand, Sarteschi reports that pinealectomized hens dislike to copulate. Izawa gives tables showing the exact weight and size of the various organs and parts of the animals experimented on, and of the controls. From the statistical side it should be borne in mind that the results obtained by Izawa, striking as they appear to be, were based on only three cases, two male and one female, and that the controls were individuals matched with regard to age and weight with the experimental animal rather than of average size and weight.

Positive results following pinealectomy have also been recorded by Urechia and Gregoriu, Hoffmann, Zoia, Clemente, Izawa, and Yokoh in young rats and chickens, namely, general increase in the growth of the body and increase in the size and weight of the genital glands in both males and females. Hoffmann also found in three pinealectomized rats a decided enlargement of the vesiculæ seminales.

Horrax, 1916, experimenting with rats and guinea-pigs, found acceleration of spermatogenesis in the pinealectomized animals.

Pinealectomy Resulting in Negative or Regressive Effects

Kolmer and Loewy destroyed the pineal gland by cauterization in immature rats weighing 50 grm. They obtained negative results and verified histologically that the destruction of the organ was complete.

Cristea practised epiphysectomy in 30 male chicks, 12 of which survived, and in place of increased growth showed a rapid retardation of both general development and of secondary sexual characters.

Foa's experiments, previously mentioned, were negative with respect to chicks of the female sex.

Dandy, who experimented on dogs, came to the following conclusions :

1. Following the removal of the pineal he observed no sexual precocity, or indolence ; no adiposity or emaciation ; no somatic or mental precocity or retardation.
2. The experiments seemed to yield nothing to sustain the view that the pineal has any active endocrine functions of importance either in very young or adult dogs.
3. The pineal is not essential to life and seems to have no influence on the animals' well-being.

Demel performed epiphysectomy on rams aged 4 weeks, of which four survived. These showed a diminished growth, they became timid, their fleece was poor and diminished in amount, their horns grew very slowly and in two of them the horns were shed. The testicles were as large as those of the healthy rams or definitely larger (positive change). The hoofs were defective and there was an increase in the body temperature, which was raised by more than $1°$ C.

As a counter-test, Demel fed these animals for three months with " epiglandol." They rapidly recovered, attained the weight of the control rams, and developed the normal amount of fat and their horns. Demel came to the conclusion that the pineal played a rôle in the regulation of temperature and in producing hypertrophy of the testicles. He considered that it had no effect on the secondary sexual characters. But, since as is well known, the development of these is associated with the development of the genital organs, it is difficult to believe that the one system could be affected without the other. It is possible also that the rise of temperature and poor condition of the experimental animals might have been due to concomitant injury of the meninges and other important parts, and the subsequent improvement in their condition to recovery from this, quite apart from the action of epiglandol.

Negative results were also obtained in lower vertebrates, e.g. frog tadpoles, by Atwell and E. R. Hoskins and M. Hoskins. In those animals which survived complete destruction of the pineal body by means of a thermocautery, nothing abnormal was observed in their development.

In one of the most recent publications on the effects of pinealectomy, namely, by L. G. Rowntree in the *Practitioners' Library of Medicine and Surgery*, 1938, Chapter 5, this author summarizes the general results of this operation in the following words : " Pinealectomy in the hands of many investigators has led consistently to negative results ; in the rat (Foa, Horrax, Kolmer, Loewy, del Castillo, Renton and Rushbridge, Anderson and Wolf) ; in the rabbit (Exner and Boese) ; in the dog (Dandy) ; and in the chick (Badertscher). Positive results have been claimed in the rat by Izawa and Yohoh ; in the guinea-pig (Horrax and Clemente) ; and in the chick (Foa, Zoia, and Clemente). The most common results of pinealectomy are said to be : premature development of secondary sexual characters in the male ; enlargement of the gonads, overgrowth of the body, and obesity. Anderson and Wolf, after a critical analysis of the several papers submitted, expressed the opinion that the data submitted do not justify the conclusions reached."

The Effects of Feeding with Pineal Substance and the Injection of Pineal Extracts

Precocious sexual and mental development and early somatic development when occurring in the human subject are usually interpreted as indicating pineal deficiency or hypopinealism. If this opinion is correct, one would expect that feeding with pineal substance or the injection of pineal extracts would produce a condition of retarded sexual and mental development and deferred somatic maturity. The effect of feeding experiments, however, appears in many instances to be just the reverse, namely, in place of inhibition of growth of the sexual organs and of the body, there is often a rapid sexual and somatic development. There are, however, a considerable number of experiments which have given results which appear to confirm the general opinion of the restraining influence of the pineal and which may, according to Calvet, be regarded as positive in nature, whereas the accelerating and stimulating influence may be regarded as negative.

Positive Effects.—Sisson and Finney obtained a retardation of growth in young rats by feeding with the epiphysis of the calf. Priore found that repeated injections of pineal extracts produced a definite retardation of development in young male rabbits. M‘Cord and Allen dissolved the desiccated powder of the pineal in water containing living Amblystomes [1]

---

[1] The type of this group of tailed amphibians is the Mexican axolotl, which is the permanent larval form of a salamander from the United States, *Amblystoma tigrinum*.

and obtained a retardation of metamorphosis. This result is, however, counterbalanced by the results of experiments published by M‘Cord in 1917, in which he states that : " In unicellular organisms (paramœcia) pineal extract increases the rate of reproduction to more than double that of the controls " ; and " in larval forms (*Ranidæ*) both growth and differentiation are hastened."

Berblinger, experimenting on young rats, injected alcoholic and watery extracts of the epiphyses of oxen subcutaneously, and also administered the pineal by way of the alimentary tract. He obtained positive results in most, but in some there was an increase in size.

Calvet also experimented on immature white rats, using epiphyseal extracts obtained, fresh, from entire horses, geldings, and mares. These were ground aseptically in a mortar and mixed with equal parts of physiological serum. The animals received daily injections of this solution for 8 days, and were killed two days after the injections had been discontinued. The testicles were slightly smaller than those of the controls, but the size of the animals remained practically the same as the controls.

Negative Results.—M‘Cord fed young chickens and guinea-pigs with food containing a mixture of desiccated pineal gland and lactose. The control animals received a similar food containing the same amount of lactose but without the pineal. In both cases there was an acceleration of growth in the experimental animals. At the end of two weeks the guinea-pigs fed with pineal substance showed an increase in weight of 100 per cent., as compared with an increase of 77 per cent. in the controls. The author, however, noted that the action was variable (Fig. 283), and that if young animals were fed with epiphyses obtained from aged oxen, there was a diminution in weight.

Negative results, namely, acceleration of development and increase of weight, have also been obtained by Roux in frog tadpoles, Calvet in tadpoles of *Alytes*, M‘Cord (previously mentioned) in *Ranidæ*, by feeding with desiccated epiphysis, and also by Calvet with daily injections of Epiglandol into immature rats, 1 c.c. of Epiglandol being equal to 0·02 grm. of the fresh gland. The injected animals killed three weeks after weighed 34 grm., while the largest of the controls weighed only 31 grm. Notwithstanding this somatic increase, the testicles were not hypertrophied and macroscopically appeared even smaller than those of the controls ; moreover, microscopical sections showed no appreciable change in structure.

In discussing the various results of these experiments depending on the use of desiccated epiphysis or extracts of the epiphysis, Calvet puts forward the suggestion, based on the biochemical researches of Fenger and Roux, that since phosphoric acid, calcium, magnesium, sodium, and other inorganic elements are present in the desiccated epiphysis it is possible that the power to influence growth may be due to the action of these chemical constituents rather than on the supposed action of a hormone.

Robinson reports further feeding experiments carried out by M'Cord on young animals using fresh pineal glands, with resulting early precocity and adiposity ; Hoskins' results were almost completely negative. Kozelka also obtained negative results with pineal implants in chicks ; whereas increased rate of growth has been claimed by Dobowik ; and in the rat

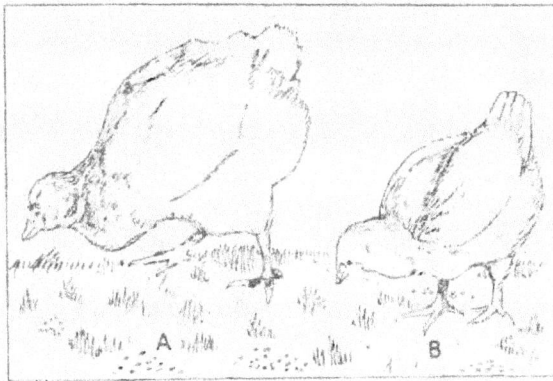

FIG. 283.—A—CONTROL BIRD, AND B—EXPERIMENTAL CHICK NOURISHED WITH A DESICCATED EXTRACT OF THE EPIPHYSIS, OBTAINED FROM YOUNG OXEN.

The experimental chick is diminished in size ; feeding with the extract has, therefore, in this instance retarded growth.

(Redrawn from Calvet, after M'Cord.)

Lahr found no influence on body-growth in either sex, but retardation of gonadal development in both male and female animals. Robinson further records the experimental work of Hanson on the effects on the offspring of intraperitoneal injections of pineal extracts in successive generations of parent rats. In succeeding generations up to the fifth he obtained increasing retardation of growth, with acceleration in gonadal development, precocity, " dwarfism," and macrogenitalismus præcox being the outstanding results.

Incidentally it may be mentioned here that observations on the human subject seem to indicate that in those cases in which excessive premature growth of the body has been associated with mental and sexual precocity, the ultimate stature and body-weight of those individuals who have lived to adult life is below the average height and weight.

In an interesting article by H. Lisser in *Bedside Diagnosis*, 1928,

W. B. Saunders, Philadelphia, the author, refers to certain cases of hyper-genitalism in preadolescent males combined with premature union of the epiphyses of the long bones. The principal signs being : premature and excessive development of the genital organs ; premature change of voice, associated with rapid and excessive development of the body in general ; the mental development, although somewhat precocious, not keeping pace with the general precocity, and in addition to the above-mentioned well-recognized group of symptoms, under the heading of skeletal changes, Lisser states that " the boy is large for his age, as if he were becoming a giant, but the excessive output of testicular secretions hastens epiphyseal unification, and the premature union of the epiphyses transposes a mis-leading and transitory gigantism into a final height which is not excessive and which may indeed incline to a mild form of dwarfism. Roentgeno-grams on such boys will reveal a bone age in advance of their chronological age as an additional proof of precocity."

It seems possible that this explanation of premature bodily growth associated with excessive testicular secretion and premature union of the epiphyses may account for some of the apparently contradictory results of experimental work on the effects of feeding with pineal substance or extracts, or injections of pineal extracts, namely : in some retardation or arrest of growth, " dwarfism," while in others there has been excessive growth. It must be borne in mind, however, that in a large proportion of the clinical cases that have been recorded in which these symptoms have been present there is no proof of their having been connected either directly or indirectly with the pineal organ.

The Influence of Pineal Grafts

Calvet experimented on three rats belonging to the same litter. These animals received every second day one-half epiphysis of an entire adult horse, which was introduced into the subcutaneous tissue of the dorsal region with aseptic precautions. The control animal received a portion of muscle or cerebral substance of equal weight from the horse and suffered the same traumatism as the experimental animals. The grafts commenced on the 15th November, 1932, and ceased on the 10th December. The weight of the control rat, which at the commencement of the experiment was 38 grm., reached 62 grm. The others treated with the epiphysis weighed 40 grm. at the commencement, decreased 3 grm. from their original weight. The normal rat increased 3 cm. in length, while the size of the grafted animals remained stationary.

Moreover, the migration of the testicles was arrested in the grafted animal, and microscopic sections of the testicle showed a true atrophy, whereas the testicles of the normal rat had migrated into the scrotum and showed active spermatogenesis. Calvet repeated the same experiment on a number of rats and young guinea-pigs and obtained practically the same results.

Grafts carried out on adult males were without effect on either growth or the testicles.

Hölldöbler and Schültze obtained acceleration of metamorphosis with increase of weight after implantation of a small piece of the epiphysis of the ox at the root of the tail in the larva of the toad, their results are opposed to those of Calvet and are classed by him as negative. On the other hand, the same experiment was repeated by Romeis, who was unable to confirm the result of the last-mentioned observers.

Correlation of the Pineal Gland with the Genital Glands and other Endocrine Organs

An interesting observation which appears to indicate an interrelationship of the pineal organ and the genital glands was made by Jean Calvet, namely, that the parenchyma cells in the pineal gland of the bullock are less numerous than in that of the bull, and also that the neuroglial tissue is relatively more abundant in the castrated than in the entire animal. This observation is of considerable importance and if confirmed by subsequent investigations on similar lines with a detailed record of the age of the animals from which the epiphyses were obtained would be of real value in establishing the existence of a definite interrelationship between the pineal gland and testicles.

Biach and Hulles (1912) found in cats which had been castrated when very young that 7–8 months after there was an atrophy of the parenchyma of the pineal, and he also stated that the epiphysis of the ox was smaller than that of the bull. Calvet also weighed the epiphyses of geldings and oxen and compared these with the weights of the pineal body in stallions and bulls. The results were variable, the glands being sometimes larger in the castrated than in the entire animals, but the weight of the pineal glands of the stallions and bulls was on the whole greater than in the castrated animals and they were more developed.

Aschner (1918),[1] moreover, has confirmed the observations of Calvet with regard to the predominance of neuroglial fibres and fewer nuclei of the parenchyma cells of the pineal gland in the ox as compared with the bull, and has noted the same differences in dogs, cats, rabbits, and guinea-pigs.

---

[1] Aschner, B., *Die Blutdrüsenerkrangungen des Weibes*. (Wiesbaden, 1918.) Physiologie der Hypophyse. Handbuch der inneren Sekretion, II, Liefkabitzsch.

CHAPTER 29

PATHOLOGY OF PINEAL TUMOURS

THE various pathological conditions which arise in and around the pineal gland can be discussed in relation to the actual lesion itself, in relation to the local changes produced inside the cranium, and in relation to the somewhat variable general skeletal and endocrine changes which are sometimes associated with such pathological conditions.

General Pathology.—The pineal gland may undergo simple hypertrophy. This was described by Virchow as occurring in an infant. It has also been observed in association with other pathological conditions, such as myxœdema and polyglandular dysfunctions, and has also been described in a case of general cerebral hypertrophy.

Laignel has observed and described a case in which atrophy of the gland was found.

The other pathological conditions arising in and in the region of the pineal may be classified as follows : (1) cysts ; (2) cholesteatomata ; (3) teratomata ; (4) pinealomata ; (5) pineoblastomata.

1. *Cysts.*—Cysts of various types have been described in relation to the pineal. They are usually simple cysts without any associated tumour growth. Often they may be found to project into and obliterate the third ventricle and to compress the corpora quadrigemina. They almost invariably give rise to hydrocephalus by blockage of the aqueduct.

No rule can be formulated as to the age incidence of such growths, since they have been described both in the new-born and in the aged. Such cysts are commonly single, but may be multiple. They are lined with flattened cells and contain fluid which is occasionally discoloured from recent hæmorrhage. These cysts are very seldom accompanied by any changes of the pubertas præcox type.

2. *Cholesteatomata.*—These tumours occur in the region of the pineal ; they are firm in consistency, the cut surface being yellowish-white and waxy in appearance. On section they can be seen to be composed of lamellated waxes or scaly material enclosed in a wall of stratified squamous cells concentrically arranged. Such cells may be multinucleated. The waxy material consists of desquamated cells and cholesterol crystals.

Cholesteatomata occur anywhere in the brain, but more especially do they occur near the midline. They are regularly connected with the meninges. Bostroem concludes that all cholesteatomata arise from embryonal epidermal inclusions.

3. *Teratomata.*—These tumours arise exclusively in young males from 4 to 16 years of age, and are associated with precocious sexual development, hirsutes, and sometimes with adiposity and general overgrowth.

These complex teratomata are of moderate size ; they may be solid or cystic, and are usually circumscribed. They give rise to marked pressure signs. They may consist almost entirely of hair, sebaceous material, epidermoid cysts, cartilage, calcific grains, fat tissue and non-medullated nerve-fibres, and smooth muscle.[1] A small layer of normal pineal tissue may be found beside and unusually compressed and displaced by the tumour. They are firm in consistency, irregular and knobbly on the surface, often with elongated shreds of tela choroidea adherent to the upper and posterior surface.

Their nature and origin is obscure, but of interest ; they are probably derived from embryonic vestiges. The dermal structures, such as hair and sebaceous glands, require an ectodermal tissue for their development, which may possibly reach the pineal gland by the same developmental disturbances that give rise to cholesteatomata. It must also be remembered that in certain reptiles and fishes the pineal is a well-developed organ which passes through a minute foramen in the skull and reaches the surface. Alternatively these may develop by pseudogestation from a fertilized filial polar body.

4, 5. *Pinealomata and Pineoblastomata.*—Tumours arising from the pineal gland tend to resemble the structure of the developing pineal at some definite stage of its development. The more primitive the type that is found in these tumours, the more rapidly growing and more invasive is the growth. The primitive type of such tumours is termed pineoblastoma. The course is usually short. If the tumour cells resemble more the adult type of pineal structure, they are slow growing, less invasive, are less liable to hæmorrhage, and less vascular, and the tumour is termed pinealoma.

Pineoblastomata : these tumours are usually soft, with a tendency to

---

[1] Transversely striated muscle fibres have also been found in teratomata of the pineal gland, and very occasionally in the normal gland, more especially in the ox, as described by Nicolas and Dimitrowa (Fig. 284). Striated muscles fibres have, moreover, been observed by Hammer in the epiphysis of a human fœtus aged 5 months, and cells which have been described as "myoid" in the adult human organ. They have been found chiefly in the vascular connective tissue septa or trabeculæ, and usually appear as isolated fibres, as in the specimen described by Dimitrowa. In some cases the nucleus is central and the general appearance of the fibres is intermediate between that of the striped and unstriped types of muscle-fibres.

infiltrate into the surrounding tissue—the hemispheres, the cerebellum, and the third ventricle—and tend to obliterate the aqueduct. Cysts are often present and areas of hæmorrhage occur. The surface is irregular and lobulated ; cysts may be seen on the cut surface.

Microscopically there is a marked variation in the type and arrange-

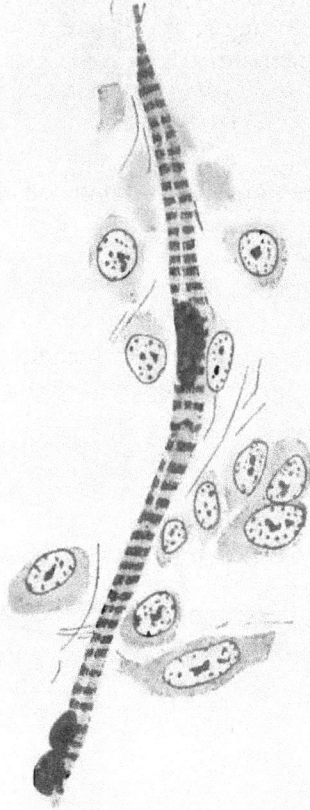

FIG. 284.—A TRANSVERSELY STRIATED MUSCLE-FIBRE FROM THE EPIPHYSIS OF BOS TAURUS. (AFTER DIMITROWA.)

ment of cell found. The cells are arranged in a mosaic with streams of small cells deeply staining in character and enclosing nests of larger cells with vesicular nuclei and larger masses of clear cytoplasm, bearing a strong resemblance to the parenchyma cells of the mature pineal body. Giant cells are not an uncommon feature in various areas of these tumours ; they are more common in the vicinity of the calcified plaques, which are a frequent feature of such growths.

Pinealomata : the other main type is that which more closely approximates to the adult or mature type of pineal. They are slower in growth and less invasive. Hæmorrhages and cysts are less common. Microscopical section shows an alveolar pattern ; the cells are chiefly of the large vesicular type, and are separated by strands of fibrous tissue.

Thus we see the importance of recognizing the developmental stages

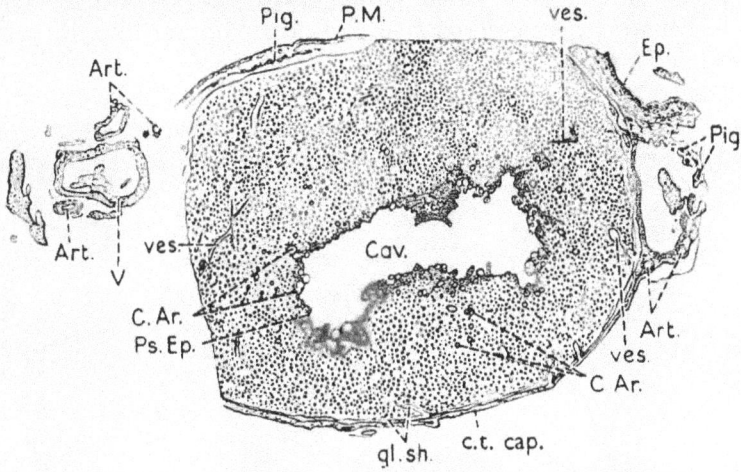

Fig. 285.—Section through Pineal Body showing a Central Cavity, the Wall of which is stained Deeply and contains numerous Corpora Arenacea.

Art. : artery.	*Pig.* : pigment.
Cav. : central cavity.	*P.M.* : pia mater.
C. Ar. : corpora arenacea.	*Ps. Ep.* : pseudo-epithelium.
c.t. cap. : connective tissue capsule.	*V.* : vein.
Ep. : ependyma.	*ves.* : vessel.
gl. sh. : glial sheath.	

(Drawn from a specimen in Professor Barclay-Smith's collection at King's College, London.)

through which the pineal passes when attempting to understand the histology of these tumours.

General Changes.—The associated changes in the brain are due to direct displacement and invasion of the brain substance. The cerebellum is often invaded. The growth extends beneath the tentorium and invades the cerebellum both in the midline and in either of the lateral lobes.

The midbrain is pressed upon, and especially the corpora quadrigemina. This distortion gives rise to the characteristic eye signs and may also occlude the aqueduct of Sylvius. Occlusion of the aqueduct may also be brought about by direct invasion of the third ventricle by the growth. The outcome of these changes is that the whole ventricular

28

system above the aqueduct becomes distended and internal hydrocephalus results. Pressure on the vein of Galen by the growth may also play a part in the development of the hydrocephalus.

The floor of the third ventricle is depressed. The hypophysis is pressed upon and the hypothalamus distorted. It is this change as well as the direct invasion which occurs which probably accounts for the changes in growth and sexual development and other hypothalamic signs which are sometimes seen. Extension may occur into the cerebral hemispheres by direct invasion.

Hæmorrhage occurs into these growths, and terminally hæmorrhage into the ventricles is not an uncommon finding. Changes are also found around the medulla, there usually being a very well-developed pressure cone.

CHAPTER 30

SYMPTOMATOLOGY OF PINEAL TUMOURS

ENLARGEMENTS of the pineal gland usually present clinically a well-defined syndrome. Owing to the anatomical position, enlargements of the gland cause pressure on structures which give rise to clear-cut clinical symptoms and hence are quite early recognizable.

The symptoms can best be considered under three headings : (1) Focal

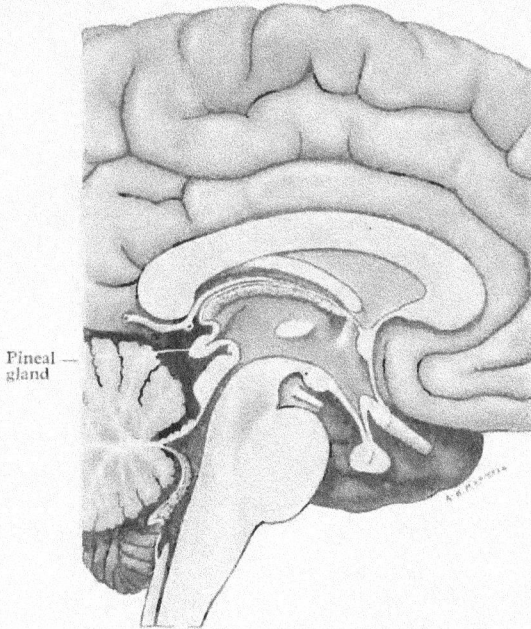

FIG. 286.—ANATOMICAL RELATIONSHIPS OF THE PINEAL GLAND.

—those due to the lesion itself. (2) Local—the changes brought about within the central nervous system. (3) General—the somatic changes which sometimes accompany such enlargements.

1. **Focal Signs.**—The focal signs which may be produced by tumours are due in the main to the anatomical position of the gland (see Fig. 286). It is because of its relationship to the superior corpora quadrigemina that the eye signs produced are so characteristic.

The aqueduct of Sylvius lying below the gland is very liable to be occluded and produce a severe degree of internal hydrocephalus when pressed upon by a pineal tumour.

The cerebellum lies immediately posterior to the pineal and is often invaded by growths arising in that neighbourhood.

A contributory factor in the production of the internal hydrocephalus is the fact that the vein draining the choroid plexuses—the vein of Galen—is very liable to be compressed, with the result that engorgement of the

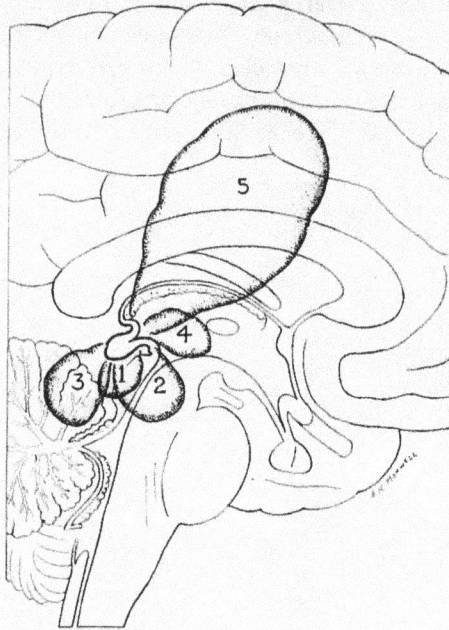

FIG. 287.—SCHEMATIC REPRESENTATION OF THE VARIOUS WAYS IN WHICH A PINEAL TUMOUR MAY EXTEND AND CAUSE PRESSURE SYMPTOMS : (1) ON THE CORPORA QUADRIGEMINA ; (2) ON THE AQUEDUCT OF SYLVIUS AND MIDBRAIN ; (3) DOWNWARDS ON THE CEREBELLUM, CAUSING CEREBELLAR SYMPTOMS ; (4) ON THE MIDBRAIN THALAMIC AND SUBTHALAMIC REGIONS ; AND (5) ON THE CEREBRAL HEMISPHERE.

choroid plexuses is produced and possibly an increased secretion of the cerebrospinal fluid.

Tumours which arise in the pineal may extend in various directions, and Fig. 287 illustrates the common methods of extension.

Eye Signs.—Tumours may extend into the corpora quadrigemina and oculomotor region and produce a clinical syndrome which is characterized by loss of pupillary reaction to light, reaction to accommodation, and upward, downward, and lateral movement of the eyes, in that order of development.   It is extremely common to find that the light reflex is absent and the patient unable to look upward.

To understand this clearly it is necessary to visualize the arrangement of the oculomotor nuclei (Fig. 288).   It will be remembered that the nuclei of the IIIrd, IVth, and VIth nerves lie in about one continuous line on either side of the aqueduct just below the corpora quadrigemina, together with the medially placed nuclei.   Various functions have been mapped out for the several parts of the nucleus.   In Fig. 288 it will be seen that the Edinger-Westphal nucleus (A) is the most anterior, and is concerned with control of the pupillary and ciliary muscles ; the dorsi-

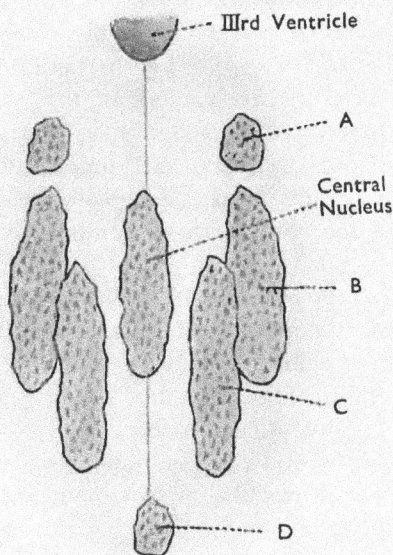

FIG. 288.—DIAGRAM SHOWING ARRANGEMENT OF OCULOMOTOR NUCLEI.

lateral nucleus (B) is concerned with upward movements ; the ventro-medial nucleus (C) is concerned with downward movement ; the central nucleus with movements of divergence.   The small caudal nucleus (D) may be concerned again with pupillary reaction.

Thus it will be seen that pressure exerted from in front and above the nuclei will give rise first to absence of light reflex, then to loss of accommodation and loss of upward and downward movement.   In clinical practice it is the lateral movements which persist for the longest period.

Ear Signs.—Should the inferior corpora quadrigemina be pressed upon, then deafness, unilateral or bilateral, complete or partial, may result.

Cerebellar Signs.—Extension occurs into the cerebellum. This may be into either hemisphere or directly in the midline.

Nystagmus is very common ; there is often giddiness and incoordination, with a tendency to swerve to the side most affected, or, if in the midline, a tendency to fall backward. There is weakness, adiadochokinesia, intention tremor in the arms, and usually a grossly ataxic gait. Rombergism may be present. The cerebellar involvement will in some cases also give rise to a dysarthric speech, usually staccato in type.

Other cerebellar signs may be present. On extension of the hands there is a tendency to fall away on the side of the lesion. The pastpointing test may show deviation.

The reflexes may be diminished or absent on one or both sides and the limbs atonic, but usually the pyramidal involvement predominates.

Pyramidal and Sensory Signs.—The pyramidal tracts and medial lemnisci may be affected. Involvement of the pyramidal tracts gives rise to increase in tone on the affected side, weakness, increased deep reflexes, absent abdominal reflexes, and an extensor plantar response. The sensory changes take the form of a hemianæsthesia, as all the sensory fibres at the level of the corpora quadrigemina have joined the medial lemniscus.

Signs of Third Ventricle Involvement.—The somatic changes sometimes associated with pineal tumours have been referred to involvement of the hypothalamus and third ventricle.

Disturbed temperature regulation has been reported in a few cases of pineal tumour. The hypothalamus is probably concerned in the control of body temperature, and the case reports show that there may be rise of temperature of an irregular type without any apparent source of infection and with no corresponding rise in pulse-rate. The controlling centre in the hypothalamus itself or its efferent pathway may be damaged. Polyphagia, polyuria, and glycosuria have also been observed, and are probably due to hypothalamus involvement.

Signs of Involvement of the Cerebral Hemispheres.—As a pineal tumour grows, extension occurs upwards into the hemispheres. It is of necessity a deep extension, and the motor cortex and sensory cortex are not usually involved. The optic radiations, however, pass near by on their way to the occipital cortex, and these may be cut through and a right or left homonymous hemianopia result.

2. Local Signs.—Owing to the site of the lesion, signs due to raised intracranial pressure manifest themselves early in the course of the tumour growth. Headaches are severe and continuous, and are associated with vomiting. Mental lethargy and reduction in mentality may be early signs, as may also giddiness. Loss of vision occurs from the effects

of papilloedema, which is usually very marked and presents itself as a very early sign. Epileptiform fits also occur.

Signs are produced in the cranial nerves as the result of the raised intracranial pressure. The third ventricle is commonly affected, and double vision and strabismus are frequently present. The VIth nerve is also involved. There is paralysis of the external rectus on either or both sides, with a convergent strabismus. The olfactory nerve is not affected. The Vth nerve may be affected, giving rise to a weakness of the muscles of mastication and sometimes sensory loss on that side of the face.

Facial paralysis is seen quite commonly, and is either produced by the local extension of the growth or from damage to the nerve resulting from the raised intracranial pressure.

Deafness is common, and has already been mentioned.

The nerves IX, X, XI, and XII are not usually affected ; only if the cerebellum is extensively invaded will they be pressed upon and give rise to their characteristic physical signs.

3. **General Signs.**—Pineal tumours associated with general somatic changes are almost confined to the male sex. The disturbances of growth associated with pineal tumours affect chiefly the genital organs, but are often associated with adiposity and sometimes with general and symmetrical overgrowth.

Hypertrophy of the penis and testes, with growth of pubic hair and precocious sexual instinct, have been observed with most tumours classed as teratomata, as well as with simple, benign, and malignant tumours. The testicles show a marked increase in the size and number of the interstitial cells. The breasts enlarge, and one case has been reported of a secretion of colostrum in a boy aged 4, associated with testicular enlargement.

Increase of hair occurs also on the lips and chin and in the axillæ. Deepening of the voice may take place.

The adiposity which occurs has been observed with all varieties of pineal tumours, and cannot be distinguished clinically from hypophyseal obesity—probably because, as already pointed out, it is in both cases due to hypothalamic involvement. The adiposity is proximal in distribution ; it is marked over the shoulders and pelvic girdles, with considerable enlargement of the breasts. The buttocks, thighs, and abdomen also show heavy deposits of fat.

Physiological experiments seem to point to the fact that injection of pineal extracts in chicks and guinea-pigs causes a general increase in size, with genital overgrowth and sexual precocity, but the evidence is still not completely convincing.

The possibility is that the pineal gland normally facilitates growth in general, and sexual development in particular. Acceleration of these functions occurring in the course of pineal tumours may therefore be interpreted as hyperpinealism. In the absence of further data, obesity and hypertrichosis may be considered as part of the general and sexual overgrowth, but the hypophyseal failure must be considered as a possible contributing factor in the adiposity.

A close relationship evidently exists between the pineal and testicular functions, which are probably not antagonistic in nature, but as yet there are insufficient data to define the relationship between the pineal organ and the ductless glands, and hence of its relationship to the gonads. Moreover, in quite a number of cases there are no signs whatever of any sexual abnormality.

CHAPTER 31

OPERATIVE TECHNIQUE

ALTHOUGH it is possible to operate on the pineal using local infiltration of the scalp and some scopolamine and morphine, yet it is preferable, in the author's opinion, to use rectal avertin, local infiltration of the scalp with $\frac{1}{2}$ per cent. novocain, and to follow with intratracheal gas and oxygen. The reasons for using intratracheal gas and oxygen are that it is desirable to have the patient completely quiet while the deep approach to the pineal is proceeded with, and that if the patient stops breathing, oxygen or

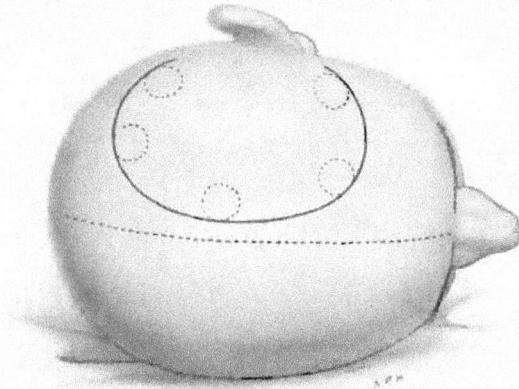

FIG. 289.—DRAWING SHOWING THE SKIN INCISION AND SITE FOR THE BURR HOLES IN THE BONE SO AS TO EXPOSE THE POSTERIOR TWO-THIRDS OF THE CEREBRAL HEMISPHERE.

carbondioxide can be given, a very desirable precaution when operating near the brain-stem, where slight deflections in either direction may press or drag upon the respiratory centre.

There are only two approaches to the pineal gland which are of any practical value, and both demand a large right occipito-parietal osteoplastic flap.

1. **Dandy's Operation.**—This is the method of choice, and is based on experimental operative procedure performed on dogs. After preliminary infiltration of the scalp with novocain, a large occipito-parietal scalp flap is fashioned (Fig. 289) and bleeding controlled. Some five

burr holes are made in the skull at the periphery of the scalp incision and
these burr holes are joined by means of a Gigli saw, which is inserted
by a special curved introducer (Fig. 290).   After the saw has been introduced, the bone between the burr holes is cut on the bevel, the intro-
ducers acting as a protector to the underlying dura mater and brain
(Fig. 291).   When all the burr holes have been united with the exception
of the lowest two, the osteoplastic flap can be elevated and fractured
across its narrow and thinned-out base ; it is then hinged outwards on
the temporal muscle.   Bleeding vessels in the dura mater are underrun

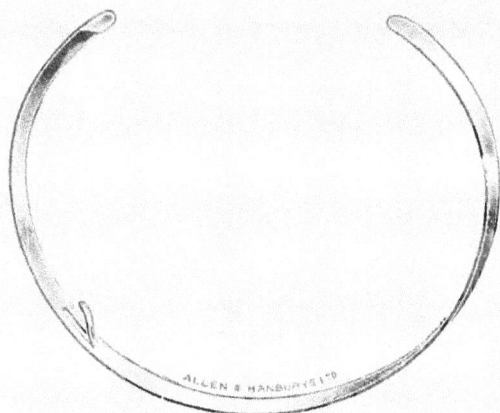

FIG. 290.—USEFUL GIGLI SAW
GUIDE.

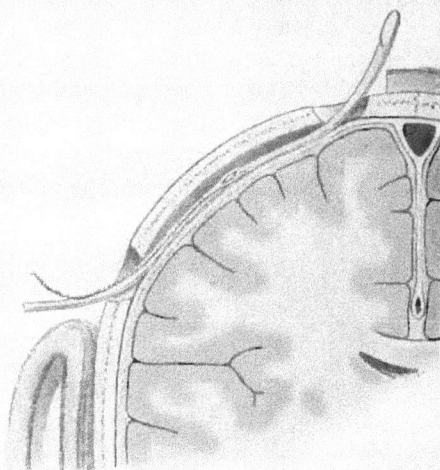

FIG. 291.—THE METHOD OF INTRODUC-
ING A GIGLI SAW BETWEEN TWO
BURR HOLES.

with silk sutures, while those occurring in the bone are controlled with
Horsley's bone wax.   If there is a considerable increase of the intracranial pressure this can be diminished by the administration of 20 c.c.
of hypertonic saline (15 per cent.) at the commencement of the operation,
but as a rule this is not necessary because adequate reduction of the intracranial pressure may be produced by tapping the lateral ventricle.   It is
a remarkable fact that although an internal hydrocephalus causes gradual
destruction of cerebral tissue, yet this hydrocephalus is advantageous to
the surgeon when removing a pineal tumour ; otherwise it would be
impossible to retract the posterior part of a normal hemisphere without
causing some permanent damage.   When the fluid from the ventricle
is withdrawn in a case of internal hydrocephalus, the flattened-out hemisphere can be retracted without further damage ensuing.

A flap of dura mater is turned outwards on top of the osteoplastic flap (Fig. 292) and bleeding from the cut surface of the dura is controlled with silver clips. As the mesial margin of the flap extends almost to the superior sagittal sinus, there are numerous bleeding vessels which will require ligature ; some of the smaller ones may be dealt with by silver clips. The lateral ventricle is then tapped at the junction of its body and descending horn, the cerebrospinal fluid being allowed to flow away over the brain ; the needle is left in situ for as long as possible to ensure complete evacuation of the ventricle.

The next step is to divide any cerebral veins which may be running

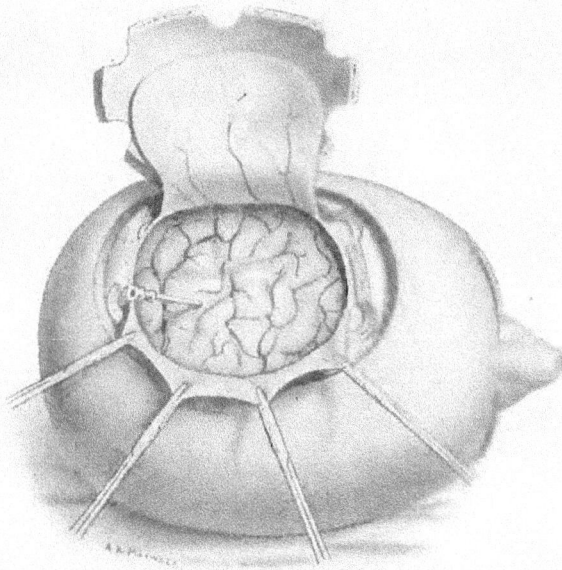

FIG. 292.—THE METHOD IN WHICH THE OSTEOPLASTIC FLAP IS RAISED AND TURNED OUTWARDS : FLAP OF DURA MATER IS THEN TURNED OUTWARDS AND THE LATERAL VENTRICLE TAPPED.

from the upper part of the hemisphere into the superior sagittal sinus. There are five or six of these veins, and they can be secured between fine ligatures or silver clips. Care should be taken to avoid injury to the vein which drains the Rolandic area of the brain, otherwise a transient hemiplegia may result.

After the cerebral veins have been divided the whole of the posterior extremity of the hemisphere is to be retracted to such an extent as to expose the falx cerebri (Fig. 293). Continued retraction will bring the inferior longitudinal sinus into view, and beneath it the corpus callosum (Fig. 294). To obtain an adequate exposure of the splenium of the corpus callosum, it is often advisable to divide the inferior longitudinal sinus between silver clips, and then slit up the lower border of the falx for half an inch or more with a curved tenotomy knife (Fig. 295). The splenium of the corpus callosum is then incised in the midline and the tumour exposed. Any bleeding that may be encountered in this procedure is checked by the diathermy point. The most important structure in relation to the tumour is the great vein of Galen, which lies under the fornix. This vein and its tributaries should be carefully preserved.

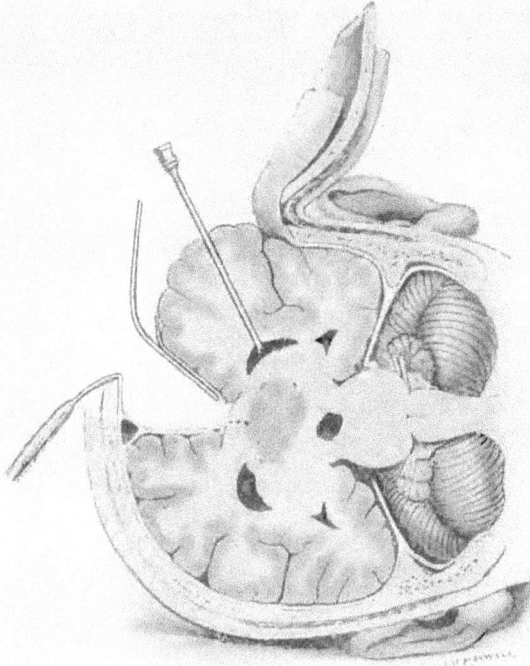

FIG. 293.—THE EXPOSURE OF THE CORPUS CALLOSUM. THE LIGATED CEREBRAL VEINS CAN BE SEEN AS THEY ENTER THE SUPERIOR SAGITTAL SINUS.

The tumour is carefully prised out of its bed by means of a curved dissector, such as Adson's. It may be that the third ventricle is opened while the tumour is dissected out of its bed, but this does not matter (Figs. 294, 296). Absolute hæmostasis is essential, and all bleeding points are controlled by the application of silver clips or the use of the diathermy point.

The tumour bed must be quite dry before completing the operation. The posterior part of the cerebral hemisphere is allowed to fall back into place, and the dura mater united with one or two tethering sutures. Drainage by means of a fine corrugated rubber dam is often necessary

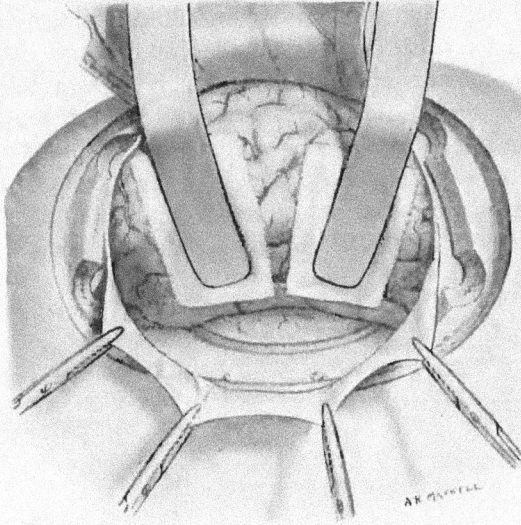

FIG. 294.—THE POSTERIOR PART OF THE CEREBRAL HEMISPHERE IS RETRACTED
SO AS TO EXPOSE THE CORPUS CALLOSUM.

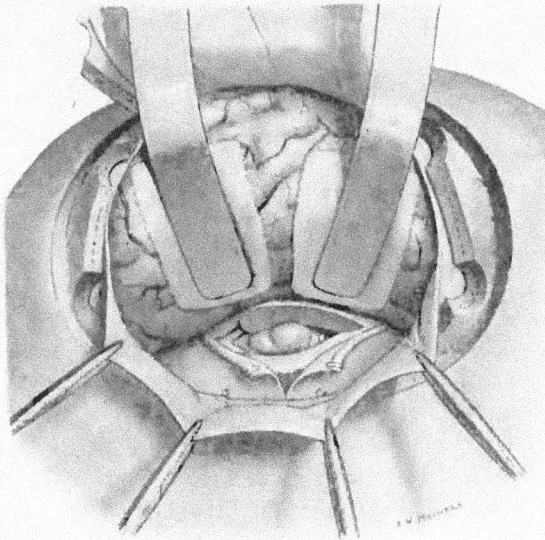

FIG. 295.—THE INFERIOR SURFACE OF THE FALX HAS BEEN DIVIDED, TOGETHER
WITH THE INFERIOR SAGITTAL SINUS. THE POSTERIOR END OF THE CORPUS
CALLOSUM HAS BEEN DIVIDED, EXPOSING THE PINEAL TUMOUR.

for a day or so. The osteoplastic flap is replaced and the scalp approximated by two layers of sutures. The head is covered with a firm bandage,
and the patient nursed flat for the first three days and then allowed a

pillow. With the depletion of cerebrospinal fluid during the operation, it is necessary to balance this by an adequate intake, and therefore after the operation a continuous rectal saline infusion is instituted. A purge is given on the second day after operation, and if there is much headache a lumbar operation is performed. The stitches are removed on the tenth day, and the patient is subsequently allowed to get out of bed.

2. **Van Wagenen's Operation.**—The second method of surgical approach is that devised by van Wagenen, in which the tumour is attacked

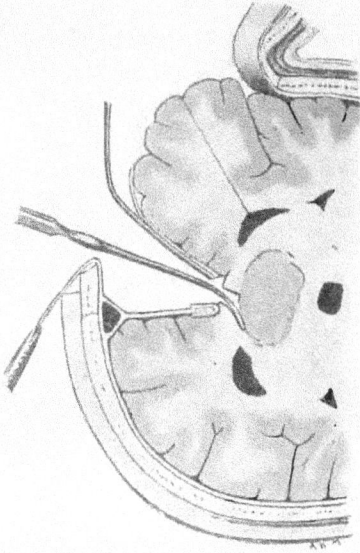

FIG. 296.—SECTION THROUGH THE BRAIN SHOWING THE EXPOSURE AND INCISION OF THE CORPUS CALLOSUM.

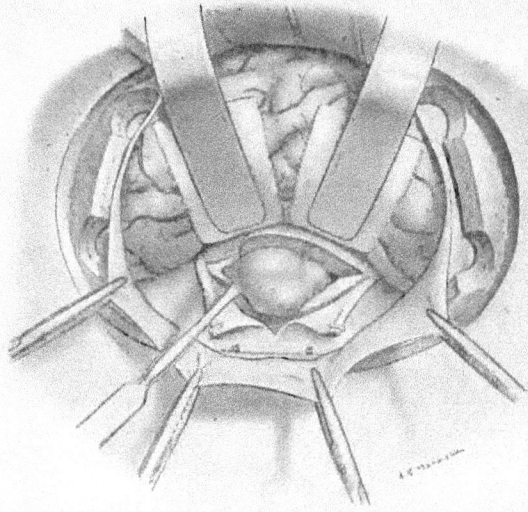

FIG. 297.—THE ACTUAL REMOVAL OF A PINEAL TUMOUR.

through the median wall of the lateral ventricle. It is an easier method and the route is less vascular, and the tributaries of the great vein of Galen can be more easily seen and dealt with. The disadvantage, however, is that it leaves some permanent disturbance of function in the form of hemiplegia and homonymous hemianopia.

The first part of the operation is very similar to Dandy's approach—an osteoplastic flap is fashioned and turned outwards (Fig. 298). The dura mater is incised and a flap turned downwards. A reversed L-shaped incision about 6 cm. in length is made in the cortex, extending from the posterior end of the superior temporal lobe gyrus upward and slightly backward, ending in the lobus parietalis superioris. This incision is gradually deepened by means of the diathermy cautery, using the cutting and coagulating currents alternately, and its edges retracted by small flange retractors covered with moist lint. The incision is deepened until the dilated lateral ventricle is opened (Fig. 299). The wound can now be retracted sufficiently to enable the surgeon to see the bulging medial wall of the ventricle covered in part by the choroid plexus. If the choroid plexus is well developed and extends over the medial wall of the ventricle

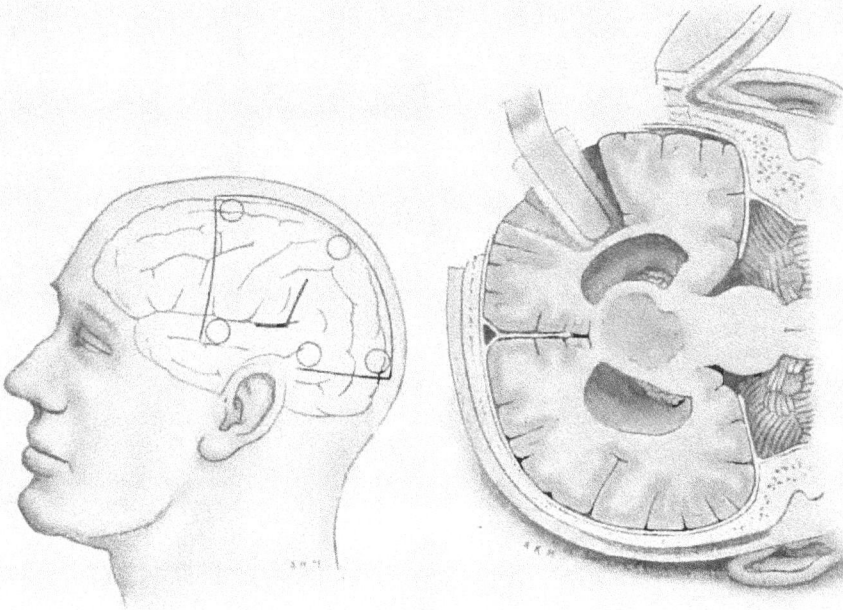

FIG. 298.—VAN WAGENEN'S APPROACH TO THE PINEAL SHOWING THE OUT-LINE OF THE OSTEOPLASTIC FLAP AND THE SITE OF THE INCISION IN THE CORTEX.

FIG. 299.—SECTIONAL VIEW OF THE APPROACH TO A PINEAL TUMOUR THROUGH A DILATED LATERAL VENTRICLE.

in the region of the bulging pineal tumour, it may be coagulated with the diathermy point. The medial wall of the ventricle is then gently incised and the pineal tumour exposed and gradually separated from its connections (Fig. 300). Absolute hæmostasis is procured, and a small piece of rubber dam is inserted into the incision in the brain for drainage. The dura mater is replaced and held in position by a few anchoring stitches. The osteoplastic flap is accurately put back in its original position, and the scalp united by a double layer of interrupted sutures, and a firm dressing then applied. The drainage wick is removed after twenty-four hours and the stitches on about the tenth day.

Whichever method of operation is adopted, it is a wise precaution to give the patient some post-operative X-ray therapy, as it is impossible to be quite sure that every particle of the tumour has been removed, and pineal tumours for the most part are radiosensitive.

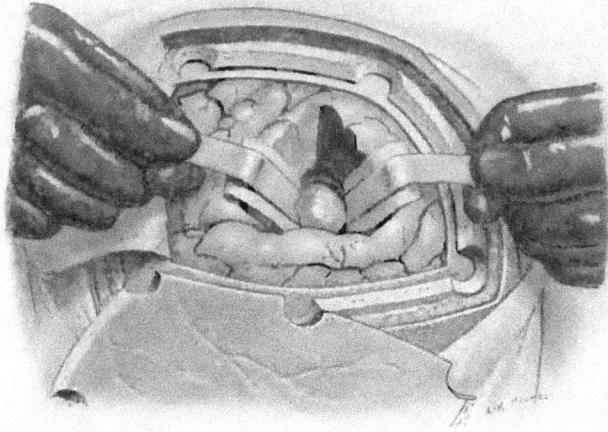

FIG. 300.—ACTUAL EXPOSURE OF A PINEAL TUMOUR THROUGH THE LATERAL VENTRICLE.

Ventricular puncture may be necessary during convalescence if the intracranial pressure becomes increased.

In some cases where the pineal tumour is very large it may be advisable to perform a partial lobectomy of the occipital lobe in order to give the surgeon a better method of approach.

CHAPTER 32

CLINICAL CASES

THE following clinical cases have come under observation and treatment since 1919.

Case 1.—Elsa B., aged 26, was admitted to hospital under the late Sir David Ferrier, in May, 1919, complaining of headache and vomiting. Up to a year prior to admission the patient was a cheerful individual who was employed in a laundry, and was very keen on tennis. Gradually she lost interest in her work and gave up all games. For a month previous to her admission to hospital she had attacks of vomiting, and was unsteady while walking.

On Examination.—The patient appeared rather depressed, but was quite keen to cooperate in the hope that something could be done to relieve her symptoms. She walked with a staggering gait, but there did not seem to be any tendency to fall to either side. She had a good sense of smell. The visual fields were complete. Bilateral papillœdema was present, more marked on the right side—right, four diopters ; left, three diopters. The pupils were dilated and did not react to light or accommodation. There was loss of conjugate upward movement of the eyes. There was weakness of the right VIth nerve and bilateral nerve deafness. The other cranial nerves appeared normal. There was a fine lateral nystagmus to the right. Ataxia was marked and Romberg's sign was positive. The diagnosis of a pontine or pineal tumour was made, and a subtentorial decompression advised.

Operation.—On 15th May, 1919, a large subtentorial decompression was performed under ether anæsthesia ; there was marked increase of the intracranial pressure, but no tumour was discovered. The wound was closed without drainage. Healing was sound and the stitches were removed after ten days. The patient rapidly improved after the operation, the vomiting stopped completely, and the papillœdema subsided. However, a month after the operation the decompression area began to bulge (Fig. 301), and the papillœdema returned. The patient began to go downhill and died two months after her operation.

An autopsy was performed and the brain removed entire and hardened. No obvious tumour could be seen. After the hardening process was complete, several sections were made through the entire brain, and a pineal tumour was discovered.

Pathology.—The tumour was situated between the splenium of the corpus callosum and the quadrigeminal plate of the midbrain, both these parts being invaded by an ingrowth of the tumour (Fig. 302). Its maximum transverse diameter in the section examined was 17 mm. and its vertical measurement

29 449

15 mm. There was no definite capsule, the growth being limited by the tissues with which it came into contact. Thus it was covered laterally by vascular

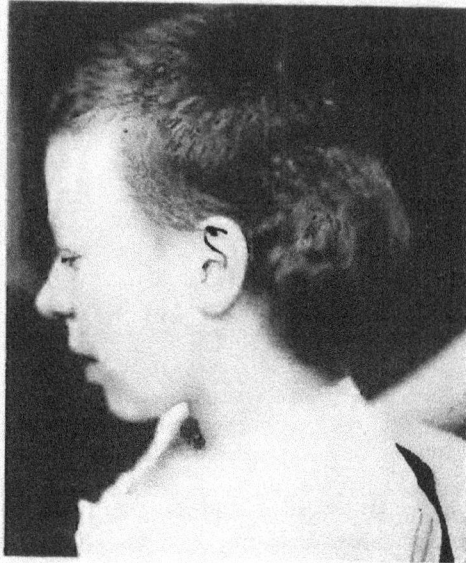

FIG. 301.—PHOTOGRAPH OF CASE 1, SHOWING BULGING THROUGH A SUB-TENTORIAL DECOMPRESSION.

pia mater, and where it was invading nerve-tissue this was pushed aside and compressed, the original covering having been either partially or completely destroyed. The aqueductus cerebri had been flattened by pressure, its roof

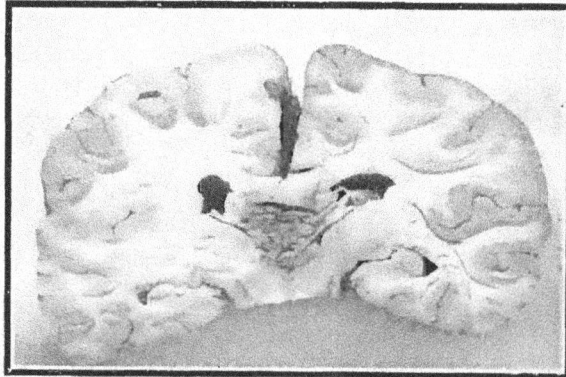

FIG. 302.—CASE 1. BRAIN AFTER REMOVAL, SHOW POSITION OF PINEAL TUMOUR.

being almost in contact with the floor except in the centre, where in the position of the median groove in its floor the section showed a triangular space with the apex directed downwards. The single layer of cubical epithelium which lines the duct was retained on the right side, but had disappeared for the most part on the left side, where it was replaced by an ingrowth of vascular glial tissue. In the nerve-tissue of the splenium and quadrigeminal plate which surrounded the growth there was a considerable increase in the number and size of the blood-vessels. Many of these contained thrombi, in which there was a relatively very high proportion of lymphocytes as compared with red blood-corpuscles. The walls of the vessels were thickened, and there was a considerable nuclear proliferation in surrounding glial tissue.

The surface of the tumour was very irregular and in places lobulated. The central parts were broken down, an irregular cavity being present in the lower part of the section, with spaces running out from the main cavity into the central axes of the lobules, where the destruction of tissue was less complete. The

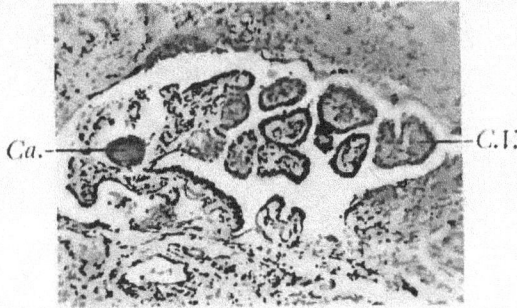

FIG. 303.—CASE I. SMALL CYST IN BASE OF TUMOUR CONTAINING CHOROIDAL VILLI.

Ca. : calcareous body. *C.V. :* choroidal villus.

central axes of the lobules showed a canal which was in some places lined by flattened epithelial cells, external to which was a layer of condensed glial tissue continuous with that of the tumour. These spaces were for the most part empty, but occasionally contained a small amount of cell debris or degenerated blood-corpuscles. They probably represent remnants of the lumen of the original pineal outgrowth which had become cystic.

The tumour cells were loosely arranged in a lobular manner around these cystic spaces, the lobules being separated by vascular ingrowths from the surface. Two principal types of cell were present : the majority had spherical nuclei, deeply stained with hæmatoxylin, and surrounded by a small amount of feebly stained cytoplasm. Among these were larger cells with a feebly stained round or oval nucleus. They appeared to belong to the supporting glial tissue, which in some places formed a trabecular network similar to that seen in the normal gland. No mitotic figures appeared to be present, though in some parts the cells were of small size and closely packed together, suggesting an active proliferation. In the upper part of the tumour there were extensive areas of necrosed tissue showing an irregular fibrinous network containing degenerated red blood-corpuscles and leucocytes, which were intersected by strands of degenerated glial tissue.

A small cyst lined by ependyma and containing choroidal villi was present at the base of one of the lobules in the lower part of the tumour (Fig. 303).

This was probably a remnant of the dorsal diverticulum, which was present during fœtal life and projects backwards over the pineal body from the posterior part of the roof of the third ventricle. This figure should be compared with Fig. 304, which represents a small cyst, lined by cylindrical ependymal cells, found in the substance of the epiphysis of an ox.

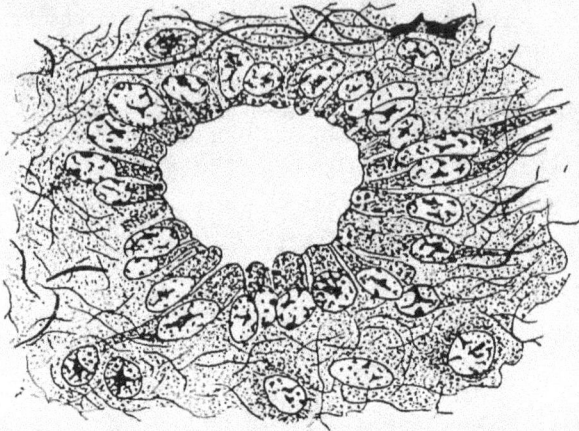

FIG. 304.—SMALL CYST, LINED BY CYLINDRICAL AND IRREGULARLY SHAPED EPENDYMAL CELLS, IN AN EPIPHYSIS OF BOS TAURUS.

Some of the ependymal cells send processes outward towards the periphery.

(After Dimitrowa, 1901.)

Case 2.—Harry P., aged 12, was admitted to hospital in October, 1923, with a history of constant headaches for nearly two years. He had been fitted with various glasses without any benefit. Four months before admission he had his tonsils and adenoids removed, as it was thought that this treatment might alleviate the headaches.

On Examination.—The patient was thin, and inclined to be irritable. There was no sign of pubertas præcox. The pupils reacted sluggishly to light and accommodation, and there was bilateral papillœdema of 4·5 diopters in each eye. The visual fields were normal. There was complete paresis of upward gaze and some weakness of the right VIth nerve. The hearing on the right side was somewhat diminished. The other cranial nerves were normal. There was a slight lateral nystagmus to the right. The gait was somewhat ataxic and Romberg's sign was positive. There was very slight weakness of the right arm. All the deep reflexes were normal.

Radiographs revealed a calcified pineal body and some opening up of the sutures of the skull. After the boy had been in hospital for a week attacks of vomiting and sweating commenced, and it was thought that the condition might possibly be due to a tuberculoma. This diagnosis was supported by the fact that although the boy had a good appetite, he put on no weight and remained exceedingly thin. However, owing to the very definite paresis of upward gaze, it was decided that the more probable diagnosis was that of pinealoma.

Operation.—Under rectal ether and local anæsthesia a large osteoplastic flap was turned down over the right parieto-occipital region. The lateral ventricle was tapped, but owing to the poor condition of the patient no further exploration was carried out. The patient never really rallied, and died three days later.

At autopsy the pathologist unfortunately cut into the brain, and exposed a large but somewhat fragmentary vascular pineal tumour. Microscopically there was a definite mosaic arrangement of the cells, with one or two giant cells surrounded by a definite layer of small cells. It was unfortunate that the brain was not hardened before it was sectioned.

Case 3.—Hilda H., aged 25, was admitted to hospital on 30th October, 1930, complaining of headaches, sickness, and occasional attacks of double vision. The headaches were not continuous, but occurred spasmodically, the patient being quite free from them for several weeks at a time. The headaches first commenced about two years previously. A month before admission to hospital she became unsteady in her gait and could not see to mend her clothes. She was seen as an out-patient, and was found to have bilateral papillœdema, and admission was recommended.

On Examination.—The patient was found to be well-nourished and quite cheerful and very keen to get well in order that she could go back to her work.

There was bilateral papillœdema, four diopters of swelling in the right eye, and three diopters in the left. The pupils reacted sluggishly to light and accommodation. The visual fields were full. There was weakness of both VIth cranial nerves. There was limitation of upward gaze, which increased while under observation in hospital. An X-ray examination showed some increase in the meningeal grooves in the skull, which was significant of increased intracranial pressure. There was no sign of calcification of the pineal gland. There was some ataxia on walking, but this on the whole was slight. There was a fine lateral nystagmus to the right, and slight deafness in the right ear. Rombergism was present. The deep reflexes were slightly increased on the right side of the body. There were no other neurological symptoms. The diagnosis of tumour of the pineal gland was made, and a supratentorial approach was advised.

Operation.—On 21st November, 1930, under intratracheal gas and oxygen anæsthesia combined with local infiltration, a large occipito-parietal osteoplastic flap was turned down on the right side. The dura mater was very tense, and to relieve the intracranial pressure the right lateral ventricle was tapped. The dura mater was incised and the cerebral hemisphere was carefully retracted ; several cerebral veins required to be secured by silver clips, as they entered the superior longitudinal sinus. On exposing the falx cerebri, a little more retraction brought the corpus callosum into view. Two silver clips were placed on the inferior longitudinal sinus and the falx was divided between them. The corpus callosum was then divided longitudinally, and a large tumour of the pineal gland was exposed. An attempt to remove this with the diathermy knife failed owing to excessive bleeding from the great vein of Galen and its tributaries. When the bleeding was more or less under control the condition of the patient was so very poor that the osteoplastic flap was replaced and the scalp wound closed. A blood transfusion of 400 c.c. of citrated blood was given immediately the patient returned to the ward. The condition of the patient rapidly improved and next day she was talking quite happily. There was well-marked lateral nystagmus to the left and right.

Thirty-six hours after the operation the patient became drowsy and then unconscious, with a pulse-rate of 50. The upper part of the scalp wound was opened, the bone flap removed, and the lateral ventricle tapped. Some 40 c.c. of cerebrospinal fluid were withdrawn. The patient rapidly improved after this, but by the tenth day after operation, when the stitches were removed, there was considerable bulging of the scalp in the region of the wound ; 200 c.c. of a 15 per cent. sodium chloride solution were given intravenously. This worked like a charm, and the bulge completely disappeared for four days, when it became more tense again. As a further operation for the complete

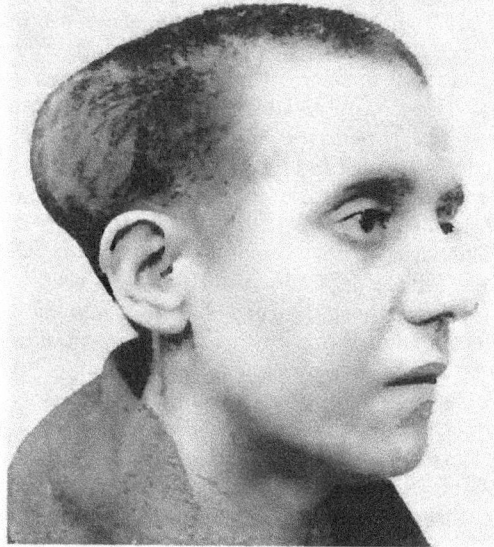

FIG. 305.—CASE 3.   SHOWING BULGING OF DECOMPRESSION AREA IN THE RIGHT OCCIPITO-PARIETAL REGION.

removal of the tumour was refused by the patient, it was decided to give a course of X-ray treatments. Four treatments were given at two-weekly intervals, the applications being given over the decompressed area. This kept the patient quite fit, the papillœdema subsided, and the patient was able to go home.

On re-admisson.—She was readmitted in May, 1931, with bulging of the decompression area and an increase in the papillœdema (Fig. 305). Operation was again refused and a further course of X-ray treatment was given. The patient was discharged in June, 1931, in an improved condition ; the papillœdema was subsiding again and the cerebral hernia was less. She died quite suddenly in August, 1931, but no autopsy was obtainable.

Case 4.—Albert P., aged 23, was admitted to hospital under the care of Dr. Worster-Drought, on 9th October, 1931, complaining of headaches, drowsiness, dizziness, and a constant " vacant " feeling. He was quite well until three months ago, when he first complained of occipital headache, which had persisted ever since. Soon after the headaches began he became drowsy and had attacks of " vacancy," during which he would sit or stand motionless for as long as half an hour. He slept well and ate well. Apart from headaches he did not feel ill. He had noticed dimness of vision on occasions. He had had several attacks of giddiness, in one of which he fell downstairs. He had only vomited once prior to admission. He had grown fatter during the last three months.

On Examination.—The patient was found to be somewhat slow in his movements. He weighed 12 st. 1 lb. A considerable amount of subcutaneous fat was noticeable (Fig. 306).

Cranial nerves.—The pupils were equal, but reaction to light and accommodation was slow. The visual fields were normal to rough tests. Bilateral papillœdema was present ; five diopters in the right and four in the left. There was no nystagmus, and the ocular muscles were normal. Speech was slow, and ponderous, and the whole attitude was slow and heavy ; he never smiled, and the facial expression seemed lost.

Sensation to cotton-wool and pin-pricks was quite normal. The cold tube felt hot on the right side of the trunk from the acromion process to the midline nearly down to the umbilicus. All limb reflexes were normal. The gait was slow, but with no obvious defect. Co-ordination, finger-nose test, was poor. Rombergism was slight. The heart, lungs, etc., were normal, and the blood-pressure 100 85. An X-ray examination made on 16th October, 1931, showed that the sella turcica was enlarged and eroded, and the pineal body calcified. Cushing's thermic reaction was negative. The blood-sugar curve was normal. The visual fields were constricted. The cerebrospinal fluid showed : total protein 0·03 per cent. ; globulin, no excess. The Wassermann reaction was negative.

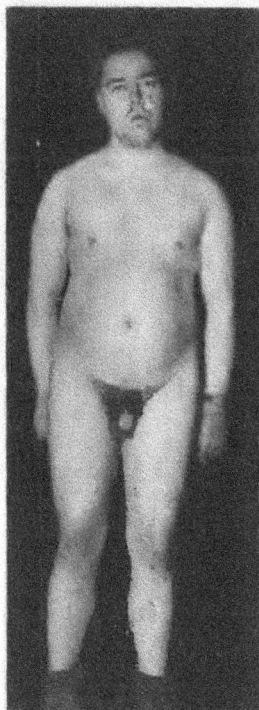

FIG. 306.—CASE 4. PHOTO-GRAPH OF PATIENT SUFFERING FROM A PINEAL TUMOUR.

The vacant expression in this patient is well marked.

First Operation.—Air ventriculography was carried out on 31st October, 1931, under local anæsthesia. A small trephine was made in the right parietal bone and a cannula passed into the ventricle ; 200 c.c. of ventricular fluid were withdrawn and 140 c.c. of air introduced (Fig. 307).

The ventricular fluid was clear and colourless, cells 1 per c.mm. There were no red corpuscles. Total protein was 0·015 per cent. There was no excess of globulin, and the Wasserman reaction was negative. The patient was very drowsy after the ventriculography.

Second Operation.—On 5th November, 1931, a right subtemporal decompression was carried out under local anæsthesia. Considerable intracranial pressure was found. The patient stood the operation well, but afterwards became more drowsy and gradually got weaker. He suddenly collapsed and died on 21st November, 1931. He had been running a high temperature for three days. The wound had quite healed and was healthy.

Pathology.—A post-mortem examination was carried out by Dr. Carnegie Dickson. The body was that of a well-nourished, well-developed young adult male, with little of note externally except that the figure showed a tendency to the female type. There was marked general flattening of the convolutions, more especially of the left hemisphere, which appeared to be slightly larger

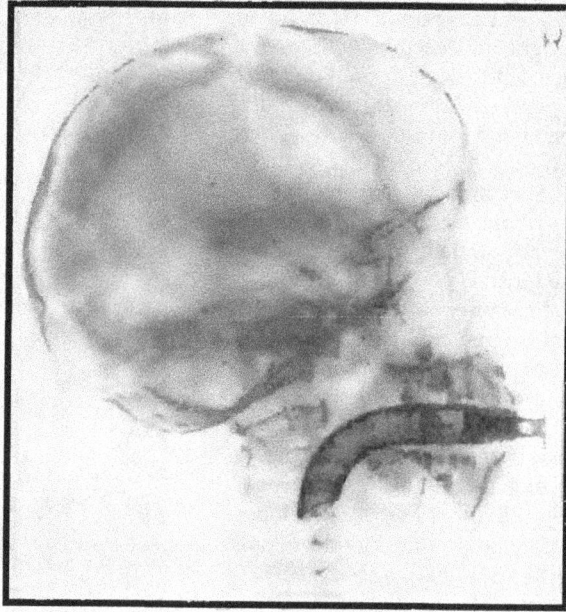

FIG. 307.—CASE 4. RADIOGRAPH AFTER VENTRICULOGRAPHY, SHOWING DILATED LATERAL VENTRICLES AND AREA OF PINEAL TUMOUR JUST BENEATH THE CORPUS CALLOSUM.

than the right. The larger surface veins were somewhat dilated and the Pacchionian bodies about the vertex were numerous and prominent. Over the central portion of the base, e.g. over the pons and the interpeduncular space and dilated infundibulum, there was some thickening of the pia arachnoid.

On horizontal section of the brain at the level of the upper surface of the corpus callosum, the lateral ventricles were found to be very considerably dilated, especially the left, and the section at this level passed through a pearly " epidermoid " or " cholesteatomatous " tumour to the left side of the middle line, just posterior to the central point of the hemisphere, and occupying roughly the normal position of the left optic thalamus, which was displaced by the tumour forwards and outwards. This tumour had evidently arisen from the pineal region, the tumour lying mostly to the left side of this, pushing downwards the corpora quadrigemina and lamina quadrigemina and compressing the subjacent aqueduct of Sylvius, thus producing the hydrocephalus. The body of the pineal gland was still present, about the size of a small cherry-stone, and apparently more or less independent of the tumour, which, however, was in contact with its upper and left surface. The central portion of the pineal was removed for section, and the remaining sides of the gland sewn together to preserve the continuity of the specimen. The tumour was about the size of a large walnut or small plum, and it reached and pushed downwards and backwards the upper and anterior part of the cerebellum.

On the right side of the brain, just external to the dilated posterior ventricular horn, there was considerable softening and hæmorrhage due to the compression, and the cerebrospinal fluid had evidently ruptured outwards at this point during the removal of the specimen. The right optic thalamus showed considerable bulging into the dilated right lateral ventricle, suggesting the possibility that this also contained tumour, but on cutting into it, this was disproved and it was found to be due merely to pressure displacement by the tumour to the left side, pushing it towards the right and upwards. Sections of the tumour itself had a glistening, pearly white iridescence, suggestive of the presence of cholesterol. Horizontal sections at a lower level showed much the same appearance, with dilatation of the ventricles, including the third ventricle, thus producing the prominent infundibulum as seen from below.

Histological Examination —Sections from various parts of the pearly tumour showed it to be a typical epidermoid consisting of a series of cysts or tumours, showing a concentric laminated appearance due to the production from the periphery inwards of squamous epithelium   The outer or formative layer in most of these cysts is much degenerated or has largely disappeared, i.e. is now more or less inactive. Where it persists it shows a tendency to the production of multinucleated plasmoidal squamous cells. Here and there, however, the formation of outward budding and the production of further small cysts at the periphery of the main mass persist. The central portions of the cysts consist of desquamated epithelial cells and debris, including cholesterol crystals.

Sections of the pineal itself show at some parts more or less normal pineal structure, but at others there is distinct proliferation, with the production of what may be considered a simple pinealoma, involving more especially the larger pineal cells, and with little or no proliferation of the so-called " small lymphocyte-like " cells.

The adenomatous cells are somewhat loosely arranged, the stroma varying in amount and in some parts being scanty and containing numerous thin-walled blood-vessels.

Case 5.—George W., aged 32, came under observation in March, 1932, complaining of giddiness and some difficulty in walking. The patient was a bank clerk, and was able to do his work until February, 1932, when he had an attack of influenza which kept him in bed for three weeks. On getting out of bed he found he was very unsteady on his feet and could not stand alone. He was treated with tonics and massage, but did not improve.

On Examination.—When seen on 10th March, 1932, he appeared to be somewhat dull and listless. His pupils were dilated and reacted sluggishly to light. There was bilateral papillœdema, there being five diopters of swelling in the right eye and four in the left. Except for slight bilateral deafness, the other cranial nerves appeared normal. There was a slight lateral nystagmus to the right. Rombergism was marked, and the patient was quite ataxic. The deep reflexes were normal, and there was no impairment to sensation.

Lumbar puncture revealed a clear colourless cerebrospinal fluid under pressure ; there were no abnormal constituents. The day following the lumbar puncture the patient was incontinent three times, and there was a well-marked lateral nystagmus. Also for the first time there was limitation of upward gaze and a definite weakness of the right sixth cranial nerve. Both lower limbs became spastic two days later. Radiographs of the skull revealed a midline calcified pineal shadow. This case was looked upon as a typical pinealoma, and removal was advised.

Operation.—On 21st March, under avertin and local anæsthesia, a large

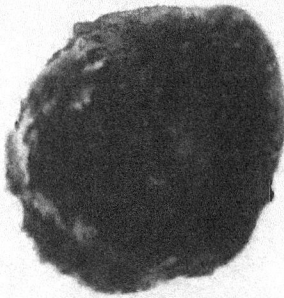

FIG. 308.—CASE 5. ACTUAL SIZE OF PINEAL TUMOUR AFTER REMOVAL.

right occipito-parietal osteoplastic flap was turned down, the lateral ventricle tapped, and the dura mater opened. Bleeding was reduced to a minimum by the application of silver clips and the use of the diathermy knife. The falx was exposed and the inferior longitudinal sinus severed between the clips. The inferior border of the falx was divided to the extent of half an inch. The splenium of the corpus callosum was split with a curved diathermy knife and a large pineal tumour exposed. Large veins could be seen surrounding the tumour. An incision into the tumour was made with the diathermy knife, and a definite capsule appeared to cover the tumour. With a curved dissector the tumour was shelled out of its capsule. The bleeding, which was not great, was controlled by the use of diathermy. The retracted cerebral hemisphere was replaced and covered by dura mater. A small piece of corrugated rubber tubing was inserted into the region of the tumour and brought out through the upper part of the wound. The bone flap itself was removed, as it was thought that as the capsule had been left behind it would be advisable to give a course of X-ray treatment later. The patient stood the operation very well.

The following day the right ventricle was tapped and 30 c.c. of blood-stained cerebrospinal fluid were withdrawn. The drainage tube was removed after forty-eight hours. The fifth day following operation lumbar puncture was performed—the fluid was under slight pressure and blood-stained. From this day recovery was uneventful, and the patient left hospital a month after the operation.

The tumour was about the size of a plum (Fig. 308) and was quite hard in consistency. Histologically the tumour was a typical pinealoma.

Subsequent History.—At the end of May, 1932, the patient was given a course of X-ray treatment ; he seemed very well, and was able to go back to his office in September, 1932 ; he was able to walk quite well. There was no papillœdema, but still some lateral nystagmus to the right. The patient had a bad attack of influenza in December, 1932, which was followed by pneumonia which proved fatal in four days. Every effort was made to obtain an autopsy, but this was refused by the relatives.

Case 6.—Harry F., aged 27, was admitted to hospital on 5th February, 1935, complaining of headaches. The duration of the present headache was about three weeks, but he had had a similar bout of headaches one year previously. The headaches were mostly occipital, but sometimes were on top of the head, mostly on the right side. They lasted for a quarter of an hour, and were worse in the morning. On two occasions he had vomited in the last three weeks, and frequently was nauseated without vomiting. He had double vision for moderately distant objects, which was getting worse. Movement of the eyes was painful. He suffered from giddiness two or three times a week, mostly when standing. There was no tendency to fall to one side more than to the other. There was no deafness, no noises in the head, no loss of power in any part of the body, and no unconscious attacks. There was no difficulty in speech, but he experienced difficulty in swallowing. There was no urinary trouble. He sometimes had numbness at the back of the head, but did not suffer from pins-and-needles in the extremities.

There was no previous history of ear trouble or of trauma. The patient had fainted once five years ago, and had had Vincent's angina three years ago.

On Examination.—On examining the fundi on 12th February, 1935, the edge of the left disc was less distinct than that of the right. Papillœdema on the left side was in sharp contrast to a lesser amount on the right. The veins in both fundi were distinctly enlarged.

On 19th February a stereoscopic X-ray examination of the skull showed a small rounded shadow of calcified pineal, a linear shadow situated at a certain distance from the rounded shadow and quite close to the right temporal bone.

On 24th February examination of the fields showed no abnormality. The patient continued to complain of severe headaches, and diplopia was still present.

Operation.—Ventriculography was performed on 7th March. Both lateral ventricles were very dilated (Fig. 309). The patient was given avertin anæsthesia with gas, oxygen, and ether. A large flap was turned down over the right occipito-parietal region. The dura was quite tense, and the lateral ventricle was therefore tapped and some 80 c.c. of fluid withdrawn. The dura mater was then incised and the occipital pole of the brain was retracted outwards. The inferior border of the falx was now incised after having clipped the inferior sagittal sinus by means of silver clips. The splenium of the corpus callosum was pushed upwards by the underlying tumour ; the splenium was cut through with a knife and the tumour exposed. It was a vascular tumour and a portion was removed with punch forceps. It was considered impossible to remove the tumour owing to the great vascularity, and therefore the occipital pole of the brain was replaced and the dura held together by three interrupted sutures ; the bone flap was removed and the scalp united by a double row of interrupted sutures. The patient stood the operation very well, and after three weeks deep X-ray therapy was given through the defect in the skull made by removal of the bone flap.

The portion of tissue removed showed a typical pineal tumour, with plenty of large cells (Fig. 310).

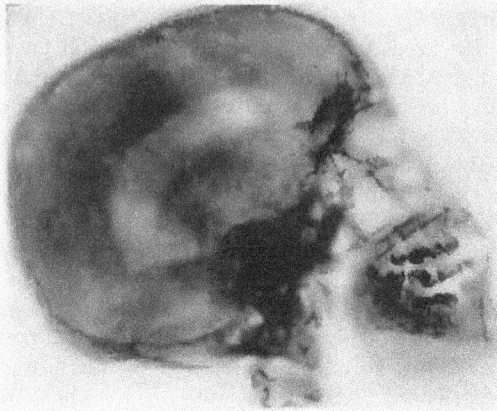

FIG. 309.—RADIOGRAPH AFTER VENTRICULOGRAPHY, SHOWING DILATED LATERAL VENTRICLE.

Subsequent progress.—The patient was discharged from hospital two months later, but the stigmata of the pineal tumour, due to pressure on the corpora quadrigemina, still persisted.

The patient was admitted on 19th October, 1935, for a second course of deep X-ray therapy ; but this did not have a very beneficial effect, and the

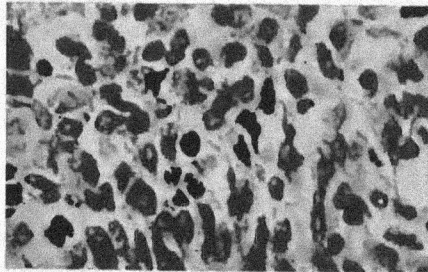

FIG. 310.—CASE 6. HISTOLOGICAL APPEARANCE OF PINEAL TUMOUR (× 32).

patient left hospital very little improved by this treatment. We were informed that he died a month afterwards at his home, no autopsy being obtained.

Case 7.—Herbert O., aged 23, was admitted to hospital on 4th March, 1935, complaining of double vision, which was first noticed some six weeks prior to admission. The onset had been gradual and seemed to follow a series of headaches. The patient blamed his left eye, as he said the false image was to the left of the real one. There had been no vomiting or blurring of vision. His speech was normal and memory good. He had had no fits.

On Examination.—The pupils were equal and reacted to light. There was absence of accommodation and of the upward and downward movements of the eyes. There was some slight ptosis of the left eye and some rotary nystagmus.

The cranial nerves appeared normal, with the exception of some weakness of the right VIIth, IXth, and XIIth. There was no sensory loss in the arms, but some slight intention tremor. Reflexes were increased in the arms, but were equal on the two sides. There was no weakness of the legs and no sensory loss. Knee and ankle-jerks were brisk and the plantars were extensor in type. There was bilateral papilloedema—right three diopters, left four diopters.

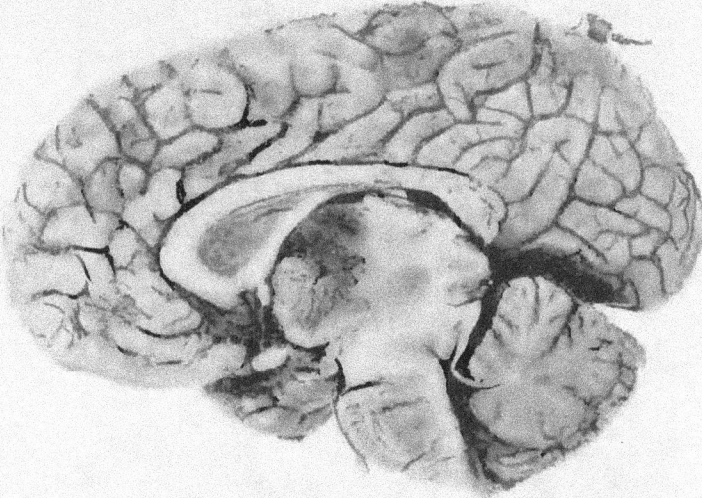

FIG. 311.—CASE 7. PHOTOGRAPH OF BRAIN, SHOWING POSITION OF PINEAL TUMOUR.

Lumbar puncture gave a clear, colourless fluid with a pressure of 270 mm.

Cells	..	..	..	..	10 per c.mm.
Protein	..	..	..	..	50 mg. per 100 c.c.
Chlorides	..	..	..	..	710 mg. per 100 c.c.
Globulin test	..	..	..	..	Negative
Sugar	..	..	..	..	Within normal limits
Culture	..	..	..	..	Sterile
Wassermann reaction	..	..	..	Negative

A radiograph of the skull was normal except for some erosion of the posterior clinoid processes. The visual fields were normal.

The patient gradually became comatose and paralysed down the right side of the body, and died on 10th March, 1935, some six days after his admission, without any operation being contemplated.

Post-Mortem Examination.—At autopsy there was bilateral pulmonary collapse and enlargement of the heart. A very large tumour was found in the pineal region (Fig. 311). The photograph reveals the right half of the brain, showing a tumour 2½ in. in diameter occupying almost the whole of the third ventricle, and extending forwards to the anterior commissure and below to the tuber cinereum. The tumour is infiltrating the superior corpora quadrigemina

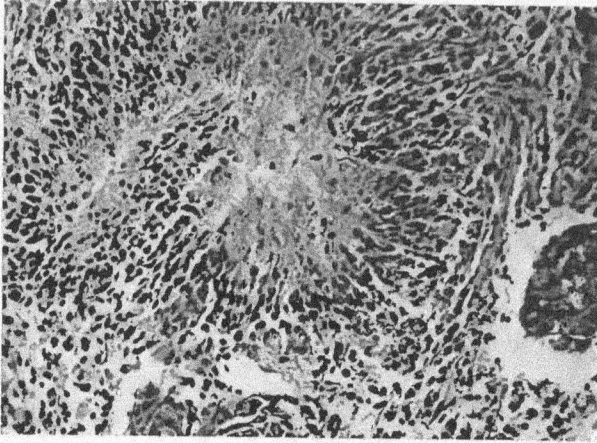

FIG. 312.—CASE 7. LOW-POWER PICTURE OF HISTOLOGICAL SECTION OF THE PINEAL TUMOUR.

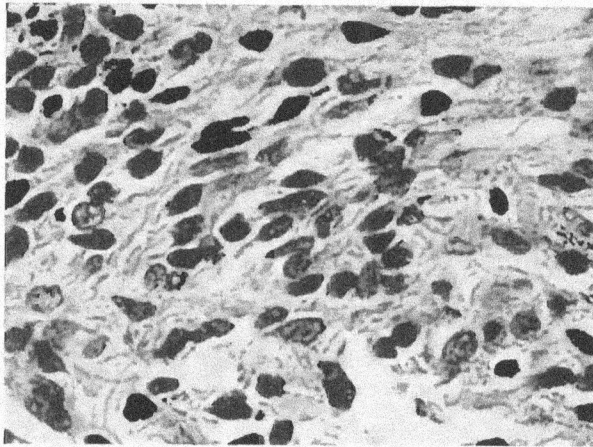

FIG. 313.—CASE 7. HIGH-POWER PICTURE OF HISTOLOGICAL SECTION OF THE PINEAL TUMOUR.

and the midbrain, extending to the interpeduncular space and the upper border of the pons. The point of origin of the tumour is not obvious, but from the mode of extension forwards into the third ventricle, and the direction of infiltration downwards and forwards into the midbrain, it would seem that the tumour arose in the pineal gland, which is no longer distinguishable.

Histology.—Sections show a cellular tumour intersected by numerous capillaries. Some areas show the characteristic carrot-shaped cells arranged in circles, with their long, protoplasmic processes forming a fibrillary network in the centre (pseudo-rosettes) (Figs. 312, 313).

Case 8.—Henry B., aged 11, came under observation on 4th July, 1935, with a history of more or less constant headaches for two years. However, he was free for some weeks at a time. A week prior to admission he had repeated vomiting attacks which could not be stopped with any kind of treatment.

On Examination.—He was a well-built and well-nourished boy, and quite intelligent. He complained of double vision and inability to look upwards beyond the horizontal plane. The pupils did not react to light, but reacted quite well to accommodation. The visual fields were normal. There was slight weakness of the right external rectus. There was bilateral papilloedema, more marked on the right side. The rest of the cranial nerves appeared normal. There was no loss of sensation in the body and the deep reflexes were normal. The cerebrospinal fluid was under tension, the manometric reading being 250. The fluid was clear and colourless and did not contain any abnormal constituents.

A radiograph of the skull (Fig. 314) revealed definite hammer markings owing to the increased intracranial pressure. The Wassermann reaction in the blood and cerebrospinal fluid was negative.

Four days after admission the patient was found to develop skew deviation of the eyes on looking at objects in front of him, and the double vision became constant.

Operation.—A ventricular puncture was performed and 100 c.c. of air injected into the lateral ventricle. Ventriculography revealed bilateral dilatation of the lateral ventricles. A diagnosis of pineal tumour was made, and a large osteoplastic flap was turned down over the right occipito-parietal region. The lateral ventricle was tapped and the occipital pole of the brain retracted outwards through the opening in the skull. The splenium was cut through revealing a large pineal tumour. A portion was removed for examination and the operation was terminated. The general condition of the patient improved somewhat and the wound healed well.

The microscopical examination revealed an undifferentiated form of pinealoma (Fig. 315).

Subsequent Progress.—After three weeks, deep X-ray therapy was given to the pineal region through three ports of entry, some nine treatments being given, and the boy was discharged on 1st September with very slight papilloedema and slight ataxia. On writing to the patient three months later from the follow-up department it was found that the boy had died in his sleep six weeks after leaving hospital and no post-mortem examination was held.

Case 9.—The specimen was obtained from a brain supplied to the Anatomy Department of King's College, London. No history of the case was available. A median longitudinal section of the brain showed a cyst which occupied the centre of the pineal body and compressed the quadrigeminal plate of the midbrain. The aqueductus cerebri was also compressed, but it was not completely obstructed, and there was no marked distension of the third or lateral ventricles (Fig. 316). The pia mater around the pineal body and neighbouring parts was considerably thickened.

The pineal cyst was removed for microscopical examination and serial longitudinal sagittal sections were cut and stained with hæmatoxylin and eosin and with picro-indigo-carmine.

These showed that the cavity of the cyst was formed by the breaking down of the central part of the pineal body. Its wall showed, in a modified form, the structure of the pineal gland (Fig. 317, A). There was a pseudo-epithelial stratum lining the cavity, the tissue immediately bounding the lumen being fibrillar and glial in nature. A middle zone, which formed the major part of

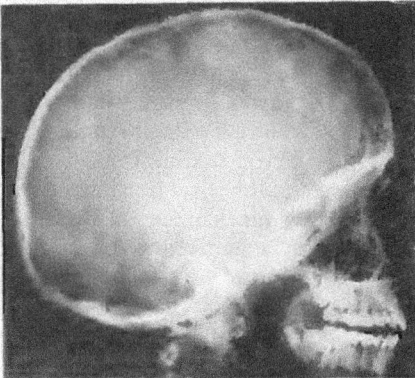

FIG. 314.—CASE 8. RADIOGRAPH DEMONSTRATING HAMMER MARK-ING OWING TO THE INCREASED INTRACRANIAL PRESSURE DUE TO A PINEAL TUMOUR.

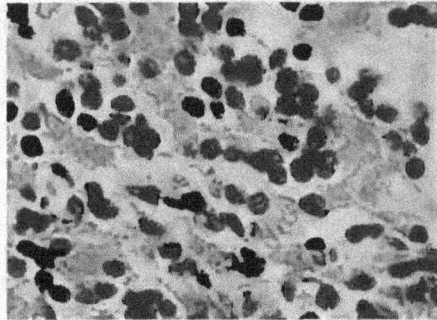

FIG. 315.—CASE 8. HISTOLOGICAL PICTURE SHOWING APPEARANCE OF A PINEAL TUMOUR (× 320).

the thickness of the cyst wall, showed typical parenchymatous pineal cells. These were of small size, but had relatively large nuclei ; they were imbedded in a loose glial network, which forms the supporting tissue throughout the whole thickness of the cyst wall.

There were some irregular plaques of calcareous deposit in the wall of the cyst, and corpora arenacea were abundant in the surrounding membranes, but were not present in the actual wall of the cyst.

Lying dorsal to the pineal body was a tubular diverticulum of the ependyma, which extended the whole length of the pineal body (Fig. 318). It opened into the third ventricle at the suprapineal recess, and contained groups of choroidal villi, which projected into its lumen (Fig. 317, B). This represents the persistent dorsal sac which is present in fœtal life, and is formed as a tubular outgrowth from the roof of the posterior part of the third ventricle. It would probably have contributed to the secretion of the cerebrospinal fluid. Should its opening have become blocked, it might have given rise to a thin-walled cyst, which would have differed from the pineal cyst described above in having

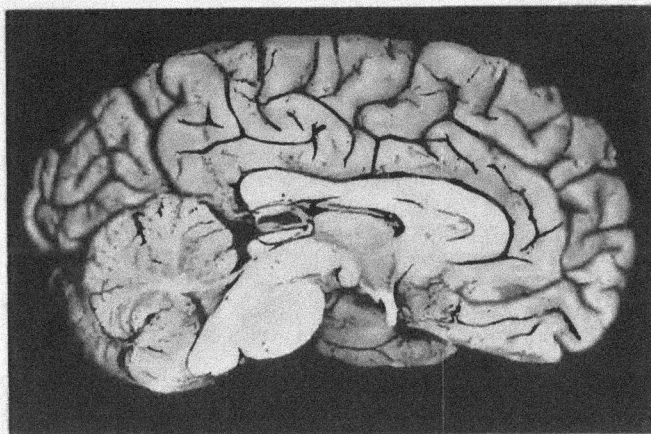

FIG. 316.—MESIAL SECTION OF THE BRAIN, SHOWING LARGE PINEAL CYST LYING BETWEEN THE SPLENIUM OF THE CORPUS CALLOSUM AND THE CORPORA QUADRIGEMINA.

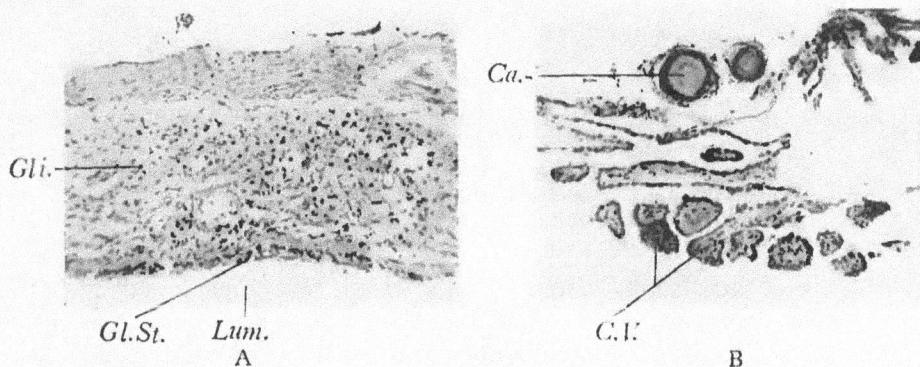

FIG. 317.—CASE 9.

A—Section through the wall of the pineal cyst shown in Fig. 316. The lumen of the cyst lies below ; it is lined by a layer of condensed glial tissue, no ependymal epithelium being visible. The middle zone is formed of a degenerate tissue containing few parenchyma cells and showing numerous spaces. In the upper part of the section is the fibrous capsule.

Gli : glial tissue. *Gl. st.* : glial stratum. *Lum.* : lumen.

B—Portion of the wall of the dorsal diverticulum or suprapineal recess which lay above the pineal cyst. It shows sections of corpora arenacea and choroidal villi.

Ca. : corpus arenaceum. *Cv.* : choroidal villi.

a wall lined with ependymal epithelium, and most probably containing tufts of choroidal villi projecting into its lumen.

Pineal cysts lined by ependyma also occur, and vary in size from small microscopic cysts such as that shown in Fig. 304, in which the lining

30

epithelium is columnar in type, to larger cysts which are formed, as is indicated by septa projecting into the lumen, by the coalescence of adjacent smaller cysts. The lining membrane in the larger cysts, found in old

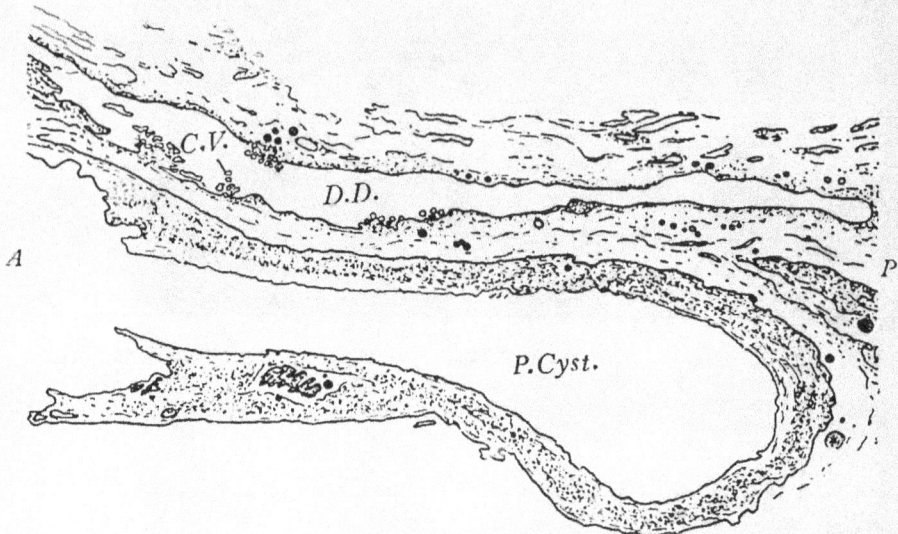

FIG. 318.—CASE 9. DRAWING OF A LONGITUDINAL SECTION OF THE PINEAL CYST, AND THE SUPRAPINEAL RECESS ABOVE IT, D.D. (R. J. G.)

A. : anterior end.

C.V. : choroidal villi projecting into the lumen of the diverticulum.

P. cyst. : lumen of the pineal cyst.

P. : posterior end.

subjects, is formed by flattened cells which have been described as "pseudo-ependymal." Whether these cells are responsible for the secretion of the fluid which fills the cyst or whether this fluid is derived from the vessels supplying the gland appears to be undetermined.[1]

[1] Further information on the development and nature of pineal cysts will be found in an article by Eugenia R. A. Cooper in the *J. Anat.*, **67**, 1932 3, p. 28.

CHAPTER 33

GENERAL CONCLUSIONS

THE surgery of the pineal organ, although yet in its infancy, may be said to be advancing rapidly owing to the fact that neurological diagnosis becomes more established and more accurate each year.

The symptomatology tends to be more definite : there is usually a severe degree of raised intracranial pressure, associated with headache, vomiting, papillœdema, epileptiform fits, and some cranial nerve paralysis. The eye signs are definite, with loss of pupillary reaction and failure of upward movement of the eyes.

Operations for the removal of pineal tumours have become standardized ; and even if the complete removal cannot be undertaken, a postoperative course of deep X-ray therapy will complete the cure, as the majority of pineal tumours are radio-sensitive.

Morphology

1. The pineal system, including the parietal eye, its nerves, and the related cerebral ganglia is one of the most ancient sensory systems of the vertebrate phylum. The existence of a parietal sense-organ being plainly indicated in certain of the primitive ostracoderm fishes by the presence of a pineal plate, showing either a complete pineal canal or a pineal pit on the inner surface of the plate. The canal and plate are well seen in the examples of Anaspida and Cephalaspida, which are found in strata ranging from the lower Silurian[1] to the Devonian eras and in specimens of Pterichthys and Bothriolepis belonging to the Order Antiarchi, found in upper Devonian strata.

2. In these fishes there is definite evidence that the parietal eye coexisted with other sensory organs of the head, namely : the lateral eyes, the olfactory organs, and the vestibular or static organs ; and also that these had approximately the same relative positions to each other and the parietal foramen or pit that they have in the heads of living cyclostomes and other vertebrates.

3. The closure of the outer or superficial end of the parietal canal by a thin plate of bone in certain examples indicates that in these specimens

[1] The Silurian Epoch has been estimated by Barrell to embrace a period from 390,000,000 to 460,000,000 years ago.

467

regression of the organ had already commenced, and that it had ceased to function as a visual organ.

4. In some palæozoic fishes, e.g. *Pholidosteus*, *Rhinosteus*, and *Titanichthys*, bilateral pineal impressions are visible, either (*a*) on the dorsal or outer aspect of the pineal plate, or (*b*) on its inner or intracranial surface. Moreover, evidence of the bilateral nature of the pineal system is also present in existing species. Thus in some species in which two separate parietal eyes are present, e.g. *Petromyzon* or *Geotria*, each eye is connected by its own nerve with the habenular ganglion of the same side ; and when the two parietal organs differ in size there is a corresponding difference in size of the habenular ganglion and also of the fasciculus retroflexus of Meynert of the two sides.

5. In those animals in which there is normally only one parietal sense-organ or an unpaired epiphysis, the normal connections of the basal part of the stalk of the parietal organ or of the epiphysis with the right and left habenular ganglia and posterior commissure are bilateral. Moreover, the occasional occurrence of accessory parietal sense-organs and indications of coalescence of two retinal placodes, or of two lenses in a single eye, may also be regarded as evidence pointing to a primary bilateral origin of the system. Bifurcation of a single pineal stalk into two terminal vesicles has also been observed as a variation in different classes of vertebrates, more particularly in fishes (Cattie) ; in amphibia (Cameron) ; in reptiles (Spencer, Klinckowstroem) ; in birds, e.g. *Emys europea* (Nowikoff) ; and among mammals several instances in human embryos.

6. The development of two separate pineal diverticula, in the median plane and in the interval between the habenular commissure and the posterior commissure, seems to be a rare occurrence, although two terminal vesicles which have arisen from a common stalk may lie one behind the other. If one parietal vesicle only is developed and it is later cut off from its stalk of origin, the latter is usually displaced backwards so that the epiphysis lies behind the parietal eye. Apart from the paraphysis, which originates anterior to the velum transversum, diverticula arising from the roof of the third ventricle in front of the habenular commissure are developed from the dorsal sac or postvelar arch, and give rise to the suprapineal recess or are an outgrowth from the choroid plexus. Neither the paraphysis nor diverticula originating from the postvelar arch are epiphyseal in nature.

7. The parietal eye, which seems to have attained its maximum development in certain extinct amphibia, reptiles, and mammal-like reptiles, and the epiphysis or pineal body usually show signs of regression in specimens of mature living species. The most important of these indications are : (1) the frequent absence or disappearance during the later stages of development of the nerve or nerves connecting the parietal eye or epiphysis with the central nervous system ; (2) excessive development of pigment in or around the retinal cells, or development of pigment in the lens or cornea ; (3) degeneration of the retinal epithelium of the parietal organ ; in the epiphysis of anamniota degeneration of the lining epithelium of the pineal stalk ; or in the pineal organ of adult birds, degeneration of the epithelium lining the follicles, accompanied in some cases by obliteration of the lumen of the follicles ; and in the pineal organ of adult mammals frequent degeneration of the parenchyma cells. The degree of degeneration of the parenchyma cells in adult mammals varies both in different individuals and in different parts of the organ in the same individual. In the latter case it is common to find areas in which the parenchyma cells have disappeared altogether and been replaced by neuroglial plaques or bands. These often break down in the centre to form cysts, and deposits of calcareous salts are frequently seen in the walls of the cysts or in the trabeculæ or capsule. See Figs. 221, A, B, C, 285, 317, and 318.

8. In addition to the evidence in some extinct and living vertebrates of a single pair of pineal organs which are united, either partially in the stem of a Y-shaped organ bearing two terminal vesicles, or completely fusion having taken place throughout the whole length of the stalk which terminates in a single composite vesicle, there are indications, according to certain authors, of the existence of two pairs of parietal organs arranged serially, one pair lying in front of the other. Thus in the Palæozoic fish *Bothriolepis* (Fig. 319), Patten describes, in addition to the median eye tubercle situated on the pineal plate between the two orbital cavities, a pair of bilateral impressions which are visible only on the internal aspect, and are present on the deep surface of the post-orbital plate (Fig. 320). These he believed lodged a pair of posterior median or parietal eyes. The three impressions or pits form a triangular group disposed in a similar manner to the median eyes of many invertebrates, and, more particularly, the triplacodal entomostracan eye which is found in certain Branchiopods, e.g. *Apus* and *Branchipus* (Figs. 248, 250), and in the " carp louse " *Argulus foliaceus*, which is typical of many other crustaceans. Another interpretation of the meaning of these two impressions is given on p. 472 by Stensiö, who suggests that they are produced by the attachment of paired muscles of the lateral eyes. The existence and exact position of two pairs of retinal placodes which will give rise to the median eyes of vertebrates and which lie one in front of the other on each side of the open medullary plate, has not, we believe, been definitely established, nor is there agreement with respect to their exact position

relative to the pair of placodes which give origin to the lateral eyes. Thus, Patten assumes that two pairs of retinal placodes which become incorporated in the roof of the third ventricle and give rise to the parietal eyes of vertebrates lie in front of those for the lateral eyes in a position which he describes as typical, in the development of Arachnids (Figs. 257, 258, 259), whereas Locy in his account of two pairs of "accessory" or pineal eyes in *Acanthias*, figures these as lying behind the placodal pits, which will develop into the optic vesicles of the lateral eyes (Fig. 143). Moreover, the intermediate stages between the first appearance of the two pairs of rudiments for the accessory eyes and the outgrowth of the pineal diverticulum in the later stages do not appear to have been definitely established by Locy. The appearance, however, of symmetically arranged sensory placodes or pigment spots formed in series around the margin of the medullary plate (Figs. 257, 258, 259), or head region (Fig. 19) in invertebrates suggests the possibility that one pair of a series of simple eyes being more favourably placed for the reception of visual impressions than the others—e.g. at the antero-lateral margins of the

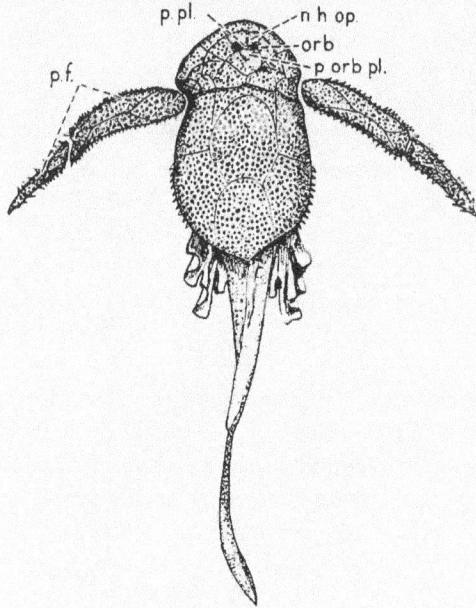

Fig. 319.—Dorsal Aspect of Bothriolepis Canadensis, showing the Nasohypophyseal Opening, Lateral Orbits, Pineal and Post-orbital Plate, and the Cephalic Appendages which have recently been shown to be True Pectoral Fins. (After Patten.)

n.h. op. : naso-hypophyseal opening.
orb. : orbital cavity.
p.f. : pectoral fin.
p. orb. pl. : postorbital plate.
p. pl. : pineal plate.

head on each side—becomes more highly evolved than those in front of or behind this pair The more favourably situated pair, it may be assumed, gains the ascendancy over the others and becomes the principal pair, whereas the less favourably situated ocelli retain their primitive simple character and tend to degenerate. If this is the case, and if as is commonly believed both the lateral and median eyes of vertebrates have been evolved from the simple eyes of a lowly organized type of invertebrate, the discrepancy which exists with regard to the position of the median or accessory placodes relative to the optic pits for the lateral eyes in vertebrates may be readily explained.

The presence of the two impressions on the deep aspect of the postero-median plate of *Bothriolepis* described by Patten has recently (1929–1930) been confirmed by Stensiö, who gives an illustration (Fig. 321) of the same two pits in *Asterolepis*, an allied genus. He suggests that the pits are produced by the attachment of one or several of the recti muscles of

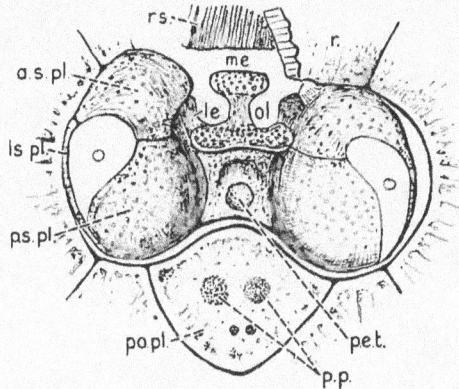

FIG. 320.—DORSAL ASPECT OF THE OCULAR AND OLFACTORY PLATES OF BOTHRIO-
LEPIS ENLARGED. (AFTER PATTEN.)

A part of the olfactory and rostral plates has been removed on the left in order to expose the deeper-lying sclerotic plates. Between the lateral eyes is the quad-rangular parietal plate, nearly perforated by a deep conical pit opening inward and covered externally by a thin, lens-like tubercle, beneath which was the parietal eye. On the deep aspect of the post-orbital (post median) plate are two similar pits, which Patten believed were occupied by a pair of posterior parietal eyes.

a.s. pl. : anterior sclerotic plate.
le. : lateral ethmoid.
ls. pl. : lateral sclerotic plate.
me. : mesethmoid.
o. : corneal opening.
ol. : site of primitive olfactory organ.
p.e.t. : parietal eye tubercle.

po. pl. : postorbital plate.
p.p. : position of paired pits on inner aspect of *po. pl.*
p.s. pl. : posterior sclerotic plate.
r. : rostrum.
rs. : shelf plate on inner surface of rostrum.

the lateral eye on each side ; a supposition which appears much more probable than Patten's hypothesis ; more especially since the investiga-tions of Stensiö and others into the general anatomy of these fishes have definitely proved that the cephalic appendages of *Bothriolepis*, *Asterolepis ornata*, and allied genera—which were at one time thought to closely resemble the cephalic appendages of the Merostomata, e.g. *Eurypterus* —are true pectoral fins, consisting of two segments, each of which contains inside the *dermal bony exoskeleton*, an axial *cartilaginous endoskeleton*, which in *Bothriolepis* was provided with a perichondral layer of lime-bearing tissue, intermediate between true bone and calcified cartilage. The endoskeleton in the specimen described did not participate either in the axial articulation or in the articulation between the two segments of the fin, since both these articulations were formed solely by the dermal bones. In the proximal articulation the inner ends of the dermal bones embraced the neck, of the processus brachialis of the anterior ventro-lateral plate ; the opening in the dermal bones of the appendage which surrounded the process is called the axial foramen, and besides enclosing the head or condyle of the processus brachialis transmitted vessels and nerves to the appendage. The intermediate position in a direct line of descent between fishes and the invertebrate Merostomata, which was claimed for the Antiarchi (*Bothriolepis*,

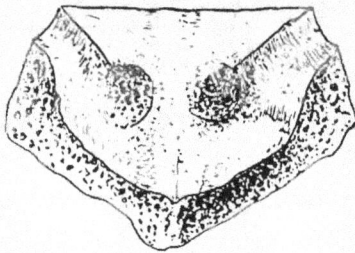

FIG. 321.—INTRACRANIAL SURFACE OF POSTMEDIAN PLATE OF ASTEROLEPIS ORNATA. (AFTER STENSIÖ.)

Pterichthys), is thus not confirmed by recent work. This Order being now considered to belong definitely to the fishes, their appendages being true pectoral fins and their resemblance to the large paddle-like appendages of the Merostomata (*Eurypterus* or *Pterygotus*) being functional rather than structural.

9. The theory that a higher race of animals which was " predominant " arose directly from a lower race in the geological period which immediately preceded it, must, in the light of modern knowledge, be radically modified, since it is evident that the common ancestor of two highly differentiated and in many respects divergent classes must have been of a much simpler type than either of the two classes under consideration. Moreover, the divergence of the two classes must have taken place long before dominance of one class over the other could have existed as a factor in their evolution. Certain points of similarity in particular organs or systems seem to have been preserved in the two divergent classes, although even these when critically examined are found to present modifications in detail ; and the modifications or divergences are in general more pronounced in the phylogenetically older races and in adult animals as compared with their larval or embryonic stages. To take a concrete instance, the difference between the compound faceted eye of an arthropod and the inverted eye of an adult vertebrate is very great, and since the upright faceted eyes of certain arthropods were already highly evolved in some trilobites which were living in the Upper Cambrian period and since median eye tubercles have been found in both larval and adult specimens of *Trinucleus* and

other closely related forms of trilobites, it is evident that the distinction between median eyes and lateral eyes had occurred at a very early date and that the time required to produce the differentiation of the complex faceted eyes must place the actual origin of the lateral eyes of arthropods at a still earlier period.

The degree of differentiation of the lateral eyes of invertebrates varies greatly in different classes, and the divergence from the simpler types is greater in the adult animal than in the larva and in the more highly organized types of animal than in the more primitive.

Now the earliest known fossil vertebrates, the ostracoderms, agree with the invertebrate Eurypteridæ in possessing both lateral and median eyes, and they were contemporary with each other, living in the sea under much the same conditions and in the same geological period. Comparisons were therefore made between the ostracoderms and the eurypterids, and between the living representatives of these two extinct classes, the cyclostomes, which are the direct descendants of the ostracoderms and certain of the more primitive types of cartilaginous fishes on the one hand, and the land scorpions, spiders, *Limulus*, and certain of the Crustacea on the other ; all of which resemble each other in possessing lateral and median eyes in the same relative positions with regard to each other and other organs in the head.

It will be unnecessary to refer to more than two or three of the more salient points which have recently been settled by a critical examination of the alleged similarities between the ostracoderm fishes and the eurypterids. One of these apparent similarities was the possession in Cephalaspid fishes of an exoskeleton which seemed to closely resemble the chitinous exoskeleton of eurypterids and Xiphosura. Now the exoskeleton of the fishes, whether it consists of denticles, scales, scutes, or " armour plating," consists of an outer layer of epidermal bone or of enamel, which covers a dermal bony stratum, or osteodentine ; and it will be recalled that in the development of a tooth the formation of the enamel is at the inner or deep end of the enamel cells or ameloblasts ; further, the increase in thickness of the enamel is by the laying down of new layers on the superficial surface of those which have already been deposited ; and also that the dentine which is formed on the surface of the dermal papilla by the odontoblasts is layed down in the reverse direction to the enamel, namely, from without inwards, the increase in thickness of the dentine being due to its formation at the outer or superficial ends of the odontoblasts. The shields or plates forming the armour plating of the ostracoderm fishes are of the nature of a vaso-dentine, and the rhombic scales on the posterior part of the body, in some examples, e.g. *Pteraspis* (Fig. 322), were coated on their superficial aspect by an enamel-like layer. In the formation of the chitinous exoskeleton of an arthropod, however, there is a secretion of a cuticular nature from the *outer* ends of the columnar hypoblast cells or deric epithelium, this becoming condensed forms a hard chitinous shell on the surface of the hypoblast. The shell thus consists of a thickened and hardened cuticle and differs both structurally and chemically from enamel and osteodentine. Chitin is a nitrogenous and carbohydrate substance allied in its composition to horn ; it may be impregnated with lime salts, but no true Haversian systems, such as those present in bone, are found in it. Increase in size of the animal including its appendages is obtained by a series of moults (ectdyses) in which the hardened cuticle undergoes softening and is cast off ; the

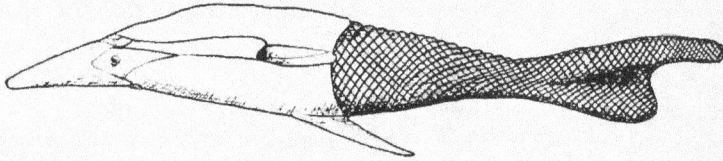

FIG. 322.—LATERAL ASPECT OF PTERASPIS ROSTRATA, AN OSTRACODERM FISH CHARACTERIZED BY THE ABSENCE OF PECTORAL OR PELVIC FINS, A HYPOCERCAL TAIL, LARGE PLATES OR SCUTES COVERING THE HEAD AND ANTERIOR PART OF THE BODY, AND RHOMBIC SCALES COVERING THE REMAINING PART OF THE BODY AND TAIL.

The pineal plate is not perforated in *P. rostrata*, but in some specimens a pit is present on its internal surface. In *P. monmouthensis* a complete perforation is found. (E. Ivor White.)

growth of the animal taking place chiefly in the intervals between the moults ; whereas the increase in size of vertebrates which possess an exoskeleton is similar to that of the skull, a continuous process, taking place partly along the lines of suture between the plates and in the case of dermal bones which have sunk beneath the surface of the skin also by deposit of new bone on the surface of the old, and absorption of bone on the internal surface.

Another important distinction between the fishes and the palæostracan arthropods is the existence of median dorsal and caudal fins in the former, as compared with the long, tapering caudal spine of the Xiphosura, as well as the presence in some, e.g. *Asterolepis, Remigolepis, Bothriolepis*, of a cartilaginous endoskeleton, having the structure of a true pectoral fin inside the bony plates forming the exoskeleton. Finally the existence of a notochord (Fig. 238, p. 341), and the vertebrate position of the heart and main blood-vessels relative to the alimentary canal are fundamental differences which serve to place the ostracoderms definitely among the fishes, and not, as was formerly supposed, in an intermediate position within the direct line of descent of the vertebrates from a highly differentiated ancestral arthropod, such as *Limulus*, or a species resembling any other of the living arachnids.

Summary of Observation on the Development and Structure of the Human Pineal Organ

1. The pineal diverticulum first appears in human embryos of approximately 15 mm. length.

2. The apex of the diverticulum is primarily directed forwards.

3. The pineal outgrowth lies a short distance in front of the posterior commissure, and sometimes presents a constriction subdividing it into an anterior and posterior segment.

4. The whole thickness of the neural wall participates in the formation of the pineal evagination.

5. In some specimens there is an indication of the anterior segment being subdivided into right and left lobes.

6. The " anterior lobe " first described by Krabbe appears in embryos of about 22 mm. length as several neuro-epithelial buds which grow forward into the surrounding connective tissue.

7. A well-marked supra-pineal recess (dorsal sac) is present at the 22-mm. stage.

8. Transverse grooves, which are produced by folding of the roof of the aqueductus cerebri in the region of the posterior commissure, represent temporary infrapineal recesses.

9. Between the third and fourth months of fœtal life there occurs an active proliferation of cells derived from the inner or ependymal zone of the pineal diverticulum. These grow outward in the form of cords, the component cells of which are arranged radially round a central axis which is destitute of nuclei. This is accompanied by a simultaneous ingrowth of vascular processes of mesenchyme.

10. A special mass of proliferating cells growing from the anterior wall of the main diverticulum gives rise to the solid anterior lobe of Krabbe, whereas the cords which grow from the fundus of the diverticulum form the principal solid part of the posterior lobe. The cavities at the base of the stalk and that of the posterior diverticulum appear to open out, and their lumina thus become incorporated in the cavity of the third ventricle, whereas the cavity of the main or anterior diverticulum, which may be cut off as the " cavum pineale," usually disappears.

11. The neuro-epithelial cells give rise to (1) the glia lining the fibrous capsule and covering the trabeculæ, (2) the parenchyma cells, and (3) the neuroglial cells (astrocytes). The surrounding connective tissue and ingrowing vascular mesenchyme form the fibrous capsule and the connective tissue basis of the septa and finer trabeculæ, including the contained vessels. Many of the sinusoidal vessels in the central part of the pale vascular areas, which are seen in the earlier stages of development, disappear, leaving only a very fine capillary plexus in the parenchymatous tissue of the lobules.

12. The parenchymatous tissue in the adult consists of a reticulum of branched pineal cells, among which are a few neuroglial cells, chiefly of the astrocyte type. The " alveolar " appearance which is sometimes seen in adult specimens is due to the persistence of primary neuro-epithelial cords, cross-sections of which appear as rosettes.

13. Cells and nerve-fibres belonging to the sympathetic system accompany the vessels entering and leaving the pineal organ ; and medullated nerve-fibres connect the habenular and posterior commissures with the parenchymatous tissue, but the exact mode of termination of their axons with regard to the pineal cells is not certain. True ganglion cells belonging to the central nervous system and having an axis cylinder process, although described by some authors, appear to be very rarely seen in the human pineal gland, but transitional forms exist, which are intermediate between true nerve cells and parenchymatous cells. These are described as " neuronoid."

The experimental and clinical evidence with respect to function of the mammalian pineal body is at the present time too conflicting to allow of any definite conclusions being drawn. We know that before the age of puberty, more especially in boys, pineal tumours have sometimes been associated with premature growth in size of the body, precocious development of the genital organs, and the early appearance of secondary sexual characters. But it seems probable that certain other factors have been involved in the production of these symptoms—more particularly pressure, either direct or indirect, of the pineal tumour on neighbouring parts of the brain, such as the hypothalamus and pituitary region, combined with the irritative reflex effects produced by increased intracranial tension—and that the symptoms are not directly attributable to disturbance of any special function possessed by the pineal body itself. Moreover, a considerable number of cases have been reported in which sexual precocity and macrogenitosomia have been present but there has been no pineal tumour, and the reverse condition in which a pineal tumour has been present in young boys but unaccompanied by the Pellizzi syndrome. Further, that although some cases of premature development of the breasts in girls and gynæcomastia in males have been reported, these conditions appear to have been absent in the majority of cases of pineal tumour.

An accurate knowledge of the immediate anatomical relations of the pineal body, is essential in order to clearly distinguish the symptoms due to implication of neighbouring parts and those due to a supposed special function of the pineal gland. Some of the structures in close relation with the pineal body are : the aqueduct of Sylvius, the quadrigeminal plate, the geniculate bodies, the nuclei and nerve tracts of the ventral part of the midbrain, the thalamencephalon, the hypothalamus and " portal system " of vessels supplying the pituitary gland, the cerebellum, and the related intracranial nerves and blood-vessels. The mere enumeration of these parts which are liable to be involved in a growth of the pineal body will indicate that when the pressure symptoms are eliminated from the total " symptom complex " accompanying the growth of such tumours there is little left in support of the contention that the human pineal gland has a regulating influence on the normal development of the body and the genital organs, and more especially in the direction of inhibiting or retarding their growth.

In Fig. 323 we have tried to show in a diagrammatic manner the general distribution of the different types of median and lateral eyes in the animal kingdom. We have not attempted to include in this scheme any of the aberrant forms of eye such as those met with on the back of the *Chitons*, or " coat-of-mail shells," or invertebrate eyes with inverted retinæ such as those on the back of *Oncidium* or at the edge of the mantle in *Pecten*, since these are not specially concerned in the phylogeny of either the paired median or paired lateral eyes of vertebrates, and although of great interest in showing how special organs are sometimes evolved in anomalous situations in adaption to special needs, they do not assist in tracing the general evolution of the eyes of vertebrates. We hope that the diagram will be of some assistance in showing graphically how very far removed the more highly organized classes of living vertebrates are from the highly organized living invertebrates ; and, although the form and dimensions of the " tree " are not intended to accurately represent the periods of time which have elapsed since the divergence of the various classes took place in the course of evolution, that it will give some indication of the way in which certain of the simple types have persisted to the present day without, it may be presumed, having undergone marked modifications in general form and structure, while others have diverged from the primary simple type, but have nevertheless retained some of their older traits, which appear either in a simple form in the early larval condition, or may be present in the adult, in a modified and highly differentiated form. We have limited the term " parietal eye " to the parietal sense-organ of vertebrates, and designated the median eyes of invertebrates as such, or as frontal, triplacodal, or entomostracan eyes. We do not, however, wish it to be inferred that we consider the parietal sense-organ of vertebrates has arisen quite independently of the median eyes

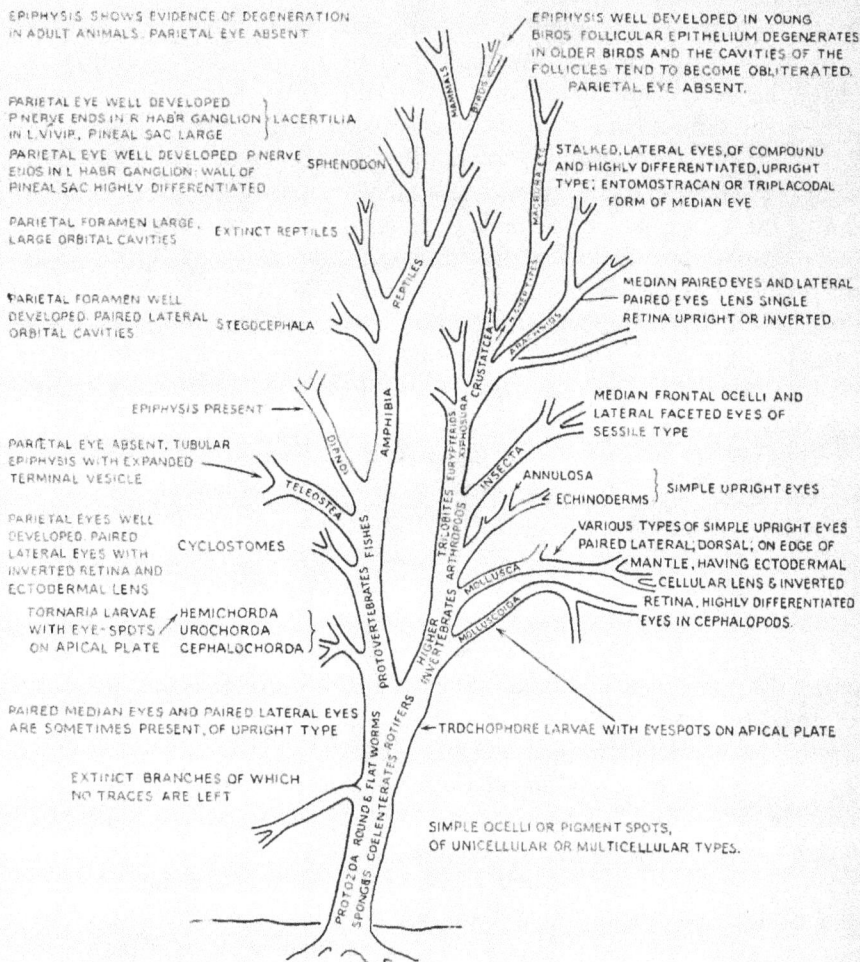

EPIPHYSIS SHOWS EVIDENCE OF DEGENERATION IN ADULT ANIMALS. PARIETAL EYE ABSENT

EPIPHYSIS WELL DEVELOPED IN YOUNG BIRDS. FOLLICULAR EPITHELIUM DEGENERATES IN OLDER BIRDS AND THE CAVITIES OF THE FOLLICLES TEND TO BECOME OBLITERATED. PARIETAL EYE ABSENT.

PARIETAL EYE WELL DEVELOPED P.NERVE ENDS IN R.HAB'R.GANGLION } LACERTILIA IN L.VIVIP. PINEAL SAC LARGE

PARIETAL EYE WELL DEVELOPED P.NERVE ENDS IN L.HAB'R GANGLION: WALL OF PINEAL SAC HIGHLY DIFFERENTIATED   SPHENODON

STALKED, LATERAL EYES, OF COMPOUND AND HIGHLY DIFFERENTIATED, UPRIGHT TYPE; ENTOMOSTRACAN OR TRIPLACODAL FORM OF MEDIAN EYE

PARIETAL FORAMEN LARGE, LARGE ORBITAL CAVITIES   EXTINCT REPTILES

MEDIAN PAIRED EYES AND LATERAL PAIRED EYES LENS SINGLE RETINA UPRIGHT OR INVERTED.

PARIETAL FORAMEN WELL DEVELOPED. PAIRED LATERAL ORBITAL CAVITIES   STEGOCEPHALA

MEDIAN FRONTAL OCELLI AND LATERAL FACETED EYES OF SESSILE TYPE

EPIPHYSIS PRESENT →

ANNULOSA } SIMPLE UPRIGHT EYES
ECHINODERMS

PARIETAL EYE ABSENT. TUBULAR EPIPHYSIS WITH EXPANDED TERMINAL VESICLE

VARIOUS TYPES OF SIMPLE UPRIGHT EYES PAIRED LATERAL; DORSAL; ON EDGE OF MANTLE, HAVING ECTODERMAL CELLULAR LENS & INVERTED RETINA. HIGHLY DIFFERENTIATED EYES IN CEPHALOPODS.

PARIETAL EYES WELL DEVELOPED. PAIRED LATERAL EYES WITH INVERTED RETINA AND ECTODERMAL LENS   CYCLOSTOMES

TORNARIA LARVAE WITH EYE-SPOTS ON APICAL PLATE   HEMICHORDA / UROCHORDA / CEPHALOCHORDA

PAIRED MEDIAN EYES AND PAIRED LATERAL EYES ARE SOMETIMES PRESENT, OF UPRIGHT TYPE

← TROCHOPHORE LARVAE WITH EYESPOTS ON APICAL PLATE

EXTINCT BRANCHES OF WHICH NO TRACES ARE LEFT

SIMPLE OCELLI OR PIGMENT SPOTS, OF UNICELLULAR OR MULTICELLULAR TYPES.

Tree labels: MAMMALS, BIRDS, REPTILES, AMPHIBIA, DIPNOI, TELEOSTEA, FISHES, PROTOVERTEBRATES, HIGHER INVERTEBRATES, CRUSTACEA, ARACHNIDA, MEROSTOMATA, INSECTA, EURYPTERIDS, TRILOBITES, XIPHOSURA, ARTHROPODS, MOLLUSCA, MOLLUSCOIDA, ROTIFERS, ROUND & FLAT WORMS, COELENTERATES, SPONGES, PROTOZOA

FIG. 323.—SCHEME INDICATING THE GENERAL DISTRIBUTION OF DIFFERENT TYPES OF MEDIAN AND LATERAL EYES IN THE ANIMAL KINGDOM.

of invertebrates. Further, we have used the term " parietal eye " in the singular although, as explained elsewhere, it may represent in some cases one member of a pair of median eyes or in other cases be formed by the fusion of the right and left members of a pair of primarily bilateral organs.

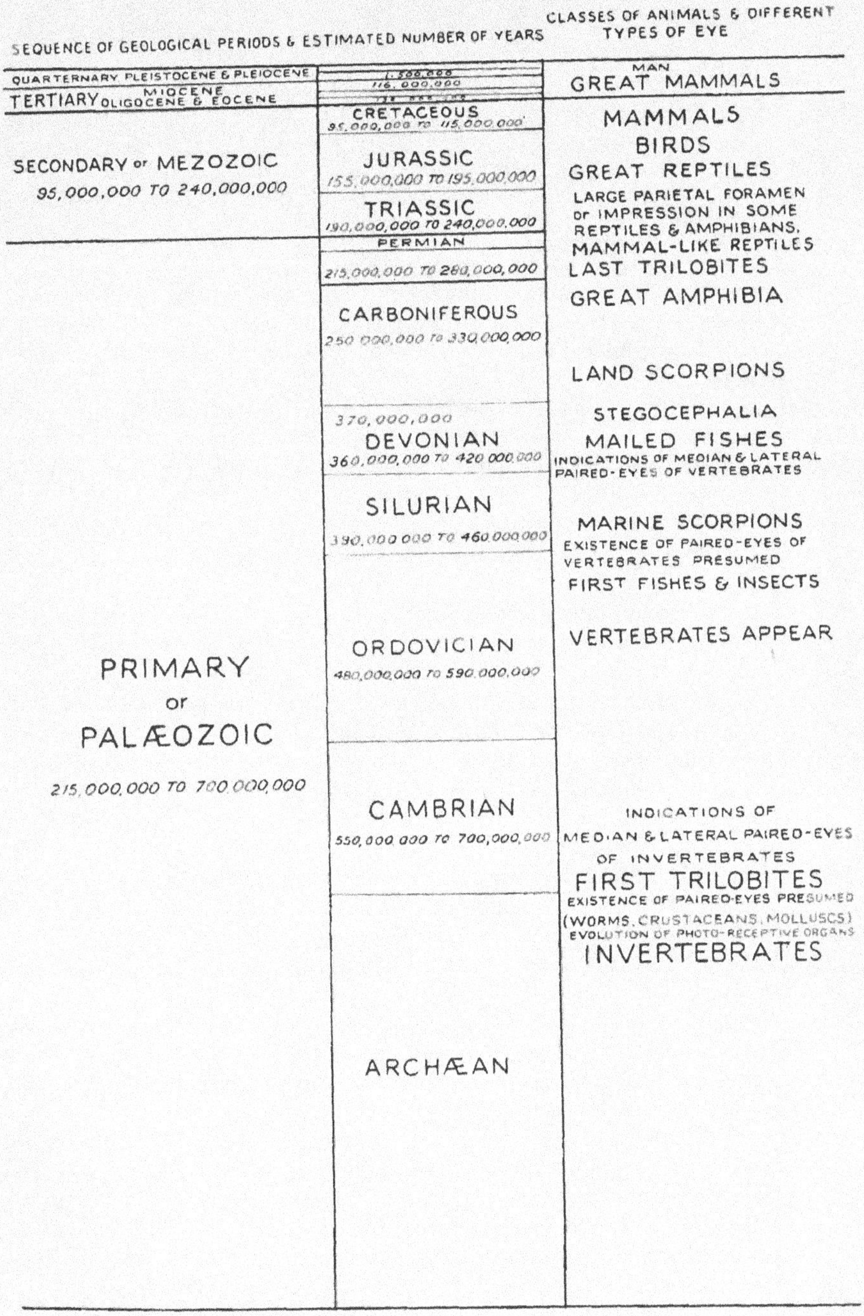

SEQUENCE OF GEOLOGICAL PERIODS & ESTIMATED NUMBER OF YEARS

CLASSES OF ANIMALS & DIFFERENT TYPES OF EYE

QUARTERNARY PLEISTOCENE & PLEIOCENE	1,500,000 / 116,000,000	MAN
TERTIARY MIOCENE / OLIGOCENE & EOCENE	735,000,000	GREAT MAMMALS
	CRETACEOUS 95,000,000 TO 115,000,000	MAMMALS / BIRDS
SECONDARY or MEZOZOIC 95,000,000 TO 240,000,000	JURASSIC 155,000,000 TO 195,000,000	GREAT REPTILES / LARGE PARIETAL FORAMEN or IMPRESSION IN SOME REPTILES & AMPHIBIANS. MAMMAL-LIKE REPTILES
	TRIASSIC 190,000,000 TO 240,000,000	
	PERMIAN 215,000,000 TO 280,000,000	LAST TRILOBITES
		GREAT AMPHIBIA
	CARBONIFEROUS 250,000,000 TO 330,000,000	
		LAND SCORPIONS
	370,000,000	STEGOCEPHALIA
	DEVONIAN 360,000,000 TO 420,000,000	MAILED FISHES / INDICATIONS OF MEDIAN & LATERAL PAIRED-EYES OF VERTEBRATES
	SILURIAN 390,000,000 TO 460,000,000	MARINE SCORPIONS / EXISTENCE OF PAIRED-EYES OF VERTEBRATES PRESUMED / FIRST FISHES & INSECTS
PRIMARY or PALÆOZOIC 215,000,000 TO 700,000,000	ORDOVICIAN 480,000,000 TO 590,000,000	VERTEBRATES APPEAR
	CAMBRIAN 550,000,000 TO 700,000,000	INDICATIONS OF MEDIAN & LATERAL PAIRED-EYES OF INVERTEBRATES / FIRST TRILOBITES / EXISTENCE OF PAIRED-EYES PRESUMED (WORMS, CRUSTACEANS, MOLLUSCS) EVOLUTION OF PHOTO-RECEPTIVE ORGANS / INVERTEBRATES
	ARCHÆAN	

FIG. 324.—GEOLOGICAL CHART INDICATING THE ORDER IN WHICH ORGANS SENSITIVE TO LIGHT AND VARIOUS TYPES OF EYE HAVE BEEN EVOLVED, AND ALSO THE ESTIMATED AGE IN WHICH THE DIFFERENT CLASSES OF ANIMALS HAVE BEEN FOUND. (MODIFIED FROM SCHEME AND DATA PUBLISHED BY GASKELL AND BARRELL.)

GLOSSARY

ACANTHIAS (Gr. *acantha*, spine) : a genus of sharks including the spiny dogfish, so named from the spines on the dorsal fins.

ACANTHOPTERYGII (Gr. acantha, spine ; *pterux*, wing or fin) : fishes with spinous rays supporting the paired fins, e.g. perch.

ACARINA (Gr. *akari*, mite) : a division of the Arachnida, of which the cheese-mite is a type.

ACILIUS CALIGINOSUS : a beetle belonging to the family Dyticidæ, Order Coleoptera.

ACIPENSER (L.—a large fish commonly taken to be sturgeon) : genus of Ganoids including the sturgeon.

ACONE EYES (Gr. *a*, without ; *konos*, cone) : retinæ of invertebrate animals in which there are no crystalline cones, as in many insects, e.g. Coleoptera, Diptera.

ACTINOZOA (Gr. *actin*, ray ; *zoön*, animal) : a division of the Cœlenterata, of which the sea-anemones are a type, and which show a radial symmetry.

ADIADOCHOKINESIA (Gr. *a*, absence of ; *diadoche*, succession ; *kinesis*, movement) : inability to perform successive movements, such as rapid and repeated pronation and supination of the two forearms.

AGELENA LABYRINTHICA : a cellar spider belonging to the Order Araneida.

AGNATHI (Gr. *a*, without ; *gnathos*, jaw) : the branch of craniate vertebrates which includes the Ostracodermi or Cyclostomata and characterized by the absence of jaws.

AMBLYSTOMA (Gr. *amblus*, blunt ; *stoma*, mouth) : a tailed amphibian, the permanent larval form of which is the Mexican Axolotl, having a blunt nose.

AMIA (Gr. *amia*, a kind of tunny) : a bony fish allied to the mackerels.

AMMOCŒTES (Gr. *ammos*, sand ; *kētos*, fish) : the larval form of *Petromyzon*, lamprey.

AMMONITES (Gr. *ammōn*, (ram's) horn, symbol of Zeus-Ammon) : the fossil shells of the extinct Cephalopoda, usually referred to the subclass Tetrabranchiata. Their spiral shells resemble that of the living genus *Nautilus*.

AMPHIOXUS (Gr. *amphi*, both ; *oxus*, sharp) : the lancelet fish, so named on account of its being pointed at both ends. It belongs to the subclass Cephalochorda.

AMPHIPODA (Gr. *amphi*, both ; *pous*, foot) : an order of the Crustacea, comprising the sand-hoppers and fresh-water shrimps. The feet are directed both forwards and backwards.

ANAPSIDA (Gr. *a, an*, without ; *apsis*, arch) : the name applied to a primitive type of reptile in which the roof of the skull is complete, without a temporal fossa, as in the Stegocephala. See : SYNAPSIDA ; DIAPSIDA.

480

ANASPIDA (Gr. *a, an*, without ; *aspis*, shield) : an order of extinct fishes belonging to the branch Ostracodermi, characterized by the absence of a head-shield.

ANGUIS FRAGILIS (L. *anguis*, snake ; *fragilis*, brittle) : blindworm, a snake-like, limbless lizard with imperfectly developed eyes.

ANNELIDA (Gallicised form of Annulata) : ringed worms, without jointed feet, and comprising the sub-classes Chætopoda and Hirudinea.

ANNULOSA (L. *annulus*, ring) : sub-kingdom comprising the Anarthropoda and Arthropoda in which the body consists of a succession of rings.

ANOMODONTIA (Gr. *anomos*, without order or irregular ; *odous*, tooth) : an extinct order of reptiles, also called Dicynodontia, with large teeth resembling a dog's canines.

ANOURA (Gr. *a, an*, without ; *oura*, tail) : tailless amphibia, e.g. frogs and toads.

APUS CANCRIFORMIS (Gr. *a*, without ; *pous*, foot ; L. *cancer*, crab ; *forma*, shape) : a small fresh-water crustacean characterized by a dorsal shield and crab-like form.

ARACHNIDA (Gr. *arachnē*, web ; *arachnēs*, spider) : air-breathing Arthropoda, including the spiders and scorpions.

ARGONAUTA (Gr. *argos*, living without labour ; *naute*, sailor) : the female " paper nautilus," a dibranchiate cephalopod, with a corrugated spiral shell in which the animal floats idly on the surface of the water.

ARGULUS : the carp louse, an external parasitic Copepod, crustacean, having a trilobate median eye and compound lateral eyes.

ARTHRODIRA (Gr. *arthron*, joint ; *deirē*, neck) : an order of extinct fishes including Coccosteus, Dinichthys, and Titanichthys ; they are characterized by a joint separating the head-shield from the body-shield.

ARTHROPODA (Gr. *arthron*, joint ; *pous*, foot) : an invertebrate phylum characterized by jointed limbs, as contrasted with " bristle " feet.

ASCIDIA (Gr. *askos*, bottle ; *eidos*, like) : an order of the class Tunicata, with sac-like bodies, comprising the sea-squirts.

ASCIDIA MAMMILLATA (Gr. *askos*, bottle ; *eidos*, shape) : a Tunicate the free-swimming larva of which contains a single eye enclosed within the ventricular cavity of the brain.

ASTACUS FLUVIATILIS : fresh-water crayfish, belonging to the order Decapoda of the class Crustacea.

ASTROSCOPUS (Gr. *astron*, stars ; *skopeō*, look) : the American star-gazer. An electric ray in which the eyes are situated close together and directed upwards. The electric organs are on the dorsal surface of the head just behind the eyes.

AUCHENASPIS (Gr. *auchēn*, narrow, neck ; *aspis*, shield) : an extinct palæozoic fish belonging to the class Ostracodermi. It had paired lateral orbital cavities, between which are two small pineal canals.

AURELIA AURITA (L. *aureolus*, golden colour ; *aurita*, long-eared) : the common jelly-fish, so named on account of its colour and the ear-shaped form of its oral arms.

AXOLOTL : the persistent larva of Amblystoma, which retains its external branchiæ throughout life.

31

BALANOGLOSSUS (Gr. *balanos*, acorn ; *glossa*, tongue) : a worm-like animal, having a tongue-like proboscis and rudimentary notochord, belonging to the class Hemichorda, of the Protochordata. The larval form, or *Tornaria*, closely resembles the trochophore larvæ of certain invertebrates.

BDELLOSTOMA (Gr. *bdella*, leech ; *stoma*, mouth) : a genus of the Myxinoidei, including the hag-fishes, so named on account of the leech-like mouth.

BELONE (Gr. " sharp "—fish with pointed nose) : the gar-pike and bony-pike, *Lepidosteus*.

BIBIONIDÆ : a group of insects in which the males possess two pairs of compound eyes—an upper, larger with coarse facets, and lower, smaller with fine facets. The two larger eyes are contiguous or united. Carrière considers that the small lower eye of the male corresponds to the whole eye of the female.

BLASTOCYST (Gr. *blastos*, bud or germ ; *kustē*, bladder, sac) : the stage of development in which the embryo consists of a single layered vesicle.

BLASTOPORE (Gr. *blastos*, germ) : the opening leading into the cavity of a gastrula.

BOMBINATOR (Gr. *bombos*, L. *bombus*, a humming or croaking sound) : a genus of European toads.

BRACHIOPODA (Gr. *brachion*, arm ; *pous*, foot) : a class of the Molluscoida having two fleshy arms, continued from the sides of the mouth. It includes the lamp-shells and barnacles.

BRANCHIOPODA (Gr. *branchia*, gill ; *pous*, foot) : a division of the Crustacea comprising the orders Cladocera, Phyllopoda, and Trilobita, and characterized by gills supported by the feet.

BRANCHIOSAURUS (Gr. *branchia*, gill ; *saura*, lizard) : a genus of extinct Stegocephala.

BRANCHIPUS (Gr. *branchia*, gill ; *pous*, foot) : a crustacean belonging to the order Phyllopoda ; the group includes the brine-shrimps ; the transparent body is unprotected by a carapace.

CÆCILIA (L. *Cæcilia*), the slow-worm or blind worm, from *cæcus*, blind. A group of limbless amphibians, with vestigial eyes, e.g. *Ichthyophis glutinosus*.

CAINOZOIC (Gr. *kainos*, recent ; *zoos*, living, life) : the Kainozoic or Tertiary period of geology, applied to recent formations in which the organic remains resemble more or less closely existing animals and plants.

CAMBRIAN SYSTEM OR PERIOD (Welsh ; Cambria, Cymry) : the earliest Palæozoic rocks, which lie below the Silurian in Wales and Cumberland. It contains marine invertebrates, including the earliest forms of trilobites.

CAPITOSAURUS (L. *caput*, head ; Gr. *saura*, lizard) : a genus of extinct stegocephalous amphibia.

CARAPACE (Gr. *cara*, head ; *karabos*, beetle ; L. *scarabæus ; carabus locusta*) : a protective covering for the head or dorsal aspect of the body.

CARBONIFEROUS (L. *carbo*, coal ; *fero*, bear) : the Palæozoic period, lying above the Old Red Sandstone (Devonian) and below the Permian. It is characterized by the presence of coal and the appearance of amphibia.

CEPHALASPIS (Gr. *kephalē*, head ; *aspis*, shield) : an extinct genus of fishes belonging to the order Osteostraci of the class Ostracodermi.

CEPHALIC APODEME (Gr. *kephalē*, head ; *apo*, with ; *demas*, body or frame) the internal skeleton of the head, present in some arthropods and molluscs.

CEPHALOPODA (Gr. *kephalē*, head ; *pous*, foot) : a class of Mollusca which includes the cuttle-fishes, squids, octopuses, and nautili.

CERATODUS (Gr. *keras*, horn ; *odous*, tooth) : a genus of the lung fishes or Dipnoi (Australia).

CHÆTOGNATHA (Gr. *chaite*, bristle ; *gnathos*, jaw) : an order of the phylum Nematohelminthes, or Round-worms, comprising the marine arrow worms (Sagitta).

CHELÆ, CHELATE (Gr. *chēlē*, claw) : the prehensile claws which are present on some of the limbs of certain Crustacea, e.g. the lobsters and crabs.

CHELONIA (Gr. *chelōnē*, a tortoise) : an order of the class Reptilia, comprising the tortoise and turtles.

CHELYDRA (Gr. *chelus*, like a tortoise ; *udor*, water) : a genus of turtles or water tortoises.

CHIMÆRA (Gr. *chimaira*, monster) : a primitive type of deep-water fish belonging to the order Holocephali.

CHITIN (Gr. *chitōn*, cuirass) : a nitrogenous horny material, which is deposited in the outer epithelial layers of certain invertebrate animals, to form a hard, protective covering, as in the exoskeleton of the Crustacea.

CHITON (Gr. *chitōn*, coat of mail) : a genus belonging to the class Amphineura of the Mollusca. The back is covered by a jointed shield.

CHONDRICHTHYES (Gr. *chondros*, cartilage ; *ichthus*, fish) : cartilaginous fishes, including the sharks and rays.

CHONDROSTEI (Gr. *chondros*, cartilage ; *osteon*, bone) : an order of Ganoid fishes comprising the sturgeons and spoon-bill, characterized by few replacing bones.

CHROMATOPHORE (Gr. *chroma*, colour ; *phoreō*, carry) : connective tissue cells found in the derma and other mesodermal tissues, which contain large pigment granules and are often branched.

CIRRIPEDIA (L. *cirrus*, a tuft or crest of curled hair or feathers ; *pes*, foot) : an order of the Ostracoda including the barnacles, in which eyes are always wanting in the adult fixed-form of the animal. Both median and lateral eyes, however, may be present in the Cypris larva, e.g. *Lepas fascicularis*.

CISTELLA (L. *cistella*, small box) : a Brachiopod in which the upper valve of the shell articulates with the lower by a horizontal hinge. It contains a shelly-loop for the support of the lophophore. The trochophore larva has one or two pairs of ocelli.

CLADOCERA (Gr. *klados*, branch ; *keras*, horn) : an order of Crustacea having branched antennæ, including *Daphnia* and *Polyphemus*.

COCCOSTEUS (Gr. *kokkos*, berry, kernel ; *osteon*, bone) : a genus of extinct fishes belonging to the order Arthrodira.

COELENTERATA (Gr. *koilos*, hollow; *enteron*, bowel): the phylum which comprises the polyps, sea-anemones, and jelly-fishes, in which there is an enteric cavity lined by entoderm.

COLEOPTERA (Gr. *koleos*, sheath; *pteron*, wing): an order of the Insecta—beetles in which the anterior pair of wings are modified to form a hard, protective covering for the posterior membranous wings.

COMPOUND EYE: a term which is applied in two senses—(1) An eye consisting of several strata of cells, e.g. (*a*) receptive (rod and cone cells), (*b*) intermediate (bipolar cells), (*c*) retinal ganglionic cells; (2) a composite or aggregate eye in which the whole is composed of an aggregate of units, each of which is called an ommatidium.

CONARIUM (Gr. *konarion*, dim. of *konos*, cone): the epiphysis cerebri, so named on account of the conical form in man and certain mammals.

CONVERGENCE: the acquisition of a similar form or structure by two or more different organisms as a result of a similar mode of life; as contrasted with resemblances which are due to inheritance from a common ancestor.

COPIOPHORA CORNUTA (Gr. *kopis*, a curved knife, sting; *phoreō*, bear; L. *cornuta*, horned): a species of locust in which there is a single, median frontal ocellus of large size.

COREGONUS: a genus of fresh-water fishes belonging to the family Salmonidæ; commonly known as " white fish."

CORNEAGEN CELLS (L. *cornu*, horn; rt. *gen*, give origin to): the epidermal cells which produce the superficial non-cellular or horny layer. When the cells form a single stratum of tall columnar cells, this layer is sometimes spoken of as the palisade layer.

CRANGON: sea-water shrimp belonging to the sub-class Malacostraca, or soft-shelled crustaceans.

CRETACEOUS SYSTEM OR PERIOD (L. *creta*, chalk): the uppermost chalky deposits of the mesozoic or secondary era, in which remains of bony fish are abundant.

CUMACEA: an order of the Malacostraca, including *Diastylis*. The eyes are sessile, close together, or fused into one. They are always poorly developed and occasionally are wanting.

CUTICLE (L. *cuticula*, the thin outer layer of the skin): the most superficial layer of an epithelial sheet, which is either secreted by the epithelial cells or formed by degeneration of the most superficial cells of the epidermis. It may be impregnated with lime salts or chitin.

CYATHASPIS (Gr. *kuathos*, cup; *aspis*, shield): an extinct Pteraspid fish belonging to the class Ostracodermi, characterized by a bowl or cup-like head-shield.

CYCLOPS (Gr. *cyclops*, the mythical one-eyed giants described by Homer: literally round-eyed): the water-flea or *Daphnia*, in which the paired lateral eyes have fused into a single organ.

CYCLOSTOMATA (Gr. *kuklos*, circle; *stoma*, mouth): a primitive class of fishes, characterized by their round mouths and absence of jaws, including the lampreys and hag-fishes.

DECAPODA (Gr. *deka*, ten ; *podes*, feet) : the division of Crustacea, which have ten walking feet ; and also the family of cuttle-fishes which possess ten " arms " or head-processes arising from the " foot " and surrounding the mouth.

DERIC (Gr. *deros*, skin) : a term used to denote a layer derived from the derma or corium, i.e. mesodermal in origin, as contrasted with ectodermal.

DERMA (Gr. *derma*, skin) : a term usually applied to denote the deeper layer of the skin, or corium.

DIBRANCHIATA (Gr. *dis*, twice ; *branchia*, gill) : a subclass of the Cephalopoda characterized by the presence of two gills or ctenidia. The foot is sub-divided into eight or ten arms, which surround the mouth. The subclass includes the cuttle-fishes, squids, spirula, and the extinct belemnites.

DICYNODONTIA (Gr. *dis*, twice ; *kuon*, dog ; *odous*, tooth) : an extinct order of reptiles having two large teeth in the upper jaw, which resemble the " canine " teeth of a dog.

DINICHTHYS (Gr. *deinos*, strange, terrible ; *ichthus*, fish) : an extinct genus of fishes belonging to the order Arthrodira.

DINOPHILUS TÆNIATUS (Gr. *dinos*, whirling movement or eddy ; *philos*, fond ; *tainia*, band) : a cylindrical worm-like animal characterized by a series of circular ciliated bands, an apical plate, and paired ocelli, belonging to the phylum Trochelminthes.

DIPLOSTICHOUS (Gr. *diploos*, double ; *stichos*, layer) : a term applied to an eye consisting of two layers of cells, e.g. the central eyes of *Limulus*, in which a single layer of hypoderm or vitreous cells lies in front of the retina.

DIPNOI (Gr. *dis*, twice ; *pnoē*, breath) : the order of fishes comprising *Ceratodus Lepidosiren* and *Protopterus*, commonly known as lung-fishes or mud-fishes. Their respiration is aquatic, by means of gills, and aërial by a single sacculated lung, corresponding to the air-bladder of Ganoids and Teleosts.

DIPROSOPUS (Gr. *diprosopos*, two-faced) : a double-faced monster, as in Duplicitas anterior.

DIPTERA (Gr. *dis*, twice ; *pteron*, wing) : an order of the Insecta having a single pair of transparent membranous wings, e.g. bugs, plant lice.

DORSAL SAC : the recess which lies between the velum transversum in front and the superior or habenular commissure behind. Its roof forms the post-velar arch.

DYTISCUS MARGINALIS (Gr. *dutes*, diver ; *dutikos*, fond of diving) : a carnivorous water beetle belonging to the group Hydradephaga.

ECHIDNA (Gr. *echidna*, adder ; monster) : the spiny ant-eater of Australia, belonging to the order Monotremata, comprising the egg-laying mammals.

ECTODERM (Gr. *ektos*, outside ; *derma*, skin) : the outer layer of cells in a multi-cellular animal. It corresponds to the term " epiblast " of the growing embryo, and gives rise to the epidermis of the adult animal.

ECTOPARIETAL-EYE (Gr. *ektos*, outside ; L. *paries*, wall) : the term applied by Patten to " the outer of the two vesicles produced by constriction of

the single terminal vesicle of the parietal organ of vertebrates." He
believed that it contains in its walls two of the four retinal placodes,
belonging to the undivided terminal vesicle. It corresponds to the
parietal eye of *Petromyzon* (Studnička).

EDRIOPHTHALMATA (Gr. *hedraios*, sitting ; *ophthalmos*, eye) : a division of the
crustacea having sessile eyes, not supported on a stalk. It includes the
Amphipoda, e.g. sandhopper (*Talitrus*), and Isopoda, e.g. fresh-water
shrimp (*Gammarus*).

ELASMOBRANCHII (Gr. *elasma*, plate ; *branchia*, gill) : an order of fishes including
the sharks and rays, having plate-like gills.

ENDOCHROME CELLS (Gr. *endon*, within ; *chroma*, colour) : pigmented cells
of the retina in which the pigment granules are deposited in the epithelial
cells composing the retina. The pigment may be deposited in one part
of a sensory or visual cell or in a specialized epithelial pigment cell.

ENDOCRINE (Gr. *endon*, within ; *krinā*, separate) : adjective used to denote the
function of internal secretion.

ENDOPARIETAL EYE (Gr. *endon*, within ; L. *paries*, wall) : term applied by
Patten to " the inner of the two vesicles produced by constriction of
the terminal vesicle of the parietal organ of vertebrates." He believed
that it contains in its walls two of the four retinal placodes belonging to
the undivided terminal vesicle. It corresponds to the " parapineal
organ " of *Petromyzon* (Studnička).

ENDOTHELIUM (Gr. *endon*, within ; *thēlē*, nipple) : a layer of cells lining a vessel
or vascular space, or the epithelial lining of a serous membrane.

ENTODERM (Gr. *entos*, within ; *derma*, skin) : the inner layer of embryonic
cells, also called endoderm and hypoblast.

ENTOMOSTRACA (Gr. *entomos*, incision, division ; *ostrakon*, shell) : a sub-class
of the Crustacea in which the shell is divided into segments. It comprises the orders Phyllopoda, Cladocera, Ostracoda, Copepoda.

ENTOMOSTRACAN EYE : the name given to the median eye-spot which is
commonly found in species belonging to the four orders which are
included in the subclass Entomostraca. It usually consists of three
single eyes joined into a triple eye, one segment of which is median and
ventral, the remaining segments being lateral and dorsal. The median
segment appears to be formed by the fusion of two primarily bilatera'
eyes.

EPIBLAST (Gr. *epi*, upon ; *blastos*, germ) : the outer or upper layer of cells in
the embryo. See ECTODERM.

EPIPHYSIS CEREBRI (Gr. *epi*, upon ; *phusis*, originate or grow from) : the diverticulum from the roof of the diencephalon, which gives rise to the pineal
body, pineal sac, or parietal sense-organ.

EPITHELIUM (Gr. *epi*, upon ; *thēlē*, nipple) : a layer of cells covering a surface
or lining a duct, canal, or vessel. It covers the nipple-shaped dermal
papillæ of the skin.

EPIZOA (Gr. *epi*, upon ; *zoon*, animal) : (1) animals which are parasitic on other
animals ; (2) a subclass of the crustaceans in which the adult animal
is usually fixed to the gills or exterior of a fish or other animal. The

young are free-swimming, and are provided with eyes and antennæ :
e.g. *Argulus*.

ERYOPS : a genus of extinct amphibia belonging to the order Stegocephala.

EUCONE EYES (Gr. *eu*, well, complete ; *konos*, cone) : invertebrate eyes in which
the crystalline cones are well developed, as in many of the compound
eyes of Crustacea.

EUPHAUSIA PELLUCIDA (Gr. *eu*, well ; *phausis*, bright ; L. *pellucidus*, clear, transparent) : an order of the Eucarida. The carapace coalesces with the
thoracic segments to form a continuous shield and there are stalked eyes.

EURYPTERUS (Gr. *eurus*, wide ; *pteron*, wing) : an extinct scorpion-like genus
belonging to the order Merostoma.

EXOCHROME CELLS (Gr. *ex*, out of ; *chroma*, colour) : pigment cells of the retina
of extraneous origin, and thought to be derived from the subepidermal
connective tissue.

FLABELLUM (L. *flabellum*, fan) : the last appendage of the prosoma of the adult
Limulus has an outer segment which is called the epipodite or flabellum.

FLUKE : an internal parasitic worm of leaf-like form (*Distoma hepaticum*)
belonging to the class Trematoda. It is frequently found in the gall
bladder or bile ducts of the sheep.

FUNDULUS HETEROCLITUS (L. *fundulus*, closed end of gut, or tube ; Gr. *hetero-
clitos*, irregularly bent) : a marine minnow, the developing embryos of
which were used by Stockard and others for the experimental production
of cyclops and other deformities.

FUSCIN (L. *foscus*, brown) : the colouring material contained in the pigment
granules of the hexagonal cells of the retina, a form of melanin.

GALEODES : an Arachnid belonging to the order Solpugidæ, and resembling
the scorpions.

GAMMARUS ORNATUS : the gadfly, belonging to the order Hymenoptera of the
class Insecta. A small median or frontal ocellus is situated between two
large faceted eyes.

GANOID (Gr. *ganos*, sheen ; *eidos*, like) : (1) A term applied to the glistening
scales or plates of certain fishes ; they are composed of a deep layer
of true bone, which is covered by a superficial layer of enamel or ganoin.
(2) An order of fishes characterized by incomplete ossification of the
endoskeleton, and an exoskeleton usually formed of rhombic, ganoid
plates, e.g. *Polypterus ; Osteolepis*, a primitive extinct genus.

GASTEROPODA (Gr. *gaster*, stomach ; *pous*, foot) : the class of Mollusca, comprising univalve forms in which movement is effected by contractions
of the foot—e.g. snails and slugs.

GASTRULA (Gr. *gaster*, stomach) : the name applied to the double-layered
vesicle formed by the invagination of one part of the wall of the blastocyst into the opposite part.

GLABELLA (L. *glabella*, smooth, bare area) : e.g. the smooth median part of the
cephalic-shield of a trilobite.

GNATHOSTOMATA (Gr. *gnathos*, jaw ; *stoma*, mouth) : the Branch of fishes
characterized by the presence of jaws in the mouth, as contrasted with
the cyclostomata in which jaws are absent.

GYMNOPHIONA (Gr. *gumnos*, naked ; *ophis*, snake) : an order of the Amphibia comprising the snake-like Cæcilia.

GYMNOTUS (Gr. *gumnotes*, naked) : the electric eel of South America.

GYRINIDÆ (Gr. *gureuō*, run in a circle) : a family of beetles which possess two pairs of compound eyes. See BIBIONIDÆ.

HATTERIA PUNCTATA or SPHENODON, a primitive type of reptile belonging to the order Rhynchocephalia, in which the parietal eye is well developed.

HELIX NEMORALIS (Gr. *helix*, twisted or coiled) : land-snail, belonging to the order Pulmonata of the Mollusca. The eyes are situated at the apex of each posterior or ocular tentacle.

HEMIASPIDÆ (Gr. *hemi*, half ; *aspis*, shield) : an extinct Palæozoic order related to the Xiphosura, and including *Bunodes*, *Hemiaspis*, and *Belinurus*.

HEMICHORDA (Gr. *hemi*, half ; *chordē*, string) : a subphylum of the chordata, comprising *Balanoglossus*. An œsophageal diverticulum in the region of the neck is regarded as a rudiment of the notochord. The tornaria, or larva, has an apical plate bearing two eye-spots.

HEMIPTERA (Gr. *hemi*, half ; *pteron*, wing) : an order of the Insecta in which the anterior wings are membranous at the tip, while the inner part is chitinous—e.g. bugs, plant lice, cicadas, lice (*Anoplura*), wingless parasites of mammals.

HEXAPODA (Gr. *hexa*, six ; *pous*, foot) : name applied to the Insecta on account of their having six legs.

HIRUDINEA (L. *hirudo*, leech) : the order of Annelida, which includes the leeches.

HOLOCEPHALI (Gr. *holos*, whole ; *kephalē*, head) : a sub-order of the Elasmobranchs which includes *Chimæra* and *Callorhynchus*.

HOLOCHROAL EYES (Gr. *holos*, complete ; *chroa*, surface) : the term used to denote a form of compound lateral eye of trilobites, in which the corneal surface was continuous ; the ommatidia not being separated as in the schizochroal type.

HOLOSTOMATA (Gr. *holos*, whole ; *stoma*, mouth) : a division of the gasteropod molluscs in which the opening of the spiral shell is entire.

HOMARUS : lobster belonging to the order Decapoda, of the class Crustacea.

HOPLOCARIDA (Gr. *hoplon*, armour ; *karis*, a small lobster) : a division of the Crustacea, comprising the squills, in which the carapace or head-shield covers only the anterior thoracic segments. Large stalked eyes are borne by the first segment of the anterior region of the head.

HYDRODROMA (Gr. *hudra*, water ; *dromos*, movement, running) : a fresh-water mite belonging to the family Hydrachnidæ and the order Acarina. It has two paired eyes and a central or median eye.

HYMENOPTERA (Gr. *humen*, membrane ; *pteron*, wing) : an order of the Insecta characterized by having four membranous wings, e.g. bee, wasp, ant.

HYPODERMIS (Gr. *hupo*, under ; *derma*, skin) : the single layer of cells which lies beneath the cuticle in invertebrates. It is also known, with reference to invertebrate eyes, as the vitreous or corneagen layer. It corresponds to the deeper cells of the epidermis of vertebrates and the tall columnar cells composing it are spoken of as palisade or epiderm cells.

HYPOSTOME (Gr. *hupo*, under ; *stoma*, mouth) : the upper lip or " labrum" of certain Crustacea, e.g. Trilobita.

ICHTHYOPSIDA (Gr. *ichthus*, fish ; *opsis*, appearance) : the division of vertebrata which comprises the fishes and amphibia ; also known as branchiate vertebrates.

ICHTHYOPTERYGIA (Gr. *ichthus*, fish ; *pterux*, wing or fin) : an extinct order of fish-like reptiles, which includes the Ichthyosauri.

ICHTHYOSAURUS (Gr. *ichthus*, fish ; *saura*, lizard) : an extinct order of reptiles belonging to the Mesozoic period.

ISOPODA (Gr. *isos*, equal ; *pous*, foot) : an order of the Crustacea in which the feet are approximately equal in size and appearance, e.g. *Asellus*, *Sphæroma*. The eyes are compound and usually sessile ; in some examples, however, they consist of a collection of simple eyes.

JURASSIC SYSTEM OR PERIOD : the oolitic and lias deposits found in the Jura Mountains and stretching across England from Yorkshire to Dorset. It belongs to the Mesozoic period and contains remains of marine animals such as the ammonites and large Saurian reptiles.

KAINOZOIC (Gr. *kainos*, recent ; *zoe*, life) : the tertiary period in geology, in which the remains of animals and plants closely resemble living species.

KIAERASPIS (Gr. *apis*, shield) : a primitive Palæozoic fish belonging to the Order Cephalaspidomorphi of the branch Ostracodermi.

KING-CRAB (*Limulus*) : a marine arachnid belonging to the order Xiphosura. It is characterized by a large dorsal-shield and plate-like " book gills."

LABIUM (L. lip) : term used to denote the lower lip of articulate animals. See LABRUM.

LABRUM (L. lip) : term used to denote the upper lip of articulate animals.

LABYRINTHODONTIA (Gr. *laburinthos*, labyrinth ; *odous*, tooth) : an extinct order of the Amphibia, also named Stegocephala. The term was employed to express the complicated structural appearance of the teeth when seen in transverse section.

LAMELLIBRANCH (L. *lamella*, plate ; Gr. *branchia*, gill) : a bivalve mollusc having lamellar gills, e.g. Fresh-water mussel (*Anodonta cygnea*) : scallop (*Pecten*). In some, the larva of which lead a parasitic existence, visual sense-organs are vestigial or absent. In others, e.g. *Pecten*, highly differentiated eyes are developed in the adult animal round the edge of the mantle.

LENS (L. *lens, lentis*, lentil) : the crystalline lens of the eye, so named on account of its being about the size and shape of a lentil seed. There are three principal types of lens, named according to their composition : cuticular, vitreous, cellular. In some instances two or all three of the constituent elements may be combined in the formation of a single lens.

LEPAS FASCICULARIS, LEPAS ANATIFERA (L. *lepas*, small shell-fish) : cirripede Crustacea, e.g. barnacle, characterized by the fixed condition of the adult animal and by passing through a free-swimming nauplius stage, which is followed by a cypris stage in which the larva is enclosed in a bivalved shell and has both simple (ocellar) and compound eyes.

LEPIDOPTERA (Gr. *lepis*, scale ; *pteron*, wing) : an order of the Insecta having four wings covered with scales, e.g. butterflies, moths.

LEPIDOSIREN (Gr. *lepis*, scale ; *surinx*, tube) : a genus of the lung-fishes (Dipnoi) of a long pipe-like form, found in South America.

LEPIDOSTEUS (Gr. *lepis*, scale ; *osteon*, bone) : genus of ganoid fishes, e.g. gar-pike.

LEPIDURUS (Gr. *lepis*, scale ; *ourus*, tail) : a crustacean belonging to the subclass Branchiopoda and order Notostraca. It has a well-developed head shield and a tail-like plate between two caudal styles.

LINGULA (L. variant of *ligula*, spatula or shoe-string) : lamp-shell, a stalked brachiopod in which the two valves of the shell are not joined by a hinge. Existing genera of *Lingula* appear first in the lower Cambrian rocks, and with other genera of the Brachiopoda, e.g. *Cistella*, it forms a striking example of persistence of type. See CISTELLA and RHYNCHONELLA.

MALACOSTRACA (Gr. *malakos*, soft ; *ostrakon*, shell) : a subclass of the Crustacea characterized by having a soft shell, e.g. the shrimps and prawns.

MANTLE : the outer covering or pallium which protects the viscera in most of the Mollusca.

MARSIPOBRANCH (Gr. *marsipos*, pouch ; *branchia*, gill) : the order of cyclostome fishes, which includes the lampreys and hag-fishes, which is characterized by pouch-like diverticula separated by septa bearing gills.

MELANOBLAST (Gr. *melas*, black ; *blastos*, bud or germ) : branched pigment cells of the epidermis. They are believed to elaborate pigment granules which pass from them into the epidermal cells.

MELANOPHORE (Gr. *melas*, pigment ; *phoreo*, bear) : a cell bearing pigment granules, also called chromatophore.

MEROSTOMATA (Gr. *meros*, thigh ; *stoma*, mouth) : an extinct order of the Crustacea, including the extinct forms *Eurypterus* and *Pterygotus* and the living genus *Limulus*. The appendages situated round the mouth act as jaws, and their free extremities serve as legs or as prehensile organs. The head-shield bears two lateral compound eyes and two ocelli placed near the median line.

MOLLUSCOIDA (L. *mollis*, soft ; *mollesco*, become soft ; Gr. *eidos*, likeness) : a subdivision of invertebrates resembling the Mollusca in possessing soft bodies, including the Polyzoa, Brachiopoda, and Phoronida.

MONOSTICHOUS (Gr. *monos*, single ; *stichos*, layer) : a term applied to an eye consisting of a single layer of cells, e.g. the larval eye of *Dytiscus* or lateral eyes of *Limulus*.

MYRIAPODA (Gr. *murios*, numerous, 10,000 ; *podes*, feet) : a class of the Arthropoda comprising the centipedes and millipedes.

NAUPLIUS (L. *nauplius*, a sea-fish) : the free-swimming larva which results from the hatching of the embryo of certain crustaceans, e.g. *Apus*.

NAUTILUS (Gr. *nautilos*, sailor) : a genus of the subclass Tetrabranchiata of the class Cephalopoda. It is a primitive type of mollusc the shell of which resembles the extinct Ammonites.

NEREIS : A marine annelid belonging to the subclass Polychæta. It has two pairs of eyes of a simple ocellar type.

NEUROPTERA (Gr. *neuron*, nerve, cord ; *pteron*, wing) : an order of the Insecta having four membranous wings, strengthened by tendinous cords or " nervures," e.g. dragon-flies.

NOTOSTRACA (Gr. *notos*, back ; *ostrakon*, shell) : an order of the branchiopod crustaceans comprising *Apus* and *Lepidurus*, so named on account of the shell-like carapace which covers the dorsal surface of the head and thorax.

NYCTIPHANES (Gr. *nuctiphanes*, visible by night) : a crustacean belonging to the order Euphausiacea, having luminous organs or photospheria on the basal joints of certain of the thoracic feet.

OCELLUS (L. diminutive of *oculus*) : the name given to a single or simple eye as contrasted with a multiple or aggregate eye. The ocellus may be a simple placode or eye-spot ; an optic pit, with open mouth ; or a closed vesicle, having a corneagen or vitreous lens. In some cases a group of larval ocelli are replaced in the adult insect (imago) by an aggregate or compound eye.

OMMATIDIUM (Gr. *omma*, eye, diminutive suffix) : one of the component units of an aggregate or compound eye of an adult arthropod, e.g. *Dytiscus marginalis*. Each ommatidium consists of an outer dioptric part, formed of the vitreous cells or crystalline-cones, and an inner percipient part called the retinula, which is composed of a central visual-rod or rhabdome, and the neuro-sensory cells. The retinulæ are separated by inter-retinular pigment cells.

ONISCUS : wood louse, a crustacean belonging to the order Isopoda. They resemble the trilobites in being able to roll themselves up into a ball, and in the feet being like one another and approximately equal in size.

ONTOGENY (Gr. *on*, *ontos*, a being or individual ; *genesis*, origin) : the life-history of an individual, including embryonic development.

ORDOVICIAN SYSTEM OR PERIOD : the geological strata between the Silurian and Cambrian found in Bala, Llandello, and Scotland. It contains remains of marine invertebrates, e.g. small ostracode Crustacea.

OSTEOLEPIS (Gr. *osteon*, bone ; *lepis*, scale) : an extinct Ganoid fish having a protective covering of closely set bony scales, and a large pineal foramen situated in a single frontal bone. See LEPIDOSTEUS.

OSTRACODA (Gr. *ostrakon*, shell) : an order of small bivalve Crustacea, including *Cypris*, in which median and sometimes both median and lateral eyes are present.

PALÆMON : prawn, belonging to the subclass Malacostraca, or soft-shelled crustaceans.

PALISADE CELLS (Fr. *palissade*, enclose with fence) : the name given to the tall columnar cells which form a single layer of cells beneath the cuticle in many invertebrate animals. They are also termed " hypoderm cells."

PARAPHYSIS (Gr. *para*, beside ; *phusis*, growth) : a branched tubular outgrowth from the roof of the third ventricle. It lies in front of the epiphysis and the postvelar arch or dorsal sac. It is well-developed in *Sphenodon* and certain fishes.

PARAPINEAL ORGAN (Gr. *para*, beside ; L. *pinus*, fir cone) : the anterior or left parietal sense-organ of *Petromyzon*. It lies beneath the right parietal sense-organ and is smaller and less differentiated than the right organ.

PARIETAL (L. *paries*, wall) :

BONE : roof-bone of skull.

EYE : visual sense-organ.

" FLECK " : white spot visible through cornea.

FORAMEN : complete parietal canal.

PIT : incomplete parietal canal.

PLATE : separate bone in pineal region.

" PLUG " : translucent tissue closing up pineal canal.

REGION : pineal region of roof of third ventricle.

SCALE : horny scale overlying pineal region of skull.

SENSE-ORGAN : terminal sensory-vesicle.

VESICLE : dilated distal end of pineal stalk.

PATELLA (L. *Patella*, a small pan or dish) : the limpet, a gasteropod mollusc having a low conical shell. The paired eyes of the adult animal are open pits, without a lens. The larva is a typical free-swimming trochophore.

PERIPATUS (Gr. *peripateō*, walk about) : an aberrant arthropod resembling a caterpillar ; neither body nor legs are definitely segmented. The eyes are of a simple ocellar type, and resemble those of *Nereis*.

PERMIAN SYSTEM OR PERIOD : the uppermost strata of the Palæozoic or Primary Era—found in the district of Perm, East Russia. It consists of sand-stone, marls, rocky salt, and magnesium limestone ; the conditions were chiefly continental and desert.

PHASCOLOSOMA (Gr. *phaskolos*, leather bag or purse ; *soma*, body) : a genus of the suborder Sipunculidæ, class Annulosa. Eyes are absent in the adult animal ; a pair of ocelli are, however, present in the trochophore larva.

PHYLLOPODA (Gr. *phullon*, leaf ; *pous*, foot) : an order of the Crustacea having leaf-like legs and comprising *Apus*, *Lepidurus*, and the fairy-shrimp or *Branchipus diaphanus*. The order resembles in many respects the extinct Trilobita.

PHYLOGENY (Gr. *phulon*, race ; *genesis*, origin) : the ancestral origin of a phylum or subdivision of a phylum.

PINEAL BODY (L. *pinus*, a fir cone) : the epiphysis cerebri, so named on account of its conical shape in man and certain animals.

PINEAL FORAMEN : the canal which contains the pineal organ ; it is usually situated between the parietal bones or in the centre of a single bone formed by fusion of the parietal bones. It may, however, be situated between the two frontals, in a single frontal bone or in a special pineal plate.

PINEAL SAC : the dilated distal end of the " epiphysis," sometimes termed the end-vesicle. It is well developed in *Sphenodon*, contains pigment, and it was believed by Dendy to represent the right member of a pair of parietal sense-organs of which the left, or pineal eye, is more highly developed and lies in the parietal foramen.

PINEAL SYSTEM (L. *pinus*, a fir cone) : the term applied to the parietal sense-organ (or organs) and the associated structures, such as the parapineal organ, pineal sac, the pineal stalk, the epiphysis, the pineal nerves, commissures, and habenular ganglia.

PLANARIA (L. *planus*, flat) : a small flat worm, showing bilateral symmetry and having paired ocelli. Phylum Plathelminthes.

PODOPHTHALMATA (Gr. *pous*, foot ; *ophthalmos*, eye) : a division of the Crustacea having compound eyes borne at the free ends of movable stalks. It comprises two Orders, Stomatopoda (e.g. *Squilla*) and Decapoda (e.g. *Astacus*).

POLYCLADA (Gr. *polus*, many ; *clados*, branch) : an order of the flat worms belonging to the class Turbellaria, so named on account of the complex branching of the intestine.

POLYPHEMUS (Gr. the cyclopean giant described by Homer) : a small crustacean belonging to the order Cladocera, in which the eyes are sessile and are joined into a single organ.

PORTHETIS SPINOSA (Gr. *porthetes*, destroyer ; L. *spinosa*, thorny) : an insect belonging to the group Acridiidæ, in which there is a coexistence of the compound and simple eyes in the imago. The three frontal ocelli are arranged in a triangle, one in front, two behind.

PTERICHTHYS (Pterychthys) (Gr. *pteron* (*pterux*), wing ; *ichthus*, fish) : an extinct fish belonging to the order Antiarchi of the class Ostracodermi. It is characterized by wing-like pectoral fins.

PTERYGOTUS (Gr. *pterux*, wing ; *ous*, ear) : a genus of the Eurypterida belonging to the order Merostomata. The antennæ ended in prehensile lobster-like claws ; the maxillipedes formed large ear or oar-like appendages which could be used as paddles.

RETINULA (L. diminutive of *rete*, net) : the inner sensitive segments of the ommatidia of an aggregate or compound eye, as contrasted with the outer, purely dioptric part. Some writers include the pigment cells, which surround the clear cells of the rhabdome, whereas others appear to limit the term to the clear central cells of the ommatidium.

RHABDITE (Gr. *rhabdion*, a little rod) : the central columnar cell of a retinula. The basal part of the cell containing the nucleus is usually expanded, whereas the distal part tapers or is prolonged as a slender refractile rod.

RHABDOME (Gr. *rhabdos*, rod) : the central clear cells of a retinula, including the rhabdite and the peripheral non-pigmented cells.

RHABDOMERE (Gr. *rhabdos*, wand or rod ; *meros*, part) : one of the constituent cells or rods of a rhabdome.

RHIPIDOGLOSSA (Gr. *rhipis*, a fan, something thrown out, as a javelin ; *glossa*, tongue) : the name given to the chameleon family on account of the rapid movement of the long tongue, which is used for catching flies.

RHYNCHONELLA (Gr. diminutive of *rhunchos*, a small beak) : an articulate brachiopod in which the dorsal and ventral valves of the shell are joined by a horizontal hinge with a beaked process. Found in lower cretaceous strata, and closely resembles the shells of certain living species.

ROMBERG'S SIGN : if the patient closes his eyes when standing with the feet together, he sways from side to side, and if not supported will eventually fall. It occurs in cases, such as locomotor ataxia, in which there is a loss of the deep reflexes, which are concerned in maintaining the erect posture.

SALPA (L. *salpa*, stock-fish) : a tunicate belonging to the order Thaliacea. A median horseshoe-shaped eye is present, and sometimes small accessory eyes.

SAURIA (Gr. *saura*, lizard) : term applied to lizard-like reptiles in general, but sometimes restricted to the crocodiles and Lacertilia.

SAUROPSIDA (Gr. *saura*, lizard ; *opsis*, appearance) : the name given collectively to the two classes Birds and Reptiles.

SCHIZOCHROAL EYES (Gr. *schizo*, cleave, separate ; *chroa*, surface) : the term applied to the type of lateral compound eye of trilobites in which the constituent units of the eye were separate, the areas between the corneal facets being occupied by an interstitial test or sclera.

SEPIA (L. *sepia*, cuttle-fish) : a mollusc belonging to the class Cephalopoda possessing ten arms or feet and highly developed eyes. The name " sepia " is also used for the black pigment which is obtained from it.

STEMMA (Gr. *stemma*, crown or wreath) : the simple eyes or ocelli of certain invertebrates, e.g. the frontal stemmata of insects.

TAPETUM (Gr. *tapē*, L. *tapētum*, carpet, many-coloured garment or tapestry) : *T. argentea*, the silvery or greenish-gold, iridescent membrane between the lamina fusca and choroid coat in certain Teleost fishes. The iridescence is due to crystals of calcium salts deposited in the cells : syn. *T. cellulosum*. *T. pellucidum*, a delicate fibrous membrane in the choroid coat next the retina. It has a metallic lustre due to the reflection and interference of light rays by the fibrillæ in the membrane. It is found in certain fishes, carnivores, and ungulates, e.g. the horse and ox. Reflecting membranes behind or external to the retina are also found in some invertebrate eyes and luminous organs, e.g. the photospheria, found on the first abdominal segments of *Nyctiphanes*.

TETRABRANCHIATA (Gr. *tetra*, four ; *branchia*, gills) : a subclass of the Cephalopoda, having four comb-like gills or ctenidia. It includes one living genus, *Nautilus*, and the extinct Ammonites are usually referred to it.

TRETASPIS (Gr. *tretos*, perforated ; *aspis*, shield) : the name given to the larval form of a genus of the trilobites characterized by " holes " or eye-spots on the glabellum.

TRIASSIC SYSTEM OR PERIOD : the lowest strata of the Mesozoic period, during which mammal-like reptiles first made their appearance. It comprised the Rhœtic, Keuper, and Bunter series.

TRILOBITA (Gr. *treis*, three ; *lobes*, lobe) : an extinct Order of crustaceans. The dorsal aspect is divided into three lobes, a median or axial and lateral or pleural. In many the labrum or hypostome supports a pair of compound eyes ; and a median eye-tubercle is present in the larval fossils of certain forms, e.g. *Trinucleus*.

TRIPLOSTICHOUS (Gr. *triploos*, threefold ; *stichos*, layer) : an eye consisting of three layers : preretinal, retinal, and postretinal, e.g. the median eyes of the larval scorpion, in which the retina is inverted. The post-retinal layer may be pigmented or serve as a reflecting membrane (tapetum lucidum or argentea).

TRITON : a marine gastropod mollusc enclosed in a univalve spiral shell, and possessing two simple eyes of the upright type situated near the bases of the tentacles.

TROCHELMINTHES (Gr. *trochos*, wheel ; *helmins*, worm) : an invertebrate phylum comprising the wheel animalcules or rotifers. The free-swimming larva is known as a trochosphere or trochophore.

TROCHOPHORE (Gr. *trochos*, wheel ; *phoreō*, bear or carry) : the cylindrical, free-swimming larva of certain annelids and molluscs. It is characterized by two or more circlets of cilia, resembling those of the rotifers, and the presence of an apical plate bearing an upright tuft of cilia, and often two ocelli.

TUNICATA (L. *tunica*, cloak) : a subphylum Urochordata, which includes the ascidians or sea-squirts, so named on account of the thick, leathery coat with which they are covered.

TURBELLARIA (L. *turbo*, disturb) : a class of flat worms, mostly leaf-like in form, including the Planaria. Pigmented eye-spots are found on the dorsal aspect of the head-region.

UROCHORDA (Gr. *oura*, tail ; *chordē*, string) : a subphylum of the Chordata, in which a notochord limited to the tail region is present in the free-swimming larva.

URODELA (Gr. *oura*, tail ; *delos*, visible) : tailed amphibians, including the newts and *Proteus anguineus*.

VARANUS : a lizard of the Monitor family in which the parietal sense-organ is large and well differentiated.

VELIGER (L. *velum*, a sail ; *gero*, carry) : a stage in the development of certain Gasteropods, e.g. *Vermetus*. The preoral circlet of the trochophore larva has become bilobed, and by means of its cilia serves as an organ of locomotion. Paired lateral eyes are present at the bases of the tentacles. The term is also applied to one stage in the development of *Geotria*.

VELUM TRANSVERSUM (L. *velum*, veil or curtain) : the thin fold of the roof of the third ventricle, which forms the anterior boundary of the dorsal sac. Laterally it is continuous with the choroid plexuses of the lateral ventricles.

YUNGIA : a marine Planarian belonging to the order Polycladidæ, class Turbellaria, of the flat-worms. Ocelli are developed over the region of the apical cells of the free-swimming larva.

ZŒA (Gr. *zōon*, living being, animal) : a larval stage of the crab, characterized by the very large size of the compound eyes as compared with the size of the body.

BIBLIOGRAPHY AND INDEX OF AUTHORS

ABEL, O. (1920). *Lehrbuch der Palæozoologie.* Gustav Fischer, Jena.

ACHÚCARRO, N., and SACRISTAN, J. D. (1913). Zur Kenntniss der Ganglienzellen der menschlichen Zirbeldrüse, *Trab. del lab. de inv. biol.,* 11.

—— (1912). Investigaciones histologicus e histopatologicus sobre la glandula pineal humana, *ibid.,* 10.

AGDUHR, E. (1932). Choroid Plexus and Ependyma. E. V. Cowdry, *Cytology and Cellular Pathology of the Nervous System.* W. Penfield. Vol. II, pp. 535–74.

AHLBORN, F. (1883). Untersuchungen über das Gehirn der Petromyzonten, *Z. f. wiss. Zool.,* **30,** 191–294.

ALMEIDA DIAS, A. (1930). Ueber einen Pinealtumor mit multiplen Fliomen, *Mschr. Psychiat. Neurol.,* **86,** 9.

ALTMANN, F. (1930). Ueber ein Dermoid der Zirbeldrüse Wien, *Klin. Wschr.,* **43,** 108.

AMPRINO, R. (1935). Transformazioni della ghiandola pineale dell uomo e degli animali nell accressimento e nella senescenza, *Arch. Ital. Anat. Embr.,* **34,** Fasc. 4, 446.

ANDREWS, E. A. (1891). Compound Eyes of Annelids, *J. Morph.,* **5,** 271.

ASCHNER, B. (1918). *Die Blutdrüsenerkrangungen des Weibes.* Wiesbaden. Physiologie der Hypophyse. Handbuch der inneren Sekretion, II., Liefkabitzsch.

BAILEY, P. Pinealomas, *Intracranial Tumours,* 1933, Ch. 16, p. 331. Chicago.

BAILEY, P., and JELLIFFE, S. E. (1911). *Arch. intern. Med.,* **8,** 851.

BALADA, M. (1927). Tumores de la Epifisis, *Arch. argent. Neurol.,* **1,** 10.

BALFOUR, F. M. (1885). *Comparative Embryology.* Vol. II, pp. 432, 498.

BAUDOUIN, A., L'HERMITTE, J., and LEREBOULLET, J. (1932). Un Cas de Pinealome : Absence de Macrogenitosomie précoce. Le Probleme de la Cachexie hypophysaire, *Rev. neurol.,* **1,** 388.

—— (1932). Un Cas de Pinéalome : Absence de Macrogenitosomie précoce. Le probleme de la Cachexie Hypophysaire, *ibid.,* No. 3.

BEARD, J. (1889). The Parietal Eye of Cyclostome Fishes. *Q. J. Micr. Sc.,* **29,** N.S., 55.

—— (1889). The Development of the Peripheral Nervous System, *Q. J. Micr. Sc.,* **29,** 153–223.

—— (1887). The Eye of Vertebrates and the Third Eye of Reptiles. *Nature,* 21st May, 246.

BEDFORD, T. H. B. (1934). *Brain.* Part I, 57.

BENECKE, E. (1936). Über die funktionelle Bedeutung der Zirbelgeschwülste. *Virchows Arch.,* **297,** 26–39.

32   497

BÉRANECK, E. (1892).   Sur le nerf pariétal et la morphologie du troisième oeil des vertébrés, *Anat. Anz. Jahrg.*, 7.

BERBLINGER, W. (1928).   Die Theorien über die Zirbelfunktion und ihre anatomischen Grundlagen. *Arch. f. Psychiatr.*, **85**.

—— (1929).   Pineal Form of Pubertas Præcox; Pineal Hypertrophy of Genitalia in Adults, *Deutsche Med. Wochenschrift*, 55, 1926.

—— (1921).   Zur Frage der Zirbelfunktion, *Virchows Arch.*, 237, 144.

BERGER (1878).   Untersuchungen über den Bau des Gehirns und der Retina der Arthropoden, *Arb. a.d. Zool. Institut. Wien.*

BERNARD, H. M. (1896).   An Attempt to deduce the Vertebrate Eyes from the Skin, *Q. J. Micr. Sc.*, 39, N.S.

BERTKAU (1886).   Beiträge zur Kenntniss der Sinnesorgane der Spinnen. I. Die Augen der Spinnen, *Arch. f. mikr. Anat.*, 27.

BIENSTOCK (1926).   Tumour of Pineal Gland, *Schweiz. med. Woch.*, 56, 502 (abstr. *J. Amer. med. Ass.*, 87, 284).

BRAEM, F. (1898).   Epiphysis und Hypophysis von Rana, *Zeitschr. f. wiss. Zool.*, 63.

BROOM, R. (1930).   *The Origin of the Human Skeleton.*   H. F. and G. Witherby, London.

BROWN, R. S. (1938).   The Anatomy of the Polychæte *Ophelia cluthensis*, *Proc. Roy. Soc. Edin.*, 58, Part II, 135.

BUCHANAN, L. (1907).   *Notes on the Comparative Anatomy of the Eye*, 27, 262.

DE BUSSCHER, J. (1936).   Tumour épiphysaire : envahissement des ventricules cérébraux, *J. belge de neurol. et de psychist.*, 36, 373–85.

CALVET, JEAN (1934).   *L'Epiphyse (Gland Pinéale)*.   J. B. Baillière et Fils, Paris.

CAMERON, H. (1902–3).   On the Origin of the Pineal Body as an Amesial Structure deduced from a Study of its Development in Amphibia, *Proc. Roy. Soc. Edin.*, 24.

—— (1903–4).   On the Origin of the Epiphysis Cerebri as a Bilateral Structure in the Chick, *ibid.*, 25.

—— (1903).   On the Origin of the Pineal Body as an Amesial Structure, deduced from a Study of its Development in Amphibia, *Anat. Anz.*, 23.

CATTIE, J. T. (1882).   Recherches sur la gland pineale, *Arch. de Biol.*, 101–194.

CLARKE, J. M. (1888).   The Structure and Development of the Visual Area in the Trilobite *Phacops rana*, Green.   *J. Morphology*, II.

COOPER, EUGENIA, R.A. (1932).   *J. Anat.*, 67, 28.

CUNNINGHAM, J. T., *vide* VALLENTIN, R. (1888).   The Photospheria of Nyctiphanes Norvegica, *Q. J. Micr. Sc.*, 28, N.S., 321.

CUSHING, H. (1914).   Studies on the Cerebrospinal Fluid, *J. Med. Research*, 31, 1–20.

—— (1925).   The Cameron Lectures : I. The Third Circulation and its Channels, *Lancet*, 2, 851.

DANA, C. L., and BERKELEY, W. N. (1913).   The Functions of the Pineal Gland, *Med. Rec.*, 83, 835.

DANDY and BLACKFAN (1914).   *Amer. J. Dis. Child.*, 8, 406.

DANDY, W. E. (1919).   *Ann. Surg.*, **70**, 129.

—— (1929).   *J. Amer. Med. Ass.*, **92**, 2012.

—— (1915).   Extirpation of the Pineal Body, *J. Exp. Med.*, **22**.

—— (1921).   *Surg., Gynec., and Obstetrics.*

—— (1921).   Operation for Removal of Pineal Tumours, *Surg., Gynec., Obstet.*, **33**, 113.

—— (1936).   Operative Experience in Cases of Pineal Tumour, *Arch. Surg.*, **33**, 19–46.

DARKSCHEWITSCH, L. (1886).   Zur Anatomie der Glandula pinealis, *Neurol. Zbl.*, **5**.

DEAN, A. (1895).   *Fishes, Living and Fossil.*   Colombia University Biological Series.   New York.

DENDY, A. (1907).   On the Parietal Sense-organs and Associated Structures in the New Zealand Lamprey (*Geotria australis*), *Q. J. Micr. Sc.* **51**, 1.

—— (1911).   *Phil. Trans. Roy. Soc.*, Ser. B, **201**, 227.

—— and NICHOLLS, G. E. (1910).   On the Occurrence of a Mesocoelic Recess in the Human Brain and its Relation to the Subcommissural Organ of Lower Vertebrates with Special Reference to the Distribution of Reissner's Fibre in the Vertebrate Series, *Proc. Roy. Soc.*, Ser. B, **82**.

DEXTER, F. (1902).   The Development of the Paraphysis in the Common Fowl, *Amer. J. Anat.*, **2**.

DIMITROWA, MLLE. Z. (1900–1).   *Recherche sur la structure de la glande pinéale chez quelques mamifères.*   Thèse de Nancy.

—— (1901).   *Le Nevraxe.*

DUKE-ELDER, S. (1934).   *Recent Advances in Ophthalmology*, J. and A. Churchill, London.   " Origin of Melanin," pp. 170 *et seq.*

DYES, O. (1936).   Verlagerungen den verkalten Zirbeldrüse auf dem seitlichen Röntgenbild des Schädels, *Nervenarzt.*, **4**, 11–14.

EGAS MONIZ, PINTO, A., and ALMEIDA LIMA (1930).   " Tumeur de la Glande pinéale irriguée par un Seul des Groupes sylviens.   Diagnostic par L'Epreuve encéphalographique," *Rev. Neurol.*, **2**, 51.

ELKINGTON, J. ST. C. (1932).   Calcified Pineal Tumour, *Proc. Roy. Soc. Med.*, **25**, 1533.

ENGEL, P. (1936).   Die physiologische und pathologische Bedeutung der Zirbeldrüse.   *Ergebn. d. inn. Med. u. Kinderh.*, **50**, 116–71.

EXNER, A., and BOESE (1910).   *Dtsch. Z. Chir.*, **107**, 182.

EYCLESHYMER, A. C. (1892).   Paraphysis and Epiphysis in Amblystoma, *Anat. Anz.*, 7 Jahrg., 215.

FAVARO, C. (1904).   Le fibre nervose prepineali e pineali nell' encefalo di mammiferi, *Arch. di Anat. e di Embriol.*, **3**, fasc. 3.

FLEISCHMANN, W., and GOLDHAMMER, H. (1936).   Zur Frage der hormonalen Wirkung der Zirbeldrüse, *Klin. Wschr.*, **15**, 1047–8.

FOA, C. (1912).   *Archives italiennes de Biologie*, 233.   R.N. **1**, 675.

—— (1928).   Pineal Gland in Fowls.   *Arch. di Sc. biol.*, **12**, 300.

—— (1929).   *Arch. ital. de Biol.*, **81**, 147–158.

FRORIEP, A. (1906).   Ueber die Herleitung des Wirbelthierauges von Auge der Ascidienlarve, *Verh. Anat. Gesellsch.* (Rostock), *Anat. Anz.*, Suppl., **29**, 145.

GASKELL, W. H. (1908). *Origin of Vertebrates.*

—— (1890). On the Origin of Vertebrates from a Crustacean-like Ancestor, *Q. J. Micr. Sc.*, **31.**

—— (1910). Discussion on the Origin of Vertebrates, *Proc. Linnean Soc. of London*, Session 122.

GAUPP, E. Zirbel, Parietal organ und Paraphysis. *Ergebnisse der Anat. und Entwicklungsgeschichte*, von Merkel und Bonnet.

VAN GEHUCHTEN, P. (1936). Un cas de tumeur de l'épiphyse, *J. belge Neurol, Psychiat.*, **36,** 69–72.

GLADSTONE, R. J. (1910). A Cyclops and Agnathic Lamb, *Brit. Med. J.*, **2,** 1159.

—— and DUNLOP, H. A. (1927). A Case of Hydrocephalus in an Infant with Comments on the Secretion, Circulation, and Absorption of the Cerebrospinal Fluid, *J. Anat.*, **61,** 366.

GLADSTONE, R. J., and WAKELEY, C. P. G. (1920). A Cyclops Lamb (*C. Rhinocephalus*), *ibid.*, **54,** 196.

GLASER, M. A. (1929). Tumours of Pineal, Corpora Quadrigemina, and Third Ventricle : Inter-relationship of their Syndromes and their Surgical Treatment, *Brain*, **52,** 226.

GLICK, D., and BISKIND, G. R. (1936). Studies in Histochemistry : Relationship between Concentration of Vitamin C and Development of Pineal Gland, *Proc. Soc. Exper. Biol. U. Med.*, **34,** 866–70.

GLOBUS, J. H., and SILBERT, S. (1931). Pinealomas, *Arch. Neurol. Psychiat.*, **25, 937.**

—— (1932). Pinealoma with Supratentorial Extension, *Libman Anniv. Vols.*, **2, 491.**

GRENACHER, H (1879). *Untersuchungen über das Sehorgan der Arthropoden*, **76,** 100. Göttingen.

HALDEMAN, K. O. (1927). Tumours of Pineal Gland, *ibid.*, **18,** 724.

HANSON, A. M. (1937). Histology of the Pineal Gland and its Probable Physiologic Function, *Minnesota Med.*, **20,** 78.

—— (1936). Biologic Effects of Active Thymus and Pineal Extracts : Brief Review, *ibid.*, **19,** 1–4.

HANSTRÖM, B. (1926). Eine genetische Studie über die Augen und Sehzentren von Turbellarian, Anneliden und Arthropoden, *Kungl. Swenska Vetenskapsakademiens*, Hardlinger Tredje Serien, **4,** No. 1. Upsala.

HARRIS, W., and CAIRNS, H. (1932). Diagnosis and Treatment of Pineal Tumours, with Report of Case, *Lancet*, **1,** 3.

DEN HARTOG JAGER, W. A., and HEIL, J. F. (1935). Über die Epiphysefrage, *Acta brev. Neerland.*, **5,** 32–4.

HEIDER, *v.* KORSCHELT.

HEINTZ, A. (1932). The Structure of Dinichthys. The Bashford Dean Memorial : *Archaic Fishes*, No. IV, New York.

HERRING, P. T. (1927). The Pineal Region of the Mammalian Brain, its Morphology and Histology in relation to Function, *Quart. J. exp. Physiol.*, **17,** 125.

HERTWIG, O. (1880). *Die Chaetognathen.* G. Fischer. Jena.

HESSE, R. (1898). Untersuchungen über die Organe der Lichtempfindung bei niederen Thieren. Die Sehorgane des Amphioxus, *Z. f. wiss. Zool.*, 63.

HEWER, EVELYN, *v.* LUCAS KEENE.

HILL, CHA. (1891). Development of the Epiphysis in *Coregonus albus*, *J. Morph.*, 5, 503.

—— (1894). The Epiphysis of Teleosts and Amia, *ibid.*, 9, 237.

—— (1900). Two Epiphyses in a Four-day Chick, *Bull. North-Western Univ. Med. Sch.*, Chicago, Nov. 1900.

HILLS, E. S. (1933). On a Primitive Dipnoan from the Middle Devonian Rocks of New South Wales. *Annals and Magazine of Nat. History*, Ser. 10, 11, 634.

HOCHSTETTER, F. (1921). *Verhandl. d. anat. Ges. a.d. 30 Vers. in Marburg*, 193–212.

HOFFMANN, C. K. (1891). *Bronns Klass. und Ord. Thierreichs*, 6, Abt. 3, 1891. Epiphyse u. Parietalauge.

HOFSTATTER, R. (1936). Organotherapeutische Versuche mit Hilfe von Zirbelextrakten, besonders bei sexueller Uebererregbarkeit, *Wien. klin. Wschr.*, 49, 136–7.

HORRAX, G., and BAILEY, P. (1925). Tumours of Pineal Body, *ibid.*, 13, 423.

HORRAX, G. (1927). Differential Diagnosis of Tumours Primarily Pineal and Primarily Pontile, *Arch. Neurol. Psychiat.*, 21.

—— (1936). Further Observations on Tumour of Pineal Body, *ibid.*, 35, 215–28.

—— (1927). " Differential Diagnosis of Tumours Primarily Pineal and Primarily Pontine," *ibid.*, 17, 179.

HOWARD and BELL (1916). Hyperplasia of the Pineal Body, *J. Nerv. Men. Dis.*, 44, 481.

HOWELL, C. M. Hinds (1909–10). *Proc. Roy. Soc. Med.* (Neurol. Sect.), 3, 65.

IMMS, A. D. (1925). *A General Textbook of Entomology, including the Anatomy, Physiology, and Classification of Insects.* Methuen and Co., London.

IZAWA, Y. (1922). On the Experimental Removal of the Pineal Body in Chickens. *Trans. Japanese Path. Soc.*, 12, 139.

JAENSCH, P. A. (1931). " Doppelseitige Trohlearisparese als einzige Motilitatsstörung bei Zirbeldrüsentumor," *Z. Augenheilk.*, 75, 58.

JOHNSON (1901). Contributions to the Comparative Anatomy of the Mammalian Eye, chiefly based on Ophthalmoscopic Examination, *Phil. Trans. Roy. Soc.*, B, 194, 70.

JOSEPH, H. (1904). Ueber eigentümliche Zellstrukturen im Zentralnervensystem des Amphioxus, *Anat. Anz. Ergänzlingsheft z*, 25 (Verg. d. anat. Ges, 1904).

KEIBEL, F. (1906). Die Entwicklungsgeschichte des Wirbelthierauges, *Klin. Monatsbl. Augenheilk*, 44, N.S., Bd. II, 112.

KIAER, J. (1924). Downtonian Fauna of Norway. I. Anaspida, *Videnskaps. Skr. Mat. Naturw. Kl. Cristiania.*

KINGSLEY, J. S. (1886). Development of the Compound Eye of Crangon, *Zool. Anz.*, 9, 597.

KISHINOUYE, K. (1891). On the Development of Araneina. *J. Coll. Sci.*, *Imp. Univ. Japan*, 4, 82.

—— (1894). Notes on the Eyes of *Cardium nuticum*, *ibid.*, 6, 279.

KLINCKOWSTRÖM, A. de (1893). Le premier développement de l'œil pariétal, l'épiphyse et le nerf pariétal chez Iguana tuberculata, *Anat. Anz.*, Jahrg. 8, 289.

—— (1893). Die Zirbel und das Foramen parietale bei Callichthys (asper. und littoralis), *ibid.*, Jahrg. 8, 561.

KLIPPEL, M., WEIL, M. P., and MINVIELLE (1920). Un cas de Tumeur epiphysaire, *Rev. Neurol.*, 27, 1202.

KÖBCKE, H. (1936). Über den heutigen Stand der Epiphysenforschung, *Dtsch. med. Wschr.*, 62, 1134–7.

KORSCHELT UND HEIDER (1890). *Lehrbuch der vergleichenden Entwicklungsgeschichte der wirbellossen Tiere*, 1, Jena.

KRABBE, K. H. (1915). (Abstract) : 62, *Rev. Neurol. Psychiat.*, Edinburgh, 13, 300.

KRABBE, Kund. (1916). *Anat. Hefte*, 54, 191.

KROCKERT, G. (1936). Die Wirkung der Verfütterung von Schilddrüsen und Zirbeldrüsensubstanz an Lebistes reticulatus (Zahn karpfen), *Z. ges. exper. Med.*, 98, 214–20.

KUP, G., and VEGHELYI, F. (1935). Effect of Castration on Pineal Body of Pigs, *Magyar Orv. arch.*, 36, 303–7. (In Hungarian.)

VON KUP, J. (1936). Wirkung der Kastrierung auf die Zirbeldrüse, *Wien klin. Wchnschr.*, 49, 915–7.

LANGWORTHY, O. R. (1930). *Contributions to Embryology*. No. 120. Johns Hopkins University.

LANKESTER, E. R., and BOURNE, A. G. (1893). The Minute Structure of the Lateral and Central Eyes of Scorpio and Limulus, *Q. J. Micr. Sc.*, 23, N.S.

LEREBOULLET, P., et BRIZARD (1921). Tumeur de L'Epiphyse : Autopsie, *Bull. Soc. Pediat. Paris*, 19, 324.

LEREBOULLET, P., MAILLET, and BRIZARD (1921). Un Cas de Tumeur de l'Epiphyse, *ibid.*, 116.

LEYDIG, F. (1891). *Das Parietalorgan der Amphibien und Reptilien Abhandlungen der Senckb. (naturf.) Gessellschf*. Frankfurt a. M., 19, 441–552.

LIEBERT, E. (1929). Ueber Epiphysentumoren, *Dtsch. Z. Nervenheilk.*, 108, 101.

LOCY, W. A. (1894). The Derivation of the Pineal Eye, *Anat. Anz.*, 9, 169.

—— (1894). The Optic Vesicles of Elasmobranchs, *J. Morph.*, 9, 115.

LOWNE, B. T. (1883). On the Structure and Function of the Eyes of Arthropoda, *Proc. Roy. Soc. London*, 35, No. 225, 140–7.

—— (1893–5). *The Anatomy, Physiology, Morphology, and Development of the Blowfly*. London. pp. 510–82.

LUCAS KEENE, M. F., and HEWER, E. E. (1931). Some Observations on Myelination in the Human Central Nervous System, *J. Anat.*, 66, 1.

LUCE, H. (1921). Zur Diagnostik der Zirbelgeschwülste und zur Kritik der cerebralen Adipositas, *ibid.*, 68–9, 187.

MacBride, E. W. (1914). *Textbook of Embryology.* Vol. I. Invertebrata. (Apical plate and Eyes of Tornaria Larvæ (Morgan). Macmillan & Co., London. p. 575.

McCord, C. P. (1917). *Trans. Amer. Gyn. Soc.*, 41.

Mann, Ida C. (1928). *The Development of the Human Eye,* Camb. Univ. Press.

Marburg, O. (1920). Neuer Studien über die Zirbeldruse, *Arb. Neurol., Inst. Wien. Univ.,* 23.

—— (1928). Adipositas cerebralis, *Wien med. Wschr.*

—— (1909). Zur kenntniss der normalen u. path. Histologie der Zirbeldrüse, *Arb. Neurol. Inst. Wien. Univ.,* 12.

Meyer, R. (1936). Das Verhalten mehrerer nucleolärer Blasen im Kernstoffwechsel der Pinealzellen des Menschen und die Entstehung der Kernfalten, *Z. Zellforsch. mikr. Anat.,* 25, 173–80.

—— Uber den morphologisch fassbaren Kernstoffwechsel der Parenchymzellen der Epiphysis cerebri des Menschen, *ibid.,* 25, 83–98.

Minot, C. S. (1901). On the Morphology of the Pineal Region, based upon its Development in Acanthias, *Amer. J. Anat.,* 1, 81.

Moeller, J. v. (1887). *Arch. f. Anthropologie,* 17, s. 173.

—— (1890). Einiges uber die Zirbeldrüse des Chimpanse, *Verhandl. der Naturuf. Ges. in Basel.*

Müller, W. (1874). *Ueber die Stammesentwickelung des Sehorgans der Wirbelthiere.* Festgabe, C. Ludwig, Leipzig.

Nowikoff, M. (1910). Untersuchungen uber den Bau, die Entwicklung und die Bedeutung des Parietalauges von Sauriern, *Z. f. wiss. Zool.,* 96, Heft 1.

Orlandi, N. (1922). Lo stato altnale delle nostre connoscenze sulla ghiandola pineale, *Osp. maggiore,* 10.

—— (1929). Richerche istologiche su 107 pineali de bambini, *Rev. sud-amer. Endocrin.,* 2, No. 6, Ref. en Pathologica.

Parhon, C. I., Stefanescu-Dragomireanu, M., and Marculescu, A. (1936). Action d'un extrait epiphysaire sur quelques constituants biochemiques du sang. Augmentation de la potassemie, *Bull. Acad. Med. Paris,* 116, 104–6.

Parker, G. H. (1886). The Eyes in Scorpions, *Bull. Mus. Comp. Zool.,* 13, No. 6, 173.

—— (1889). Studies on the Eyes of Arthropods, *J. Morph.* 1 and 2 (1887, 1889).

—— (1891). The Compound Eyes in Crustaceans, *Bull. Mus. Comp. Zool.,* 21, 45.

—— (1899). The Photomechanical Changes in the Retinal Pigment of *Gammarus, ibid.,* 25, 143.

Patten, W. (1888–9). Studies on the Eyes of Arthropods, *J. Morph.,* 2, 97–190.

—— On the Morphology and Physiology of the Brain and Sense Organs of *Limulus, Q. J. Micr. Sc.,* 35.

—— (1890). On the Origin of Vertebrates from Arachnids, *Q. J. Micr. Sc.,* 31, N.S., 317.

—— (1912). *The Evolution of the Vertebrates and their Kin,* J. and A. Churchill.

PELLIZZI (1910).   La sindrome epifisaria " macrogenitosomia precoce," *Rio. ital. Neurol., Psich. Elettrot*, 3, 193 e 250.

PENFIELD, W. (1928).   *Cowdry's Special Cytology*, Hoeber, N.Y.

PINES (1927).   Über der Innervation der Epiphyse, *Z. ges. Neurol. Psychiat.*, 3.

PRENANT, A. (1893-4).   Sur l'œil parietal accessoire, *Anat. Anz.*, 9, 103.

QUAST, P. (1930).   Beitrage zur Histologie und Cytologie der normalen Zirbeldrüse des Menschen, *Z. mikrs. anat. Forsch.*, 23, 335.

—— (1931).   Beitrage zur Histologie und Cytologie der normalen Zirbeldrüse des Menschen, *ibid.*, 24.

RADOVICI, A. (1936).   Le syndrome pseudo-épiphysaire.   Macro-génitosomie précoce d'origine post-encéphalopathique, *Bull. Acad. Méd. de Roumanie*, I, 194-9.

DEL RIO HORTEGA, *v.* PENFIELD, W. (1928).   *The Pineal Gland.*

ROBINSON, MARGARET (1892).   On the Nauplius Eye persisting in some Decapods, *Q. J. Micr. Sc.*, 23.

ROWNTREE, L. G. (1938).   The Pineal in Health and Disease, *The Practitioner's Library of Medicine and Surgery*, 13, Chap. V, 46.

—— (1936).   Abstract: Biologic Effects of Pineal Extract (Hanson), *Science*, 83, 164-5.

—— (1936).   Biological Effects of Pineal Extract (Hanson); Accruing Retardation in Growth and accruing Acceleration in Development in Successive Generations of Rats under Continuous Treatment with Pineal Extract, *Endocrinology*, 20, 348-57.

—— and OTHERS (1936).   Further Studies on Thymus and Pineal Glands, *Pennsylvania M. J.*, 39, 603-6.

——, CLARK, J. H., STEINBERG, A., and HANSON, A. M. (1936).   Biologic Effects of Pineal Extract (Hanson); Amplification of Effects in Young, resulting from Treatment of Successive Generations of Parent Rats, *J. A. M. A.*, 106, 370-3.

RÜCKHARD, R. (1886).   Zur Deutung der Zirbeldrüse, *Zool. Anz.*, s. 405.

—— (1882).   Zur Deutung und Entwickelungsgeschichte des Gehirns der knochenfische, *Arch. f. Anat. und Physiol.*

RUSH, H. P., BILDERBACK, J. B., SLOCUM, D., and ROGERS, A. (1937).   Pubertas Præcox (Macrogenitosomia), *Endocrinology*, 21, 404.

SCHACHTER, M. (1936).   Nos connaissances actuelles concernant l'épiphyse, *J. Med. Paris*, 56, 343-5.

—— (1936).   Troubles somato-psychiques post-encephalique prenant l'allure de syndromes epiphysaires, *Z. Kinderphychiat.*, 3, 37-42.

SCHAEFFER, DE MARTEL, T., and GUILLAUME, J. (1936).   Les tumeurs de la glande pineale sans signes focaux.   *Rev. Neurol.*, 65, 346-51.

SCHEPERS, G. W. H. (1938).   The External Morphology of the Brain of *Testudo geometrica, J. Anat.*, 72, 535.

SCHMIDT, W. J. (1909).   Beitrage zur Kenntniss der Parietalorgane des Saurier, *Z. f. wiss. Zool.*, 92.

SCHWALBE, E. (1906).   *Die Morphologie der Missbildungen des Menschen und der Tiere.*   Jena, G. Fischer.   Cephalothoracopagus, 175-219; Duplicitas anterior. 283-7; Zyclopie, II, 29-32.

SEDGWICK, A. (1888). A Monograph on the Species and Distribution of the Genus Peripatus, *Q. J. Micr. Sci.*, **28.**

—— (1888). The Development of the Cape Species of the Peripatus, Part IV, *ibid.*, **28.**

SEMPER, K. (1883). The Natural Conditions of Existence as they affect Animal Life : Dorsal Eyes of Onchidium, *International Scientific Series*, **31,** 371.

SHELDON, LILIAN (1889). On the Development of Peripatus Novæ-Zealandiæ, *Q. J. Micr. Sci.*, **29,** N.S., 283.

SMITH, G. ELLIOT (1896). The Brain of a Fœtal *Ornithorynchus*, *ibid.*, **39,** 181.

SMITH, H. M. (1936). Lizards of the Torquatus Group of the Genus Scleroporus, *Univ. Kansas Sci. Bull.*, **24.**

SPENCER, B. (1887). On the Presence and Structure of the Pineal Eye in Lacertilia, *Q. J. Micr. Sci.*, **17,** 165.

STENSIÖ, ERIK-A-SON (1927). On the Heads of Certain Arthrodira, *Kungl. Swenska. Oetenskapsakademiens*, Hardlingar Tredge Series, **13,** No. 5.

—— (1927). Downtonian and Devonian Vertebrates of Spitzbergen (Cephalaspidæ), *Norske Videnskaps- Akad. Oslo*, No. 12.

—— (1929–30). Upper Devonian Vertebrates from East Greenland, *Meddelelser om Gronland*, **86,** No. 1.

—— (1932). *The Cephalaspids of Great Britain.* British Museum (Natural History). London.

STORMER, L. (1930). Scandinavian Trinucleidæ with Special Reference to Norwegian Species and Varieties, *Skrifter utgitt av det Norske Videnskaps-Akademi i Oslo*, No. 4.

STOPFORD, J. S. B. (1926). *Brit. Med. J.*, **2,** 1207.

—— (1928). *Brain*, **5,** 485.

STRAHL, H., u. MARTIN, E. (1888). Die Entwicklung des Parietalauges bei Anguis fragilis und Lacerta vivipara, *Arch. Anat. Physiol.*, *Anat. Abt.*, **146,** 164.

STUDNIČKA, F. K. (1905). Die Parietalorgane. *Lehrbuch der vergleichenden Mikroskopischen Anatomie der Wirbelthiere.* Oppel. Teil, V.

STÜRMER, R. (1913). Die corpora amylacea des Zentralnervensystems. *Histologische u. histopathologische Arbeiten*, **5,** Heft 3, 417.

TAKACS, L. (1935). Der Einfluss der Zirbeldrüse auf das Wachstum, *Z. ges. exper. Med.*, **97,** 204–6.

TILNEY, F., and WARREN, L. F. (1919). The Pineal Body. Part I. Morphology and Evolutionary Significance, *Amer. Anat. Mem.*, *Wistar Inst. Anat. Biol. Philadelphia.*

VALLENTIN, R., and CUNNINGHAM, J. T. (1888). The Photospheria of Nyctiphanes Norvegica, G. O. Sars. *Q. J. Micr. Sci.*, **28,** N.S. 321.

VAN WAGENEN, W. P. (1931). A Surgical Approach for the Removal of Certain Pineal Tumours, *Surg. Gyn. and Obstetr.*, **53,** 216.

WAKELEY, CECIL P. G. (1934). Development of Pineal Gland, *Med. Press and Circ.*, **188,** 145, 189.

—— (1938) Surgery of the Pineal Gland. *Brit. Journ. Surj.*, Jan., 561

WAKELEY, CECIL P. G., and GLADSTONE, R. J. (1925).   Development and
    Histogenesis of the Human Pineal Organ, *J. Anat.*, 69, 427.

WALDSCHMIDT, J. (1887).   Beitrag zur Anatomie des Zentralnervensystems und
    des Geruchorganes von Polypterus bichir, *Anat. Anzeiger*, 11.

WALTER, K. (1922).   Zur Histologie und Physiologie des menschlichen Zir-
    beldrüse, *Z. ges. Neurol. Psychiat.*, 74.

WARREN, J. (1918).   *J. Comp. Neurol.*, 28, 75–135.

WARREN, L. F., *v.* TILNEY, F.

WATASE, S. (1890).   On the Morphology of the Compound Eyes of Arthropods,
    Q. J. Micr. Sci., 31, 143.

WATSON, D. M. S. (1914).   On the Skull of a Pariasaurian Reptile, *Proc. Zool.
    Soc.*, 1, 155.

—— (1914).   The Deinocephalia, an order of Mammal-like Reptiles, *ibid.*, 2,
    749.

WHITE, E. J. (1935).   The Ostracoderm *Pteraspis Kiaer*, and the Relationships
    of the Agnathous Vertebrates, *Phil. Trans. R. Soc.*, Series B, 225, No.
    527, 381.

WILLEY, A. (1897).   Letters from New Guinea on *Nautilus* and Some Other
    Organisms, *Q. J. Micr. Sci.*, 39, 145.

WOODWARD, A. S. (1922).   Observations on Crossopterygian and Arthrodiran
    Fishes, *Proc. Linnean Soc. London*, Sess. 134, 27.

VON ZITTEL, K. A. (1900).   *Textbook of Palæontology.*   Translated by C. R.
    Eastman.   Macmillan & Co., London.

ZONDEK, H. (1935).   *The Diseases of the Endocrine Organs*, 3rd ed.   Translated
    by C. Prausnitz.   E. Arnold & Co., London.

INDEX OF AUTHORS

The numbers refer to the page on which the author's name is quoted, the thick type indicates an illustration.

INDEX

The numbers refer to pages, the darker figures indicate illustrations

Printed in Great Britain by William Clowes & Sons, Limited, Beccles, for
Baillière, Tindall & Cox